COMPLETE FAMILY HEALTH GUIDE

New
Medicine

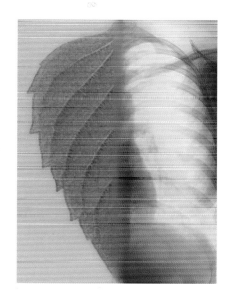

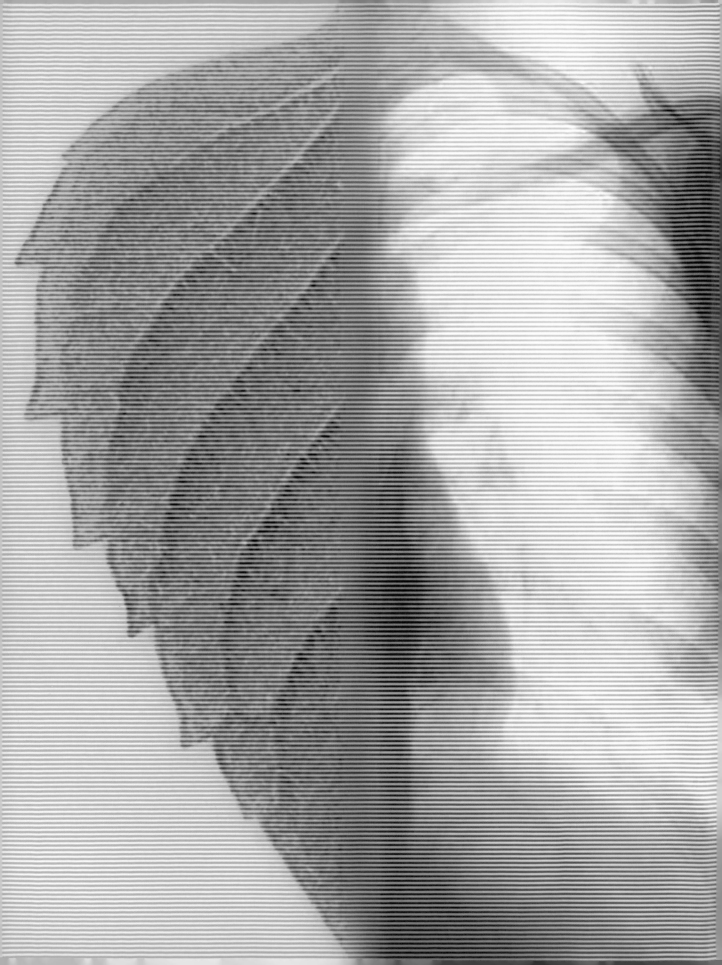

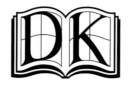

COMPLETE FAMILY HEALTH GUIDE

New Medicine

Integrating complementary, alternative, and conventional medicine for the safest and most effective treatment

EDITOR-IN-CHIEF Professor David Peters
MB, ChB, DRCOG, DMSMed, MF Hom, FLCOM

CONSULTING EDITOR Dr. Kenneth R. Pelletier
PhD, MD

LONDON, NEW YORK, MUNICH, MELBOURNE, DELHI

For my colleagues at the University of Westminster

Project Editors Kathy Fahey, Pip Morgan
Science Writer Erica Bower
US Senior Editor Jill Hamilton
US Editorial Assistants Puja Telikicherla, Nicole Turney
Picture Research Suzanne Williams
Picture Librarian Romaine Werblow
Illustrator Philip Wilson
Senior Art Editor Rosamund Saunders
Design Schermuly Design Co.
Managing Editors Penny Warren, Stephanie Farrow
Managing Art Editor Marianne Markham
Art Director Carole Ash
Publishing Director Corinne Roberts
DTP Designer Sonia Charbonnier
Production Joanna Bull, Stuart Masheter

First published in the United States in 2007 by DK Publishing
375 Hudson Street, New York, New York, 10014

07 08 09 10 9 8 7 6 5 4 3 2 1

> **IMPORTANT**
> If you have symptoms of illness, do not diagnose the problem yourself from this book. It
> is essential that you also consult your doctor. If you use complementary therapies, do not
> stop taking prescribed medication without first seeking medical advice. Always inform
> both your doctor and your complementary practitioner of all the treatments, remedies,
> and nutritional supplements you are taking or using. See also pp.46, 69, and 111.

A CIP catalog record for this book is available from the Library of Congress.
ISBN 978-07566-0933-7

Color reproduced by GRB, Italy
Printed and bound in Singapore by Star Standard

Discover more at
www.dk.com

Editor-in-Chief

Professor David Peters MB, ChB, DRCOG, DMSMed, MFHom, FLCOM is a highly respected practitioner in the field of integrated medicine. A medical doctor who is trained in osteopathy and homeopathy, he is currently Chair of the British Holistic Medical Association. He is also the Clinical Director of the School of Integrated Health at the University of Westminster.

Consultant Editor

Dr. Kenneth R. Pelletier MD PhD is a Clinical Professor of Medicine in the Department of Medicine, University of Arizona School of Medicine, the Department of Family and Community Medicine, and in the Department of Psychiatry, University of California School of Medicine, San Francisco (UCSF). He is also Chairman of the American Health Association, and is the author of ten books, including the international bestseller *Mind as Healer, Mind as Slayer*.

Contributors and Consultants

- **Dr. John Briffa**, nutrition and well-being columnist

- **Leon R. Chaitow**, consultant naturopath and osteopath, Honorary Fellow at University of Westminster

- **Dr. Andrew Chevallier**, Senior Lecturer in herbal medicine, Middlesex University

- **Dr. Peter Fisher**, Clinical Director of Research and Consultant to the Royal London Homeopathic Hospital

- **Dr. Adriane Fugh-Berman**, Associate Professor, Complementary and Alternative Medicine, Department of Physiology and Biophysics, Georgetown University School of Medicine

- **Dr. Adrian Hemmings**, psychology lecturer, University of Sussex

- **Dr. Randy Horwitz**, lecturer at the Program in Integrative Medicine, University of Arizona

- **Dr. Mark Hyman**, Hyman Integrative Therapies

- **Dr. David Kiefer**, fellow at the Program in Integrative Medicine, University of Arizona

- **Dr. Yoon Hang Kim**, Acupuncture and Integrative Medicine College, University of California at Berkeley

- **Professor George Lewith**, acupuncturist and Senior Research Fellow at University of Southampton

- **Dr. Michael McIntyre**, former chair, European Herbal Practitioners' Association

- **Dr. Pam Pappas**, Desert Institute School of Classical Homeopathy, Phoenix, Arizona

- **Dr. Kenneth R. Pelletier**, Clinical Professor of Medicine at the University of Arizona School of Medicine and the University of California School of Medicine, San Francisco (UCSF)

- **Dr. Penny Preston**, family doctor and full-time writer

- **Dr. Martin Rossman**, Department of Medicine, University of California San Francisco Medical School

- **Dr. Elad Schiff**, Bnai-Zion Medical Center, Haifa, Israel

Contents

Foreword

Conventional Western medicine used to mean taking the body apart and analyzing it down into ever smaller components. But examining a piston can't tell you how an engine works. We cannot explain the mind by dissecting the brain, nor understand a person by doing chemical tests. And living organisms are quite different from mechanisms: they self-assemble, and the whole has a huge effect on its parts. The healthy body is an infinitely intricate three-dimensional jigsaw puzzle that is continually breaking itself apart, even down at the molecular level, and then reconstructing itself.

A new medicine is emerging that realizes that you cannot predict how a complex system functions just by studying its parts. So it aims to work with the body as a whole, to trigger the awesome capacity for self-healing. This means tapping into a spectrum of complementary and conventional treatments and mind–body medicine to maintain health and well-being. Medical science is rediscovering the power of self-healing processes, an area where traditional systems, such as acupuncture, massage, or herbal medicine, may have a lot to offer.

We should consider health as having three "realms": structural, biochemical, and psychological (*see p.14*). Conventional medicine tends to focus on one or other of the three dimensions. For example, drugs target biochemical aspects, surgery focuses on the body's structure, and counseling on the mind. But since many health problems are complex, conventional medicine can offer no single "magic bullet," and its existing treatments have limited success or cause side effects. In painful, stress-related illnesses such as migraine, or in recurring disorders like arthritis, psoriasis, and eczema, single-level approaches fall short. In chronic fatigue or persistent pain syndromes where standard tests detect no changes in body tissues, drug treatment alone often proves unsatisfactory. New medicine comes into its own where there is no single well-defined cause, and various factors — biochemical, structural and pyschosocial — are involved. Avoiding single solutions, new medicine adopts a holistic approach, looking at temperament, bodily tension, breathing, coping style, lifestyle, and diet, and exploring complementary therapies' potential to trigger vitality.

New medicine is increasingly driven by patients' needs. Doctors, though, realize that self-care and patient choice are crucially important. Increasing collaboration between conventional and complementary practitioners and the rise of mind–body therapies are supported by promising research results. We present some of them in this book. While doctors are catching up with new medicine, individuals need to make a special effort to stay well and understand the spectrum of treatments available. This book has been written to support all those who share these aims.

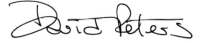

Integrated

Medicine

WELL-BEING AND HEALTH

DR. DAVID PETERS

When we are healthy, we can adapt to change. If our bodies and minds get what they need and are not overwhelmed, they can successfully meet challenges. Like a spinning gyroscope, we stay upright provided we have enough energy, but lose our balance if we are pushed too far. So what do we mean by "energy," how do we get and keep it, and how does the body manage to maintain the balance and harmony that add up to well-being?

These are the questions that new medicine has to ask. They are different from the questions medical science has asked until now, and they are important because medicine is in crisis. The crisis has to do with rocketing costs and a widespread disillusionment among the public with scientific medicine's obsession with molecules, drugs, and technology at the expense of serving the whole person. It is an aspect of a worldwide concern with sustainability and the side effects, whether global or medical, of technological solutions to complex problems. Fortunately, science is becoming more holistic as it realizes the limitations of a fragmented approach to solving problems and starts to understand complexity. Curiously, the scientific picture emerging today has a lot in common with truths known to the world's oldest healing traditions. The new medicine will integrate this timeless knowledge about self-healing and whole-person care with 21st-century science. It is even possible, as complexity is further explored and understood, that traditional notions such as "life-force" and "energy-body" could find their way into mainstream medicine.

The Body in Flux

The new medicine requires a new way of thinking about the body. The body is alive and constantly on the move, constantly changing. The body is also constantly healing and renewing itself — cells die and are replaced, food is processed, and oxygen pours in to fuel the biochemical furnaces that give us energy. Physical and mental demands are met by continual adjustments in our internal systems. On the one hand, these demands may be as straightforward as those involved in taking this book off the shelf, sitting down with a cup of coffee, and reading; or they may be

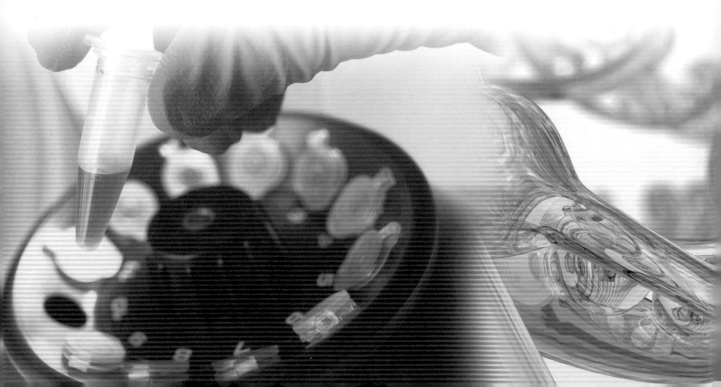

demands that the body finds difficult to handle. These difficult challenges could involve something as tiny as abnormal genes, chemical toxins, or disease-causing germs, or something much larger, such as the constant strain of an uncomfortable working position, the effects of an injury, or widespread hardening of the arteries. More subtle kinds of distress, such as the emotional strain of a difficult relationship, financial pressures, or the death of a loved one, can also present the body with challenges.

Common sense tells us that how well we feel must influence our approach to life, and that when negative influences outweigh the natural resilience of our body and mind, we become ill. Science bears these ideas out. The latest research shows that the connection between mind and body is complete; one influences the other. It is also clear that the mind–body has built-in healing responses of its own that we can tap into. Many scientists and doctors suspect that natural healing techniques can mobilize this self-healing response to prevent illness and promote better health and well-being, even in someone who has a chronic disease. Some people are convinced that the future of medicine depends on our learning how to make use of the response. Modern medicine, although skilled in waging war on disease, has lost its knowledge of self-healing. Various people have compared medical science to war: weapons can backfire and wars tend to increase the enemy's aggressiveness. Looking at medicine today, we can see how the "arms race" between science and disease has led to overreliance on technology, high costs, and side effects, and more resistant infections.

What is missing is a way of building up the mind–body's natural defenses. This is something the world's traditional medical systems know about. These systems have had to rely not on scientific research but on their traditional knowledge and skills to trigger self-healing through touch, words, movement, art, the products of nature, food, exercise, and harmonious living.

Three Mind–Body Levels

We can think of the human mind–body as composed of three interdependent levels: biochemical, structural, and psychosocial (*see box, p.14*). These levels provide a framework for thinking about aspects of our health. They are interrelated, so an impact on one level affects the others. The holistic nature of complementary medicines aims to encompass all three levels, although clearly some types of therapy are directed at a particular level: herbal medicines and nutritional supplements are more biochemical in their effect than structural therapies, such as chiropractic and massage, while cognitive behavioral therapy and other talking therapies act mainly on the psychosocial level.

In regulating itself, the body draws on all three levels: the biochemical level that fuels body processes; the structural level that supports the organs and body systems; and the psychosocial level that governs thoughts, desires, actions, and emotions. For example, after an exhausting and stressful day, a good night's sleep allows the biochemical furnace to cool down, the body's structures to rest and relax, and the mind to assimilate the day's events. If challenges become intense, unrelenting, or too frequent, the body and mind's extraordinary capacity to adapt can be overwhelmed. Coping relies on energy and order, but

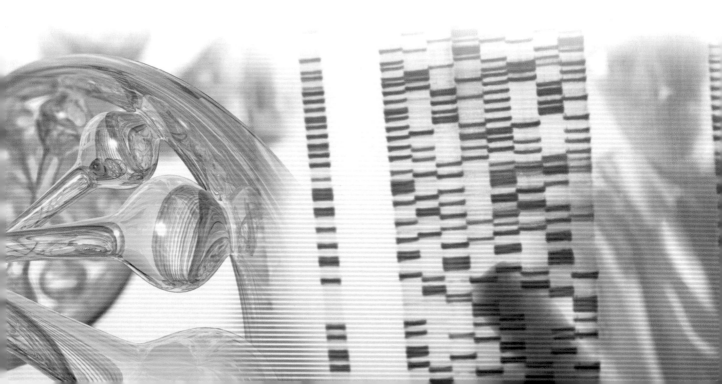

REALMS OF BODY AND MIND

Integrated medicine seeks to encompass the whole person when treating a disease or disorder. Instead of looking only at symptoms and a specific disease, integrated medicine practitioners take into account a patient's lifestyle, personality type, and social environment as well as his or her general health and medical history. This holistic approach makes treatment of many diseases more effective.

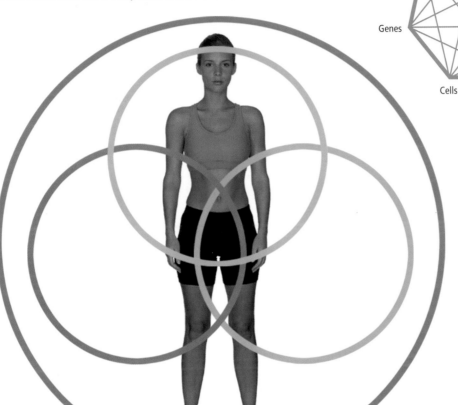

Biosphere

Molecules

Community

Genes

LIVING PERSON

Emotions

Cells

Organs

Our body, and therefore our health, is intimately connected at every level not only to cells, organs, and our living processes but also to the external influences around us. For example, our genes influence the way we respond to pollutants in the biosphere, our emotions alter the way we interact with people in our community, and our emotions affect our immune cells.

Health is controlled by three interdependent "realms" — psychosocial, structural, and biochemical. They are under-pinned by a fourth realm, "life force" or "energy."

"LIFE FORCES"

Encompassing and acting on all three realms, this concept is variously described by therapists as "regulatory forces," "vital forces," "energy," and "Qi."

Treatments include high-potency homeopathic remedies, traditional Chinese acupuncture, traditional herbalism, and spiritual healing.

PSYCHOSOCIAL

The psychosocial realm includes thoughts and feelings, relationships, social environment, community, workplace, and culture.

Treatments include psychotherapy, behavioral approaches, health promotion information, social work, hypnotherapy, and meditation.

STRUCTURAL

The structural realm includes muscles, bones, nerves, blood vessels, movement, and the physical environment.

Treatments include physical therapy, osteopathy, chiropractic, massage, medical acupuncture, and surgery.

BIOCHEMICAL

The biochemical realm includes cells, hormones, enzymes, chemical processes, digestion and respiration, the chemical environment, and pollution.

Treatments include drugs, nutritional supplements, low-potency homeopathic remedies, dietary changes, and herbal medicines.

if a person's resources are depleted, the ability to maintain balance is undermined. Defense and repair systems may begin to fail if the integrity of cell chemistry, body structures, and mind are threatened.

The underlying factors upsetting self-regulation can be obvious or subtle, intense or diffuse, short-lived or prolonged. They can include a short-term, severe injury, for example from a car accident, a bereavement triggering depression, a spell of rushed working lunches resulting in bouts of indigestion, or flu caught from exposure to an infected person. In their own important ways, the resulting ill-effects tell us something vital about how well we are adapting to the demands placed on us; they are a message about things we need to attend to, and changes that we might have to make.

Challenges affect all three levels — psychosocial, structural, and biochemical — and, since they are entwined, when there is a problem in one, it can affect how the other two work. For example, a biochemical disorder such as a nutritional deficiency or food sensitivity may have psychological consequences, such as depression. Loneliness, depression, bereavement, and inner conflicts can undermine immune system defenses, while a structural injury might cause pain that undermines well-being and relationships.

The implications are obvious: give your body what it needs to work well and avoid the things that harm it. This may include taking up yoga, meditation, or dance; giving up smoking; seeing friends; or making dietary changes. Do whatever you need to do to nourish yourself intellectually, emotionally, and spiritually.

Complexity and Medicine

Complexity is the name for the universal tendency of parts to organize themselves into more complex wholes. We humans are so much a part of our world that we often take many of its properties and qualities for granted. We fail to remember that weight, water, light, and warmth, although totally familiar to us, are also rather mysterious. Complexity can be seen at the most basic level: who could predict, for instance, that bringing the gases hydrogen and oxygen together would give you something to drink! Complexity operates too on the biggest scale of all. After the Big Bang, when time and space first began, our pattern-forming universe produced stars and galaxies; planets formed. Life — miraculously it seems, but also quite naturally — emerged out of this universal process. Organisms are alive precisely because the whole is always greater than the sum of its parts.

Medical scientists until now have tried to understand life by isolating its biochemical properties in a test tube or by examining dead tissues. While this approach has certainly proved very useful in understanding how the human body works, it can only reveal our chemical nature. Modern technology now lets us see into the intricate design and workings of the living body. As science discovers how the parts communicate, form wholes, and self-organize, medicine will change profoundly. It is too soon to know what medicine would look like if it were based on mind–body connectedness and the flow of information that keeps us well, but there are similarities between such an approach and the traditions that gave birth to complementary medicine. These traditions all include notions of mind–body wholeness, energy flow, harmonious living, and therapeutic relationships, along with knowledge of how to encourage self-healing. Science is becoming increasingly interested in this territory and the possibility that complementary therapies might provide us with further clues about human health.

Complex processes are not like sequential ones, where A causes B, which causes C. Whole system processes are networked; they happen all at once, and communication is across the whole system in all directions, so C influences A even as B influences Z — and back!

New medicine views the body as a complex system through which information flows. A school of fish is an excellent example of this type of complexity. Although each is a separate animal, when fish come together in a school they behave as a single entity.

This realization has enormous practical implications: scientists developing artificial intelligence, or predicting weather patterns or ecological consequences, need to know how to predict whole-system behavior. It is of even greater relevance for medicine to understand how the processes of life interweave, and how the whole and the part continually reshape one another.

The Intelligent Body

We tend to think of the brain as being intelligent, and that the brain controls the body, while the body is just dumb flesh. Indeed, the brain is a network of almost infinitely interconnected neurons; it has been called the most complex object in the known universe. But the whole body is a network too, which is why the psychologist Michael Hyland has put forward his "intelligent body" hypothesis. Dr. Hyland takes further the idea that there is no strict division between brain and the rest of the body. He proposes that intelligence is not confined to the brain, but rather it is distributed throughout the body in an extended network.

Medicine, if it is to get to grips with health rather than just confront disease, must comprehend the living body's extraordinary ability to maintain conditions stable enough for life to happen at all. Too hot or too cold, too acid or too alkaline, too many waste products or not enough nutrients, and we die. The same goes for the body's internal architecture and outer form, for they are not fixed, but are constantly broken down and rebuilt. The sense of self, too, although it seems stable, is formed out of a whirl of sense impressions and memories.

At a biochemical level, the properties that emerge from the network provide its ability to self-organize, control the myriad chemical reactions that provide energy and produce the living tissues. At the structural level, these so-called "emergent" properties allow the body to move through space and constantly reconstruct itself; at the level of awareness they give us the ability to sense, respond to, and reflect on our experiences.

When systems go wrong

Moderate challenges to the mind–body generally lead to recovery and even to improved resilience. Challenges that are successfully met result in better immunity, improved fitness, and more appropriate coping styles.

However, the information system can go wrong and develop less efficient modes of working. These states of "dys-regulation" prepare the ground for disease to take hold. They may arise because the challenge to the body is too great or too persistent, or the person is vulnerable psychologically (various styles of thinking and feeling can undermine recovery), biochemically (due to genetic, nutritional and ecological factors), or structurally (because

of deep patterns of tension, a lack of fitness or flexibility). The system may be overwhelmed because a person fails to notice the body's messages of distress and change habits that prevent recovery. It is the seamless mind–body network — not just brain-based intelligence — that adapts to changing internal and external conditions. The new medicine will recognize this. Faced with an illness, an injury, or a social crisis, the new medicine, which aims to unite the best of complementary therapies and conventional medicine, will aim to re-establish balance.

Michael Hyland's theory that disease begins as an information error suggests a new and important way of thinking about health. There are two kinds of "error" in the mind–body. One is the type that conventional Western medicine deals with when it looks at the body as a biological machine, identifying a biological disease such as diabetes, cancer, heart disease, or arthritis. Conventional treatment involves fixing the "broken part" or removing it. This might involve replacing a missing hormone, killing bacteria with antibiotics, reducing blood pressure with a drug, suppressing inflammation with steroids, replacing a blocked artery with an artificial graft, or cutting away a cancerous tumor.

There is another type of error affects the information in the whole network. In this case, no single organ or biochemical system can be targeted and repaired, because the information that produces health and healing processes is spread over the entire network.

In the case of the latter error, approaches that aim to create health or to trigger healing responses by acting on the mind–body as a whole are most likely to be effective. And, just as networks can take in many different kinds of information, so the mind–body can respond to diverse kinds of input — diet, botanical medicines, movement and touch. So too can it pick up more refined information — from art, communication with a therapist, and perhaps even the subtle information conveyed by a homeopathic medicine or the effect of an acupuncture needle. The entire mind–body could be influenced by lifestyle choices that have an impact on the biochemical, structural, and mental information systems.

We can imagine the whole system of information flow — the body's intelligence — as a choir of myriad voices. But it is a choir without a score or a conductor. The parts sing themselves and each voice hears the entire chorale and responds more or less harmoniously. The voices are biochemical and electrical messages, structural impulses, communications from the conscious and unconscious mind. This is an example of complexity in action: the information flow emerges from the interweaving of biochemical, structural, and mental information systems, but it simultaneously forms and shapes them all.

Perhaps the information flow that makes complexity possible is what the traditional healers refer to as "life force." If this is the case, then the body's intelligence may

TWELVE STEPS TO WELL-BEING

There are many things you can do to improve the quality of your life. Some of them are material things, such as eating well and getting exercise, but many of them are psychological. Learning to treat yourself well and to interact well with the people around you can improve the quality of your life immensely.

THE STEPS	WHY TRY THEM?	PUT THEM INTO PRACTICE
1 Eat fresh food; it's a better source of vitamins and minerals than even the best supplements.	Antioxidants mop up free radicals (super-reactive chemicals) that can damage the body's cells.	Get serious about healthy eating and choose a diet high in fiber and antioxidants and low in fat.
2 Incorporate exercise into your daily routine — you'll feel better.	Exercise makes bones and heart stronger and lifts mood.	Take the stairs rather than the elevator; walk as much as you can; find a sport you enjoy and do it regularly.
3 Relax regularly and take time to appreciate the good things you have in your life.	Relaxation prevents the body from staying in "emergency mode" due to stress.	Make time to relax each day, even if only for 15 minutes. Use a relaxation tape or try yoga or massage.
4 Be aware of stress in your life and minimize it as much as you can.	Stress puts strain on body systems and contributes to many health problems.	Keep a stress diary to help you identify where your stress is coming from. Then work to minimize or eliminate it.
5 Appreciate yourself. Dwell on your positives, not on your negatives.	People with high self-esteem cope better with life's challenges.	Try positive affirmations, such as "I am peaceful" and "I can organize my life." Sounds corny, but it works.
6 Think positively.	Optimism and humor have been shown scientifically to benefit health.	Let go of old hurts, which can drag you down psychologically. Use counseling to do this if necessary.
7 Make yourself understood. Clear communication is important in all spheres of life.	Communicating your needs and thoughts clearly can prevent stressful misunderstandings and conflicts.	Say what you think, as pleasantly and politely as possible. Listen fully to what the other person actually says.
8 Build your confidence. Believe your contribution is of value.	Being confident gives you control. People also feel more comfortable with confidence than insecurity.	Try acting with assurance, which often brings real self-confidence.
9 Build close relationships. You don't need many but you do need a few.	Having a sense that you value others and are valued yourself is essential to mental well-being.	Be open with people. Don't allow distance to grow between you and the people you love.
10 Find things to appreciate every day. It's often the little things that make life enjoyable.	Small things can be very uplifting and can help you get through difficult days.	Observe the world around you and appreciate giving and receiving kindnesses.
11 Be generous. Generosity and compassion feel better than selfishness and cynicism.	Science has shown that altruism is healthy.	Be charitable and try not to let the pace of modern life make you unkind.
12 Be thankful.	You are a living miracle and you have a right to be here, as do all people.	At the end of each day, count its blessings, no matter how small. Let the bad things go and give tomorrow another chance.

correspond to complementary medicine's "energy body," but it would probably be more accurate to call it the "information body."

Expectation, relationships, and healing

The information body may be particularly affected by the relationship between practitioner and patient. Positive belief and expectations on the part of both the therapist or caregiver and the patient can have a strong influence on the course of a condition, regardless of the type of treatment involved. This effect has been attributed to the placebo effect (*see Clinical trials, p.23*). A positive relationship between therapist and patient fuels this effect and can be a powerful force for healing. This healing effect was demonstrated in a famous study at Massachusetts General Hospital in Boston in 1964. Patients undergoing surgery who received a preoperative visit from a warm and sympathetic anesthetist had far less postoperative pain, and therefore needed fewer analgesics, than other patients undergoing similar surgery who were not visited.

It also seems that patients have responsibilities to cultivate a good relationship with their caregivers. In another Boston study, patients with chronic illnesses such as diabetes, rheumatoid arthritis, and high blood pressure were coached to ask relevant questions of their doctor. Afterward they reported more satisfaction with their visit and even enjoyed better health than those who had not been coached to ask questions.

The strong healing forces triggered by expectation can also work in a negative way. People who have insensitive treatment from nurses, doctors, or other practitioners often complain of feeling worse. This is known as the "nocebo" effect — the opposite of the placebo. The power of a positive therapist–patient relationship is the key reason why you should choose a therapy (and a therapist) that you trust.

How the Mind Influences the Body

Future research into mind–body processes will reveal a great deal more than we know now about how mind–body differences — differences in temperament, for instance — affect individual susceptibility to illness and response to treatment. Research shows that emotional states such as loneliness and grief can depress the immune system, leaving people susceptible to disease. When psychologists, immunologists, and endocrinologists began to pool information in the 1980s, they found they could track chemical pathways linking brain activity to physiological processes in the body. It had long been understood that the stress hormones epinephrine and cortisol suppressed the production of antibodies, the body's defense against disease.

But studies in 1977 and 1983 showed how white blood cells (a key part of the body's immune system) were temporarily paralyzed in bereaved men, possibly accounting for deaths from so-called "broken-heart syndrome."

The brain and central nervous system are control centers for both conscious and automatic life processes. In evolutionary terms we have three brains. The first, the cortex, is the most recently developed and allows us to engage in rational thought and language. Traditional psychotherapy or talk therapy aims to influence this "conscious" brain. The left side of the cortex processes information in a linear fashion and coordinates aspects such as language and numerical skills; the right side of the cortex is more concerned with nonlinear spatial relations, metaphor, and music. Recent research has hinted that emotional closeness in the first months of life triggers the development of an area in the forebrain called the neocortex, which allows us to deal with emotion, respond sensitively to others, and experience feelings of pleasure and beauty.

Beneath the forebrain is the second, older brain, which we share with other mammals and which is involved with nonlinear and nonrational aspects, emotions, memory, and feelings. This part of the brain is a rich source of what Candace Pert (who discovered the endorphins and enkephalins) calls "molecules of emotion." These "molecules of emotion" are not confined to the brain, though, because all the body's cells are coated with receptors that constantly scan for them, while also sending out their own messenger molecules to communicate with sites in the brain.

We share the third brain with the reptiles. The medulla oblongata, which is found at the base of the skull, is the seat of instincts and unconscious body-control processes such as breathing.

Science is realizing that well-being is not just "all in the mind" and that the mind is not confined to the brain. So individual temperament is physical as well as psychological, because both brain and body play their crucial part. But is temperament something we inherit or do we learn to be the way we are? A study was done in which 2,000 people were asked to rate their levels of well-being. It showed that people with high well-being ratings usually said they had a happy childhood, are usually optimistic, feel that others think well of them, and that they have life under control. Are people born this way, or does upbringing and learning mold their sunny outlook? Both factors probably come into play. Yet curiously, the science of well-being is revealing how even happiness has its physical components. The way we respond to life's demands and how we express feelings depends at least partly on genetic makeup, body makeup, and brain chemistry. It is not simply that genes program our personality, but rather that our personal style of dealing with the world around us — how we think, feel, learn — has a definite bodily basis.

Neuroscientists now say there's a biological foundation for the temperaments, based on how the brain works and the amounts of different chemical messengers there are. The latest evidence shows how positive feelings boost activity in the left frontal lobe of the brain — if you offer someone an incentive this part of the brain starts to work harder; even small babies show this pattern when they gaze at their mother. The current theory sees this part of the brain as a sort of psychological accelerator pedal, which psychologists call the behavioral approach system — BAS for short. It's more active in people who are extroverted, impulsive, and sensation-seeking, but much quieter in the brain scans of more introverted people. So if temperament is shaped by the way individual brains work and how the body responds, this will influence what we need for our own individual style of well-being.

The Cellular Level

The entire body is built from cells and connective tissue. Each cell is an incredibly complex structure carrying out the processes of life. Cells turn food molecules into energy and building materials; they deal with toxins, enlarge and divide to make your body grow, heal wounds, and replace cells that have died. The various kinds of cell have different natural lifespans, a natural limit to the number of times they can divide and reproduce. For example, red and white blood corpuscles can divide millions of times, but most nerve cells do not reproduce at all. Once a cell has reached its natural limit, it withers and dies. When enough of our cells die, so do we. Some kinds of cell do not age; bacteria keep on dividing forever, unless killed by some outside event. Cancer cells are immortal too, dividing endlessly, unless treatment kills them or the person dies.

Cells communicate with one another by chemical messengers in the intracellular fluids, but they are also intricately connected to the spinal cord and brain through the finest filaments of the nerve fibers that reach each one of them. Inside the cell specialized zones in the outer layer (the cytoplasm) produce energy, or secrete specific molecules that give an organ a specialized function. For example, liver cells produce large amounts of enzymes, catalysts that speed up the chemical processes of detoxification, while fibroblasts produce the skin's supportive matrix of collagens and elastin and have a role in healing wounds. As new and ever more powerful microscopes probe the minute detail of cells' internal architecture, science has realized that each cell has its own cytoskeleton. This acts as a

scaffolding, steadying the nucleus (the cell's central control system) and holding up the cell membrane. The cytoskeleton also provides a communication web within the cell, through which physical forces (pressure and stretching) are transmitted to the nucleus. The cytoskeleton's extension links with those from other cells.

The old idea was of the body as a stack of separate cells awash in fluids; the new image is of a network of cells intricately connected and interpenetrated by fibrils and nanofibers, all embedded in connective tissue that positively hums with vibrant energetic and chemical messages. In addition to involving the brain, nervous, and endocrine systems, this information flow takes place in the connective tissues that hold the organs in place and gives the body its flexible firmness.

Genes, chromosomes, and health

In recent years, medical science has come to recognize the vital role that genetic makeup plays in human health. The human genome, or complete set of genes, has now been mapped and further genetic research will no doubt provide insight into many health problems. But what are these somewhat mysterious things called genes? A gene is one stretch of DNA that contains instructions for making a

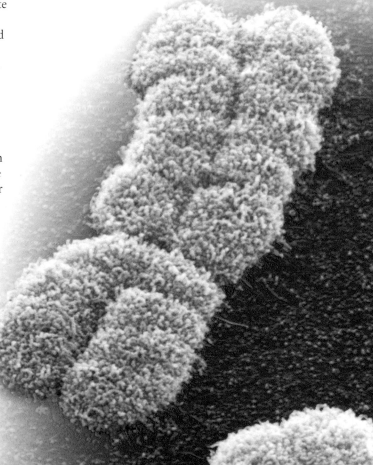

Chromosomes, such as this X-chromosome, are made up of genes — segments of DNA that code for many of our physical and psychological characteristics, such as eye color, stature, gender, and possibly some aspects of personality. Human cells each contain 23 pairs of chromosomes.

particular protein, one of the key molecules that make up your body. Genes store and process biochemical information that evolved as Earth itself was changing from a cloudy swamp into a blue planet. For eons, genes have evolved both as parts of whole organisms and in response to the organisms' relationship with the environment.

Thus, our genes record not only our parents' heredity but also our evolutionary past. Just as our threefold brain connects us to our reptilian ancestors, so too do our genes contain the immense accumulated biochemical intelligence of the evolutionary process. The information they carry is an important aspect of the intelligent body.

Genes are arranged along chromosomes — neatly packaged strings of DNA that hold the genetic instructions controlling your biochemical makeup and determining many physical aspects of who you are. The nucleus of each cell that makes up your body contains 46 chromosomes — 23 inherited from each parent. This set of chromosomes, which each of us has, is estimated to contain about 90,000 pairs of genes. Inheriting 23 chromosomes from each parent means that we have two copies of most genes. This has a bearing on our health, because if one gene is defective, we usually have another to fall back on.

However, in some cases we may have just one copy of a gene. Only 22 of the 23 pairs of chromosomes in each cell are matching. The sex chromosomes may be different. Women have two "X" chromosomes, one inherited from their mother and one from their father. Men, on the other hand, have just one "X" chromosome, inherited from their mother, and a "Y" chromosome, inherited from their father. For this reason, many of the genes on the "X" chromosome have no backup copy in men, and accounts for the fact that genetic conditions due to faulty genes on the "X" chromosome, such as red–green color blindness and hemophilia, are more common in men than women.

An Integrated Approach to Health

Most diseases do not have a single specific cause. For example, smoking may cause lung cancer, but there are smokers who live into their 90s without any apparent ill-effects. Whether or not we succumb to illness and our recovery rate are dependent on a multitude of interrelated factors that affect our self-regulation.

Sickness is not the same as disease. Someone with a headache may feel sick without having a diagnosable disease. A doctor makes a diagnosis based on the patient's story and clinical signs (observable changes) and then prescribes treatment. Complementary and alternative practitioners consider signs and symptoms differently and may suggest treatments to stimulate the self-healing processes. The integrated approach seeks to use conventional treatments if a clear diagnosis and safe, effective treatments are available, and to explore the role of alternative and complementary treatments depending on their appropriateness and availability. Often, this approach will explore what triggered the problem, made you susceptible, or undermined your resilience, and what may be preventing you from getting better. An integrated approach may require motivation to change something: diet, exercise, or a way of thinking; or learning a self-healing practice.

The risks of integrated medicine

As natural products — herbs and nutritional supplements — become more popular, there has been much publicized concern about their side effects and interactions. Experts are advising caution when prescribing natural products

MAKING A DIAGNOSIS

	CONVENTIONAL DIAGNOSIS	ALTERNATIVE DIAGNOSIS	THE INTEGRATED APPROACH
Conventional and alternative practitioners both diagnose illness, but they tend to take different approaches. Conventional practitioners rely on symptoms and signs, possibly with tests, to make a diagnosis. Alternative practitioners spend more time discussing your lifestyle and medical history.	● A doctor asks you about symptoms and refers to your medical record. ● He or she examines you for clinical signs of disease, such as a raised temperature, a rash, lumps, enlarged liver, or abnormal heartbeat. ● You may have blood and urine tests and X-rays. ● You might be referred for further tests, such as ultrasound or MRI. ● Depending on the diagnosis, treatment might include drugs, physical therapy, surgery, etc.	● A practitioner takes a full case history and asks about your lifestyle. ● Depending on the therapy type, the practitioner may run diagnostic tests. ● The explanation given may bear no relationship to conventional medical diagnosis. ● The diagnosis will usually imply certain biochemical, structural, or psychosocial causes. ● Treatment is likely to be tailored to suit the individual.	In integrated medicine, diagnosis and treatment is based on both conventional and alternative or complementary approaches to treat the whole person.

alongside conventional drugs. So, should we be concerned about herb–drug interactions? Yes, we should, because they may be more common than we know; reporting systems for alternative therapies are not yet very effective. However, so far, many nutritional supplements and herbs have excellent safety records, while there are sizable known health risks associated with many medications. Vitamin E, omega-3 fatty acids, and ginkgo, for instance, all have a slight anticoagulant effect, so they could in theory increase the blood-thinning effects of aspirin and warfarin. Their interaction could therefore increase the tendency to bleed. Perhaps further research will confirm that these interactions are truly significant. However, the greatest risk of adverse interaction with conventional medicines comes from food, rather than from vitamin supplements or herbs. Grapefruit enhances the effects of many drugs, among them certain antihistamines, calcium-channel blockers (for reducing blood pressure) and some statin drugs (also used to reduce blood pressure). Some vegetables, including garlic, onions, and broccoli, have the opposite effect, enhancing drug breakdown by boosting the liver's detoxification enzymes.

St. John's wort, which has a similar effect on the liver as these vegetables, reducing the effectiveness of certain drugs, particularly oral contraceptives, some antidepressants, digoxin, and cyclosporin. Coenzyme Q_{10} and hawthorn (*Crataegus*) improve heart function and, consequently, heart patients may need to check with their health-care practitioner about adjusting prescribed heart medicines, such as digoxin (*see Using herbs safely, p.69*).

There are also risks associated with other alternative and complementary therapies. The biggest one is the danger that a harmful but conventionally treatable condition might be missed. This is far less likely to happen when conventional doctors and alternative or complementary practitioners work together. Other rare risks include stroke and damage to arteries in the neck after manipulation of the cervical spine. Massage has few adverse effects, although it would be best avoided where deep vein thrombosis, burns, skin infections, eczema, open wounds, bone fractures, advanced osteoporosis, and lymphoma are involved. Acupuncture is extremely safe when performed by a skilled practitioner, even though it involves needles. One survey of doctors and physical therapists who performed acupuncture reported no serious adverse events and only 671 minor adverse events per 10,000 consultations. Only 14 of these minor events were said to have been significant. The danger of cross-infection through needles is negligible if disposable needles are used, as they always should be.

Integrating conventional medicine and alternative and complementary therapies

Alternative and complementary therapies can work well in conjunction with conventional ones, to reinforce effectiveness of conventional treatments, to strengthen the body and aid recovery, or to ease symptoms or side effects of treatment. However, you may often find that therapists have totally different approaches to your health care.

Differences in use of language and concepts can cause communication problems. Conventional medical practitioners tend to have a highly scientific approach, which treats the body or the symptoms as a set of separate, discrete entities. Disease is usually ascribed to a fault in one or more measurable physical or biochemical systems. On the other hand, alternative and complementary therapists tend to make their diagnosis using a very different interpretation of the patient's body, the patient's experiences, and the illness. For example, an acupuncturist might attribute a certain type of headache to "stagnation in the gallbladder meridian"; this is clearly not a diagnosis that any conventional doctor would understand.

Such different approaches can make it difficult to see compatible therapeutic aims between your conventional doctor and alternative or complementary practitioner. Perhaps you have found a practice where they are working together. If so, you are fortunate indeed, for such projects are still rather unusual. However, there is a powerful trend toward collaboration, driven by promising research results in some areas, particularly acupuncture, nutrition, herbal medicine, and mind body medicine. For most people, taking an integrated approach to health will mean that you as the patient will have to coordinate the various therapies you are using. This entails taking responsibility for communicating between therapists and ensuring that your treatments are compatible.

Integrated medicine in practice

Taking an integrated approach to managing your health care involves thinking and working on several levels. The three key factors are: maintaining self-regulation and building up resilience; using self-help and conventional medicine when it is necessary; and using alternative and complementary approaches appropriately.

Although many medical practices provide access to some form of alternative therapy, the availability of integrated treatment, and the amount that you may have to pay for it, varies widely among regions. The most commonly used alternative therapies available within the US are acupuncture, aromatherapy, chiropractic, homeopathy, hypnotherapy, and osteopathy. There are also more than 30 colleges and medical schools that offer training in alternative and complementary therapies.

Hospitals, hospices, palliative-care services, and some pain clinics are increasingly using alternative and complementary therapies to give patients a wider choice of treatments. Many charities and community health services, such as those for people with alcohol or drug-related problems, mental health issues, cancer, or HIV, also offer these therapies as part of their program.

Most alternative therapists run their own private practices. They may work from home or be based in alternative health clinics. Information on associations and regulatory bodies can easily be found on the internet (*see Useful Websites and Addresses, p.486*).

Choosing a therapy and a practitioner

In choosing a therapy, you need to examine your attitude to health. Do you believe in making an effort to stay in good health, or do you prefer not to think about it? It is also important to consider your attitude to the treatment itself and what it will involve. For example, do you dislike being touched? Are you organized enough to take pills regularly? Are you comfortable talking about your life with someone else? All of these things have a bearing on the type of therapy that might work for you.

Once you have chosen the therapy/therapies that you think are most likely to help your condition, it is important that you also find a practitioner with whom you feel comfortable. You should be sure to check that he or she has appropriate training, qualifications, and facilities to help you with your condition (*for details of regulatory bodies, see Useful Websites and Addresses, p.486*).

If you do not feel well and are planning to see an alternative therapist, it is also important that you see your doctor first. The doctor can rule out any dangerous or life-threatening conditions and can discuss treatment options

Doctors may send blood or tissue samples to a laboratory, where they will be examined to determine the nature of a disease.

with you. You should always try to discuss your decisions about using alternative therapies with your conventional practitioners (internist, midwife, etc.).

Questions you may want to ask include the following:
- Is the practitioner regulated by a professional body?
- What does he or she charge for a treatment? Does the first appointment cost more?
- Is the treatment covered by your health insurance company?
- Has he or she treated people with your condition before?
- How many treatments might be needed?
- Is there anything you should do before treatment, such as fasting for a short time, or wearing special clothes?
- How will you feel after treatment? Are there any precautions you should take right after a treatment?
- Are there any possible side effects or risk factors? If you are not entirely happy, say so.
- Tell your doctor and practitioners about any over-the-counter medication or alternative remedies or treatments you are taking.
- Tell your practitioner and your doctor whether a treatment worked. Feedback is always appreciated.

Managing health and illness

Research shows that when people take responsibility for their health care, symptoms often improve and quality of life is enhanced. The first stage involves gaining knowledge, so it is important to learn as much as possible about all the factors that influence your health. If you are prone to, or already have, a health problem, understanding how you can compensate for this susceptibility will help minimize its impact. Knowing about causes, symptoms, and the range of available treatment options is obviously empowering. You can begin your research by looking up your condition in the relevant section of this book and then doing some further reading or research on the internet.

Overly optimistic expectations about your condition can lead to a roller coaster of emotional highs and lows that does nothing to aid your recovery from illness. Beware of practitioners who say they have a definite cure for a chronic condition, or of advertisements for products that make exaggerated claims; you should even be cautious of reports of scientific breakthroughs (whether made or about to be), for they rarely turn out to be the desired "magic bullet"; all too often the silver lining comes with a gray cloud of side effects. Particularly for people with chronic disease, it is crucial to have realistic expectations and it helps to develop an understanding of these claims and how research is conducted (*see p.23*) so that you can make judgments about the quality of the information that you are presented with. However, bear in mind that even if many useful therapies can only control or ameliorate symptoms, their value in improving quality of life should not be underestimated.

Research and Evidence

Any treatment that you receive should be safe and effective; therefore, there should be evidence for its safety and efficacy. However, the general understanding of the safety and efficacy of treatment options is not always as good as it could be. For example there is a widespread belief that "chemicals" are bad, while "natural" is good for you. (Snake poison is entirely natural!)

Research to obtain this evidence is not always straightforward and easy to conduct, and interpreting the results from research can be equally complex. Even when good experiments have been conducted, getting the information in an appropriate and unbiased form to patients and practitioners can be slow and difficult. One of the key difficulties facing a medical researcher is that all people are different. Not only do we look different from those around us, we also respond differently as a disease progresses, and to the treatments that we might be using. This means that even if you have the same disease or condition as your neighbor, it may not follow exactly the same course, and a treatment that works for your neighbor may not work for you. Researchers have to use large numbers of people in their studies to untangle real effects from this background variation. Another factor to be taken into account is that patients have "good days" and "bad days." A researcher also needs to know if an improvement in a condition is the result of treatment, or just part of this natural variation. Therefore, large numbers of patients in a study, and an appropriate timescale for the tests, may be important factors when testing for efficacy.

Alternatives to research and evidence do not provide proof that treatments are safe and effective. Anecdotes (stories) of cures may be coincidences or due to natural variability of conditions and people. People also have a natural tendency to report only positive stories ("miracle cures") rather than those where not much happened. Even less reliable is "knowing" or a "gut feeling" that something works. What is "known" to be true by one person can just as easily be "known" to be false by another. Long-term use of a therapy (e.g., over centuries) does instill confidence in its effectiveness, but safety issues may be harder to establish, especially where problems occur over many months or years, making it difficult to pinpoint their true cause.

Medical research attempts to distinguish real effects from random events, to tease out bias and detect unexpected or unwanted outcomes.

Clinical trials

The principal method for testing a treatment is the clinical trial. These were originally devised to test pharmaceutical drugs and treatments in conventional medicine, and now they are also being used to investigate alternative therapies such as herbal medicines.

A clinical trial aims to test whether a treatment works, but one of the main problems with testing any therapy is that providing the therapy (or even talking about it in positive terms) can cause a person's condition to improve, whether the therapy has any true activity or not. This natural and widely documented response is the placebo effect.

Placebo-controlled trials are conducted to distinguish between the placebo effect and a true response. In a placebo-controlled trial, the therapy that is being tested is compared with a seemingly identical treatment. The patients are split into two groups and one is given the test therapy (e.g. the medication in pill form) while the other group is given a "control" (e.g., an inactive sugar pill that looks the same as the test pill). For the treatment to be deemed to have worked, patients in the experimental group must perform significantly better than those taking the placebo.

For ethical reasons, particularly in life-threatening conditions, the "control" is often the best medication currently available, because patients who are given a nonactive treatment could experience a worsening of symptoms The "control" can also be the current standard treatment, or the drug of a competing pharmaceutical company, depending on what the researcher is trying to demonstrate. In clinical trials, enough people are tested to minimize bias due to natural variation in people and their illness. Further risks of bias are ruled out by assigning patients at random to the groups.

More recently research has demonstrated that even subtle cues given unconsciously by therapists or experimenters can influence the outcome. To counteract these subtle effects, researchers use double-blind methods (where a clinician randomly assigns patients to either group, then codes the treatments so that neither the patient nor the experimenter knows who is getting which treatment). This makes the randomized double-blind trial the ultimate test.

However, testing alternative therapies using standard randomized controlled methods can be difficult, since it can be hard to provide a realistic control. Some alternative therapies have been tested using placebo-controls, for example, acupuncture methods have been tested by using needles on patients either in the correct acupuncture locations or at sham nonacupuncture sites. But if you want to test the benefits of massage, how do you give the control group a dummy treatment that is convincingly similar to massage? Clinical trials must be carefully adapted to fit the personalized nature of many alternative therapies.

Finally meta-analyses or systematic reviews are useful tools. These are ways of collecting and analyzing the results of a number of studies in the same area to give a more accurate picture of the total research evidence available.

Throughout this book the authors have endeavored to base treatment recommendations on reliable scientific evidence, combined with practitioner experience of what is particularly effective (*see p.111 for how treatments are rated*).

CONVENTIONAL MEDICINE

DR. PENNY PRESTON

Conventional medicine views the body as a number of interdependent systems that can be affected by a variety of diseases. The aim of conventional medicine is to treat existing medical conditions while also promoting a healthy way of life. Health care providers often make recommendations on lifestyle and other measures with the aim of reducing the risk of developing diseases. In addition, screening, for example for precancerous changes of the cervix through cervical smears, is part of the responsibility of conventional medicine.

Physicians and Diagnosis

Different medical specialities tend to focus on particular systems. Thus, apart from the family practitioner, there are specialists such as obstetricians and gynecologists, who specialize in pregnancy and female reproductive health; pulmonologists, who specialize in respiratory problems; cardiologists, who specialize in treating problems with the heart; and so on. Some specialities, such as neurology, deal only with specific systems, such as the nervous system, while others, such as geriatrics or pediatrics, concentrate on one age group. In some instances, the combined expertise of several specialists may be needed to treat a condition or an injury. Specialists are often associated with hospitals.

In addition to specialists, many other medical professionals deliver health care. These include nurses, midwives, physical therapists, occupational therapists, and counselors.

The role of the family practitioner

The family practitioner plays a key role in the delivery of medical treatment, being the usual first port of call for people who are ill. These doctors have a broad knowledge base and expertise in a wide range of diseases. In many cases they can recommend appropriate treatment, whether it is lifestyle measures (such as reducing stress), medicines, or other treatments. Sometimes, a family practitioner will recommend referral to a specialist or to another member of the medical team, such as a counselor or speech therapist.

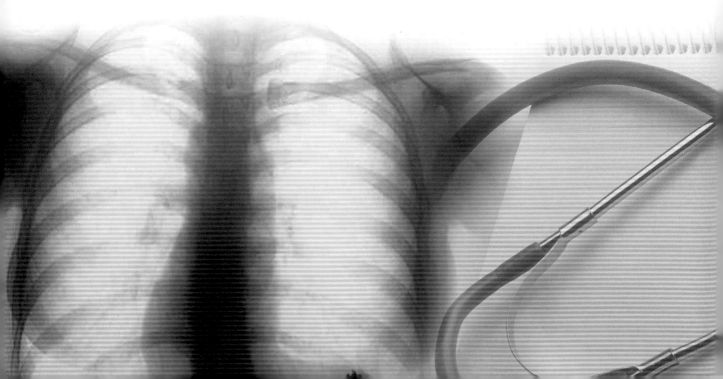

Complementary and alternative therapies

The value of complementary and alternative therapies is gaining acceptance and a family practioner may incorporate them into the treatment plan. The relative roles of the treatments may depend on several factors, including the condition, the patient's wishes, and the available treatment options. For certain conditions, such as cancer, schizophrenia, or coronary artery disease (CAD), the physician will generally recommend that conventional drugs and procedures take a predominant role, but for other disorders complementary and alternative therapies may be a preferred first option. Complementary therapies can often work hand in hand with conventional treatments to relieve symptoms, reduce underlying stress, and improve general well-being.

Making a diagnosis

Key to making appropriate recommendations for treatment is making a diagnosis whenever possible. The physician will look for patterns of symptoms that may suggest particular disorders. For example, certain types of chest pain may be characteristic of coronary artery disease. He or she will take your medical history, which involves not only asking about your symptoms but also about other issues. This may include a discussion of any previous illnesses, lifestyle habits (such as alcohol intake, exercise, and whether you smoke) and the health of relatives. If stress may be contributing to or causing your symptoms, the physician will ask about work, conflicts, concerns, relaxation, and sleep patterns. He or she may then carry out a physical examination. All of this information will help the physician make a diagnosis and select appropriate treatment, or to recommend further tests or referral to a specialist if necessary.

Specialists

Some physicians are specialists, with additional training in their chosen area, and most are associated with a particular hospital. For example, an oncologist specializes in cancer and an urologist in disorders of the urinary tract. In some cases, the physicians "super-specialize," concentrating on one aspect of a speciality. For example, an endocrinologist (a specialist in diseases affecting the hormone system) may have a particular interest in diabetes mellitus.

Visiting a specialist can seem daunting, but it is worth remembering that his or her aims are the same as your physician's: to make a diagnosis, which may involve ordering some tests, and to recommend treatment that will cure or relieve your condition while causing the fewest possible side effects. Be as open as possible; feel free to ask any questions you have and discuss any concerns.

In some cases, specialists will prescribe drugs or recommend a treatment and then hand the patient's care back to the regular physician; in other cases, they will wish to see the patient on a regular basis to monitor progress and to make changes to the treatment plan as necessary.

Tests and investigations

Where further tests or investigations are required, your physician may arrange them or refer you to a specialist, who will organize the appropriate procedures. Tests and investigations can range from simple blood tests to highly sophisticated imaging tests, such as MRI and radionuclide scanning. The tests you will have depend on the nature of the condition that is suspected. Some of the common tests and investigations are described on the following pages.

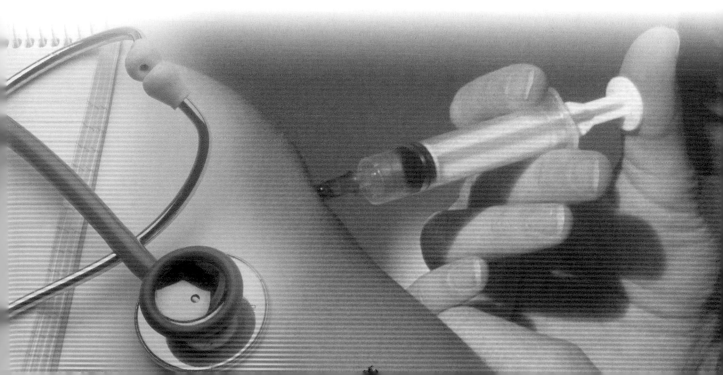

COURSE OF TREATMENT

Your family practitioner is usually the first person you contact when you or a member of your family is sick. He or she will ask you about your symptoms and may examine you physically if necessary. The course of treatment may go something like this:

- Visit to the family practitioner's office.
- Examination by physician.
- The physician may prescribe a drug or a treatment, such as an NSAID gel for muscle pain or an antifungal drug for vaginal yeast.
- The physician may order further tests, such as blood tests, urine tests, X-rays, or ultrasound scans. Some may be done in the office.
- Alternatively, the physician may refer the patient to a specialist for further examination.
- The consultant (or a member of his team) will examine the patient and may arrange tests from simple blood tests to more sophisticated procedures, such as CT scans, MRI, or endoscopy.
- The patient's care may then be handed back to the physician, or be arranged and monitored at the specialist's office.

Blood tests

These are among the most frequently and easily performed medical tests. The composition of the blood can tell a great deal about the state of someone's health. Blood cell tests look at the number and composition of red and white blood cells and platelets in the blood. They help physicians diagnose diseases of the blood, such as anemia. Blood cell tests can also show evidence of infection because it causes the white blood cell count to rise.

Tests on blood chemistry measure the levels of certain chemicals and minerals in the blood and are particularly used to check the functioning of the kidneys and the liver.

Finally, blood lipid tests measure the levels of certain fatty substances (known as lipids) in the blood. High levels of some lipids cause fatty deposits to develop on the lining of the artery walls, a condition known as atherosclerosis (*see p.252 for more information*).

Urine tests

The substances that are usually checked in a urine analysis include glucose, proteins, some electrolytes, and creatinine (a product of protein metabolism). The presence of certain hormones in the urine indicates pregnancy. Testing a urine sample may also reveal blood cells, bacteria, or other substances that indicate an underlying problem.

Biopsies

Tests performed on tissues, often called biopsies, involve taking a small sample of tissue from the body for examination under a microscope. Biopsies may be done for a number of reasons, including confirmation of a diagnosis or in order to investigate a suspicious lump or area of tissue. In the case of cervical smears, a few cells from the cervix are removed so that they can be examined for precancerous changes.

Patch tests

A dermatologist or allergist can carry out patch tests on the skin to look for evidence of allergic reactions. In these tests, small, diluted amounts of potential allergens are placed on strips or disks, which are then taped to the skin for 48 hours. When the strips or disks are removed, the skin underneath is examined. Skin that is reddened or inflamed indicates an allergic reaction to the substance. Tested areas that show no reaction at first are examined again after a further 48 hours for any delayed reaction.

X-rays

These use radiation to form an image on film placed on the other side of the body. Hard structures in the body, such as bones, block the radiation and show up on the film as white areas. X-rays are useful for imaging hard structures but are not very useful for imaging most soft tissues, including liver tissues, since soft tissue does not effectively block the radiation. However, a type of X-ray known as a contrast X-ray may be used to image certain soft tissue structures, such as those in the digestive tract.

Ultrasound scanning

This type of scanning uses sound waves to produce images. The image is formed by the "echo" of the sound waves as they bounce off different parts of the body. The echoes differ in their wavelength according to the density of the area examined. Ultrasound has become an important diagnostic tool, for example to investigate breast lumps in young women and to look for a cause of abdominal pain, such as gallstones. Ultrasound scanning also plays an important part in prenatal testing. A specialized form of ultrasound scanning, known as echocardiography, may be used to assess heart structure and function.

Computerized tomography (CT) scanning

In this technique, X-rays in conjunction with a computer produce images that build up a cross-sectional view of the body. CT scanning makes it possible to gather detailed information about organs and tissues. CT scans are most often taken of the head and the abdomen.

Magnetic resonance imaging (MRI)

Like CT scanning, MRI provides detailed cross-sectional images of internal organs and structures. These images are created using information received from a scanner. Unlike X-rays or CT scanning, MRI does not involve radiation; instead, it uses a magnetic field and radio waves. MRI may distinguish abnormal soft tissue more clearly than CT scanning, and may be used at a greater range of planes through the body than is possible with CT scanning. MRI is especially useful for imaging the brain and for detecting tumors. It is also valuable for looking at the intervertebral disks and may be used to investigate low back pain.

Radionuclide scanning

In radionuclide scanning a radioactive substance called a radionuclide is introduced into the body (usually by injection) and is taken up by the organ or tissue to be imaged. A counter outside the body detects the radiation that is emitted and this information is in turn transmitted to a computer, which transforms it into images. Radionuclide scans may be used to detect abnormal levels of activity in organs such as the thyroid gland and the kidneys

and is useful for detecting tumors and other disorders in these organs. Another type of scanning, known as thallium scanning, may be used to investigate heart function.

Endoscopy

This procedure allows physicians to look inside the body. A tubelike instrument is inserted into the body. Endoscopes are very fine fiberoptic instruments that allow physicians to view organs and other structures on a monitor. Depending on the area to be viewed, access may be through a natural opening, such as the mouth or anus. Alternatively, it may be through a small incision, which may be made into a joint or the abdominal cavity. Many endoscopic procedures are performed under a general or local anesthesic.

BLOOD TESTS

When a physician takes a blood sample from you, it can be used for a range of tests. The blood is usually separated into its different components before testing.

Plasma

White cells and platelets

Red blood cells

How blood separates in a centrifuge

BLOOD COMPONENT	TEST	RESULTS
Plasma The liquid portion of blood that carries dissolved chemicals	Electrolyte (salt) levels	Abnormal: impaired kidney function
	Blood urea nitrogen levels	
	Creatinine levels	
	Liver enzyme levels	Abnormal: impaired liver function
	Blood protein levels	
	Blood sugar levels	High: diabetes
White blood cells Part of the immune system, these cells are involved in the body's defense against disease	Number and type	High: infections, injury or burn, leukemia, cancer
		Low: impaired bone marrow function. May be a side effect of certain medications
		Regular cell counts show progress of a condition
Platelets Cell fragments which clump together to initiate blood clotting	Quantity	Low (bleeds too easily and profusely): autoimmune diseases, or leukemia, viral infections, chemotherapy, and some medicines
		High (blood clots too easily): suggests conditions involving the bone marrow such as leukemia
Red blood cells Contain hemoglobin — the chemical that carries oxygen around the body	Volume (hemocrit value), measured by spinning the sample very fast in a centrifuge. The red cells are the heaviest, so they sink to the bottom.	Low: anemia High: bone marrow conditions, dehydration
	Microscopic examination	Strange shape: e.g. sickle-cell anemia Abnormal size: e.g. pernicious anemia
Whole blood	Microscopic examination	Parasites, visible in cases of sleeping sickness or malaria
	Blood culture	Bacteria present: blood poisoning
	Antibody testing	Present: may indicate diseases such as hepatitis

Treatment

Prescribed treatment, such as drugs or physical therapy, is not always necessary. For some conditions, a family practitioner's important FDA role may be to offer reassurance that a symptom is not a cause for concern. Many minor health problems cure themselves. In long-term illness, a family physician can provide crucial support and understanding, often based on a relationship built over years. However, in many cases drug treatment will be recommended, either on a short-term basis to relieve an acute problem (such as antibiotics for a bacterial infection), or for a longer period for a chronic condition (such as drugs for high blood pressure). Other treatments may be recommended to complement prescribed medicines; for example, physical therapy may be prescribed in combination with nonsteroidal anti-inflammatory drugs (NSAIDs) to treat a muscle problem. Sometimes surgery may be necessary to treat a condition and in most cases this involves referral to a hospital, unless the surgery is very minor (such as wart removal).

Sometimes, despite many investigations, a definitive cause cannot be found to explain a patient's symptoms. In these circumstances, the physician may recommend measures to relieve symptoms and to address factors that may be contributing to the problem, such as stress.

Why medication is prescribed

Drugs may be given for different reasons. Some cure or control diseases, others relieve symptoms. In addition, there are drugs, including vaccinations, which are given to prevent diseases from developing in the first place. Another example of using drugs for prevention is the prescription of lipid-lowering drugs to reduce blood lipids, thereby lowering the risk of developing coronary artery disease and stroke.

Research continues into improving existing medicines and developing new ones, particularly in key areas such as cancer, HIV, and mental health. Drugs are tested extensively before they are marketed. In the US, for example, all drugs must be approved and licensed by the Food and Drug Administration (FDA). However, side effects can still be a problem: although drugs are given to produce specific effects, they all have the potential to cause unwanted effects as well. These adverse reactions may cause 140,000 or more deaths per year. If such effects are found to be unacceptable or unnecessarily risky, the FDA can withdraw a drug from the market.

How drugs work

Drugs can have a variety of effects. Some can replace or supplement a substance that is lacking. For example, levothyroxine is prescribed to treat an underactive thyroid gland (*see chart opposite*). Some drugs eliminate or prevent the spread of infective organisms, such as bacteria and viruses. Others target a specific type of cell. For example, certain cancer treatments destroy the rapidly dividing cells of a tumor. Nonsteroidal anti-inflammatory drugs (NSAIDs) reduce the production of prostaglandins, chemicals that are released in response to tissue injury and result in inflammation. Certain other medications are used to oppose unwanted processes, such as muscle spasm and high blood pressure.

Some drugs mimic or block the effect of certain chemicals in the body. Cells have receptors on their outer surface, which are activated by specific chemicals, triggering activities within the cell. Some drugs, called agonists, attach themselves to these receptors and trigger a response by the cell. Agonists often mimic the action of a naturally occurring substance. For example, the analgesic morphine is an agonist that mimics endorphins and works by preventing transmission of pain signals in the brain.

Others drugs, known as antagonists, attach themselves to receptors but block the action of the chemicals, thereby preventing the particular process. Antihistamines are antagonists. The chemical histamine is released by the body in susceptible individuals in response to a substance such as pollen, triggering an allergic reaction. Antihistamines attach themselves to some of the histamine receptors on the surface of certain cells, reducing the action of histamine and dampening down the allergic response.

Finally, some drugs are useful because of their effect on the nervous system, where impulses are passed from one nerve to another by chemicals called neurotransmitters. Some of these chemicals are reabsorbed into the nerve endings and stored ready to be used again. In depression, the levels of the neurotransmitter serotonin, which acts on brain cells involved in thoughts and mood, are low. Certain antidepressants called selective serotonin reuptake inhibitors (SSRIs) block some of the reabsorption of serotonin and increase the amount available to stimulate nerves.

Drug delivery

Drugs can be delivered in various ways. Most are taken orally, but other preparations, such as eye drops, skin creams, and inhalers for asthma, bypass the digestive system and deliver the drug to the particular part of the body affected. If rapid effects are required, some drugs can be given by injection directly into the bloodstream. Patches applied to the skin and implants inserted beneath the skin deliver drugs slowly for a more prolonged effect.

Side effects and interactions

Every drug has the potential to cause side effects. For example, in addition to lowering blood pressure, beta-blockers may cause fatigue, cold hands and feet, and sleep disturbances. Chemotherapy drugs, in addition to targeting the rapidly dividing cells of a tumor, can affect other rapidly dividing cells in addition, resulting in hair loss and other side effects. Drugs may also cause allergic reactions;

for example, some people are allergic to the antibiotic penicillin and must use other antibiotics instead. Most drug side effects are not serious but in some cases physicians have to decide whether the overall benefit outweighs the risk of harmful effects.

Some drugs interact with each other. For this reason, physicians ask about medicines already being taken when prescribing new medication. It is also important to check that any over-the-counter drugs you buy do not interact with your existing medication and to remember that conventional drugs can sometimes interact with nutritional supplements and herbal remedies (*see also pp. 46 and 69*). If you plan to use herbs or nutritional supplements and you are on medication, check with your physician first. You should also make sure that your complementary therapist knows which drugs you are taking.

Tolerance and dependence

If certain drugs are taken on a long-term basis, the body may grow accustomed to them in a process known as tolerance. Sometimes, tolerance can be beneficial if some of the side effects experienced with a drug reduce as the body

TYPES OF DRUG AND THEIR ACTIONS

Different types of drugs can be categorized according to their mode of action.

TYPE	EXAMPLES	ACTION
Replacement	Insulin	For diabetes: replaces the insulin that the body no longer produces.
	Levothyroxine	For thyroid deficiency: replaces the thyroxine that an underactive thyroid gland is unable to produce.
	Iron	For anemia: replaces the body's reserves of iron lost through bleeding, poor diet, or when the body fails to absorb iron from food.
Suppression	Anti-inflammatories	Suppress the body's inflammation response (a natural response to tissue damage). Nonsteroidal examples include ibuprofen and diclofenac; corticosteroids include hydrocortisone.
	Antihistamines	Suppress the action of histamine, a chemical that the body releases in an allergic response (e.g. cetirizine, diphenhydramine).
	Analgesics	Prevent pain signals from being produced, or alter the way in which the brain perceives pain. Opioid analgesics include codeine and morphine, nonopioid analgesics include acetaminophen and aspirin.
Elimination	Antibiotics	Kill susceptible bacteria or halt their multiplication, e.g. penicillin.
	Antivirals	Stop viruses from reproducing, e.g. acyclovir.
	Cytotoxics	Kill body cells; used for cancer because the rapidly dividing cancer cells are more susceptible than most of the body's other cells.
Opposition	Sedatives	Either slow mental activity by reducing the signals between brain cells (e.g. benzodiazepines), or block the action of stress hormones (beta-blockers). Used for anxiety disorders.
	Relaxants	Reduce muscle spasms by reducing transmission of nerve signals from brain and spinal cord to muscles (e.g. baclofen), blocking transmission of nerve signals from nerve endings to muscles (botulinum toxin), or making muscles less sensitive to nerve signals (e.g. dantrolene).
Immunotherapies	Vaccines	Infectious organisms that have been modified or killed are injected into the body to stimulate the immune system to produce its own antibodies, or antibodies are given.
	Allergens	Substances that can cause an allergic reaction, e.g. grass pollen or bee sting venom. To desensitize an allergy sufferer, he or she may be injected with the allergen at intervals, initially with tiny amounts then with a gradually increasing dose.

becomes accustomed to it. However, with a small number of drugs, it means that the drug becomes less effective over time and therefore an increasing dose will be needed to achieve the same effect. In some cases, a person develops a physical or psychological need for a drug. This is known as dependence. Sometimes, unpleasant symptoms may develop if the drug is suddenly withdrawn. Various drugs can cause dependence. Benzodiazepines (found in some antianxiety drugs and sleeping tablets) have particular dependency-producing potential and can cause dependence within as little as two weeks.

The choice of drug

When considering the choice of prescribed drug, the physician will discuss the patient's medical history and any existing medication, as well as talking about the potential side effects of the drugs. When prescribing, the physician will balance the drug's possible side effects against its potential benefits. In the ailments section of the book, we mention the side effects of a few drugs, but it is not possible to give a comprehensive list. It is essential that you discuss possible side effects with your physician.

When a physician makes a recommendation it will be backed up by information from various sources, including information gained from personal experience of use in patients, information from colleagues, and data from clinical trials, which may be found in journals, discussed at conferences, or presented on recognized websites on the internet, such as the Cochrane Library or the Food and Drug Administration.

Contraindications and cautions

Many drugs are contraindicated (i.e. should not be taken) in certain circumstances, such as during pregnancy or when breast-feeding because they affect the fetus or can be passed via the breast milk to the baby. Sometimes there are insufficient study data to back the use of the drugs during these times so physicians err on the side of caution and do not prescribe them.

Drugs may also be contraindicated in certain medical conditions. For example, NSAIDs should be avoided by people who have peptic ulcers. In some medical conditions there may be some drugs that are not contraindicated, but caution may be advised. This means that the drugs are not suitable in some circumstances or that special monitoring is required. An example would be the use of anticonvulsants for epilepsy during pregnancy, when the risk of the drug to the baby must be weighed against the risk of seizures.

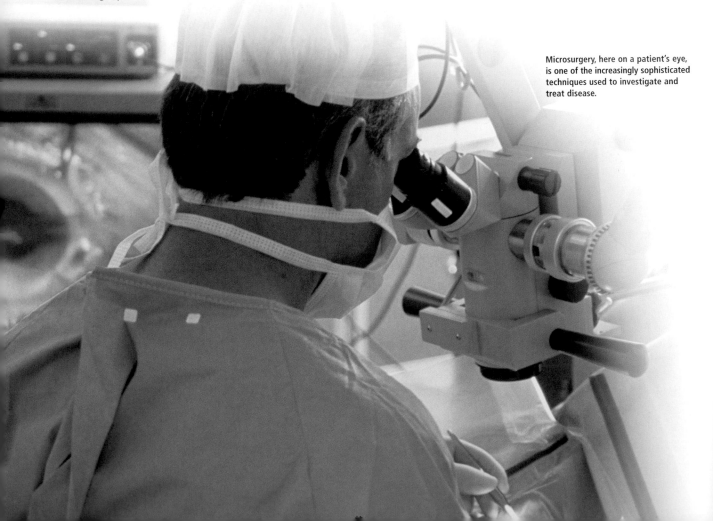

Microsurgery, here on a patient's eye, is one of the increasingly sophisticated techniques used to investigate and treat disease.

It is important to bear all of this in mind when purchasing over-the-counter drugs and to take advice from the pharmacist if you are pregnant or breast-feeding, or if you have any medical conditions. Great care must also be taken when giving medication to children. Often the dose of medication is calculated on the basis of a child's weight but it is not precise. Always ask your physician or pharmacist before giving medicines to children. Many drugs are not licensed for use in children.

Surgery

For some conditions, surgery is the most appropriate treatment. Some very minor surgery may be carried out by a family practitioner, but in general it is necessary to go to a hospital. Certain operations can be done on an outpatient basis, so that patients are able to go home the same day, but in other cases a hospital stay is necessary.

Open surgery
In open surgery, an incision is made in the skin large enough to see clearly the internal body parts that require treatment and the surrounding tissues. Open surgery is usually performed under a general anesthesic and may leave an obvious scar.

Endoscopic surgery
Endoscopic, or "keyhole," surgery is a relatively new technique that enables various surgical procedures to be performed without making large incisions in the skin. The surgeon makes small incisions and introduces the viewing instrument and surgical instruments into the body through these. Endoscopy on joints (arthroscopy) is often done under local anesthetic, whereas abdominal endoscopic surgery is usually performed under a general anesthetic. The length of hospital stay and recovery time are usually shorter for endoscopic surgery than for open surgery.

Microsurgery
This relatively new form of surgery makes it possible for physicians to operate on extremely small and delicate tissues within the body that are otherwise hard to view. Micro-surgeons use binocular microscopes to view the operating site and specially adapted small operating instruments. Microsurgery can be used to operate on nerves and blood vessels and on small structures in the eye, middle ear, and reproductive system. Depending on the operation, it may be performed under a general or a local anesthetic.

Other treatments

There are many other treatments that a physician may recommend. Sometimes these are in addition to drug treatment or surgery; for example, physical therapy may be necessary after an knee or shoulder operation in order to restore a full range of movement to the joint. Psychological therapy may be recommended on its own to treat depression or may be given to patients in combination with antidepressant drugs. In all cases, for the best possible outcome the aim is to put together a treatment package that is appropriate to the individual, taking into account various factors, including patient choice.

The role of complementary and alternative therapies in conjunction with conventional medicine is evolving all the time. Many family practices now have psychotherapists, hypnotherapists, osteopaths, acupuncturists, and other alternative practitioners working alongside their teams providing health care. Also, many hospital pain clinics use medical acupuncture as well as drugs. As the medical profession's understanding and knowledge of alternative and complementary therapies grows, many therapies are likely to play a more prominent role in the care of patients.

Gene therapy and future treatments

New approaches to treating diseases are being researched all the time, some of which are radically different from the treatments we have known in the past. Gene therapy is a good example of an approach that may offer a new way of treating people with a range of conditions.

Genes are made of DNA (deoxyribonucleic acid), which codes for the proteins that make up the body. To a large extent, genes determine who you are. Errors in the genes are responsible for diseases such as some types of cancer and cystic fibrosis. Gene therapy is a technique in which DNA, rather than drugs, is administered to the patient. The new DNA can correct or replace faulty genes, or change the way that genes behave. The most common way for the new DNA to be introduced into the body is through viruses. Viruses normally package and deliver DNA into body cells as part of the infective process. Gene therapists take disease-causing viruses, inactivate them, and put therapeutic genes inside them. The patient is infected with the modified virus so that the new genes will reach body cells and be activated.

Gene therapy is still experimental and is likely only to be appropriate for a few types of diseases. By 2004, over 300 patients had been involved in clinical trials using gene therapy. There have been a number of successes, but also some failures that have highlighted a range of problems. It works best for genetic diseases in which only a single gene is at fault, such as Severe Combined Immunodeficiency Syndrome ("baby in the bubble" syndrome), hemophilia, cystic fibrosis, and some cancers. Many common diseases, such as heart disease, arthritis, and Alzheimer's disease, have genetic components, but they involve more than one gene and are therefore more difficult to target.

As with any experimental technique, it will take years of trials before it can be made available to the public. However, gene therapy, new drugs, and other technical advances offer real hope for people with as yet unconquered diseases.

NUTRITIONAL THERAPY

DR. JOHN BRIFFA

The body is in a state of constant renewal: millions of cells die every second, while others multiply to compensate. Food provides the raw materials for building and regenerating the body. Clinical experience and many studies show that dietary changes and nutritional supplements can restore and maintain health and well-being, as well as helping treat a range of everyday conditions. Nutritional approaches can also be effective in preventing and treating serious conditions such as coronary artery disease, stroke, cancer, and diabetes.

Dietary Carbohydrates

Carbohydrates — sugars, starches, and fiber — are made of the elements carbon, hydrogen, and oxygen. Their main role is to provide a source of energy for the body.

Sugars

The basic building block of all carbohydrates is a single sugar molecule, such as glucose or fructose, known as a monosaccharide. A disaccharide is two monosaccharides joined together — sucrose, for example, contains glucose and fructose. Sugars in fruit and vegetables are "intrinsic" because they are incorporated into the structure of foods, often hidden within cell walls. In some foods, such as cookies and sweetened cereals, the sugar is not bound into the structure of food so these are called "extrinsic" sugars. Generally, foods with intrinsic sugars are healthier than those with extrinsic sugars; an apple is healthier to eat than a piece of cake. Foods containing intrinsic sugar tend to release energy more slowly into the bloodstream compared to foods rich in extrinsic sugar.

Starches

Also referred to as complex carbohydrates, dietary starches are made up of chains of sugar molecules. Starch-based foods include vegetables, bread, pasta, rice, potatoes, beans, legumes, and breakfast cereals. Starches come in two main forms. Refined starches, as found in white bread, white rice, and most commonly available types of pasta, have lost much of their fiber, vitamin, and mineral content.

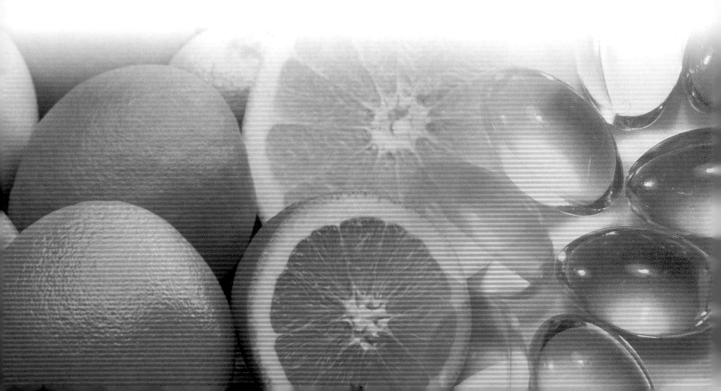

Unrefined starches are richer in fiber and nutrients than their refined counterparts and are therefore considered nutritionally superior. They also tend to give a slower, more sustained release of sugar into the bloodstream, which may be important for health in both the short and long term. Examples of unrefined starches include whole-grain bread, whole-wheat pasta, brown rice, and rolled oats.

Fiber

Fiber is plant material that is indigestible and is sometimes referred to as nonstarch polysaccharide (NSP). Fiber comes in two main forms. Soluble fiber dissolves in the digestive tract to form a thick gel-like substance that slows down the release of some nutrients, particularly sugar, into the bloodstream. It appears to help control the levels of cholesterol in the blood, which may help reduce the risk of coronary artery disease.

Insoluble fiber does not dissolve in the digestive tract and therefore adds bulk to the feces. It is useful for preventing constipation and there is evidence that a high-fiber diet is associated with a reduced risk of cancer of the colon. A diet that is rich in insoluble fiber may also reduce the risk of other conditions, including hemorrhoids and diverticular disease (abnormal pockets on the lining of the colon that can become infected and cause bleeding or perforation of the gut wall).

Good sources of soluble fiber include fruit, vegetables, beans, oats, barley, and rye. Good sources of insoluble fiber include whole-grain (unrefined) cereals, such as whole-wheat bread or pasta and brown rice, as well as beans and legumes, nuts, seeds, and fibrous vegetables, such as carrots, celery, and cabbage.

Dietary Proteins

Dietary proteins, like all proteins, are composed of amino acids and play a role in the manufacture of many structures and tissues, such as bone, muscle, skin, and hair. They are essential for normal growth and development in children. In adults, proteins provide the raw materials needed for cell repair. Cells use amino acids from the diet to make DNA and enzymes — molecules with key roles in maintaining healthy structure and function within the body.

Of the 21 amino acids, many can be made in the body and therefore do not, strictly speaking, need to be eaten. However, eight cannot be made in the body and must be provided in the diet. They are the "essential" amino acids.

Adults need about 0.75–1g of protein for each kilogram of body weight per day. Meat, fish, eggs, and dairy products are very good sources of protein, as are nonanimal foods, such as beans, peas, and nuts. Some grains, such as rice, wheat, and corn, can also supply significant quantities of protein. In general, animal-derived proteins are more "complete" in terms of their component amino acids than vegetable sources. Vegetarians should eat a broad range of protein-containing foods, including beans, legumes, nuts, seeds, and grains, to ensure amino acid intake.

There is some evidence that too much protein can pose hazards. Excess protein is believed to cause the loss of calcium from bone, predisposing a person to osteoporosis and increased risk of fracture. In one study, women who ate more than 95g of protein a day were found to be 20 percent more likely to have broken a wrist over a 12-year period when compared to women who ate an average amount of protein (less than 68g a day)

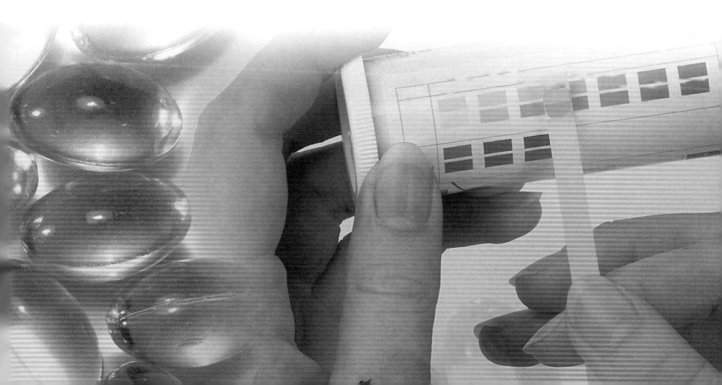

Dietary Fats

Fats provide energy and components for some structures, such as cell membranes and certain hormones. The basic building blocks of dietary fats are fatty acids, which consist of chains of carbon atoms with hydrogen atoms attached. There are three main natural forms of fatty acid. Saturated fatty acids have as many hydrogen atoms as they can hold. Monounsaturated fatty acids lack a pair of hydrogen atoms per molecule. Polyunsaturated fatty acids lack four or more hydrogen atoms per molecule.

Saturated fatty acids

These are found in animal products, such as butter, cheese, whole milk, ice cream, and meat, and in some vegetable oils, such as coconut and palm oils. It is often said that eating a diet rich in saturated fatty acids can raise levels of cholesterol in the blood. However, more than one study has found that this may not be the case. Even the belief that such a diet is a major risk factor for coronary artery disease may be overstated, partly as a result of misquoting and misinterpretation of research studies. Saturated fatty acids may be a factor in weight gain and obesity, although a comprehensive review of the subject concluded that dietary fat is not a major determinant in body weight, and eating less fat is unlikely to bring lasting weight loss.

So, on balance, it appears that saturated fatty acids might be less harmful than is often believed, and that eating them in moderate amounts may not be damaging to health.

Monounsaturated fatty acids

Food rich in monounsaturated fatty acids include olive oil, avocados, nuts, and seeds. These fatty acids can lower blood levels of low-density lipoprotein (LDL) cholesterol, the type of cholesterol that is believed to increase the risk of heart disease. They can also raise blood levels of high-density lipoprotein (HDL) cholesterol, which is thought to protect against heart disease. A high intake of mono-unsaturated fatty acids is believed to be one of the reasons certain populations, such as the southern Italians and the Greeks, have relatively low levels of heart disease.

Polyunsaturated fatty acids (PUFAs)

There are two main groups of PUFAs in the diet: omega-6 and omega-3. The major omega-6 fatty acid is linolenic acid — rich sources include plant oils, such as hemp, pumpkin, sunflower, safflower, sesame, corn, walnut, and soy oil. Other sources include gamma linolenic acid (GLA), dihomogamma linolenic acid (DGLA), and arachidonic acid (AA). The major omega-3 fatty acids are alpha-linolenic acid (from plants, such as flaxseed), eicosatetraenoic acid (ETA), eicosapentaenoic acid (EPA), and docosahexaenoic acid (DHA). EPA and DHA are mainly found in oily types of fish. Within the body, these fatty acids can be converted into other substances that may affect health.

The omega-6 and omega-3 balance

The omega-3 and omega-6 fatty acids have important roles in many body systems, including the brain, nerves, immune system, cardiovascular system, eyes, and skin. They are converted into hormonelike substances called eicosanoids.

Eicosanoids derived from omega-6 fatty acids tend to encourage inflammation, blood-vessel constriction, and blood clotting. Therefore, they increase the risk of coronary artery disease, stroke, and inflammatory conditions such as arthritis. Eicosanoids derived from arachidonic acid are particularly potent. Those from omega-3 fatty acids, such as EPA, are less likely to encourage inflammation; some are actually anti-inflammatory. They tend to reduce the risk of clotting and help relax blood vessels, thereby helping reduce the risk of coronary artery disease, stroke, and inflammatory conditions, such as arthritis.

The roughly opposing actions of omega-3 and omega-6 fatty acids mean that it is important to balance their intake. A ratio of 1:1 is believed to be ideal. Over the past 40 years, however, the proportion of omega-6 to omega-3 in the average diet has increased to roughly six to one. This may be an important factor in the development of many chronic diseases, such as cardiovascular disease and cancer.

To reduce your intake of omega-6 fatty acids and increase your intake of omega-3 fatty acids:

- Limit the intake of vegetable oils, such as sunflower oil, corn oil, and rapeseed oil, which contain omega-6 fatty acids. Processed foods labeled as containing "vegetable oil" contain these oils.
- Sprinkle flaxseeds on cereals and take flaxseed oil, which is a rich source of omega-3 fatty acids.
- Eat three portions a week of oily fish, such as mackerel, herring, salmon, trout, and sardines.
- Take a fish oil supplement each day.

Partially hydrogenated and trans fatty acids

Some margarines and vegetable shortenings (the fats added to many processed foods) are manufactured using a process known as hydrogenation. This can change the structure of fats, creating what are known as trans fatty acids. These are believed to have harmful effects on health, particularly with regard to heart disease. While trans fats do occur naturally in some foods (such as butter), there is evidence that it is only industrially produced, and not naturally occurring, trans fats that have a detrimental effect on heart health. You should consider avoiding margarines and processed foods listing partially hydrogenated oils (or trans fatty acids) as an ingredient.

Water

The body is made up of about 70 percent water. Water is vital in most of the processes that are integral to health. Even mild dehydration (losing about 70ml of fluid for a

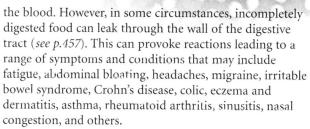

Fats are moved around the body as lipids bound with proteins, to form particles of low-density lipoprotein (LDL). LDLs transport cholesterol (a steroid) from the liver to the tissues of the body. High cholesterol levels are linked to cardiovascular disease, but some cholesterol is vital for the functioning of body cells.

150lb/70kg adult) can impair essential body processes and cause symptoms such as light-headedness, headaches, muscle weakness, appetite loss, fatigue, and dry eyes and mouth.

Keeping well hydrated also seems to help reduce the risk of chronic disease. Research indicates, for instance, that low levels of fluid consumption are associated with increased risk of cancers of the kidney, bladder, prostate, and testes. Other research has found that increasing fluid intake seems to reduce the risk of bladder and colon cancer. Evidence also suggests that drinking water may reduce the risk of heart disease. In one study, women drinking five or more glasses of fluid each day had a 41 percent reduced risk of dying from a heart attack compared to women drinking two or fewer glasses each day, and for men the risk was reduced by 54 percent.

As a rough guide, drink about 0.5 fl.oz (15ml) of water for each pound (0.1kg) of body weight. For most people, this equates to 1.6–2.6 quarts (1.5–2.5 liters) of water a day. However, individual needs can vary with factors such as outside temperature and activity. A good guide to the state of hydration is the color of the urine. The aim is to drink enough water to keep the urine pale or very pale yellow during the day.

The quality of the drinking water is important, too. Tap water contains chlorine. This can induce chemical changes which, at least in theory, should increase cancer risk. It seems sensible to drink filtered tap water or mineral water. (*See also Environmental Health, p.86*).

Imbalances and Treatments

The body can be subject to a variety of imbalances that may cause health problems. This section explores the most common ones and explains how to deal with them.

Food intolerance and exclusion diets

Food intolerance occurs when the body has difficulty digesting and using a certain food or group of foods. It is different from food allergy, in which a certain type of food causes an abnormal immune response, such as a rash or swelling. Intolerance, although not usually as dangerous as allergy, can still cause a great deal of discomfort.

Most of what we eat must be broken down by digestion before it can be absorbed through the intestinal wall into

the blood. However, in some circumstances, incompletely digested food can leak through the wall of the digestive tract (*see p.457*). This can provoke reactions leading to a range of symptoms and conditions that may include fatigue, abdominal bloating, headaches, migraine, irritable bowel syndrome, Crohn's disease, colic, eczema and dermatitis, asthma, rheumatoid arthritis, sinusitis, nasal congestion, and others.

If a nutritional therapist suspects a food intolerance, the following tests can help with the diagnosis.

Prick testing
The prick test checks for an allergic response. It involves breaking the outer layer of the skin and introducing a tiny amount of the food or other substance (such as animal hair or pollen). If the skin becomes inflamed, it is likely that you have an allergy to the food, not an intolerance.

IgG and IgE blood testing
Antibodies are proteins made by the immune system in response to proteins or other compounds that the body recognizes as "foreign." One type, the IgG antibodies, are thought to be involved in food reactions. IgG antibodies to specific foods can be detected using biochemical techniques, of which there are two basic types — RAST (radioallergosorbent test) and ELISA (enzyme-linked immunoserological assay). An IgE blood test can measure the levels of a specific form of antibody (Immunoglobulin E) in the blood and also check for an allergic response.

Neither prick tests nor IG tests are particularly useful for forms of food intolerance or allergy. Allergies involve the immune system, which recognizes food molecules as foreign and attempts to label or attack them with IG antibodies. As food intolerances do not tend to involve an immune reaction, different tests are needed.

THE MICRONUTRIENTS

The diet provides the body with a range of vitamins and minerals that have important roles to play in health and well-being. The major nutrients, along with their dietary sources, key effects, and recommended daily amounts (also known as the reference nutrient intakes) are summarized here.

NUTRIENT	MAIN SOURCES	KEY EFFECTS	CURRENT RNI*
Vitamin A	Milk, butter, egg yolk, liver, oily fish As beta-carotene (a precursor of vitamin A) in carrots, tomatoes, dark green/yellow vegetables	• Believed to be cancer-protective • Important for night vision • Important for cell growth and development • Important for the health of the skin	600mg per day (women) 700mg/d men
Vitamin B_1 (Thiamine)	Cereals, nuts, legumes, whole grains, green vegetables	• Supplementation may enhance mood and mental alertness • Important for carbohydrate metabolism • Important for nervous system maintenance	0.8mg/d women 1.0mg/d men
Vitamin B_2 (Riboflavin)	Liver, milk, eggs, green vegetables, yeast extract	• Important for metabolism • Important for all cell growth and development	1.3mg/d
Vitamin B_3 (Niacin)	Liver, beef, pork, fish, fortified breakfast cereals, yeast extract	• Important for metabolism • Essential for the formation of red blood cells • Important for the nervous and digestive systems	13mg/d women 17mg/d men
Vitamin B_5 (Pantothenic acid)	Animal products, cereals, legumes	• A constituent of coenzyme A — essential for metabolism • Coenzyme A is important for the immune system	No RNI
Vitamin B_6	Meat, fish, eggs	• May be important in reducing the risk of heart disease (in combination with folate and vitamin B_{12}) by lowering homocysteine levels • Is required for the efficient functioning of the immune and nervous systems • Supplementation may be beneficial in the treatment of premenstrual syndrome	1.2mg/d women 1.4mg/d men
Vitamin B_{12}	Liver, meat, eggs, milk, yeast extract	• May be important in reducing the risk of heart disease (in combination with folate and vitamin B_6) by lowering homocysteine levels • Is important for production of red blood cells • Supplementation may be beneficial in the treatment of premenstrual syndrome	1.5mg/d
Vitamin C	Fresh fruit especially citrus fruit, blackcurrants, kiwi fruit, and green vegetables	• Supplementation has been associated with a reduced risk of heart disease (especially in combination with vitamin E) • Some evidence exists to suggest that vitamin C may be important in cancer prevention	40mg/d
Vitamin D	Oily fish, e.g. mackerel; egg yolk, fortified margarine	• Important for regulating calcium in the body and for bone health • Evidence suggests that vitamin D supplementation may play a role in cancer prevention (especially colon and breast cancers) • Evidence suggests that vitamin D supplementation may help prevent heart disease	No RNI for those aged 19–50. After the age of 65 RNI is 10mg/d

*(for those aged 19–50)

THE MICRONUTRIENTS CONTINUED

NUTRIENT	MAIN SOURCES	KEY EFFECTS	CURRENT RNI*
Vitamin E	Nuts, vegetable oils, vegetables, whole-grain cereals, oily fish	• Appears to enhance immune function • Associated with a reduced risk of heart disease in people who do not have diabetes or clogged arteries • May reduce the risk of prostate cancer • May slow the progression of Alzheimer's disease • Evidence suggests that supplementation (particularly in combination with vitamin C) lowers the risk of developing Alzheimer's disease	No RNI
Vitamin K	Dark green leafy vegetables e.g. spinach	• Evidence suggests supplementation may prevent fractures	No RNI
Folic acid	Liver, orange juice, green vegetables, nuts	• Proven to reduce the risk of neural tube defects such as spina bifida • Supplementation lowers plasma homocysteine levels — believed to reduce risk of heart disease • Supplementation may be important in cancer prevention (especially cancers of the colon and breast)	200mg/d
Calcium	Milk, canned fish, dark leafy greens	• Necessary for the formation and maintenance of strong bones and teeth • Important for the proper functioning of nerves and muscles	700mg/d
Magnesium	Nuts, legumes, whole-grain cereals	• Important for nerve and muscle function • May be used to treat cardiovascular disorders • Supplementation appears to reduce blood pressure • Supplementation may reduce the risk of stroke • Supplementation may be associated with better lung function • Supplementation may be useful in reducing the symptoms of PMS	270mg/d women 300mg/d men
Zinc	Meat, eggs, milk, fish, whole-grain cereals, legumes	• Important for immune system function • Supplementation may modulate testosterone levels in men (especially in men who are mildly deficient)	7mg/d women 9.5mg/d men
Selenium	Brazil nuts, fish, liver	• Appears to be cancer-protective • Supplementation may be protective against asthma • Supplementation may improve immunity • Supplementation may improve mood	60mg/d women 75mg/d men
Iron	Red meat, cereals, legumes	• Essential for formation of red blood cells • Important for the immune system • Essential for brain function • Essential for the proper functioning of the thyroid	14.8mg/d women 8.7mg/d men
Iodine	Seafood, seaweed, eggs, milk	• Essential for the synthesis of thyroid hormones, which regulate metabolic activity	140mg/d
Copper	Meat, whole grains, nuts, seeds	• Important for the immune system • Promotes normal formation of red blood cells	1.2mg/d
Potassium	Widespread in food	• Needed for proper nerve function • Aids in the maintenance of blood pressure	3,500mg/d
Sodium	Widespread in food	• Important for nerve and muscle activity	1,600mg/d

*(for those aged 19–50)

Cytotoxic and ALCAT tests

The cytotoxic test mixes white blood cells with individual food extracts and then ascertains which foods caused reactions in the cells. The ALCAT test (ALCAT stands for antigen leucocyte cellular antibody test) is similar except that assessing the reaction of the white cells requires a sophisticated piece of laboratory equipment.

Electrodermal testing

Practitioners of Chinese medicine believe that energy flows down channels known as meridians in the body. Electrodermal testing involves measuring the electrical current that flows through an acupuncture point on a meridian, then detecting any changes in the current as the body is challenged with individual foods. Extracts of those foods

DIGESTIVE SYSTEM

The digestive system consists of the digestive tract, which is a tube about 24 ft (7 meters) long from mouth to anus, and its associated organs. Food is digested and the macronutrients (carbohydrates, proteins, and fats) are broken down into their constituent components.

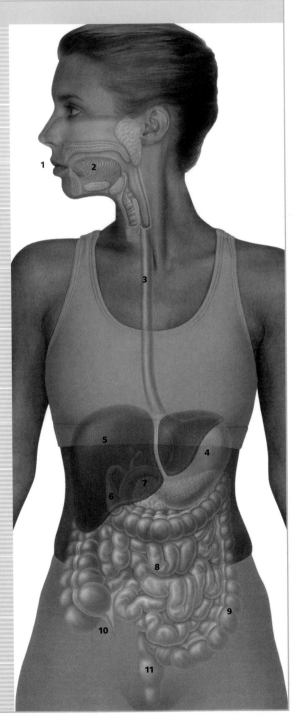

ORGAN	FUNCTION
1 Mouth	The teeth and tongue mash food, mixing it with saliva.
2 Salivary glands	Three pairs of salivary glands release saliva. Salivary enzymes begin the digestion process, breaking down starch into simple sugars.
3 Esophagus	This muscular tube connects the throat to the stomach. At the bottom is a ring of muscle (a sphincter) that relaxes to let food into the stomach.
4 Stomach	The stomach is a muscular bag. Stomach (gastric) juices contain acids and enzymes. The acid kills most bacteria, and enzymes begin to digest protein into amino acids.
5 Liver	The liver produces bile, a digestive juice made from old blood cells. The liver is also where nutrients are modified or stored, and alcohol and other toxins are broken down.
6 Gallbladder	The gallbladder stores bile and releases it into the duodenum.
7 Pancreas	The pancreas produces juices that are powerful digesting agents. Pancreatic juices also neutralize the stomach acids.
8 Small intestine	This is the longest section of the digestive tract, at 17 ft (5 m), and consists of the duodenum, jejenum, and ileum. This narrow, tightly packed tube has a very convoluted lining with millions of microscopic projections that together give a huge surface area for absorption.
9 Large intestine	This section of the digestive tract is about 5 ft (1.5 meters) long, and consists of the cecum, colon, and rectum. The tube is wider than the small intestine, and the internal surface is not as wrinkled.
10 Appendix	A blind-ending tube coming off the cecum. In humans it appears to have no digestive function.
11 Rectum	Stools collect in the rectum before being excreted through the anus.

may be put in the same circuit as the subject tested — if it changes the current there is a problem with the food.

However, in one reliable study this form of testing failed to identify genuine IgE-type acute food allergy. It has not been fully studied as a way of identifying food intolerance.

The elimination diet

Many practitioners of nutritional medicine regard this as the most accurate way of testing for food sensitivity. Once identified, problem foods can be eliminated for good. Many individuals whose health issues are linked with food intolerance find they experience a sudden improvement in their condition, along with increased energy, enhanced mental clarity, and improved digestive function. Foods generally eliminated on such a diet include:

- Wheat (a very common problem food), found in breads, pasta, pastry, pizza, cookies, cakes, wheat-based breakfast cereals, wheat crackers, breaded food, battered food, and anything containing wheat flour.
- Milk, cheese, and yogurt.
- Foods or drinks that are consumed repeatedly, say on four or more days each week (the more often a food is eaten, the more likely it is to be a problem).
- Foods or drinks that are craved (cravings for a particular food can be a sign of intolerance to that food).
- Foods and drinks that are suspected because they seem to induce symptoms.

All likely problem foods are removed from the diet for two to three weeks. If a food sensitivity is at the root of the symptoms, and the problem food has been eliminated, improvement can generally be expected in this time. A good amount of a specific food should be eaten in the morning. Over the next few hours, look out for a return of the original symptoms. Other problems may include headache, itching, depression, fatigue, irritability, and foggy thinking. A note should be made of any food that seems to bring on an unwanted reaction and it should be eliminated again from the diet. Foods that do not provoke a reaction after breakfast should be eaten at lunch and dinner. If by the following morning there are still no symptoms, this food can be provisionally added to a list of "safe" foods.

For the next three days, the food should be eliminated again and a watchful eye kept for any symptoms that suggest a food reaction. It is possible that the symptoms of a reaction may come on two or three days after a food or drink is consumed. If there are no symptoms after three days, it is likely that the food being tested is safe to eat. This process can be repeated for all the eliminated foods.

In normal circumstances, it is wise to exclude problem foods for a month, although two or more months may be better. Abstaining from a food for a period of time can make the body more tolerant to it in the long term. However, initial food reactions can be worse, not better, than before — a phenomenon that is referred to as "hypersensitization." Care should be taken when foods are reintroduced, particularly if the condition being treated has an allergic component, such as asthma. When a food is reintroduced, it is best not to eat too much of it too frequently, as this can increase the risk of the original problem recurring.

Improving digestion and food combining

Making sure that foods are fully digested can help reduce food intolerance. Simple steps that can be taken to improve digestion include the following:

Thorough chewing

Chewing mixes food with saliva, which contains an enzyme that starts the digestion of starchy foods, such as bread, potatoes, rice, and pasta. It also breaks up food, increasing the surface area available for contact with the digestive juices and enzymes. Each mouthful ideally should be chewed to a creamlike consistency before swallowing.

Avoid big meals

The larger the meal, the larger the load on the digestive system. Therefore small meals eaten frequently reduce the risk of indigestion.

Avoid drinking with meals

Some people tend to drink fluid with meals in the belief that this helps "wash food down." The reality is quite the reverse. Drinking with meals dilutes the acid and enzymes that do the digestive work and does nothing to help the process of digestion. On the whole, drinking should be done between meals, not at mealtimes.

Food combining

Proteins and starches are very different chemically and are digested by different enzymes in the intestines. Initially, proteins are digested in acid, starches in alkali. An inability to cope with protein and starch combinations can lead to impaired digestion.

The aim of food combining is to avoid mixing protein and starch at the same meal. This means eating either protein or starch combined with a food that is "neutral" — neither protein nor starch. (For a list of common protein, starch, and neutral foods, see p.40.)

Examples of healthy meals include: meat or fish with salad or vegetables other than potatoes; pasta with tomato-based sauce (no meat) and salad; vegetable curry and rice; baked potato, ratatouille, and salad; meat stew with vegetables, and avocado salad sandwiches.

Eating to this pattern can bring tremendous relief to people with indigestion and increase the chances of complete and rapid food breakdown. It may also help reduce the risk of food sensitivity, and is often very effective in helping improve digestive symptoms such as bloating, indigestion, and acid reflux.

Candida overgrowth

Within the gut live about 2–4lb (1–2kg) of gut flora. These "friendly bacteria" have a variety of roles to play, including assisting in digestion, keeping unhealthy organisms at bay, and ensuring that the gut lining remains healthy. The yeast organism *Candida albicans* can also inhabit the large intestine and does not usually cause health problems.

However, under certain circumstances, it can overgrow in the small intestine, leading to symptoms that include erratic bowel habits (constipation and/or loose bowel movements); gas and flatulence; abdominal bloating; anal itching; recurrent bouts of yeast (vaginal yeast infection); other fungal infections, including athlete's foot or generalized itching around the groin and/or the inside of the buttocks; recurrent bouts of cystitis and/or problems with vaginal irritation; and cravings for sugar, sugary foods (such as chocolate, cookies, or cakes), or yeasty foods (cheese, bread, alcohol, or vinegar). *Candida* overgrowth may also cause vague, unexplained health problems, such as fatigue, pain, and mental distress. The overlap between symptoms of gut flora disturbance and depression can be confusing for patients as well as practitioners.

One of the major causes of yeast overgrowth is antibiotic therapy, which can kill the healthy gut organisms that normally help keep yeast organisms such as *Candida* under control. Other common underlying factors in yeast overgrowth include stress (which can upset the immune system), the consumption of yeast-encouraging foods, such as sugar, bread, cheese, and alcohol, and taking the oral contraceptive pill or hormone therapy (HT).

Tests for Candida

If *Candida* is suspected, a nutritional therapist may arrange one of the various tests. Yeast analysis of stool samples can be tried, although it can be misleading because *Candida* is normally present in the large intestine. The blood can be tested for the *Candida* antigen — if positive, an ongoing yeast infection may be indicated.

Antibodies are substances the immune system produces in response to antigens. Two types of antibodies, known as IgG and IgM, are usually measured in the blood. Raised levels of the antibodies specific for *Candida* may indicate a significant infection. A type of antibody known as secretory IgA is produced by the gut. Measuring the amount of secretory IgA made specifically against *Candida* can be a good guide to the presence of yeast in the gut.

Another test that examines gut fermentation is based on the principle that yeast tends to metabolize sugar into alcohol. After a blood sample is taken, a person is given a measured dose of sugar. One hour later, another sample of blood is taken. Both blood samples are then analyzed for various fermentation products. The presence of these in significant quantity can point to the presence of excess yeast in the gut.

FOOD COMBINING

PROTEIN	NEUTRAL	STARCH
Meats:	**All green and root**	bread
beef	**vegetables apart**	potatoes
lamb	**from potatoes:**	rice
chicken	asparagus	pasta
turkey	broccoli	cereal
veal	brussels sprouts	
venison	cabbage	**Foods from flour:**
pork	carrots	pastries
bacon	cauliflower	cakes
	celery	cookies
Fish:	eggplant	
mackerel	green beans	**Dried fruits:**
herring	leeks	dates
trout	mushrooms	figs
salmon	onions	currants
tuna	parsnips	raisins
cod	peas	golden raisins
plaice	spinach	
skate	turnips	**Other fruit:**
	zucchini	bananas
Shellfish:		mangoes
shrimp	**Salad vegetables:**	
cockles	avocado	**Sweeteners:**
mussels	cucumber	sugar
crabs	tomatoes	maple syrup
lobster	lettuce	honey
	peppers	
	radishes	
Dairy products:	scallions	
cheese, milk, eggs,	nuts and seeds	
yogurt		
	Fats and oils:	
	cream, butter	
Vegetable proteins:	extra virgin olive oil,	
soybeans	other vegetable oils	
soybean curd (tofu)		

The anti-Candida diet

The cornerstone of the anti-*Candida* approach is a diet that helps starve yeast out of the system. Foods to be avoided include those that feed yeast directly and those that are yeasty, moldy, or fermented in their own right.

Yeast-feeding foods to avoid include: sugar; sweetening agents, such as maple syrup, molasses, honey, malt syrup; sugar-containing foods, such as cookies, cakes, pastries, candy, ice cream, sweetened breakfast cereals, soft drinks, and fruit juice; white flour products, such as white bread, crackers, pizza, and pasta.

Yeasty, moldy, or fermented foods to avoid include: bread and other items made with yeast; alcoholic drinks, particularly beer and wine, which are very yeasty; gravy mixes (most contain brewer's yeast); vinegar and vinegar-containing foods, such as ketchup (which also contains sugar), mustard, mayonnaise, and many prepared salad dressings; pickles, miso, tempeh, and soy sauce (all are fermented); aged cheeses, such as cheddar, Stilton, Swiss, Brie, and Camembert (cheese is inherently moldy); peanuts, peanut butter, and pistachios (tend to harbor yeast); mushrooms; dried fruits (these are intensely sugary and tend to harbor mold); and prepared soups and pre-packaged foods, which tend to contain yeast.

Foods to eat freely on an anti-*Candida* diet include meat, fish, eggs, beans, legumes, vegetables, nuts (but not peanuts or pistachios), seeds, oats, and brown rice.

Views on whether fruit can be eaten on an anti-*Candida* diet vary. Some experts recommend complete exclusion, while others say you can eat it frequently. In general, one or two pieces of fruit a day will be well tolerated, although grapes are generally best avoided because they are very sugary and usually are covered in a moldy bloom.

Supplements to overcome Candida

In addition to the anti-*Candida* diet, it may help to take specific supplements — probiotics, liver-supporting agents, and antifungal supplements — to help restore the full functioning of the digestive system.

Probiotics contain gut bacteria. Those that contain both *Bifidobacterium bifidus* (the predominant bacterium in the large intestine) and *Lactobacillus acidophilus* (the predominant bacterium in the small intestine) can help restore the balance of organisms in the gut and help combat *Candida* overgrowth.

During the initial phases of an anti-*Candida* regime, it is quite common for the condition to get worse. Lethargy, fuzzy-headedness, and flulike symptoms can start a day or so after the regime starts and generally last

Candida albicans is a type of yeast that lives naturally in the mouth, skin, gut, and vagina. One way that it reproduces is by spores. These rounded spores are connected by long threadlike filaments, called hyphae.

from a few days to a couple of weeks. Liver-supporting agents (*see p.42*) can help reduce these symptoms.

Antifungal supplements can help combat the *Candida* fungus directly. Oregano contains two important active ingredients, carvacrol and thymol. Studies have shown that oregano can inhibit the growth of *Candida*. In natural medicine, garlic is widely used in the control and eradication of *Candida*. Finally, grapefruit seed extract supplements are also useful because they have the ability to kill *Candida* in the body.

Detoxification

The body is constantly exposed to substances that have the potential to adversely affect health and well-being. Some, such as the pollutants we breathe and the herbicides and pesticides that lace our food, come from outside. Others are the result of the metabolic and physiological processes that go on within the body every day. If the toxic load on the system is large, and/or there is a problem with detoxification processes, toxins may accumulate, giving rise to fatigue, lethargy, weight gain, headaches, joint and muscle aches, acne, bad breath, body odor, and cellulite. Ensuring efficient elimination of toxins from the system is fundamental. The liver is the main organ of detoxification in the body. It contains thousands of lobules, which are tiny blood-processing units just 1mm wide. Since the liver takes blood from the digestive tract and from the general circulation it is able to neutralize toxins from the diet and the processes of metabolism, as well as pollutants from the air that are taken in through the lungs. It processes these toxins so that they can be removed from the body without causing harm.

Optimizing liver function

To improve liver function, try the following:

- Eat plenty of fresh fruit and vegetables. These do not tax or stress the liver, and contain an abundance of nutrients such as vitamin C and carotenoids (e.g. beta-carotene) that can support liver function.
- Limit the amount of dietary fat and protein, which need substantial processing by the liver. The main foods to avoid are fatty meats, such as beef, lamb, and duck; dairy products; hydrogenated vegetable oils present in margarine; and many processed, baked, and fast foods.
- Avoid artificial additives such as sweeteners, colorings, flavorings, and preservatives.
- Avoid alcohol and caffeine, both of which stress the liver and encourage toxicity.
- Drink plenty of water (1 quart/2 liters a day), which dilutes toxins and speeds their elimination from the body.
- Eat plenty of fiber to avoid constipation, which is believed to increase the risk of toxins being absorbed through the wall of the large bowel.
- Take milk thistle supplements. This herb contains a complex of bioflavonoid molecules known collectively as silymarin, which appears to have the ability to protect liver cells by reducing the takeup and enhancing the removal of harmful toxins. Silymarin also has a powerful antioxidant action and can help in the regeneration of injured liver cells.

Blood-sugar imbalance

The body keeps the level of sugar (glucose) in the blood within a relatively narrow range. Eating carbohydrate-based foods (containing sugars and starches) increases the level of blood sugar, causing the pancreas to secrete insulin, which transfers sugar from the blood into the body's cells and lowers the blood-sugar level. Other hormones, such as glucagon, help keep blood-sugar levels from falling too low (see p.314).

Some people may have trouble regulating their blood-sugar levels, so that they experience "peaks" and "troughs." Stabilizing blood-sugar levels can help to combat a wide variety of symptoms and conditions in the body.

The symptoms of fluctuating blood sugar are most obvious when blood-sugar levels are low (often referred to as hypoglycemia, although true hypoglycemia, in which blood-sugar levels fall dangerously low, usually occurs only in people being treated for diabetes). Symptoms of low blood sugar include:

- Fatigue. Low blood-sugar levels can cause energy levels to drop. The mid- to late-afternoon is a common time for fatigue associated with low blood-sugar levels.
- Loss of concentration and/or mood disturbance (especially anxiety and irritability). The brain depends on a ready supply of sugar for normal function. Low blood-sugar levels can provoke loss of concentration, low mood, anxiety, depression, and mood swings.
- Sweet cravings. When blood-sugar levels are low, people tend to crave sweet foods, such as chocolate, cookies, cakes, and candy.

High levels of blood sugar can damage the body's tissues through a process known as glycosylation; they can also cause the body to produce excessive amounts of insulin that stimulate the conversion of sugar into a starchlike substance called glycogen, which can be stored in the liver. However, when glycogen stores are full, insulin stimulates the production of fat. People who have excess insulin tend to accumulate fat around the middle (also known as abdominal obesity), which has been linked with an increased risk of conditions such as coronary artery disease and type 2 diabetes (which usually begins in middle age).

Large amounts of insulin in the circulation affects other parts of the body. It causes the kidneys to retain sodium, which can make an individual prone to high blood pressure and fluid retention over time. Insulin also stimulates the liver to make cholesterol, which is likely to increase the risk of coronary artery disease and stroke.

If the pancreas secretes excess insulin over many years, the body can become less sensitive to insulin's effects. This may lead to a condition known as insulin resistance, which may ultimately develop into type 2 diabetes.

Balancing blood sugar

Eating patterns and the types of food eaten both influence blood-sugar balance. The best blood-sugar control is achieved by eating unrefined carbohydrates in three meals a day, perhaps with healthy snacks, such as fresh fruit and nuts, in between. This can help control appetite and may prevent overeating, with its corresponding surges in blood sugar and insulin.

In addition to regular, moderately sized meals, it is important to base the diet on foods that give a controlled release of sugar in the body (See glycemic index foods, opposite). Traditional wisdom dictates that starchy foods release sugar slowly into the blood because they must first be broken down into sugar before they are absorbed from the gut. However, it appears that this is not the case for many starch-based foods, including most forms of bread, potatoes, rice, and pasta. For the best blood-sugar control, these foods, as well as those containing refined sugar, should be limited in the diet. The best diet for blood-sugar control is one based on meat, fish, eggs (high-protein foods tend to help stabilize blood-sugar levels), beans, legumes, nuts, seeds, fruits, and vegetables (other than the potato).

GLYCEMIC INDEX (GI) FOODS

The speed and extent to which a food increases blood sugar can be quantified using the glycemic index scale. In this scale, glucose (a fast-releasing sugar) is given an arbitrary glycemic index (GI) of 100. Other foods are then compared to this. Generally speaking, the higher a food's GI, the greater its tendency to upset blood-sugar balance. (Adapted from *The Glucose Revolution: The Authoritative Guide to the Glycolic Index* — Jennie Brand-Miller and Thomas Wolever.)

HIGH GLYCEMIC INDEX FOODS (OVER 50)

Food	GI	Food	GI
Glucose	100	White pita bread	57
French baguette	95	New potatoes	57
Lucozade	95	Muesli	56
Baked potato	85	Popcorn, brown rice	55
Cornflakes	83	Corn	55
Rice Crispies	82	Spaghetti made with durum wheat	55
Pretzels	81	Bananas, sweet potatoes	54
Rice cakes	77	Special K	54
Cocoa Puffs	77	Kiwi fruit	53
Doughnut	76	Orange juice	52
French fries	75	**LOW GLYCEMIC INDEX FOODS (UNDER 50)**	
Corn chips	74	Pumpernickel bread	50
Potato — mashed	73	Hot oatmeal	49
Bagel — white	72	Baked beans	48
Raisin Bran	71	Instant noodles	47
White bread	71	Grapes	46
Shredded Wheat	69	Oranges	44
Whole-grain bread	69	All-Bran	42
Croissants	67	Apple juice	41
Gnocchi	67	Apples	38
Pineapple	66	Whole-grain spaghetti	37
Cantaloupe melon	65	Pears	37
High-fiber rye crispbread	65	Chickpeas	33
Couscous	65	Lima beans	31
Rye bread	64	Dried apricots	31
Muffin	62	Soy milk	30
Muesli bar	61	Kidney beans	29
Ice cream	61	Lentils	29
Pizza with cheese	60	Grapefruit	25
White rice	58	Cherries	22

Supplements for blood-sugar balance

The trace mineral chromium seems to help to regulate the action of insulin in the body. In so doing it helps ensure that the body handles and metabolizes sugar efficiently. The normal recommended dose is 200–800mcg of chromium per day. Other nutrients believed to help blood-sugar metabolism include manganese, vanadium, and the B vitamins (particularly vitamin B_3).

Diet and the thyroid gland

The thyroid gland sits in the front of the neck just above the top of the breastbone and collarbones. It is essentially the body's thermostat, determining the speed at which it burns fuel. Each cell in the body uses oxygen and sugar to make energy, some of which is released as heat. The speed at which the cells do this, also known as the metabolic rate, is regulated by the thyroid. If, for any reason, thyroid function should falter, all the cells in the body tend not to operate as well as they should. (*For symptoms of low thyroid gland function see Thyroid Problems, p.319.*)

Thyroid blood tests

The thyroid gland produces various hormones including thyroxine (also known as T4), which is converted into a more active hormone called tri-iodothyronine (also known as T3) in the tissues. If the levels of T4 and/or T3 fall, then the pituitary gland at the base of the brain will secrete a hormone called thyroid-stimulating hormone (TSH), which stimulates the production of more thyroid hormones.

There are several tests for levels of thyroid hormones in the blood. Testing for TSH is generally the screening test for thyroid disease, with a raised TSH level generally taken to be a sign of low thyroid function (hypothyroidism).

A HEALTHY DIET

A healthy diet is one that provides the building blocks that your body needs for growth and maintenance, and in appropriate quantities and proportions. It should also be low in substances that can cause harm, or that the body finds difficult to process.

Many of the diseases that are on the increase in developed countries, such as type 2 diabetes (*see p.314*), coronary artery disease (*see p.252*), and some types of cancer, have a strong link with dietary factors. Making changes to improve the health-promoting qualities of your diet will reduce the likelihood of suffering from these conditions. A good all-round diet also gives you more energy and vitality, and improves your resistance to minor illnesses such as colds and flu.

Base your diet on natural, unadulterated foods

There is a wealth of evidence that shows the most nutritious diet is one based on whole, unprocessed foods. Some of the foods which should form the basis of the diet include meat, fish, seafood, eggs, fruit, vegetables, nuts, seeds, beans, and lentils.

Eat plenty of foods rich in healthy fats

Oils and fats are an important part of the diet. Different types of fat, though, have different effects on the body. Oily fish, nuts, seeds, olives, olive oil, and avocado are rich in fats that have a range of health-giving properties (*see p.34*).

Avoid eating too much fast and processed food

Fast and processed foods tend to be rich in dietary elements including refined sugar, salt, and food additives, which can have adverse effects on health. Other ingredients commonly found in fast and processed foods are types of fats known as partially hydrogenated and "trans" fatty acids, which have been strongly linked with coronary artery disease.

Avoid eating too many potatoes and refined grains

Potatoes and refined grains such as white bread, pasta, white rice, and many breakfast cereals generally lack nutritional value. They also tend to disrupt blood sugar and insulin levels (*see p.42*). The imbalance that these foods can induce in the body may have adverse effects for short- and long-term health.

Eat regular meals, with healthy snacks in between

Regular meals help ensure that we get the nourishment we need for optimal health. Also, snacking (on foods such as fruit and nuts) can help control appetite and help prevent overeating. Regular eating also helps stabilize blood sugar and insulin levels.

Drink plenty of water

Water makes up about 70 percent of the body. We lose water through sweating and urination, so drinking enough to maintain our hydration levels is important for maintaining general well-being and health. You should drink enough mineral or filtered tap water or juices to keep the urine pale yellow in color throughout the day. It is better to drink between meals, rather than with a meal.

Some practitioners, however, believe that certain people with low thyroid function can have normal TSH readings. Measuring T4 and T3 levels also seems to be important, although in some people with symptoms of low thyroid function, the blood tests may be entirely normal. Anyone who suspects they have low thyroid function is advised to see an endocrinologist.

Thyroid function can also be assessed using a simple home test known as the Barnes test. This involves taking the underarm temperature on waking (before rising) with a mercury thermometer (this should be left under the arm for at least 10 minutes). Because premenopausal women's temperatures tend to fluctuate with the hormonal cycle, Barnes suggested that the most accurate time to assess temperature was on the third, fourth, and fifth day of the menstrual period. For nonmenstruating women and for men, any days will do as long as there is no sign of infection (this can raise body temperature). The normal underarm body temperature in the morning is between 97.8° and 98.2°F (36.6°–36.8°C). A temperature of 97.4°F (36.4°C) or less suggests low thyroid function.

Treating a sluggish thyroid gland

Several nutrients may help support thyroid function. These include iodine, selenium (which helps in the conversion of T4 to T3), vitamin A, and the amino acid L-tyrosine. Some doctors recommend supplements that contain actual thyroid tissue. These extracts, often referred to as "thyroid glandulars," are usually made from the thyroid glands of either cows or pigs. It is believed that the range of hormones available in a glandular supplement is much more likely to have a beneficial effect on hypothyroid individuals than the single hormone conventional treatment, which centers upon thyroxin alone. Thyroid glandulars should only be taken under the supervision of a doctor experienced in their use.

Adrenal weakness

The human body has two adrenal glands. Each sits on top of a kidney and is about the size of an apricot. The adrenal glands secrete a variety of hormones that play important roles in maintaining homeostasis, or balance, in the body. They are also the chief glands responsible for the body's reaction to stress because they produce the hormones epinephrine and cortisol (*see p.409*).

In some individuals, often as a result of long-term stress, adrenal function may be weakened. This condition, which nutritional therapists call "adrenal exhaustion," can have important implications for health.

Symptoms of adrenal exhaustion

- Fatigue. Adrenally weakened individuals tend to be tired, and adrenal exhaustion seems to be a common feature in people with chronic fatigue syndrome.

- Easy fatigue. Adrenally weakened individuals often have little in the way of energy reserves and get tired quite easily. For people with adrenal exhaustion, any additional stress (of a physiological and/or emotional nature) can cause a significant worsening of the fatigue.
- Low blood pressure. Normal blood pressure is usually around 120–130/70–80mmHg. Adrenally weakened individuals often have a blood pressure of 110/70mmHg or less, which may drop on standing and cause dizziness.
- Salt craving. Some individuals will crave salt, which may reflect the body's need to raise blood pressure.
- The need to eat regularly. Individuals with adrenal exhaustion tend to need to eat regularly to keep them from feeling weak and light-headed.

Laboratory tests for adrenal function
Blood tests designed to diagnose a condition known as Addison's disease, also called "adrenal insufficiency," are available. This condition is characterized by extreme adrenal weakness, to the extent that regular doses of steroids, such as cortisol, and perhaps other drugs are necessary to maintain health. Many conventional doctors do not believe in the concept of adrenal exhaustion. However, in practice, some individuals who do not have Addison's disease nonetheless have clinical evidence of impaired adrenal gland function.

Restoring adrenal health
Rest is key to restoring adrenal gland function. Adequate amounts of sleep are important, and it may be necessary to reduce workload or strenuous activity. Techniques designed to reduce demand and promote relaxation (see p.99) will also help. In addition, certain supplements may help restore adrenal gland health, including vitamin C, vitamin B$_5$, and the herbs licorice and ginseng. However, anyone who may have adrenal exhaustion is advised to work with a practitioner experienced in this health problem.

Immune system health

The immune system is a network of specialized tissues, organs, cells, and chemicals, whose chief function is to protect the body against potentially harmful agents including microorganisms (e.g. bacteria and viruses) and cancerous cells. The lymph nodes, spleen, bone marrow, thymus gland, and tonsils all play a role in immune functions, as do blood cells known as lymphocytes and the chemicals produced by them, known as antibodies.

The immune system uses two main forms of protection: innate and adaptive. Innate immunity is present at birth and provides the first barrier against organisms. It includes the skin, the acid in the stomach, and mucus secreted in the nose and lungs. Adaptive immunity is the second barrier to infection and is acquired later in life. The adaptive immune system may retain a memory of the infecting agent, which means that one infection may be enough to ensure it never happens again (as, for example, with measles and chickenpox). However, some organisms, such as the viruses that cause colds and flu, come in a variety of forms and can infect the body repeatedly.

A weakened immune system may not repel invading organisms efficiently, which makes infections more likely. Dietary approaches to combat this include avoiding sugar and taking supplements. Sugar interferes with the ability of white blood cells to destroy bacteria, and animal studies suggest that a diet high in sucrose (table sugar) may impair some aspects of immune function. Avoiding sugar in the diet may therefore help improve resistance to infection.

Several nutrients can help increase immune function. Some doctors recommend zinc supplements for people with recurrent infections, suggesting 25mg per day for adults and lower amounts for children (depending on body weight, see p.17). Vitamin C stimulates the immune system by elevating the levels of interferon and by enhancing the activity of certain immune system cells.

Diet and mood problems

Mood problems, such as depression and anxiety, can have important links with the diet. Identifying and correcting one or more of the following common imbalances is often very effective in correcting mood-related issues.
- Food sensitivities may give rise to poor concentration, low mood, and depression (wheat is a common problem food in this respect). *Candida* overgrowth can cause the same kinds of symptoms.
- Blood-sugar imbalances may give rise to low mood, anxiety, and mood swings.
- Adrenal gland weakness can contribute to anxiety (especially when meals are skipped) and depression.
- Hypothyroidism is linked to low mood and depression.

Caffeine and mood
Caffeine is a stimulant with addictive qualities. It can also upset blood-sugar levels and stimulate the adrenal glands to produce epinephrine. One study showed the equivalent of one cup of coffee provoked nervousness and/or anxiety in some individuals prone to these problems. Caffeine may also contribute to insomnia (see p.448), which can impact negatively on mood. Reducing or eliminating caffeine from the diet may help improve mood-related disorders.

Essential fatty acids
Fats play a fundamental structural and functional role in the nervous system. Of particular importance are omega-3 fatty acids (see p.34), such as EPA and DHA. People with depression have reduced levels of omega-3 fatty acids. EPA supplements may help depressed people on conventional antidepressant therapy. Omega-3 fatty acids may also help treat ADHD, manic depression, and schizophrenia.

Anemia, iron deficiency, and mood

Iron is important for hemoglobin, the pigment in red blood cells that delivers oxygen to the tissues. A deficiency of iron leads to anemia (low hemoglobin levels), which may cause low mood, mental lethargy, poor attention span, and apathy. Iron-deficiency anemia is quite common in women, vegetarians, and vegans. People with persistent fatigue and/or mood disturbance should be tested for both anemia and for iron levels in the body. The best test for iron measures serum ferritin. If this is low, then increasing iron intake often helps enhance mood. Iron-rich foods include red meat, fish, dried fruit, nuts, and seeds. A doctor should monitor iron supplementation so that it can be adjusted according to a person's serum ferritin level.

Contraindications

The following lists the minerals and vitamins and their contraindications with conventional medications:

Biotin may improve blood glucose control in diabetics. The dose of a drug that lowers blood sugar (insulin or an oral diabetic medication) may need to be reduced to avoid episodes of low blood sugar.

Bromelain can increase absorption of amoxicillin and may have a similar effect on other antibiotics. Avoid taking bromelain with antibiotics unless supervised by a doctor.

Calcium can lower the levels of beta-blockers (for high blood pressure or heart disorders). Avoid taking calcium supplements within two hours of a beta-blocker dose.

Calcium reduces the effectiveness of ciprofloxacin, ofloxacin, doxycycline, and tetracycline. Avoid taking calcium supplements within three hours of an antibiotic.

People with kidney failure may develop high blood levels of calcium. Calcium supplements should be avoided in kidney failure unless under the supervision of a doctor.

Calcium may reduce the effectiveness of thyroxine medication (for thyroid problems). Avoid taking calcium supplements within four hours of thyroxine medication.

Coenzyme Q_{10} is structurally similar to vitamin K and may also encourage blood clotting. People on warfarin should not take CoQ_{10} unless supervised by a doctor.

Folic acid may increase the frequency and/or severity of seizures. Individuals taking anticonvulsant drugs should consult their doctor before supplementing with folic acid.

Folic acid-containing supplements may interfere with methotrexate therapy for cancer since methotrexate blocks the activation of folic acid. People using methotrexate for cancer treatment should consult their prescribing doctor before using any folic acid-containing supplements.

5-Hydroxytryptophan (5-HTP) and zolpidem (for insomnia) may increase zolpidem-induced hallucinations.

5-HTP may increase the side effects of fluoxetine, venlafaxine, fluvoxamine, and paroxetine (antidepressants) and sumatriptan (for migraines). Avoid taking 5-HTP with these drugs unless supervised by a doctor.

Iron can reduce the absorption and/or effectiveness of the drugs ciprofloxacin, oflaxacin, tetracycline, doxycycline, levofloxacin, minocycline, and penicillamine. Avoid taking iron supplements within three hours of one of these drugs. People taking deferoxamine (which binds to iron and removes it from the body) should avoid iron supplements. Iron can irritate the stomach, especially if taken with the NSAID indomethacin. Take these separately and with food to reduce this risk.

Iron may reduce the absorption of methyldopa (for high blood pressure). Take methyldopa two hours before or after iron-containing products. Iron can also reduce the absorption of risedronate (for Paget's disease, postmenopausal osteoporosis, and osteoporosis brought on by steroids). Avoid taking iron within three hours of a risedronate dose. Iron can reduce the absorption of

White blood cells called macrophages are part of the immune system. They engulf bacteria and clean up cell debris. Macrophages, like many other components of the immune system, work best when there are sufficient levels of vitamin C and other antioxidants in the diet.

sulfasalazine. Avoid taking iron supplements within three hours of taking a sulfasalazine dose.

Iron may decrease the absorption of thyroid hormone medications, such as thyroxine. People taking these prescribed medications should consult their doctor before using iron-containing products.

Iron may reduce the absorption and activity of warfarin. Avoid taking iron within two hours of a warfarin dose.

Magnesium can reduce the absorption of the antibiotic ciprofloxacin. Take ciprofloxacin two hours after eating dairy products (due to the magnesium content) or taking magnesium-containing supplements.

Spironolactone (a potassium-saving diuretic used for edema and high blood pressure) may prevent the loss of magnesium (as well as potassium) from the body. People on spironolactone should not take more than 300mg of magnesium per day unless supervised by a doctor.

Magnesium may reduce the activity of warfarin. Avoid taking magnesium within two hours of a warfarin dose.

Omega-3 supplements/Fish oils The fatty acids EPA and DHA may reduce the clotting ability of blood and the need for warfarin. People on warfarin should not take omega-3 supplements and fish oils unless supervised by a doctor.

Quercetin may reduce the breakdown of felodipine (for high blood pressure). The subsequent increased blood levels of the drug may lead to side-effects. People taking felodipine should avoid supplementing with quercetin.

Soy products may reduce the absorption of thyroid hormones when taken at the same time. Avoid taking soy products within three hours of thyroid medication.

Vitamin A – Some people undergoing long-term treatment with HMG-CoA reductase inhibitors may have raised vitamin A levels. These drugs, such as atorvastatin, fluvastatin, lovastatin, and pravastatin, block an enzyme the body needs to make cholesterol. Individuals taking the drugs with vitamin A supplements need their vitamin A blood levels monitored.

Isotretinoin and tretinoin (used to treat acne) and vitamin A are structurally similar and have similar toxicities. People taking isotretinoin/tretinoin should avoid vitamin A supplements at levels higher than typically found in a multivitamin preparation (10,000 IU per day).

Vitamin B$_3$/Niacin Niacin is the form of vitamin B$_3$ used to lower cholesterol. People taking large amounts of niacin with HMG-CoA reductase inhibitors lovastatin or atorvastatin may develop muscle disorders that can be serious. The effect is rare and may extend to other drugs of this type. People taking niacin and HMG-CoA reductase inhibitors should be monitored by a doctor.

Individuals taking niacin with an oral diabetic drug may increase their requirements for the drug.

Vitamin B$_6$ (pyridoxine) Vitamin B$_6$ supplements above 5–10mg per day may reduce the effectiveness of levodopa (used for Parkinson's disease). Combining levodopa with carbidopa prevents this, so vitamin B$_6$ supplements may safely be taken with Sinemet® (carbidopa/levodopa).

Vitamin B$_6$ may reduce blood levels of phenobarbital (used prior to surgery, to combat insomnia, and to prevent or treat seizures). Those taking the sedative should avoid taking large amounts of vitamin B$_6$ (50mg a day or more).

Vitamin C can increase the absorption of antibiotics, though this may not pose problems for the body.

Some reports suggest that vitamin C might increase the activity of the blood-thinning drug warfarin. Individuals taking warfarin should not take more than 500mg of vitamin C a day unless supervised by a doctor.

Vitamin D may interfere with the effectiveness of verapamil (used for angina, arrhythmia, and high blood pressure). People taking verapamil should consult their doctor before using a supplement containing vitamin D.

Vitamin E may increase the blood-thinning effect of aspirin and warfarin. Individuals taking one or both of these drugs should not take more than 200 IU of vitamin E supplements a day unless supervised by a doctor.

Vitamin K Warfarin inhibits blood clotting by interfering with vitamin K activity. Individuals taking warfarin should avoid a supplement that contains vitamin K unless they are specifically directed by a doctor.

Zinc Long-term zinc supplementation can cause copper deficiency. Take 1mg of copper for every 15mg of zinc.

Zinc may reduce the absorption and/or effectiveness of the drugs tetracycline and ciprofloxacin. Avoid taking zinc supplements within three hours of these antibiotics.

FINDING A PRACTITIONER

The American Dietetic Association (ADA) approves more than 600 programs across the US for the training of various categories of nutritionists and dieticians. These programs are evaluated by the ADA's Commission on Accreditation for Dietetics Education, which is recognized by the US Department of Education, and credentials of nutritionists are tested by the Commission on Dietetic Registration. Nutritional therapists are required to abide by the codes of ethics and practice established by the ADA. You can find a qualified nutritional therapist in your area by logging onto www.eatright.org or contacting ADA (*see p.486*).

BODYWORK THERAPIES

LEON CHAITOW

The musculoskeletal system is the body's largest user of energy. It is through this system that we walk, talk, run, jump, feed ourselves, paint pictures, perform delicate surgery, make music, war, and love, and generally express our human individuality. It is also the "organ" that is most likely to produce symptoms severe enough to send you to a doctor. The purpose of bodywork and movement therapies is to restore harmonious balance to the integrated structures of the musculoskeletal system and to ease restriction, pain, and dysfunction.

Structural Framework

The human body has a structural framework of bones, ligaments, tendons, muscles, and joints, all held together by connective tissue. The connective tissue framework extends down to the most microscopic level, where minute fibers support individual cells and help carry information — even into the cell nucleus.

The body's central coordination depends on the brain and central nervous system and the body's tissues are nourished and oxygenated through the circulation. The structural framework allows us to move freely and painlessly while also providing space, protection, and support for the vital organs and glands regulating the biochemical activities that fuel and repair the body.

The musculoskeletal system is organized and held together in a structure that is remarkable for its ability to absorb external forces and inner tensions in one part of the body, and to spread the load evenly to the other parts. This flexible ability comes from a quality known as tensegrity, a word derived from "tension" and "integrity" (*see p.53*).

Connective tissue

The most widespread soft tissue in the body is connective tissue, sometimes known as fascia. It forms a thin network or mesh around nerves and between muscles, and a more dense network in cartilage, ligament, tendon, and bone. It supports, divides, wraps, connects, invests, separates, and gives cohesion to all the other soft tissues of the body.

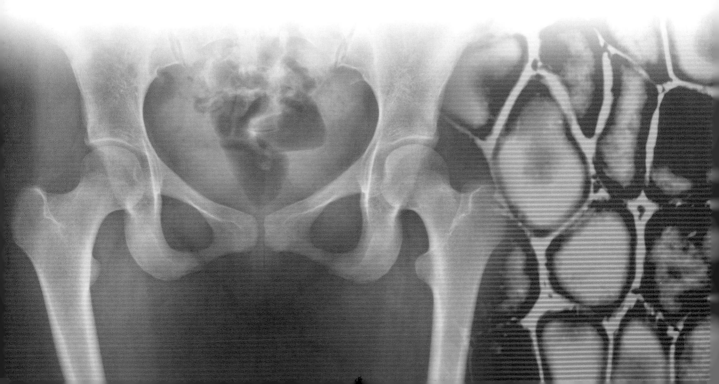

The connective tissue network is a kind of fascial web that is composed of one single continuous tensegrity structure, which reaches from the soles of the feet (plantar fascia) to the inner lining of the skull (the dura). As a result, any distortions and restrictions that occur in one part of the web can influence all the other parts, with body-wide implications. Understanding how connective tissue works helps us grasp the interconnectedness of the entire body — for example, how fallen arches in the feet can directly influence the neck and head.

Since connective tissue gives shape and cohesion to everything else in the body — including the organs, muscles, blood vessels, nerves, and cells — the fascial web can be accurately seen as a single structure. This means that the fascial "sheets" attached to the inside of the skull, such as the falx cerebri and the tentorium cerebelli (which divide different parts of the brain and give shape to the structures inside the head), merge with the lining of the skull (the dura). They are connected, without interruption, to the dura surrounding the spinal cord and the fascia of the neck, thorax, diaphragm, lower pelvis, legs, and feet. In fact, they are connected to every joint, muscle, tendon, and ligament in the body!

It is no surprise that tensions and distortions in any one part can influence the entire network. This influence may range from slight to a great extent, depending on many factors, such as the degree of distortion and the person's age and general state of suppleness and fitness. Many of the progressive changes that tighten, shorten, distort, and restrict the fascia and the associated body parts are reversible — either wholly or partially — by means of appropriate treatment and self-care.

Recent research suggests that it is through connective tissue structures — specifically the cleavage planes where the individual muscle groups are separated from each other — that many of the beneficial effects of manual therapy, as well as acupuncture, acupressure, and trigger-point deactivation, are achieved.

Form and function of cells

The body's fascial web extends into the connective tissue (cytoskeleton) inside every cell and minute protrusions (integrins) on their surfaces. These two key features have been shown to determine the overall efficiency of a cell's function, and of the way a cell expresses itself genetically.

According to recent research, the fascia of a cell becomes distorted in a gravity-free environment. This effect alters the cell's shape and modifies the way it processes nutrients. Put simply, when the structure of a cell changes, its function changes too, meaning that it cannot absorb and metabolize nutrients properly.

A cell's inability to nourish and ultimately to reproduce itself has enormous implications for the health of the whole body. We do not need to travel in outer space to create changes in our fascial structure, since the processes of adaptation (see p.53), compensation, aging, and disease, which affect us all, create localized warping, crowding, compression, and distortion of the fascia — right down to a cellular level. Over time, this is potentially harmful to normal cellular life, and therefore to general health and well-being because the changes caused restrict healthy circulation of fluids and the flow of information that organs need to stay healthy.

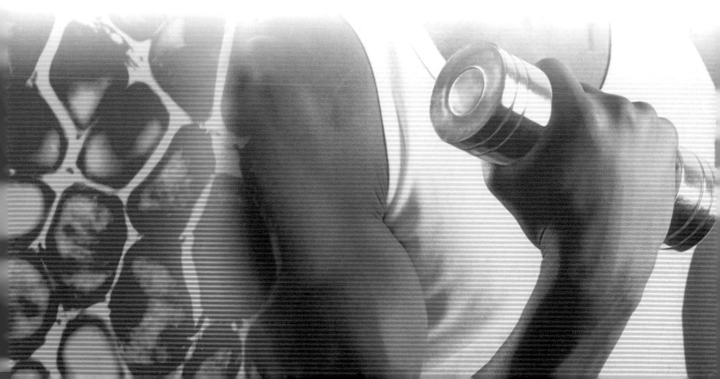

BIOMECHANICAL AND BODYWORK TISSUES

The body's framework consists of a variety of tissues that rely on biomechanical properties and information networks to perform and coordinate a wide range of movements. These are the tissues on which bodywork and movement therapists focus. in order restore health and well-being.

TISSUE	DESCRIPTION
Bone	Bone is hard and strong, but slightly flexible, with an internal structure that absorbs stresses. It is a living tissue that is constantly being rebuilt, even in adulthood.
Joints	Joints are where two bones meet. Most are moveable.
Movable joints	Movable joints include the ball-and-socket joint of the shoulder and hip, the hinge joint of the knee, and the pivot joint at the top of the neck. Movable joints are lubricated by synovial fluid.
Semimovable	Semimovable joints, such as those in the sacrum (at the base of the spine), are held together by flexible cartilage.
Fixed joints	A few joints are fixed, for example the suture joints in the skull.
Tendons	Tendons are tough, stringy connective tissues that link muscles to bones.
Ligaments	Ligaments are tough bands of connective tissue that support and bind one bone to another one at joints.
Cartilage	Cartilage has a smooth protective surface to provide ease of movement where bones meet.
Muscles	Muscle is an elastic tissue that can contract and relax. Each muscle is composed of bundles of fibers surrounded by connective tissue.
Skeletal muscle	● Skeletal muscles are attached to bones. They can be made to contract voluntarily (consciously). They contract swiftly and powerfully, but cannot sustain contractions for long periods of time. ● Different types of muscle fiber have different levels of strength and stamina, and are used in different activities. ● Type 1 fibers ("slow-twitch") have slower contractile speeds, and are used for endurance activities such as long-distance running and maintaining posture. ● Type 2 fibers ("fast-twitch") have faster contractile speeds and are used in more "high intensity" activities.
Smooth muscle	● Smooth muscle surrounds many of the tubes in the body, e.g. blood vessels and intestines. It contracts in waves (called peristalsis). It is capable of contracting for long periods of time. Smooth muscle contraction is not usually under conscious control.
Connective tissue (fascia)	● The most widespread soft tissue in the body. A thin network, somewhat like a cobweb, that surrounds nerves, runs between muscles, and connects with ligaments, cartilage, and bone. It gives cohesion to and interconnects with all other tissues in the body.
Spinal cord	● Together with the brain, the spinal cord processes information and keeps the body coordinated. The spinal cord runs down a protective tunnel inside the vertebrae (backbones). ● Spinal nerves emerge from gaps between the vertebrae and connect to all parts of the body.
Nerves	● Nerves are bundles of nerve cells. They carry messages from one part of the body to another. The fastest method is via an electrical signal, but chemicals can also be moved along nerve cells. A nerve cell has a rounded body that contains the nucleus and very long, thin extensions called axons. Nerve cells that connect the spinal cord to the toes can be over 3 ft (1 m) long.
Cytoskeleton	● Cells are the tiny units that make up all the structures in the body. Each cell contains its own "skeleton," called the cytoskeleton, which gives it its shape, holds the nucleus and other organelles ("mini organs") in place, and helps the cell move. The cytoskeleton is made of chains of protein molecules.

Cartilage, bones, and joints

The fascial web of connective tissue is anchored to the bones of the skeleton by elastic tissues (muscles, tendons, and ligaments) that form a series of interconnected "poles" and "guyline." These allow loads and tensions to be shared by the structure as a whole, of which the bones of the skeleton can be seen as the "struts." Bones seldom actually touch each other in normal conditions. Instead, they "meet" at a joint, which is held in place by ligaments and tied to muscles that move it via tendons.

The primary purpose of semimovable joints, such as the sacroiliac joint in the pelvis, is to provide stability — they are protected by pads or disks of cartilage that absorb the pressure of external loads and forces. Joints that move freely, such as the elbow and knee, offer flexibility and mobility — they are protected and lubricated by synovial membranes and fluid. To some extent, all joints provide both stability and mobility.

Wear and tear, inefficient supporting structures such as weak muscles and lax ligaments, and the aging process are the main enemies of joints. These problems are further aggravated by overuse, misuse, disuse, and abuse (see p.57). When joint surfaces become irritated, arthritic changes (see Osteoarthritis, p.289) usually begin.

The spine and the rest of the bony skeleton provide a "protective cage" that offers a safe place for the vital organs, such as the heart and liver. The health of these organs can be greatly influenced by distortions and crowding of the skeletal structures. When a slumped posture becomes a habit, for example, it can put stress on the connective tissue around the organs, negatively affecting their nerve and blood supply, as well as their lymph drainage. It may even affect how well the organs actually work.

Tendons

A tendon connects a muscle to a bone, providing the muscle with the anchorage it needs to contract and exert a force. However, tendons can become inflamed or irritated, often when the muscle to which they are attached contracts repetitively or frequently. This can lead to problems such as Achilles tendonitis and many localized painful areas close to joints, especially those prone to overuse (see p.57), such as the knees, wrists, and elbows. Trigger points (see p.55) are frequently located in the muscles associated with such irritable, overused tendons.

Ligaments

Ligaments are specialized connective tissue that support and bind joints. They are particularly important (and sometimes vulnerable) in joints that are prone to damage when excessively stressed or strained, such as the knees and ankles. Approximately one person in ten has lax ligaments (i.e. "double-jointed"), a condition known as hypermobility. In Asian and Arab women, as many as four out of ten may be born with this characteristic. Hypermobile individuals are more likely than others to develop conditions sometimes labeled "soft-tissue rheumatism" (involving muscles rather than bones or joints), as well as those involving muscle weakness, such as fibromyalgia and spinal scoliosis.

Skeletal muscles

These muscles are attached to the various bones of the skeleton and are composed of bundles of fibers that can be made to contract voluntarily. The bundles, or fasciculi, usually lie side by side in a parallel arrangement and are individually enclosed in a thin connective tissue sheath known as the endomysium.

There are two types of muscle fiber: type 1 muscle fibers will shorten when continually stressed by overuse, misuse, or abuse; type 2 muscle fibers, when similarly stressed, become weak and may lengthen. As a result, imbalances develop between opposing muscle groups, with negative effects on both the muscles and the joints they serve.

For example, the neck and shoulder muscles of someone with a slumped posture and head thrust forward are tense and tight. The deep muscles at the front of the neck (the deep neck flexors) are usually weak and inhibited, putting the joints of the neck under stress and causing awkward movements, usually involving some stiffness and probably discomfort. In time, the nerves emerging from the spine and the disks between vertebrae may become irritated, leading to painful symptoms, both locally and at a distance.

Another example of imbalance is the tight, arched low back of a person who displays a protruding and sagging abdomen. When this is chronic, symptoms of backache and abdominal and pelvic organ dysfunction are likely.

Smooth muscles

Smooth muscles form the circular walls of the bladder, blood vessels, bronchioles, and many of the hollow digestive organs, such as the gastrointestinal tract. A smooth muscle has a circular control over the tube it surrounds, often contracting in a wavelike manner — for example, in peristalsis (the action that propels food through the gut).

Tens of thousands of smooth muscle cells are also embedded in the fascial web. When they contract they increase the tension in the connective tissue, sometimes excessively, leading to body-wide stiffness and restriction.

Smooth muscles contract when the blood becomes more alkaline than normal, such as takes place during hyperventilation (see p.57). Therefore, people with a tendency to an anxious, upper-chest breathing pattern tend to have an increased degree of tone/tension in the fascia, which may affect the entire musculoskeletal system and probably encourage trigger-point formation (see p.55).

Brain and Nervous System

The brain receives a constant stream of reports (tens of thousands of messages per second) from nerve structures in the limbs, such as Ruffini nerve endings and Pacinian corpuscles, that register motion, temperature, pressure, or pain. This information relates to what is happening in the different parts of the body and answers a multitude of questions that the brain asks, such as: Is the left arm moving? If so, how fast and in what direction? What is its temperature? Is anything pressing on it? Is there any pain? In this way, the brain learns what is happening to every bone, muscle, joint, tendon, and ligament — even in the farthest reaches of the fascial web.

After interpreting the received information, the brain sends instructions, via the nervous system, that enable us to walk, talk, keep our balance, move, function, and live our lives. Some bodily functions, such as digestion, the rhythmic contraction of the heart, and breathing, are on "automatic pilot," outside our conscious control. Other functions, such as walking and talking, are directly influenced by conscious decisions.

Problems may arise as a result of various sources, for example, when the brain either receives inaccurate information from faulty nerves or misinterprets correct information; when the brain sends inappropriate instructions to the tissues and organs; and when reflex activities are either excessive or diminished.

Reflexes

Many nerve functions are reflexive in nature, which means that responses do not have to be ordered by the brain, but can take place via "short-circuit" pathways in the spine. Perhaps the most familiar example of this is the "knee-jerk" reflex reaction.

When spinal structures are injured or stressed, the normal behavior of vertebral joints may change. This may irritate or compress the nerves that emerge from it, with the potential to influence the organs and other tissues that they serve. This is known as a somaticovisceral reflex.

Similarly but in reverse, when an organ or tissue is unwell the spinal regions associated with it can become distressed, tense, and painful. This is known as a viscero-somatic reflex. A common example is the tense, sensitive region of the upper back (2nd, 3rd, and 4th thoracic vertebral areas) frequently noted in people who have heart problems. Some osteopathic and chiropractic practitioners use this knowledge in their work to attempt to modify the negative feedback pathways to the organs.

Although treatment of such spinal areas cannot "cure" organ disease, there is evidence that it brings some benefit. Awareness of these reflex pathways can also help explain the appearance of many spinal problems that do not have an obvious mechanical cause.

Axonal transportation

Nerves conduct electrical messages and carry "trophic substances," such as proteins, essential fatty acids, and neurotransmitters, to and from the target tissues and the organs they serve. This movement of substances along nerve pathways is known as axonal transportation.

According to osteopathic research, any interference with nerve function, message conduction, or axonal transport, in either direction, can cause a wide range of symptoms. Mechanical deformities, such as compression and stretching, and sustained hyperactivity of nerve cells in sensitized spinal segments can slow down axonal transport. Appropriate mobilization and manipulation of soft tissues and joints may be able to improve these functions.

Sympathetic and parasympathetic actions

The nervous system can be broadly divided into two parts. The primary role of the sympathetic nervous system is to stimulate tissues and organs, whereas the parasympathetic nervous system has the opposite effect. It primarily calms, inhibits, or damps down the activities of the tissues and organs. These stimulating and calming effects of the nervous system can be hugely affected by both emotions and biochemical factors, such as hormonal balance, diet, drugs, and allergies. The nerves of the body are therefore capable of becoming sensitized (hyperirritable), as well as being potentially inhibited, by biomechanical, psychological, and biochemical influences.

Central sensitization

Ultimately, nerves feed into the central nervous system and the brain. At times, this central control mechanism may be responsible for excessive or diminished nerve activity. Just as a local muscle area may become hyperirritable if repetitively stressed — forming a trigger point, for example — so the central nervous system, or parts of it, including parts of the brain, can become sensitized when bombarded with pain and distress messages, or when biochemically disturbed. This central sensitization can make the nerve and brain structures far more easily irritated, interfering with accurate interpretation of the messages received from the body and sending inappropriate instructions in response. Central sensitization is thought to be a major factor in many chronic pain conditions.

Entrapment and compression

Many nerves are vulnerable to mechanical interference because they pass through or around structures, such as muscles and bones, that can trap and/or compress them. Many symptoms result from such situations. Entrapment is usually the excessive pressure that soft tissues place upon a nerve. For example, when the scalene muscles in the neck or the pectoral muscles in the upper chest impinge on and crowd the nerves running toward an arm, a variety of pain and numbness symptoms can be felt in the arm. This is a condition known as thoracic outlet syndrome, or TOS.

Carpal tunnel syndrome (*see p.152*) is an example of compression. In this disorder, the arch of bones and fascia in the wrist press on the median nerve. The condition is commonly caused and always aggravated by overuse of the wrist, but it may also be partially caused by fluid retention involving swelling of the lower arm or hand.

Self-repair and Adaptation

A fundamental truth should be kept in mind as we explore the many things that can go wrong with the biomechanics of the body: there is an inherent capacity for self-repair, constantly at work, whether in response to trauma (broken bones usually heal) or to chronic patterns of overuse and misuse.

If the causes can be reduced or removed and/or the structural integrity of the biomechanical (and, of course, the biochemical and psychological) components of the body can be improved, then self-regulation processes commonly ensure a return of normal function. Many of the symptoms we experience, unpleasant as they may be, should be understood as messages of recovery and repair-in-action — for example, inflammation may be unpleasant but without it tissue repair cannot take place.

Other symptoms, such as acute pain, may be understood as vital messages, warning us not to overuse a particular area because to do so would aggravate existing damage or create a worse situation.

By learning to understand and respect these messages, and to take appropriate action, we can enhance the healing process. Ignoring the symptom's message can be disastrous. For example, inappropriate use of medication that is anti-inflammatory and analgesic can lead to overuse and therefore aggravation of already damaged structures, creating a far worse state of affairs and delaying recovery.

Does this mean that we should never use anti-inflammatory or analgesic medication? No, but it does suggest that we should only do so if we intend to respect self-healing processes that are going on in the background. The therapeutic measures used for any condition should therefore strike the balance between helping the person feel more comfortable while not creating new problems, or retarding the potential for recovery.

Adaptation

The old saying, that there are only two certainties in life — death and taxes — can be accurately expanded to include adaptation. We adapt from the cradle to the grave. We adapt to both internal and external forces as we grow, mature, develop, and interact with other people and the

TENSEGRITY

A characteristic feature of the body's musculoskeletal system is its ability to absorb the impact of external stresses and to spread the load of internal tensions without compromising the overall integrity of its structure. This flexible ability evolves from the quality known as tensegrity, which can be found in the structure of both the cell's skeleton and the geodesic dome.

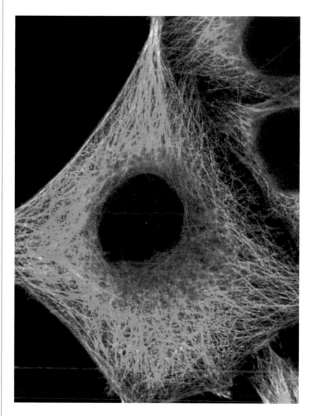

Fluorescent dyes reveal proteins in the cytoskeleton of a cell (*above*). Microtubulin (green) is the main constituent of microtubules, which are important in cell division. Actin (red) is essential to muscle contraction. Golgi protein (blue) is found in the Golgi apparatus, which plays a part in the processing and transport of proteins within the cell.

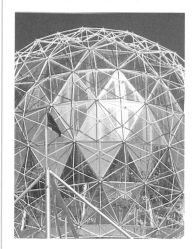

The word tensegrity was coined in 1961 by the visionary US architect Buckminster Fuller. He wanted to describe the stability that results from the interaction of rigid struts, flexible connecting fibres and filaments, and enclosed fluids under pressure. A suitable architectural example of tensegrity structure is the geodesic dome (*left*), which has no upright pillars.

environment. We adapt to the things we do, the things that happen to us and to the characteristics with which we are born. We adapt physically, biochemically, emotionally, and psychologically throughout life. And when we cannot adapt any more, problems become evident.

The pioneer researcher in this area was Hans Selye, a Canadian physiologist who identified adaptation as the main feature that characterizes and influences our development. Maladaptation largely determines whether health is good or poor and ultimately leads to our eventual collapse. On the larger stage, Selye noted that everything that calls for adaptation can be labeled as "stress." By understanding stress in this way (i.e. as an adaptation demand) we can see that it becomes harmful only when we are unable to adapt to the stress factor — i.e. when our capacity for adaptation is overwhelmed.

"As the twig is bent …"

A simple analogy clarifies what happens when we adapt to the stresses of life, and how the body compensates to the adaptive demands placed on it.

If a living, flexible branch of a tree is bent, it will adapt to the forces applied to it until it cannot absorb any more tension, torsion, or distortion — at which moment it breaks or splinters. However, if a milder force is repetitively applied, the living branch will adapt to match the "stress," and will become permanently bent. The fact that it is no longer as nature designed it means that this particular bent twig, although well adapted to the stresses imposed on it, would be unable to perform the same functions that it could when it was straight. In general, adaptation occurs at the expense of the ability to function optimally. The new situation (bent) allows the young twig to survive, but removes some of its original potential.

Research into how blood vessel walls respond and adapt to the stresses imposed on them is an example of how the "bent twig'" analogy applies to the body. Blood vessel walls adapt to the structural strain (high blood pressure), bio-chemical strain (high cholesterol), and psychological strain (hormonal instability caused by a hostile temperament) placed on them by hardening and narrowing. Gradually they become increasingly narrowed and inflexible and eventually the part of the body they supply simply does not receive enough oxygen and nutrients. Angina is the result of not enough oxygen and nutrients reaching the cardiac muscle, while if the coronary arteries are completely blocked a heart attack will probably happen.

Doctors treat the problem by attempting to lower blood pressure and the cholesterol level with drugs and, if necessary, by replacing the narrowed artery with a vein from somewhere else in the body. In the long term, however, the best medical approach is to address all the structural, biochemical, and psychological elements involved in high blood pressure and coronary artery disease in order to reduce the stresses to which the blood vessels are being forced to adapt. In parts of the US, cardiac rehabilitation programs follow up bypass surgery or a heart attack with diet, meditation, yoga, and graduated exercise. Such programs increase fitness and encourage psychological well-being, thereby improving the patient's ability to cope with stress (see Coronary artery disease & heart attack, p.252).

General and local adaptation

Selye used the terms "general adaptation syndrome" and "local adaptation syndrome." The former describes the effects of stress on the whole person and the latter the effects on a local area, such as the shoulder. Each "syndrome" follows three stages: an initial alarm phase; a period of adjustment, compensation, and adaptation, which might last for many years; and a stage of collapse, when adaptive capacity is exhausted.

Examples of local adaptation syndromes include the way specific muscles adapt to new patterns of use — as happens when you take on a new job that involves physical labor or a sustained posture. A general adaptation syndrome involves the whole body. Imagine, for instance, that you were born at sea level and relocated to live at altitude. It would take months or years for your body to adapt to the different environmental situation. The changes necessary would involve your heart, lungs, circulation, and general metabolic functioning.

Alarm and adjustment phases

Learning a new skill, such as playing tennis, places specific adaptive demands on the body. Generally, the exercise affects the whole body, bringing cardiovascular and muscular changes as the system learns to adapt to the new aerobic activity. Locally, the dominant hand, shoulder, and arm has to perform unaccustomed activities, which initially might cause muscular discomfort. This is the "alarm" phase of the adaptation syndrome.

If you continue to play tennis, the initial symptoms (soreness, stiffness) tend to lessen as the body adjusts to the new demands. However, if you play too much, too often, or too long, the compensatory demands will become excessive and the adaptive capacity overwhelmed, causing symptoms that may be severe — for example, tennis elbow or repetitive strain injury (see p.286).

Excessive training of young soccer players, gymnasts, and other athletes has been shown to produce major structural problems (including early arthritic changes), often ending careers before they begin. In these situations, it is a case of too much activity, for too long, too often, and too soon for their immature bodies.

Individual idiosyncrasies

The adaptive demands of work and leisure activities, whether mountain climbing, gardening, gymnastics, or watching TV on the sofa, affect us all in different ways.

The differences depend on various factors: your body type and constitution at birth; the nature of your health history; how "fit" and supple you are (and how you maintain this); your age; and how efficiently and nonstressfully you have learned to use the physical body.

The result is that some people adapt without problems to the demands placed upon them, but many do not. In fact, few people pass their entire working lives without discomfort and many others experience repetitive strains, aches, and pains.

Some people are also born with so-called "inborn stressors" that create adaptive demands. For example, some people have legs of unequal length; others have one side of the pelvis that is smaller than the other, leading to a "tilt" of the pelvis and spinal strain; and some people have upper arms that are shorter than usual, which leads to increased sidebending when sitting in order to gain support when resting on the arms of chair.

Finally, some people are hypermobile (*see p. 51*) and have a tendency to possess lax ligaments (they are "double-jointed"). This tendency causes muscles to overwork to protect the "loose" joints. Rehabilitation, learning new and better ways of doing things, and encouraging a more balanced state of the muscles, helps people overcome such built-in problems.

Adaptating to a deskbound occupation

The postural demands of working at a desk in front of a computer terminal for eight hours a day are likely to create adaptive stresses affecting the neck and back. Unless the seating and desk arrangements are ideal and the postural awareness is good, progressive changes occur in overused neck, shoulder, and arm muscles. Other muscles will be underused, including the stabilizers of the shoulder blade and the low back, abdominal, and leg muscles.

Progressive shortening of some muscles (hip flexors and the pectoral muscles in the upper chest) and weakness in others (abdominal muscles) lead to restrictions in overused joints and in static, underused joints. In the low back and neck, elbows, and wrists, localized areas of sensitivity and pain (trigger points) develop, particularly in the overused, shortened muscles. Eventually, background discomfort, pain, and restriction become constant, with occasional acute spells of pain whenever irritable muscles (especially in the low back and neck) get even more tense and cramped.

The solutions are obvious. They include: better seating posture and better use of the body, with particular attention to avoiding overuse; stretching and movement strategies to help compensate for being sedentary; and appropriate treatment and self-care to loosen and mobilize structures that have become tense and irritable.

TRIGGER POINTS

When cells in part of a muscle persistently receive insufficient blood and therefore oxygen (often because of excessive tension in the muscle), they become irritable. This affects the local nerve supply, producing areas of oversensitization known as myofascial trigger points ("myo" relates to muscle and "fascial" to connective tissue).

As tension builds up around this zone, calcium enters the muscle cells, but they lack the energy to pump it out again. This sets up a vicious cycle in which the muscle cells cannot loosen up and the affected muscle cannot relax. A characteristically taut band forms in the muscle, which can be located by a fingertip pressure.

TRIGGER POINT PAIN

Often, a person with trigger-point pain has not found the tender spot that is responsible. Sometimes, however, they are aware of a sore point that, when pressed, causes pain that may radiate to other areas. This is characteristic of the pain. The trigger points can cause symptoms some

distance away and they become more active when stress, of whatever type, affects the person as a whole.

Trigger points are a common feature of pain. According to leading pain researchers and renowned neurologists Patrick Wall and Ronald Melzack, there are few, if any, chronic pain problems that do not have trigger-point activity as a major part of the picture. They may not always be a prime cause, but they are almost always a factor that helps maintain the condition.

Trigger points become self-perpetuating (a cycle in which pain leads to increased muscle tension which leads to pain) and seldom disappear unless they are adequately treated, or unless the reason for their existence, such as overuse or misuse, is removed.

TRIGGER POINT FACTORS

The following factors tend to maintain and enhance trigger point activity:
- Nutritional deficiency (especially vitamin C, B-complex vitamins, and iron).
- Hormonal imbalances (for example,

low output of thyroid hormones and hormonal imbalances that occur during menopause or in premenstrual women).
- Persistent, low-grade infections (bacteria, viruses, or yeast).
- Food intolerances (wheat and dairy in particular).
- Poor oxygenation of cells and tissues (aggravated by tension, stress, inactivity or poor respiration).

TREATING TRIGGER POINTS

Ways of treating and deactivating trigger points include acupuncture, local anesthetic injections, direct manual pressure, stretching, and ice massage. These treatments will succeed in the long term only if the causes of the trigger points are removed. If muscles are stressed for long periods they tend to undergo fibrotic changes, becoming more "stringy" and less elastic, and more prone to injury when asked to perform new tasks. Regular, moderate degrees of exercise, including stretching, can help reduce this tendency.

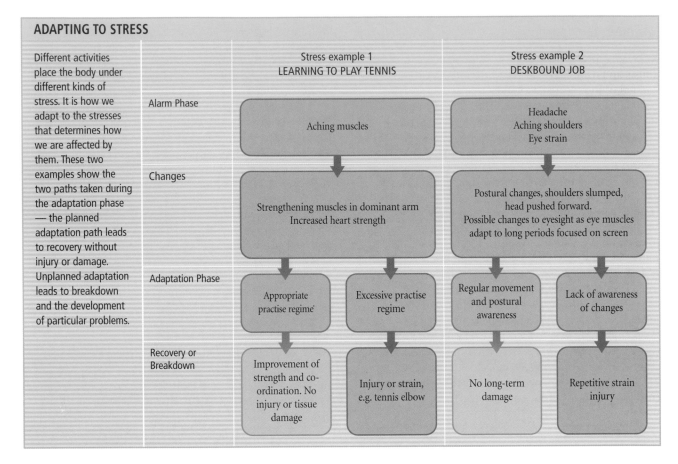

ADAPTING TO STRESS

Different activities place the body under different kinds of stress. It is how we adapt to the stresses that determines how we are affected by them. These two examples show the two paths taken during the adaptation phase — the planned adaptation path leads to recovery without injury or damage. Unplanned adaptation leads to breakdown and the development of particular problems.

	Stress example 1 — LEARNING TO PLAY TENNIS	Stress example 2 — DESKBOUND JOB
Alarm Phase	Aching muscles	Headache, Aching shoulders, Eye strain
Changes	Strengthening muscles in dominant arm, Increased heart strength	Postural changes, shoulders slumped, head pushed forward. Possible changes to eyesight as eye muscles adapt to long periods focused on screen
Adaptation Phase	Appropriate practise regime / Excessive practise regime	Regular movement and postural awareness / Lack of awareness of changes
Recovery or Breakdown	Improvement of strength and co-ordination. No injury or tissue damage / Injury or strain, e.g. tennis elbow	No long-term damage / Repetitive strain injury

Planned adaptation

Prolonged sitting results in unplanned adaptation. What happens, however, when adaptation is planned? When someone prepares for a marathon, for example, he or she does not start the process by running the full 26-plus miles! The person trains, gradually increasing the amounts of stress (running and fitness training) so that the body can adapt to the new needs — to be able to run nonstop for 2–3 hours without injury. The adaptation process develops new muscle tissue and changes in responses of the heart, lungs, and the whole biochemistry of energy production, as well as psychological adaptation to the discipline of training.

This same process of adaptation occurs in all sports, whether weightlifting or mountain climbing. Planned adaptation (training), therefore, is designed to allow us to do things — and to do them more efficiently — than before. However, just as the "bent twig" would be unable to perform the tasks of a straight twig, so the trained marathon runner could not become a sprinter. Once the body has become specialized to suit one type of sport, it is difficult to adapt to a completely different one.

Factors leading to breakdown

Adaptation leads to specialization, limiting the potential for further adaptation. This fact is critical to understanding many of the sudden pain events that occur in life. When body structures are unprepared for, or incapable of meeting unexpected demands, such as lifting, stretching, or moving suddenly, then tissues fail. Strain occurs and pain and spasm is a frequent consequence.

The limit to how much adaptation is possible is called the point of adaptive exhaustion or breakdown and is brought about by age and condition (of the person or body structure), as well as the kind and duration of stresses to which the person has had to adapt. The addition of a new adaptive demand may also be involved.

One of Selye's great discoveries was that multiple minor stresses have the same cumulative effect on the immune system and general health as one major stressful event. It is therefore extremely important to realize that adaptation is not just a response to external mechanical loads, but also a response to many internal biomechanical, biochemical, emotional, and psychological stresses.

Breakdown can cause severe biomechanical symptoms, often involving spinal, pelvic, or other joints: slipped disks, nerve impingement, inflamed tissues or other forms of dysfunction, decompensation, or maladaptation. Along with actual injuries caused by trauma, falls, etc, these are the problems that keep manipulation therapists busy, as they try in their different ways to restore functionality. However, their efforts will be in vain if the adaptive load that produced the problem is not modified or avoided.

Causes of injuries

Many adaptive changes happen because of overuse, misuse, abuse, and disuse. The sorts of problems that arise through sudden or long-term adaptation are often remediable or reversible. Treatment and self-help methods deal with the mechanical and structural changes, the functional changes, or both (*see Diagnosis, Treatments, and Therapies, p.59*).

Overuse

Repetitive movements, habitual postures, or breathing excessively use certain muscles over and over again. This leads to slow adaptation through multiple changes in the soft tissues and joints. These secondary changes produce new adaptive demands due to muscular irritation and tightness, leading to discomfort, pain, and the formation of trigger points. In breathing pattern disorders (*see right*) there is constant overuse of particular breathing muscles.

Misuse

People regularly misuse their musculoskeletal framework when sitting or standing. A slumped, or an excessively "military," posture are two examples. Using the wrong size or design of objects, such as chairs, sports equipment, shoes, and musical instruments, can all create distress in the musculoskeletal system. The mechanical strains and stresses of misuse lead to a chain reaction of secondary changes, causing pain, tension, and trigger points.

Abuse

Injuries, such as whiplash and athletic injuries (torn muscle, broken bone), and surgery can produce scar tissue and changed patterns of use. Over time, such chronic soft-tissue changes, plus joint degeneration and disk narrowing, produce pain and another round of compensation by the rest of the body. Whiplash injuries can apparently sensitize the central nervous system, and set in motion the onset of body-wide pain syndromes, such as fibromyalgia.

Disuse

Lack of exercise, immobilization, protective nonuse of an area (as in a fracture, arthritis, or a disk problem), and sedentary occupations all lead to underuse of parts of the body and the progressive weakness of disused muscles.

Remedies for overuse, misuse, abuse, and disuse

Problems caused by overuse and misuse are clearly avoidable and are often remedied by a simple change of habits. Learning to use the body more efficiently and less stressfully is a matter of reeducation and retraining, often accompanied by some form of manual treatment. These include osteopathy, chiropractic, physical therapy, occupational therapy, massage therapy (including tuina, shiatsu, Ayurvedic massage, and Thai massage), and the Alexander technique. Yoga, t'ai chi, Pilates, and athletic training can be useful in rehabilitation, too. Conditions that result from abuse may require similar rehabilitation approaches, but are more likely to require more manual and other therapeutic interventions. The after-effects of disuse also require rehabilitation. If muscles have been disused as a result of an injury, surgical operation, stroke, or other event, very specialized occupational therapy, physical therapy, or athletic training may be necessary to coax the muscles back into normal working order.

Breathing Pattern Disorders

People with a breathing pattern disorder (BPD) mainly breathe into their upper chest and do not usually use their diaphragm much. BPDs are extremely common and contribute massively to ill-health. People with a chronic BPD are often persistently fatigued and anxious; many have various musculoskeletal aches, pains, and odd sensations. BPDs are not a disease, but a habit, like poor posture. Hyperventilation is an extreme form of a BPD.

When a tendency toward upper-chest breathing becomes more pronounced (usually in stressful situations), biochemical imbalances occur. Excessive amounts of carbon dioxide are exhaled, making the blood more alkaline. This in turn produces a sense of apprehension and anxiety, reinforcing the anxious upper-chest breathing pattern. The vicious circle can lead to panic attacks and phobic behavior as the person begins to avoid situations that trigger these feelings — commonly, lines, crowds, and enclosed spaces. Recovery from this cycle may be possible only when breathing is normalized.

This breathing pattern can disturb the normal oxygen supply to the heart in three ways, at times causing it to beat abnormally. First, the smooth muscles that surround the blood vessels constrict, reducing blood supply to the heart muscles. Second, the red blood cells release the oxygen they should be delivering to the heart muscles less efficiently. Finally, the sympathetic nervous system becomes stimulated, which unbalances heart rhythms.

Consequences of increased blood alkalinity include constriction of blood vessels, thereby reducing blood supply to all tissues in general but the brain in particular. At the same time, the alkalinity of the blood discourages the release of oxygen from hemoglobin (Bohr effect), reducing further the oxygenation of tissues and the brain. This can lead to so-called "brain-fog" in which consciousness is blurred and mood swings are more likely. Peripheral nerves become more sensitive and easily irritated, thereby lowering pain thresholds. Muscles tire rapidly and a general feeling of fatigue sets in. When the smooth muscle in the walls of the digestive tract are affected, irritable bowel symptoms will get worse. Allergies and food intolerances can get worse too, due to increased circulating histamines triggered by other chemical changes.

Additionally, stresses occur in the breathing muscles themselves, purely due to "overuse," with increased tension and trigger-point activity (see p.55) that involve the chest, upper back, shoulder, and neck. A cascade of new strains follow, as tensions increase in spinal (especially neck) and rib joints, triggering head, neck, shoulder, arm, and upper back pain.

Posture and Internal Organs

The organs of the body are supported by soft tissues and the framework of the skeleton. When the body is distorted (except for a short period), there will be an impact on the way the organs function. In the first half of the twentieth century, one of the leading US physicians of the time, Joel Goldthwaite, described the effects of poor posture on the body as a whole. "When the human machine is out of balance, physiological function cannot be perfect; muscles and ligaments are in an abnormal state of tension and strain. A well-poised body means a machine working perfectly, with the least amount of muscular effort, and therefore better health and strength for daily life."

Diaphragm and abdominal muscles

Goldthwaite pointed out that the main supporting structures of the abdominal organs are the diaphragm and the abdominal muscles. If they become lax and weak, ceasing to offer support when posture is faulty, circulation to internal organs becomes disturbed. The diaphragm may also stiffen up and be unable to move freely.

Faulty body mechanics are an aspect of many chronic health problems and an important consideration when thinking of health enhancement and disease prevention. As people grow older, the abdomen tends to relax and sag, which disturbs the regular movement of the diaphragm. This can interfere with normal circulation, leading to congestion in the abdominal and pelvic organs. The congested organs put pressure on their nerve supply, which causes functional irregularities. This may contribute to many digestive problems and possibly to organ disease itself. If the abdomen and its contents sag, the chest tends to droop, the shoulders to become rounded, and the head to be thrust forward with the chin jutting out. Fortunately, the lower abdominal muscles can be trained to contract properly (achieving what is known as core stability), supporting both the organs and the lower back.

As you read through the ailments in Part 2, you will find a number of references to spinal manipulation being able, at times, to influence internal functions to improve health (see Angina, p.249, and Menstrual Pain, p.328). This is possible because of the interconnected relationship between overall posture, the functional state of the spine, and the nerve supply from the spine and the internal organs.

Mind–Body Connection

In a classic Charlie Brown cartoon, Charlie stands in a slumped position with his chin on his chest. He says to one of his friends, "This is how you have to stand when you are depressed." There is much truth in Charlie's words, because we judge people's body language all the time. If someone carries himself or herself in a dejected, "depressed" way, or in an anxious, apprehensive manner, or with an aggressive, angry posture — our instant judgment picks up on their current emotional state. Emotion changes our posture, even our breathing (see Breathing pattern disorders, p.57). If prolonged or repetitive, the adaptation to such changes then leads to new symptoms.

Long-held psychological states and repressed, unspoken emotions, such as anger and fear, can become stored (somatized) in the body. This creates a virtual armor of tension in the muscles, with consequent changes in joint and general bodily function.

"Unclenching the fist"

The osteopath Philip Latey offers a perspective on the way emotions become expressed as muscle tension in his metaphor for the different physical responses to emotional distress. He describes three key areas of the body, and the tensions in them, as the "upper fist" (head/neck area), the "middle fist" (chest area), and the "lower fist" (pelvic area). The clenched fist neatly gives an image of the tense, tight muscles of these areas, as well as the effect of release, as the fist slowly unclenches.

A question raised by Latey's work is worth considering: if the most appropriate response an individual makes is to "lock away" emotions into their musculoskeletal system, is it advisable to unlock the body and release the emotions which the tensions and contractions hold? It may well be that psychotherapy or counseling, in conjunction with appropriate bodywork, offers the best solution to "unclenching the fist," so that emotional and structural changes can occur simultaneously.

Stress and different muscle groups

One research study confirmed that specific emotions seem to affect particular muscle groups more than others. For example, the main muscles affected in agitated people are on the back of the arms; depressed individuals showed greatest activity in the sheet of muscle on the forehead (the frontalis). Another study found that careful physical examination failed in many instances to find a cause for patients' pain. There was, however, a correlation between anger and pain in the neck, between fear and abdominal pain, and between sorrow or despair and low back pain. In patients with these correlations it was rare for an organic cause to be found, even after extensive investigation.

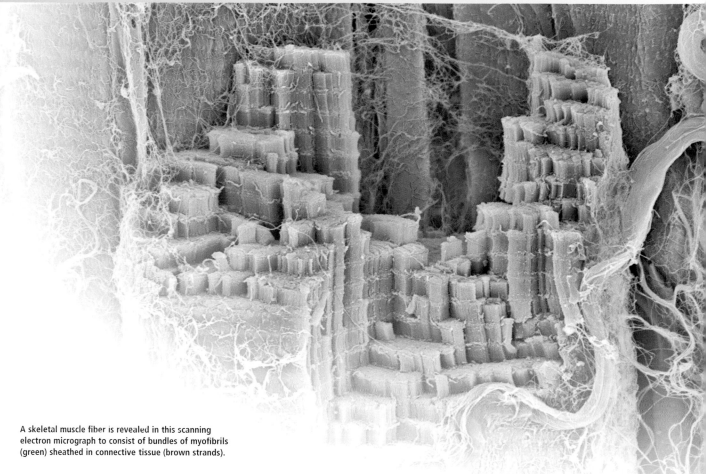

A skeletal muscle fiber is revealed in this scanning electron micrograph to consist of bundles of myofibrils (green) sheathed in connective tissue (brown strands).

Another study used electromyography to evaluate the effect that stress-inducing mental exercises had on different parts of neck and shoulder muscles. When a person was intellectually stressed and anxious, type 1 muscle fibers (which tend to shorten when stressed) became overactive. These fibers, when repeatedly activated through stressful emotions, may eventually respond with a "metabolic crisis" that produces trigger points (*see p.55*).

Emotion and psychological well-being, therefore, are key factors that influence how the musculoskeletal system behaves. At the same time, the state and functionality of the musculoskeletal system has an impact on how we experience ourselves and express our emotions.

Diagnosis, Treatments, and Therapies

Many conventional and unconventional methods can be used to assess the status of the musculoskeletal system. Some are high-tech, but most use observation and fingertip examination (palpation), requiring considerable knowledge and skill. In most instances, when you visit a bodywork practitioner (whether a physical therapist, osteopath, chiropractor, or other) a full case history will be taken,

even if the problem appears localized. This is because many apparently clear-cut conditions, such as a painful shoulder, can sometimes have serious underlying causes — digestive or cardiovascular disease, for example — that could easily be missed if the practitioner or therapist simply started treating the affected area. Questionnaires may help identify particular features of the condition — for example, the type, nature, and degree of pain.

X-rays and scans, such as MRI, may be used to search inside the area for evidence of pathology or tissue change. Chiropractors regularly take X-rays to assess the position and relationship of bones and joints. Osteopaths tend to use X-rays more rarely, and usually only to confirm, or rule out, the presence of disease processes, such as arthritis.

Practitioner tests and assessments

To make sense of how a body is adapting to the stresses of life, a therapist may turn to one of several frameworks of evaluation or grids of (relative) normality. An osteopath, physical therapist, chiropractor, or other bodywork practitioner might do one or all of the following:

- Observe your posture, looking for imbalances, asymmetries, and "crossed patterns."
- Assess your gait. What happens to your body (from the feet to the head) as you walk? An increasing number

of practitioners use computerized imaging to record a patient's posture and gait to compare images before and after treatment.

- Evaluate your respiratory function. Is your breathing unbalanced and, if so, in what ways? Sometimes questionnaires and other tests are used, but evaluating how a person breathes is normally tested through observation and palpation.
- Assess your muscles for strength or weakness — looking particularly at type 2 muscles.
- Test for relative shortness of skeletal muscles — looking particularly at the postural, type 1 muscles.
- Assess the "firing pattern" of skeletal muscles — checking to see whether the "right" muscles perform a normal, functional movement in the correct sequence, or whether some muscles have come to dominate others.
- Test the range of motion of your soft tissues and joints. Are your normal movements free from pain? Patients may be asked to perform a particular movement, or the practitioner may move the patient's tissues and joints to test for range of motion.
- Test for abnormal nerve function by looking for the presence, absence, or overactivity of neurological reflexes.
- Look for trigger points and sensitization in your spine (spinal hyperreactivity). Are trigger points feeding into the patient's symptom picture?
- Assess influences on your nutrition and lifestyle.
- Evaluate psychosocial factors.

Aims of manual techniques

The objectives of all forms of manual treatment are similar. First, to eliminate or ease pain, restriction, and patterns of dysfunction. Second, to restore flexibility, stability, strength, balance, and postural and functional integrity.

Most "conventional" bodywork therapists, for example physical therapists, rely on the same assessment methods employed in conventional medical settings. However, some complementary bodywork professions have other ways of examining the patient. Osteopaths, for example, use evidence of neurolymphatic reflexes or cranial palpation. Some chiropractors use methods known as applied kinesiology for testing the resistance of muscles. In general, however, one manual approach is usually distinguished from another by the way the practitioner interprets the examination and determines treatment.

Osteopaths tend to focus on restoring the harmonious integrated function of the whole body, with particular emphasis on the circulation. Chiropractors have a particular interest in the nervous system and in releasing what they term "subluxations," which they believe interfere with nerve function. Subluxations are essentially the same thing as the restricted joints, treated (often differently) by osteopaths and physical therapists.

Self-help during treatment

When you have a treatment, bear in mind that it will make adaptive demands on you. Afterward you may experience a "reaction" (something "feels different"), and for a day or so your muscles may ache. This is normal and to be expected and is not a cause for alarm. The condition may also temporarily get worse. Improvements may fluctuate, with minor setbacks along the way.

Normal life entails coping with a number of stressors at any one time. If you have a musculoskeletal condition, you are more likely to make progress when some of this "load" is reduced. Therefore, any self-help measures you can take, such as improving posture and breathing patterns, will speed your recovery. Remember that your body always tries to heal itself, so that removing some of the obstacles to recovery is crucial to restoring good health.

Reeducation
Recovery from long-term musculoskeletal pain and dysfunction often requires some self-education as part of the rehabilitation process. The key issues are:
- To become informed about your condition.
- To move from a passive to an active role.
- To develop effective ways of responding to your pain and the emotions associated with the pain. A key phrase to learn early on is "hurt does not necessarily mean harm."
- To develop a positive attitude toward exercise and personal health management.
- To develop a program of structured activity to reduce the effects of physical deconditioning.

Bodywork Therapies

The following is a summary of the many manipulation therapies and bodywork practices that are recommended throughout this book. Always check that the practitioner is fully trained, qualified, and registered, and inform him or her fully about your health problem and any medications you are taking before treatment starts.

If you are having treatment with one type of therapy (e.g. osteopathy), consult your therapist before embarking on treatment with another. That said, some therapies combine very well, for example the Alexander technique, Pilates, and osteopathy for back pain.

Acupressure
Part of Traditional Chinese Medicine (*see p.78*), the practice of acupressure can be summed up as acupuncture without needles. Acupressure techniques are also used in shiatsu, which is practiced in Japan. Acupressure practitioners use finger and thumb pressure on specific acupoints along meridians to stimulate the flow of *Qi* energy in order to restore harmony and health.

TREATMENT METHODS

Treatment methods vary from profession to profession (although far less than in earlier times). They include:

TREATMENT NAME	PRACTITIONER	DESCRIPTION
High-velocity, low amplitude, thrust (HVLAT)	Chiropractors Osteopaths Physical therapists	HVLAT is the main manipulation technique that chiropractors, many osteopaths, and some physical therapists use. It is a rapid "adjustment" of a joint, often accompanied by an audible "crack" or "pop" as the joint surfaces separate. It produces a nerve reflex response that relaxes all attaching muscles, usually making movement much easier afterward. Performed well, HVLAT is painless and safe. It should be used with great caution on patients with circulatory problems in the neck or on anyone with weak bones or rheumatoid disease.
Mobilization of restricted joints	Osteopaths Physical therapists Some massage therapists	Also known as articulation, this method uses rhythmic movement and stretching to relax tense soft tissue. It is used widely by osteopaths, some physical therapists, and, increasingly, by massage therapists with appropriate training.
Muscle energy techniques (MET)	Osteopaths Physical therapists Massage therapists Self-treatment	MET uses contractions against light resistance to induce relaxation in muscles so that they can then be safely stretched. They were originally osteopathic techniques, but are now also used by massage therapists and physical therapists, and can also be used on yourself at home.
Proprioceptive neuromuscular facilitation (PNF)	Physical therapists	PNF is similar to MET, but uses far greater degrees of force and effort. It improves flexibility, induces muscle relaxation, and increases range of movement in the joints. PNF is now a feature of sports therapy.
Positional release techniques (PRT)	Osteopaths Physical therapists Massage therapists Chiropractors	PRT are very gentle osteopathic manipulations, ideal for use in acute conditions and after recent injury or surgery
Myofascial release (MFR)	All manual therapists	MFR is a very slow form of manually stretching muscles and connective tissue (fascia). It helps injuries heal and increases the range of movement of joints.
Neuromuscular technique (NMT)	All manual therapists	NMT involves a combination of soft-tissue approaches that focus on normalizing trigger point activity and the reasons for the development of trigger points. It involves finger and thumb strokes or pressure. NMT has its origins in Ayurvedic (traditional Indian) massage, modified to meet 20th-century British requirements, and in American chiropractic research of the 1940s.
Direct manual pressure	All manual therapists	Direct manual pressure is also known as ischemic compression, trigger point pressure release, inhibition technique, and acupressure.
Massage methods	All manual therapists	Massage strokes such as cross-fiber friction, specific soft-tissue mobilization, and other techniques.
Moderate aerobic exercises	All manual therapists	Moderate aerobic exercises are used in a fairly standard way by all the bodywork professions. Practitioners give patients a program of appropriate aerobic, stretching, toning, breathing, balance, and other exercises.

BREATHING RETRAINING

The process of rehabilitating yourself from a lifetime of habitual breathing pattern disorders (BPDs) can take up to six months. Many research studies show the effectiveness of breathing retraining (rehabilitation) in treating this widespread, often undiagnosed problem. Breathing retraining involves relearning the mechanics of breathing (with particular emphasis on full exhalation). It also involves the release of tense muscles and joints by judicious bodywork and mobilization of the machinery of breathing.

Practice the following breathing exercise every day and whenever you feel stressed or anxious.

BREATHING EXERCISE

- Sit comfortably in a chair that has arms. Rest your arms on the arms of the chair. Relax.
- Press down on the arms with your elbows. This prevents you from using the neck and shoulder muscles while you are doing the breathing exercise.
- After a normal inhalation purse your lips (as if in an exaggerated kiss) and exhale through your mouth, counting slowly until you sense a need to breathe in.
- Close the lips, pause for a count of "one," and inhale through your nose while counting slowly.
- By exhaling fully, your inhalation will be deeper without trying.
- Your exhalation should always take longer than the inhalation.
- Repeat this sequence 20 times, morning and evening.

Alexander technique

Teachers of the Alexander technique try to show people how to avoid patterns of misusing their bodies and to relearn everyday postures, such as sitting and standing. By concentrating on moving in a balanced and fluid way, people can improve their posture, achieve a better use of their bodies, and relieve the stresses and strains that contribute to illness. The technique is usually taught on a one-to-one basis and the teacher starts by showing how to stand and sit with optimum body posture. Later, all kinds of movements are examined, to help people conduct the activities of their everyday life with minimum strain.

Chiropractic

Chiropractors use precise hand movements to manipulate the vertebrae of the spine. The therapy is particularly effective in treating low back pain and relieving muscle tension caused by stress. In correcting the alignment of the spine with the head and pelvis, chiropractors help the nervous system work normally. Treatment may involve standing, or sitting or lying on a chiropractic couch while the practitioner uses her hands to locate the source of the pain and then make the necessary adjustments.

Cranial techniques

These very gentle massage techniques focus on normalizing the tissues of the cranium (skull) and their fascial linkage with spinal and pelvic structures. Cranial osteopathy claims to balance the pressure on the bones of the cranium, correcting disturbances in the flow of cerebrospinal fluid, boosting the circulation of blood, and draining excess lymph and fluids from the head.

Craniosacral therapy is similar to cranial osteopathy, except that the focus of treatment is on the membranes surrounding the brain and spinal cord — from the cranium to the sacrum. The sacrooccipital technique is preferred by chiropractors and is a blend of cranial osteopathy and craniosacral methods.

Feldenkrais

Feldenkrais teachers employ exercises specially devised by Moshe Feldenkrais in the 1940s to reeducate people to use their bodies more efficiently. Although the outcomes are similar to the Alexander technique, the methods and exercises employed are different.

Hydrotherapy

This is an umbrella term for various spa and water therapies. Physical therapists often use a heated swimming pool where the water supports the patient's body, enabling exercise without weight-bearing. The resistance of the water can help in a strengthening program for muscle and joint rehabilitation.

Hydrotherapy can also be used as a home treatment to treat pain and inflammation. Hot packs may help treat muscle injuries and joint stiffness — they stimulate blood flow and relax muscles. Ice or cold packs help reduce swelling and relieve pain. Balneotherapy is a traditional spa therapy in which bathing improves well-being and helps heal disorders of the skin, muscles, and joints.

Lymphatic pumping and drainage

Practitioners of manual lymphatic drainage use gentle rhythmic massage to stimulate the lymphatic system to remove toxins from the body.

Massage

Massage involves kneading muscles and stroking the body with long, sweeping movements. Its main aim is to stimulate blood flow, which relieves inflammation and improves the circulation, and to encourage relaxation. There are many forms of massage, including Swedish, Thai, sports massage, shiatsu, tuina (see next page), and Indian head massage. Massage is widely available at health and sports clubs and your doctor or bodywork specialist may be able to recommend an experienced therapist. Check that a therapist has attended an accredited college (see p.486) and has completed suitable training in anatomy and physiology.

Occupational therapy

People who struggle with the tasks of everyday living because of a long-term disorder, such as arthritis or multiple sclerosis, or because they are recovering from a serious injury or a stroke, can be helped by an occupational therapist. The main aim is to help people become as independent as possible, either through the use of aids, such as a walking frame, or through practical activities that improve dexterity and coordination.

Occupational therapists take a three-year course and work in hospitals or community care alongside other health professionals. A doctor can refer you to a therapist.

Osteopathy

Osteopaths use manipulation, massage, and touch to balance tensions and remove stiffness throughout the musculoskeletal system so that the body's internal organs, circulation, digestion, and lymphatic system can function properly. Osteopathy improves mobility and is particularly good for relieving pain in the joints and soft tissues. Treatment will involve the osteopath examining the spine and alignment of structures such as the pelvis before making various adjustments.

Physical therapy

Physical therapists generally use physical techniques, such as massage, hydrotherapy, and exercise, to restore a person's muscle strength and flexibility, or to help rehabilitate their physical mobility after illness, injury, or surgery. People with arthritis can also benefit from physical therapy to help them maintain normal use of their body. Physical therapy, which can also be used to relieve pain, is often combined with drugs and occupational therapy.

Qualified physical therapists complete a three-year training. Some work alongside other medical staff in hospitals, but many work independently, outside hospitals. A doctor can refer you for physical therapy.

Pilates

Practitioners teach a sequence of "thinking and breathing" exercises that focus on improving core stability and toning the abdominal muscles in order to develop a strong and flexible body. You can learn Pilates with apparatus or without, in which case you practice the sequences on a mat. Pilates is very useful for relieving chronic back problems. Make sure the teacher you choose has completed a full course and is fully accredited.

Reflexology

Reflexologists view the feet and hands as mirrors of the whole body and believe pressure placed on specific points can stimulate the body's natural healing powers. With finger and thumb pressure, they massage particular reflex points (usually on the feet) in order to treat the corresponding areas of the body.

Rolfing

This deep-tissue manipulation loosens the connective tissue (fascia) enveloping the muscles. It releases the physical (and sometimes the emotional) stresses that cause the fascia to harden and lose elasticity, the muscles to become restricted, and breathing to be impaired.

T'ai chi

T'ai chi is an ancient Chinese practice that aims to achieve inner strength. It involves meditative sequences of slow, flowing movements (see also p.79) and is excellent for relieving stress and improving breathing.

Tuina

Tuina is a traditional Chinese massage technique that manipulates soft tissues and joints. The name, meaning "push and grasp," describes the stimulation of acupoints in order to improve energy flow around the body.

Ultrasound

Beams of high-frequency sound waves generate heat in damaged soft tissues (muscles, tendons, and ligaments) in order to combat pain and reduce inflammation.

Yoga

This ancient Indian practice has been practiced for thousands of years in India as part of Ayurveda. It combines physical postures and breathing to train the mind and body. All forms of yoga, such as hatha and astanga, can help relieve mental stress while increasing suppleness and fitness. Yoga therapists teach specific poses to treat medical complaints.

FINDING A PRACTITIONER

Practitioners of the bodywork and movement therapies listed on these pages can be found by contacting the relevant organizations, associations, unions, and professional bodies (see p.486). Your doctor may be able to put you in contact with a practitioner.

Some therapies, such as physical therapy and osteopathy, are more established than others, such as Pilates and reflexology; therefore their courses and training methods are potentially more rigorous. Before making an appointment, always make sure the practitioner is fully qualified and registered as a member with the appropriate organization.

Safety and reliability are paramount. You must be able to trust the capability of the practitioner or therapist you have chosen because, after all, you are literally placing your body and mind in their hands. If, after an appointment, you do not feel comfortable then do not hesitate to find another practitioner who suits you. This is as true for teachers of yoga, t'ai chi, the Alexander technique, and Pilates teachers as it is for massage therapists osteopaths, chiropractors, and physical therapists.

WESTERN HERBAL MEDICINE

MICHAEL MCINTYRE

The use of herbs to treat illness is as ancient as history itself and is common to all peoples of the world. In fact, in all but the last 60 years or so, humans have relied almost exclusively on plants to treat illnesses ranging from colds to malaria. The human body is geared to digesting and absorbing plant-based foods and therefore may be better suited to treatment with herbal remedies rather than with isolated chemical medicines. While conventional medicines are designed to target and reverse specific disease processes in the minimum amount of time, plant medicines provide remedies that encourage the body's capacity to regulate and heal itself by restoring disturbed physiological processes.

Herbal Medicine in History

An estimated 70,000 plants throughout the world have a medicinal use and about 500 or so are used on a regular basis in Western herbal medicine. In the distant past, sensitivity to the properties of herbs must have been vital to human survival, and using plants as medicine may be a development of instinctive herb-seeking that is found in many animals. Researchers studying chimpanzees in Gombe (Tanzania's National Park) observed that animals with fatigue and diarrhea, which are common signs of parasitic infections, searched out and ate the leaves of two plants: *Aspilia mossambicensis* and *Vernonia amygdalina*. These plants are bitter and unpleasant to eat, but they have antiparasitic, purging, and antibiotic actions that the chimpanzees seem to recognize and want to use. The same herbal medicines have been used in Tanzanian folk medicine for hundreds of years and Tanzanian farmers also use the leaves of *Vernonia* to treat parasites and other ailments both in themselves and in their lifestock. Scientists are now studying these plants as potential as sources of new medicines.

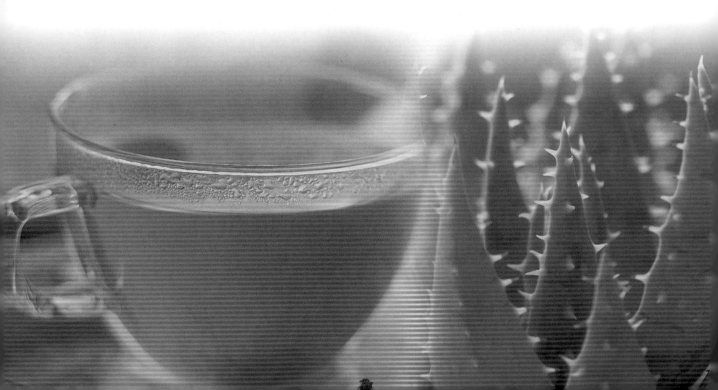

Herbs in ancient cultures

Ancient peoples valued herbal remedies and recorded their medicinal uses. For example, a manuscript dating from the 2nd century BC that listed some 224 herbal medicines was discovered in a tomb at Ma Huang Dui in Hunan Province, China, and the Egyptian Ebers Papyrus, which dates back to 1500 BC, describes more than 700 herbs, including aloes, caraway seeds, castor oil, and the hyacinth-like squill. Those who didn't have a written language passed the information orally, from one generation to the next.

The domestication of the camel, around 1200 BC, stimulated the growth of the herb trade between Egypt and Greece and eventually with Rome. Gums, resins, and spices, such as turpentine, myrrh, frankincense, and cinnamon, came through Arabia along well-established incense routes and were purchased by Mediterranean merchants. They were sold on to satisfy the increasing demands of European markets. The Greek island of Chios was the source of a prized resin called mastic, used as a chewing gum (giving the word "masticate"). Recent research shows that mastic chewing gum is a useful antiplaque agent that reduces the bacterial growth in saliva and plaque formation on teeth.

Dioscorides, a Greek doctor attached to the Roman armies of Claudius and Nero, compiled ancient and contemporary herbal knowledge in his famous herbal *De Materia Medica*, which contained descriptions of about 600 herbs and remained one of the principal medical textbooks for more than 13 centuries. The Greek herbal achieved its final form in the work of Claudius Galen, physician to the Roman Emperor Marcus Aurelius.

In the Middle Ages, much of this knowledge was brought back to Europe by Crusader doctors, who learned new skills from their Arab adversaries. The Arab doctors were expert pharmacists who had preserved and synthesized the knowledge of the ancient Greeks and Persians.

Decline and resurgence of herbs

For centuries, plant remedies were the main medicines throughout Europe, and famous herbals were published in English in the 16th and 17th centuries. Some, such as those of Culpeper and Gerard, are still well known today. However, with the dawn of the scientific age came the slow decline of herbal medicine. This decline accelerated in the 18th century as a result of the widespread introduction into medicine of mineral- and metal-based remedies such as arsenic, lead, antimony, mercury, copper, tin, and gold. In the 20th century, with the discovery of antibiotics and other major drugs that brought serious infectious diseases under control, the vast majority of herbal remedies were relegated to being mere footnotes in official pharmacopoeias.

New role for plant medicines

Recent years have seen a resurgence of interest in herbal medicine. The days when it was believed that science could deliver "a pill for every ill," and that it was just a matter of time before cures could be found for common conditions such as arthritis, migraine, coronary artery disease, and cancer, have gone. Lately, we have a more realistic under-standing of the importance of maintaining health and the prevention of disease. In many people, the realization is dawning that diet and natural plant medicines have a vital role to play in boosting the body's powers to cope with even the most serious conditions.

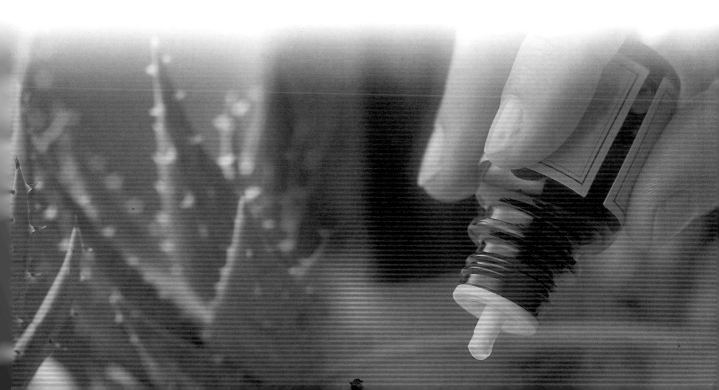

MEDICINALLY ACTIVE PLANT CHEMICALS

Plants do not have an immune system like ours to protect them from attack. Instead, they use chemicals to fight bacteria, fungi, and insects. Since these chemicals are biologically active, some also have medicinal properties.

PLANT	ACTIVE COMPOUNDS	PLANT USE	MEDICINAL USES
Garlic Allium sativum	Allyl sulfides	Antimicrobials prevent the bulb from rotting in wet soil	Antibacterial and antiviral
Ginseng Panax ginseng	Ginsenosides (triterpene saponins)	Protection against fungal diseases	Stimulates the immune system
Oak Quercus robur	Tannins	The tannins coagulate protein, so they are an effective insect deterrent	The coagulating properties of bark tannins can be used for diarrhea
Echinacea Echinacea purpurea, pallida, augustiflora	Complex mix of alkylamides, caffeic acid derivatives, palyalkynes, and polysaccharides	Antifungal compounds are a defense against fungal disease	Stimulates the immune system. Used for upper respiratory tract infections
St. John's wort Hypericum perforatum	Hypericin and pseudohypericin (naphthodianthrones)	Defense against insects that try to eat the plant	Blocks neurotransmitter reuptake. Used to treat depression
Peppermint Mentha x piperita	Monoterpene oils	Deter or prevent insect or slug attack	Provides antispasmodic action. Used for indigestion

How Herbs Work

Since the 18th century, scientists have been isolating the active constituents in plants, leading to some of the world's most powerful drugs. Not only have some of the more long-standing drugs such as digoxin, opiates, and aspirin been developed from plants, but many of the newer high-tech drugs such as the cancer drugs vincristine and toxol, and other cytotoxics (chemicals that kill cells) are also derived from plants. Some compounds have not been extracted from plants because it is not yet possible to synthesize all of them.

Herbal medicines differ from plant-derived drugs in that they consist of many chemical components. The mixture works in concert, making active constituents more easily available to the body, or buffering otherwise harmful ingredients. As a result, the total therapeutic effect of the whole plant is more than the sum of its chemical parts, since the active constituents' effects will be modified by other substances. Furthermore, the complex arrays of chemicals in even the simplest plant medicines can trigger a cascade of biochemical processes in the human body. Herbal medicines do not work in the linear cause and effect of a single chemical (drug) acting on a single receptor system — the mechanism pharmacologists know

best. Understanding plant medicines involves conceps of "complexity" and "chaos," more familiar to physicists than to biochemists, pharmacologists, or physicians.

The consequences of using the whole plant rather than an isolated component are easily illustrated by clinical studies of garlic (*Allium sativum*). Recent research has shown that because garlic can lower blood pressure and cholesterol, it may be useful to people with coronary artery disease. Yet despite their best efforts, researchers have so far failed to identify which of garlic's many chemical constituents are responsible for these medicinal virtues. Although formerly attributed to allicin, a compound found in garlic oil, it has recently become clear that the cholesterol-lowering effect of garlic results from a concerted action of several chemicals, not all of which are in the oil itself.

Research into St. John's wort (*Hypericum perforatum*) illustrates the same point. Trials have demonstrated that this ancient remedy is very effective for treating a wide range of depressive disorders, including seasonal affective disorder (SAD; *see p.432*). As effective as modern antidepressant drugs in treating mild to moderate depression, it provokes virtually none of their side effects. Researchers, however, cannot yet assign antidepressant effects to specific chemical components. Another group of chemicals with medicinal potential that is not yet well understood are flavonoids.

These compounds, which give many flowers, fruits, and vegetables their color, display a broad range of medicinal activity: improving capillary fragility and circulation, protecting the liver, and preventing heart attacks and strokes. Some are antioxidant or anti-inflammatory and antiviral; others have anticancer properties.

The recent, extensive research into plant pharmacology challenges drug-based medicine. The realization that a wide variety of herbs and other plants have many apparently minor chemical constituents with significant medicinal properties has come as a revelation.

Consulting an Herbalist

In the US, several types of health-care providers can prescribe herbal medicines. Clinical herbalists, who are trained at herbal medicine schools, are unlicensed in most states, although the American Herbalists Guild is developing a program to license herbal medicine experts. Naturopathic physicians (NDs) receive extensive botanical medicine training and clinical experience. Conventional practitioners, such as physicians (MDs), nurse practitioners (ARNPs), and physician assistants (PAs), can learn about herbal medicine from herbal medicine schools, seminars, continuing education classes, and other training. These practitioners may utilize a variety of approaches in their history-taking and/or physical examination to determine the herb(s) that would be most appropriate for you.

The herbal prescription is not a simple matter of using herbs instead of drugs to treat a particular condition. Drugs are standardized and purified single compounds, while many herbal treatments are not standardized and may contain dozens of phytochemicals that interact to produce an effect. Each prescription is unique to the patient, matching the needs of that person, supporting ailing systems or reducing overactivity when it is apparent.

Herbs are not usually given singly, but are combined for extra effect to suit the individual. St. John's wort, for example, although marketed as a remedy to treat mild to moderate depression, is commonly combined with other herbs. When St. John's wort is combined with lemon balm (*Melissa officinalis*), it is used to treat anxiety and depression; with wild oat (*Avena fatua*) and/or ginseng (*Panax ginseng*), it is given for exhaustion; with valerian (*Valeriana officinalis*), it is a treatment for bipolar disorder.

Many herbs are used to treat a variety of symptoms and conditions. For example, lemon balm can be used for anxiety and insomnia, but it is also used for calming a nervous stomach and bowel. Recently it has been found to have a significant antiviral effect and may also help in the treatment of hyperthyroidism. Herbal remedies can support and stimulate the body's healing response. The herbalist and the patient are partners in this goal, working together toward the common goal of restoring health.

Safety and Efficacy

It is clear that "natural" does not always equal "safe," and that herbal medicines, like conventional medicines, can cause adverse effects. Such adverse events may also be due to contaminants present in herbs, such as heavy metals or aflatoxins (as with peanuts), or even because of misidentification of a herb. There is a possibility of herb–drug interactions too (*see below*). Therefore herbal practitioners must be very well trained and know exactly what other medicines their patients are taking.

How safe are herbs?

Safety concerns should be put in context. Currently, an estimated 50 percent of all Americans use herbal supplements. In 1985, The World Health Organization estimated that 80 percent of the world's population used traditional therapies, which commonly employ herbs, to meet their primary health-care needs.

The incidence of herbal adverse effects is low. Until recently, studies of herbal medicine have occured far more frequently in Europe than in the US. One UK study found only 38 adverse reactions in a study of herbal supplements involving 1,297 participants. The National Institutes of Health began funding for supplement research in 1993 and has steadily increased funding since. However, the methodology for testing herbal remedies has yet to be firmly established and results are often inconclusive. In both the US and abroad, there have been a number of concerns regarding the safety of herbal medicines in the past two decades. For example, in the US, Europe, China, and Japan, the use of toxic *Aristolochia* species instead of safer herbs in some traditional Chinese medicines resulted in cases of serious kidney poisoning and cancer.

VOLATILE OILS

Volatile oils such as menthol and thymol have a pungent aromatic aroma and a range of actions because they penetrate easily through the body's tissues. Their molecules can even affect the brain directly through the nose. Herbalists have long known that the aroma of crushed mint (*Mentha*) or rosemary (*Rosmarinus officinalis*) can increase alertness and improve concentration. Internally, these oils are carminative, relaxing an overcontracted intestinal tract. They also stimulate the heart and lungs, improving circulation and deepening breathing. These oils are excreted through the lungs, kidneys, and skin, so they act as expectorants and mild diuretics, causing therapeutic sweating. The traditional germicidal properties of many volatile oils, such as from thyme (*Thymus*), tea tree (*Melaleuca alternifolia*), and garlic (*Allium sativum*), are effective to a surprising degree. Garlic has recently been shown to combat the common cold and the hospital superbug MRSA.

CONVENTIONAL MEDICINES DERIVED FROM PLANTS

In addition to being used in their own right as herbal medicines, plants are also the source of many of our conventional medicines.

Pharmaceutical companies screen plants from all over the world for chemicals that may be medicinal.

COMPOUND	CONDITION	ORIGINAL SOURCE	HISTORY
Vinblastine and vincristine	Cancers, including childhood leukemia	Madagascar periwinkle (*Catharanthus roseus*)	In Madagascar many traditional remedies are made from the plant. This alerted Western scientists to its potential.
Quinine	Malaria	Chinchona tree (*Cinchona officinalis* and others)	Quinine was extracted from cinchona bark. Now chemists can synthesize the drug.
Taxol	Cancers, especially breast cancer	Pacific yew (*Taxus brevifolia*) and common yew (*Taxus baccata*)	The bark from one Pacific yew tree only supplied enough Taxol for one treatment. Now the drug is made from a chemical extracted from clippings from common yew.
Aspirin	Pain and inflammation	Willow bark (*Salix*) and Meadowsweet (*Filipendula ulmaria*)	Willow stems were used to treat pain and fever. The chemical salicylic acid is now manufactured as acetyl salicylic acid (aspirin).
Cocaine and procaine	Local anesthetic	Coca plant (*Erythroxylum coca*)	Leaves are used by South American Indians as a stimulant and for altitude sickness. Sigmund Freud found that a small amount of the extracted drug (cocaine) placed on the tongue caused numbness. Synthetic cocainelike substances including procaine (Novocaine) are now used in medicine and dentistry.

Professor Ernst, Chair of Complementary Medicine at the University of Exeter, has recently downplayed the threat of adverse effects from herbal medicines. In an editorial in the *British Medical Journal* he comments that "Even though herbal medicines are not devoid of risk, they could still be safer than synthetic drugs. Between 1968 and 1997, the World Health Organization's monitoring center collected 8,985 reports of adverse events associated with herbal medicines from 55 countries. Although this number may seem impressively high, it amounts to only a tiny fraction of adverse events associated with conventional drugs held in the same database.... At present, the relative safety of herbal medicines is undefinable, but many of the existing data indicate that adverse events, particularly serious ones, occur less often than with prescription drugs." To put herbal medicine use in context of pharmaceutical use, approximately 100,000 people die each year in the US from the correct use of pharmaceuticals.

Only a tiny fraction of herbal medicines has been fully researched. In some cases, this has led to physicians doubting their efficacy. However, in the same editorial,

Professor Ernst sought to dispel this doubt, writing, "The efficacy of herbal medicines has been tested in hundreds of clinical trials, and it is wrong to say that they are all of inferior methodological quality. But this volume of data is still small considering the multitude of herbal medicines — worldwide, several thousand different plants are being used for medicinal purposes."

Relatively few rigorous clinical trials have been conducted on herbal therapies primarily because, compared to the pharmaceutical sector, the herbal industry can rarely afford the considerable expense of a clinical trial. Not being able to patent plant medicines and recoup the costs as drug companies are able to do puts the herbal industry at a very real disadvantage. However, many of the clinical trials that have been conducted have shown that herbal medicines do work. In a recent overview of 23 systematic reviews (which are comparative and critical analyses of many research studies) of rigorous trials of herbal medicines, 11 came to a positive conclusion, nine yielded promising but not convincing results, and only three were actually negative.

Regulation of herbal medicines

In most developed countries, herbal medicines are being subjected to increasing regulation. Most major professional herbal associations are now reporting any side effects so that this information can be shared among professionals. Herbal organizations in the US, such as the American Herbal Pharmacopoeia (AHP), the American Herbal Products Association (AHPA), and the American Herbalists Guild (AHG), collect practical herbal information from their professional members, and anyone is free to examine this information at any of their Web sites (*see p.486*). In addition, the AHP and the AHPA have adopted a Code of Ethics that sets labeling and manufacturing guidelines, and is a voluntary attempt of US herbalists to self-regulate the industry. Most regulation of herbal supplements in the US is dictated by the 1994 Dietary Supplement Health and Education Act. Regulated by the Food and Drug Administration, this act specifies that supplements, including herbal medicines, entering the market after 1994 are not treated as drugs: dietary supplements must be "reasonably expected to be safe" and labeling is restricted to statements of nutritional support or "support/function statements" rather than claims about prevention, treatment, or cure.

Using herbs safely

Herbal remedies, like all medicines, must be treated with respect. There are certain conditions and combinations of treatments in which herbs may cause problems.

General cautions
During the first three months of pregnancy, avoid all medicines, herbal or otherwise, unless absolutely essential.
- Certain herbs should be avoided throughout pregnancy, so consult a qualified herbal medicine practitioner.
- Women who are breast-feeding should consult an herbal medicine practitioner before using herbal medicines.
- Do not give babies under 6 months any internal herbal (or other) medicine without professional advice.
- The elderly, because of their slower metabolism, may require less than the full adult dose.
- Do not stop taking prescribed conventional medication without first consulting your doctor.
- Some herbs interact with drugs. If you are taking a prescribed medicine, consult an herbal medical practitioner.

Herb–drug interactions
Herbs can change the way that your body absorbs and breaks down (metabolizes) drugs. They can also affect other aspects of your metabolism, e.g. heart rate and blood pressure, which can either mask or exacerbate symptoms. If herbs and drugs have similar actions, the combined effect can be too strong. This list of cautions is a guide to some of the potential drug interactions and situations when herbs should be used with care. Consult a medical herbalist about herb–drug interactions and contraindications.

Coltsfoot (*Tussilago farfara*) in large doses may interfere with blood pressure treatment. Also, avoid long-term use.

Garlic (*Allium sativum*) in medicinal doses can cause a dangerous decrease in blood-sugar levels if it is taken with diabetes medication. Although it may have an effect on anticoagulation, it may be taken with the blood-thinning drug warfarin, aspirin, or other anticlotting medication. (Culinary amounts of garlic are safe.)

Ginkgo (*Ginkgo biloba*) may have an effect on anticoagulation, but it may be taken with the blood-thinner warfarin, aspirin, or other anticlotting medication.

Ginseng, Siberian (*Eleutherococcus senticosus*) and American Ginseng (*Panax quinquefolius*) may, in rare cases, increase blood pressure.

Hawthorn (*Crataegus* spp.) may interact with other medicines, especially those prescribed for heart conditions.

Hops (*Humulus lupulus*) have a mild sedative effect and act as a depressive. Do not take if you have depression, or breast cancer or other estrogen-responsive cancers. Do not take with alcohol.

Lily of the valley (*Convallaria majalis*) contains cardiac glycosides and may interact with other heart drugs and should be prescribed by a qualified medical herbalist.

Licorice (*Glycyrrhiza glabra*) should not be taken by anyone who is anemic or has high blood pressure, nor should it be taken for long periods of time because it can cause abnormalities in potassium.

Schisandra (*Schisandra chinensis*) should possibly be avoided by those with epilepsy or hypertension.

St. John's wort (*Hypericum perforatum*) increases the rate at which the liver breaks down drugs, so that a drug taken alongside it may not be effective. Indinavir and other drugs used for HIV infection, warfarin, cyclosporin, digoxin, some antidepressants, theophylline, and possibly oral contraceptives may all be affected. St. John's wort may also cause sensitivity to sunlight, although this is unusual within normal dosage range.

WHEN TO CONSULT A PRACTITIONER

The American Herbalists Guild (*see p.486*) keep a register of trained medical herbalists who have specific continuing education requirements and follow a professional code of ethics. Your doctor may also be able to make a recommendation. You should consult a medical herbalist before taking herbal medicines if you are pregnant or have a serious condition such as diabetes, heart disease, or hypertension. Do not stop taking prescribed medication without first consulting your doctor. Some herbs and drugs interact — see the herb–drug interactions (opposite) before taking a herbal medicine.

HOMEOPATHY

DR PETER FISHER

Homeopathy is a complementary medicine based on the idea that treating "like with like" (often quoted in Latin, *Similia similibus curentur*) will stimulate and direct the body's self-healing abilities. It can be used to treat a wide range of clinical problems, but it is particularly useful if the disease is "internal" — due to a functional imbalance rather than to a deficiency, infection, or injury. For example, it is very effective for eczema and anxiety. Homeopathy can be used on its own but it also can be combined effectively with other treatments.

Key Principles

The key features of homeopathic medicine include treating "like with like," the use of the minimum dose, and the linked concepts of holism, constitution, and idiosyncrasy, which together can be summed up as "homeopathy treats people, not diseases."

For example, the homeopathic remedy *Apis mellifica* is made from crushed honey bees. In line with treating like with like, it is used to treat medical problems with similar symptoms to the effects of a bee sting, i.e. those that appear suddenly, with a severe stinging pain and swelling. These conditions are relieved by cold applications (e.g. an ice pack), but are made worse when pressure is applied — by bandaging, for instance. While not all these features need to be present for *Apis* to work, a homeopath would normally look for at least three characteristic symptoms to make a "picture" of the remedy needed. The disease's name is less important than the resemblance between the process triggered by a bee sting and the symptoms to be treated. In practice, *Apis* is often used for skin problems and arthritis.

Homeopathy is concerned with a substance's ability to cure problems similar to those it causes, not with any similarities between its appearance and its medical use. To understand the symptoms that a particular substance can cause, and what kind of person is particularly susceptible, homeopaths conduct "provings," or homeopathic pathogenetic trials. In a proving, healthy people take the substance, usually in very small doses under controlled conditions, and report any symptoms that develop.

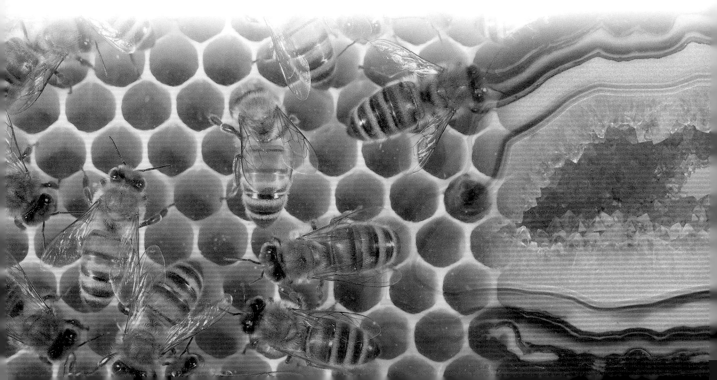

The controversial minimum dose

Although widespread and popular, homeopathy remains the most controversial form of complementary medicine because the medicines are so highly diluted. Starting from an alcoholic tincture or, in the case of insoluble substances, a "triturate," which is made by grinding the substance with lactose, medicines are made in a process of serial dilution and succussion (vigorous shaking). This process is sometimes known as potentization.

The original tincture or triturate is diluted on the decimal scale (X) with a dilution factor of 1:10 or on the centesimal scale (C) with a dilution factor of 1:100. In other words, a homeopathic medicine in the 6x potency has been diluted 1:10, six times over, giving a final concentration of one part in 1,000,000. There are also other scales of dilution, such as Korsakovian, which are prepared by slightly different methods.

Matter is composed of particles (atoms and molecules). Therefore, if you dilute a substance enough, you will eventually dilute it out altogether. Thanks to the 19th-century Italian aristocrat and scientist Count Amadeo Avogadro, we can calculate the point at which it is likely that every atom or molecule of the starting substance has been diluted out. Dilutions of homeopathic medicines above about 24X or 12C are extremely unlikely to contain a single molecule of the starting substance — such dilutions are said to be "ultramolecular."

The homeopathic medicines that are sold in most pharmacies in the US are in 6C and 30C dilutions. While the 6C dilution is likely to contain molecules of the starting substance, it is extremely unlikely that a 30C dilution does.

How does homeopathy work?

There is evidence that homeopathy does work, but if a remedy does not contain any of the original substance, how can it work? Recent scientific work has bought us closer to an answer, but the mode of action is currently unknown. Homeopaths think that the medicines contain information held by the water/alcohol mixture in which they are made (sometimes referred to as the "memory of water").

Chemically, homeopathic medicines consist of just water, alcohol, and lactose (from the pills), but there is now growing evidence that the preparation process alters the physical structure of the water and that this persists even after the solute has been completely diluted out.

This might seem bizarre, and it has even been claimed that if it were true, physics textbooks would have to be rewritten. But the evidence suggests that the change is physical, not chemical, in nature. It can be compared to a magnetic medium, such as a video tape. Chemically, these consist of vinyl and ferric oxide: one cannot determine by chemical analysis whether a video tape is blank, contains a computer virus, or records valuable data. This information is stored in physical form (the alignment of the magnetic dipoles of the ferric oxide). It is thought that water can store information in a similar way, although it is clear that the structure of liquid water is highly dynamic, not fixed like that of a magnetic medium.

Information medicine

This has given rise to the idea of "information medicine." Recently scientists at Queen's University, Belfast showed in test-tube experiments that ultramolecular dilutions of

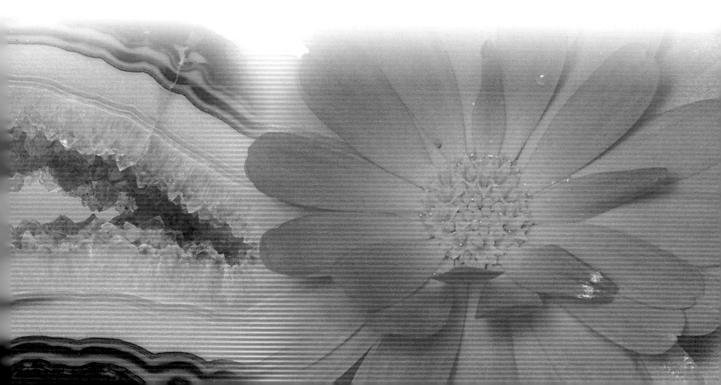

histamine, which chemically consist of pure water, reduce immune response. In addition to these laboratory experiments, there are over 200 published clinical trials of homeopathy. Overviews of these agree that homeopathic medicines are not just placebos, despite the lack of understanding of the mechanism by which they work.

The practice of using highly diluted medicines originally arose because they were safer. However, in the process, homeopaths stumbled on a different type of medical action. The process is not fully understood, but is thought to relate to the information content of homeopathic medicines. In high homeopathic dilutions, the original substance is no longer present; what remains and is transmitted to the body is information relating to it. For example, the medicine *Apis*, made from crushed bees, is thought to give a message to the body: "your problem is similar to the effects of a bee sting." Similarly, the medicine *Natrum muriaticum*, which is made from common salt (sodium chloride), transmits a message: "there is an imbalance in your sodium metabolism." The body then responds and corrects itself. This has been described as "holding a mirror up to Nature," stimulating and directing the natural healing force (sometimes referred to in Latin as "*Vis medicatrix naturae*").

Holism, constitution, and idiosyncrasy

In prescribing a medicine, homeopaths take these three principles into account. In deciding which treatment to use, a homeopath considers every aspect of a person, as well as the ailment the person has — the principle of holism. Constitution refers to the type of person as a whole (*see Constitution and constitutional prescribing, p.73*), which includes factors such as build, personality, general physical features (such as intolerance of cold and heat), and susceptibility to particular illnesses. Idiosyncrasy describes a person's unusual or atypical features or unexpected reactions to a health problem from which they suffer — homeopaths sometimes refer to the latter by the quaint phrase "rare, strange, and peculiar" symptoms.

Origins of Homeopathy

Homeopathy originates in the work of the German physician Samuel Hahnemann (1755–1843), who coined the term from the Greek word *homoios*, which means same or similar, and *pathos*, meaning disease or suffering. He became a doctor during a brutal period in medicine when treatments involved blood-letting and giving doses of medicine so large that the patient often died. Hahnemann vehemently denounced these practices, accusing his contemporaries of "killing gradually more millions than Napoleon ever slew in battle." He also condemned the chaining and beating of "lunatics," instead advocating "humanity combined with firmness."

Hahnemann grew so disillusioned that, for a while, he abandoned medical practice. The inspiration for homeopathy came as he translated a medical book by the Edinburgh physician William Cullen. He disagreed with what Cullen said about cinchona bark, the source of quinine and an effective treatment for malaria, which at that time was common in parts of Europe. Using himself as a guinea pig, he took regular doses of quinine and developed symptoms very similar to malaria, which inspired him to think of the idea of similarity. In 1796, Hahnemann launched homeopathy by publishing an article entitled "On a new curative principle."

Early homeopaths introduced many new medicines and radically changed the uses of others. Homeopathy grew rapidly through the 19th century, largely because of its success in treating epidemics, particularly of cholera. During the infamous London cholera epidemic of 1854, eventually traced to a water pump on Broad Street in Soho, the overall hospital mortality rate was 52 percent (over 500 people), but at the London Homeopathic Hospital (which was the hospital nearest the infamous pump) the death rate was only 16 percent.

In 200 years, homeopathy has become a worldwide practice. It is particularly popular in Latin America and the Indian subcontinent. In Western Europe over 50 percent of the French have used it, and usage is only slightly lower in Germany. In the UK, homeopathy is currently used by 10 percent of the population, with annual growth in sales of around 12 percent.

Homeopathy suffered a sharp decline in many parts of the world in the 20th century, but is now growing again. For example, in the US, it almost died out in the 1970s and 1980s, but sales grew by a staggering 500 percent during a seven-year period in the 1990s.

Types of Homeopathy

There are four main types of homeopathy: individualized or "classical" homeopathy, clinical homeopathy, complex homeopathy, and isopathy.

Individualized homeopathy
The practitioner builds up a "clinical picture" of the patient, often drawing on "constitutional" (*see p.73*) and psychological factors in particular (*see box, p.74*). The homeopath may also consult a "repertory" — a book or, more commonly now, a computer program, which lists symptoms. The medicine is usually given in high potency at relatively long intervals.

Clinical homeopathy
This is a more pragmatic form of prescribing. It is based on a limited number of "keynote" indications and is more often used for acute problems.

Complex homeopathy

Complex homeopathic medicines are combinations of several substances that are likely to be useful for a particular problem. They tend to target particular conditions rather than a constitutional type or symptom picture. Various brands of complexes are widely available from pharmacies for common problems such as motion sickness or insomnia.

Isopathy

Isopathy means treating the "same with the same." For instance, homeopathic dilutions of grass pollen may be prescribed for allergic rhinitis (hay fever).

Homeopathic Treatment

Although it has a wide range of uses, homeopathy should not be seen as an exclusive system of medicine. It does not necessarily provide the right treatment for every complaint or illness. For many diseases, homeopathy is best integrated with other forms of treatment, and it is important that everyone involved in the patient's care communicates with each other and works together.

Is homeopathy safe?

All homeopathic medicines are generally safe, because of the high dilutions in which they are used. A worldwide survey of adverse effects concluded that they were "minor and transient." The main risks associated with homeopathy are "indirect" — not due to the medicine itself, but to other, associated factors. For instance, factors include using homeopathic medicines to treat yourself for the symptoms of a serious disease that requires medical diagnosis. Poor advice given by inadequately trained practitioners also poses a risk.

A common indirect risk is the claim made by some practitioners that homeopathy can immunize against diseases such as pertussis or measles. There is no evidence that this is possible, and it is not recommended.

What can homeopathy treat?

Homeopathy is particularly useful when the disease is "internal" — due to an imbalance within the person rather than to an external agent, such as an infection. For instance, homeopathy is very effective for children with eczema and other allergies, and for people with anxiety, depression, sleep problems, recurrent coughs, colds and flu, arthritis, and rheumatism, and for women with PMS and menopausal problems. It can complement other treatments, too — for example, homeopathic medicines are sometimes taken alongside conventional medication to help with the side effects and symptoms of cancer.

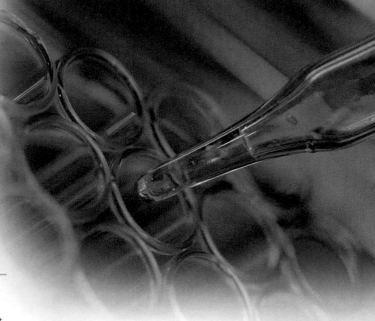

Homeopathic medicines are diluted and vigorously shaken many times in a process called succussion. As a result, the medicines are said to become more potent and more specific in the effect they have on an individual patient.

Constitution and constitutional prescribing

The constitution is the basic and essentially unalterable physical and psychological type of a person. The notion that individuals differ in their physical and psychological makeup, and that the differences predispose them to different illnesses, is found throughout medical history. The concept of constitution was known in classical Greece, where the Hippocratic doctors classified people as being of a choleric, phlegmatic, sanguine, or melancholic temperament. These were respectively dominated by one of the four traditional "humors": bile, phlegm, blood, or black bile. Similar ideas are found in the five-element theory of Traditional Chinese Medicine (*see p.78*) and in Tibetan medicine, in which practitioners believe that all aspects of a person are governed by three humors (phlegm, bile, and air).

A "constitutional medicine" is said to be the medicine that best encompasses the sum total of an individual's physical, mental, and emotional expression over an extended period of time. Constitutional prescribing is, therefore, one of the central concepts in homeopathy because, by considering a patient's constitution, the homeopath treats the person not the disease.

"Constitutional prescribing" can be contrasted with "keynote prescribing," when the prescription is based on a few characteristic symptoms of the disease (for instance, the homeopathic medicine *Magnesia phosphorica* is used for a severe pain with a cramping character, which is relieved by heat). Keynote prescribing is usually used for acute problems, while constitutional prescribing for chronic or recurrent problems.

MAJOR HOMEOPATHIC MEDICINES

A homeopathic medicine is referred to as a "constitutional medicine" when it is prescribed more for the person than the illness. It is called a "polychrest" when it can be used for different conditions providing it matches the person's constitution or the symptom picture. In practice there is a lot of overlap between the two.

This list provides details of some of the more important homeopathic medicines.

MEDICINE	MADE FROM	COMMENTS
Argentum nitricum	Silver nitrate	Most patients who respond to this medicine have marked psychological features, including anxiety with restlessness and phobias. They nearly always feel too hot. There are frequently digestive problems, particularly burping and diarrhea. *Argentum nitricum* may be indicated for headaches, vertigo, conjunctivitis, and sore throats.
Arsenicum album	Arsenious trioxide	Those who respond to this medicine tend to be anxious, tidy, and meticulous, and feel the cold greatly. They often feel weak, and may indeed be seriously ill. *Arsenicum album* may be used for many problems, including rashes, asthma, and neuralgia.
Bryonia	*Bryonia alba* (white bryony)	*Bryonia*'s keynote symptom is pain aggravated by movement. This includes headaches, chest pain due to pleurisy, and inflammation of joints and tendons. Symptoms are relieved with firm support — for instance, an elastic bandage. People who respond to it often have a dry mouth and are thirsty.
Calcarea carbonica	Calcium carbonate in oyster shells	*Calcarea carbonica* is frequently indicated for children who get recurrent coughs and colds. Adults who respond to it tend to be solid, both physically and psychologically, but this may conceal anxiety, fear of serious disease, or inability to cope. They perspire freely, especially on the head at night. *Calcarea carbonica* may help with a wide range of different illnesses when these constitutional features are present.
Causticum	A potassium compound introduced by Dr. Hahnemann	The most important mental feature of people who respond to this medicine is a strong sense of justice and sympathy. Physically, they are very sensitive to changes in the weather — for instance, they can predict when it will rain. *Causticum* may be appropriate for arthritis, hoarseness, and facial paralysis.
Graphites	Graphite (a form of carbon)	The characteristic symptom of *Graphites* people is skin eruptions, mostly in skin folds, which crack and exude when bad. The medicine can also be useful for flatulent dyspepsia, colitis, and menopausal symptoms.
Kalium bichromicum	Potassium bichromate	The most characteristic indication for this medicine is sinusitis with thick, stringy mucus. *Kalium bichromicum* is also useful for arthritis that moves from joint to joint.
Lachesis	The venom of *Lachesis mutus* (the bushmaster snake)	Some of the most characteristic features of *Lachesis* types are loquacity, aversion to tight clothes, and a tendency for the problem to be worse on the left side of the body. It is often helpful for menopausal hot flashes, migraine, and rosacea.
Lycopodium	The spores of *Lycopodium clavatum* (a kind of moss)	Individuals who respond to this medicine are often anxious and reserved. They may have stomach trouble, crave sweets, and their symptoms are often worse between 4pm and 8pm. *Lycopodium* may help headaches and many other problems.
Mercurius solubilis	An oxide of mercury	This is the most important medicine for coughs and colds if taken after the initial stage when there is a thick, greenish nasal discharge, a sore throat that makes swallowing difficult, a sore tongue with too much saliva, and sweating.

MAJOR HOMEOPATHIC MEDICINES CONTINUED

MEDICINE	MADE FROM	COMMENTS
Natrum muriaticum	Sodium chloride (common salt)	It may seem odd to make a medicine from salt, but this is one of the most commonly indicated of all homeopathic medicines. Masked depression, where depressed feelings are not expressed, is a characteristic feature of people it helps. They cope and care for everybody else, without revealing how they feel themselves. Other symptoms include cold sores and migraine.
Nux vomica	The seeds of *Strychnos nux vomica* (poison nut tree)	*Nux vomica* is the classical "stress" medicine. The stress-related problems may be triggered or made worse by overwork. The patient becomes irritable, sleeps poorly, and may develop indigestion. They may seek relief in alcohol or other drugs.
Phosphorus	The element phosphorus	Those who respond to this important polychrest are typically sensitive, both to the physical and psychological environment. They are easily tired, but recover after a short rest. They may also bruise easily. *Phosphorus* may be appropriate in hepatitis, hemhorragic conditions, and vertigo in the elderly.
Pulsatilla	*Pulsatilla pratensis* (the pasque flower)	Those who respond to this important polychrest are typically indecisive and "changeable": their moods change swiftly — they weep easily, but quickly cheer up when comforted. *Pulsatilla* may be used for nasal stuffiness, menstrual problems, circulatory problems, and arthritis in people with *Pulsatilla* characteristics.
Rhus toxicodendron	*Toxicodendron radicans* (poison ivy)	Although this medicine is good for itchy, blistering skin rashes, it is most frequently used for arthritis and rheumatism. Its most characteristic indication is restlessness and rapid stiffening up from immobility — sitting still for as little as half an hour makes *Rhus toxicodendron* patients feel uncomfortable.
Sepia	The ink of *Sepia officinalis* (cuttlefish)	This important medicine is most often indicated in women. Typically, the patient is emotionally flat, fed up, and snappy. She resents others asking what the matter is and may hide her feelings. She may lose her sex drive, but may gain a remarkable, if temporary, improvement by doing exercise.
Silicea	Sand (silicon dioxide)	Patients who respond to *Silicea* are run down and susceptible to infections. They seem to "pick up every cold," and their infections are slow to resolve. These individuals feel the cold, and have cold, clammy hands and feet. They are often thin and pale with fine hair and nails that have lengthwise ridges.
Staphysagria	*Delphinium staphysagria* (wild delphinium)	*Staphysagria* is indicated for people who are seething with anger, and who may have outbursts of rage. It is also used for genitourinary problems and styes.
Sulphur	The element sulfur	People who respond to this polychrest are often extroverted and untidy. They nearly always feel too hot and often have hot feet. They tend to have skin trouble, such as intensely itchy eczema.
Thuja	A coniferous tree, *Thuja occidentalis*	Those who respond to *Thuja* often have warts and moles, and may have strange, fixed ideas. *Thuja* may be useful for chronic nasal stuffiness, bladder and prostate problems, and neuralgia.

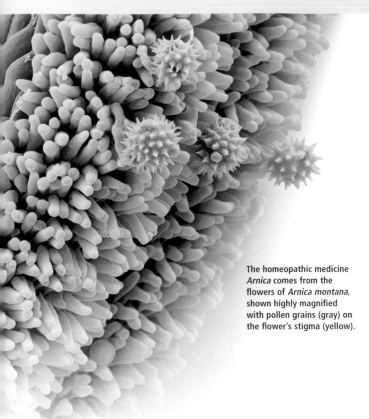

The homeopathic medicine *Arnica* comes from the flowers of *Arnica montana*, shown highly magnified with pollen grains (gray) on the flower's stigma (yellow).

Constitutional features

In deciding on a constitutional prescription the homeopath looks at the patient's physical type: for instance, patients whose constitutional homeopathic medicine is *Calcarea carbonica* or *Graphites* tend to be of solid build, inclined to be overweight, while those of *Silicea* or *Phosphorus* constitutional type are typically of slight build.

Constitutional features can be positive and adaptive, but a person who comes under strain has a negative and maladaptive side that determines how he or she will break down. For example, patients whose constitutional medicine is *Calcarea fluorica* are usually very supple and may be "double jointed." They are often talented gymnasts or dancers when young, but when they strain their joints, and later in life, they are predisposed to joint pain and arthritis.

The underlying psychological and emotional makeup also has adaptive and maladaptive aspects. For instance, *Lycopodium* constitutional types are typically reserved, intellectual, and conscientious. Consequently, they often occupy senior and responsible jobs, but when they get sick, these characteristics become maladaptive and they feel they are failing and become anxious, tyrannical, and depressed.

Similarly, *Natrum muriaticum* types are often found in the caring professions — they feel greatly for others, and sometimes seem better at dealing with other people's problems than their own. When stressed beyond the limit of adaptation, they can become very depressed and have great difficulty telling anyone how they feel.

The extroverted, garrulous *Sulphur* constitutional types become Nature's politicians and trade unionists. This sort of personality, combined with a tendency to develop itchy skin problems as a feature of almost any illness (even if they are not the main problem), suggest *Sulfur* as the constitutional medicine.

Recent research using psychological questionnaire methods and sophisticated statistical analysis supports the proposition that at least some of these constitutional types can be identified scientifically.

Building the picture

A homeopath will take a detailed case history, asking questions about medical health, lifestyle, moods, likes and dislikes to build the "clinical picture." Traditionally, the clinical picture is divided into three parts:

"Locals"

These are the particular symptoms — for instance, a pain or a rash — of which a person complains. The precise details of the quality of the symptoms are important (whether the rash is itchy or sore, for example). The homeopath will also ask what factors make the symptoms better or worse. These indicate the symptom's "modalities" and can be of great importance in determining the treatment.

"Mentals"

In addition to taking account of the patient's medical problem, the homeopath also notes the patient's "mentals": whether he or she is extroverted or introverted, assertive or unassertive, for example. Their emotional reactions to their illness, e.g. depression or anxiety, and the exact form they take, are important, as are any fears and phobias.

"Generals"

The homeopath takes into account a person's "generals" when building a picture. These are general features, including their build, what they like and dislike to eat, their reaction to temperature, and their quality of sleep.

Prescribing homeopathy

Having built up a picture of the person, a homeopath tries to match it to a "medicine" picture — i.e. the medicine that most resembles the disease and sensitivity of the patient. The homeopathic practitioner will also decide on the dilution and frequency.

The dilutions most commonly available in the US are 6C and 30C. Homeopaths usually advise taking two pills of the 6C strength two or three times daily. Higher dilutions (e.g. 30C) are usually taken less frequently, although in an acute situation they may also be used several times per day. In general, the regime corresponds to the pace of the illness — for acute conditions the treatment is repeated frequently, while for long-standing problems the patient usually takes the medicines less frequently.

Taking Homeopathic Medicines

Homeopathic medicines come in a range of strengths that are sometimes called "potencies." The potency routinely stocked by pharmacies is 6C.

For self-treatment it is usually best to start with a 6C potency. Avoid touching the medicines with your hands and fingers. Instead, tip the pills or tablets into the bottle cap then into your mouth. They should be sucked or chewed, not swallowed whole. The pills should be taken "on a clean palate," at least ten minutes before or after eating or drinking, brushing your teeth, or smoking.

Homeopathic medicines have an "all or nothing" effect: the number of pills or tablets taken is not critical. Four pills of a 6C medicine have the same effect as two 6C pills, not two 12C pills. A dose of two pills or tablets is usually recommended for safety.

Potencies

A good general-purpose potency is 6C, but others, most often 30C, are also prescribed by homeopathic practitioners. A higher potency may be necessary in the following circumstances: when a lower one seems to have stopped working; when the problem is psychological or functional, without structural changes; or when the "fit" between the patient's symptom picture and that of the medicine is very good.

Some medicines, such as *Natrum muriaticum*, work better in higher potencies. However, the main objective is to find the right medicine — the right medicine in any potency will do something, and the potency can always be adjusted later in treatment.

It is sometimes said that higher dilutions are "stronger" than lower ones. This is not true, at least not in a simple sense, although different dilutions do vary in their range and duration of action.

Homeopathy for babies and young children

Homeopathic medicines are safe for babies and young children. Getting a baby to take homeopathic medicines is not difficult. The easiest method is to crush two pills or one tablet between two clean teaspoons, and put a small amount into the baby's mouth on the tip of a spoon. They taste sweet and babies usually take them quite happily. Since the effect is all or nothing, it does not matter if the baby does not swallow the whole dose.

Lactose intolerance

Homeopathic pills and tablets are usually made of lactose (milk sugar), which may contain tiny amounts of cows' milk protein. This means that, theoretically, the tablets might upset people with lactose intolerance (lactase deficiency), a condition that is quite common in people of

East Asian descent, or children who are intolerant of cows' milk. In fact, the amounts of lactose and cows' milk protein are so small that they rarely cause problems. However, if they do, you can buy homeopathic medicines that are made with saccharose (cane sugar) or that come in liquid form (these contain some alcohol).

Precautions

Some people develop an "aggravation," or healing reaction (a temporary flareup of their symptoms), when they start a course of homeopathic treatment. This is nothing to worry about. In fact, it is a good sign because aggravations are usually associated with a promising long-term response. If you do develop an aggravation, however, stop taking the medicine until it has settled completely.

Coffee has a reputation for being an antidote to homeopathic medicines, but in fact interferes with only a few, such as *Nux vomica*. Very strong, penetrating smells, such as menthol and camphor, seem to interfere with the action of most homeopathic medicines, so you should avoid preparations such as Vicks® and Tiger Balm® while you are on homeopathic treatment. You can use mint toothpaste for brushing your teeth, but you should not take homeopathic remedies immediately afterward.

FINDING A PRACTITIONER

In general, homeopathy can safely be used to treat yourself or your family for minor or acute complaints. For chronic or complex problems, which may require "constitutional" treatment, it is best to consult a practitioner.

If you want to reduce your conventional medication, you should do so under the supervision of a competent practitioner who understands both homeopathy and your conventional medication. However, since there is no legal regulation of who can call him- or herself a homeopath, it is not always easy to identify a reliable homeopath — and some are medically trained, while others are not.

Certification and licensing requirements for homeopaths vary between countries and even states. The certification offered by The Council for Homeopathic Certification, The Homeopathic Academy of Naturopathic Physicians, and North American Society of Homeopaths indicates that the practitioner has reached a certain level of competence. However, only states can license a homeopath. Not all states grant licenses to homeopaths and those that do, require medical licensure such as MD, DO, or ND. At the other end of the spectrum, Minnesota and California allow any certified practitioner of alternative medicine to practice without being licensed.

When you are looking for a homeopath, get recommendations from friends, colleagues, or your family doctor. It is always wise to ask at the first session about his or her training, certification, experience of treating your condition, and insurance. *(For useful websites and addresses, see p.486.)*

TRADITIONAL CHINESE MEDICINE

PROFESSOR GEORGE LEWITH

Traditional Chinese Medicine (TCM) is an ancient healing system that includes acupuncture (*see p.82*), herbal medicine, dietary therapy, massage (tui na), relaxation, and special exercises, such as t'ai chi and qigong. Practitioners view the individual as an integrated whole whose health or ill-health is determined by the flow of *Qi* (energy), and they consider symptoms to be signs of a pattern of disharmony and not the result of a particular named disease.

Chinese Medicine

The *Huang Di Nei Jing* (The Yellow Emperor's Classic of Internal Medicine) is the first record of the teachings that form the foundation of Traditional Chinese Medicine. Written between 200 BC and 100 AD, the teachings appear to be transcripts of discussions between the Yellow Emperor and his disciple, Ji Buo. The book emphasizes three of the ideals of Taoist philosophy — balance, harmony, and moderation in all things.

According to TCM practitioners, the main external causes of disease ("pathogenic factors") are the following environmental factors: Wind, Cold, Summer Heat, Dampness, Dryness, and Fire. The main internal causes of disease are the "Seven Emotional Factors": Joy, Anger, Sadness, Worry, Grief, Fear, and Fright. Each of these, if excessive, can cause disease and tends to affect a particular organ. Other causes of disease include a weak constitution, incorrect diet, lack of physical exercise, overexertion, excessive sexual activity, pollution, and trauma (accidents).

Traditional Chinese diagnosis

Chinese diagnosis takes note of a broad range of symptoms and signs, many of which would not be considered especially significant in Western conventional medicine. The pattern of the symptoms and signs of an ailment are the outer manifestations of "dis-ease" and are considered to reflect the condition of *Qi* and the Internal Organs. Analysis of the symptoms and signs leads to identification of a "pattern of disharmony," which is quite different from a conventional Western diagnosis. Examining the tongue and making a detailed pulse diagnosis are important procedures. Observation of the color and shape of the

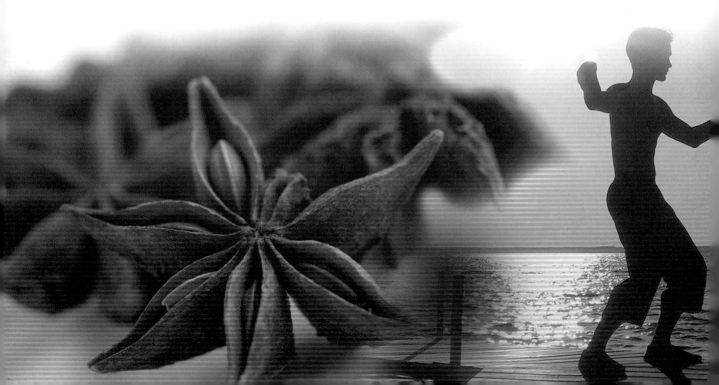

tongue body, as well as the tongue's coating, can reveal the state of the Internal Organs and the presence or absence of various pathogenic factors.

Pulse diagnosis is a complex technique and involves a high degree of subjectivity. The radial pulse is felt with the index, middle, and ring fingers at three different regions in the wrist, and the pulse characteristics are noted at three different levels (superficial, middle, and deep). The various pulses are said to reflect the state of the *Qi*, blood, *yin* and *yang*, and Internal Organs, as well as the presence of pathogenic factors.

Consulting a practitioner

At first, the TCM practitioner will look at the condition of your tongue and hair, the tone of your skin, and the way you move. He or she will listen to the sound of your breathing and voice and will note any distinctive odors. You will be expected to give details of your family history, habits, bodily functions, and symptoms of ill-health. Finally, the practitioner will feel your radial pulse, checking for strength, rhythm, and quality, and will explore your body for hard or tender areas. Treatment can involve herbal medicines, acupuncture (*see p.82*), dietary regimes, and movement therapies, such as t'ai chi.

Herbal remedies

The Chinese herbal practitioner can choose from about 6,000 herbs, a few mineral and animal sources, and hundreds of different formulas. Herbal remedies are used to restore the *yin–yang* balance within the body and to work in specific organs and channels (meridians, *see p.84*) to correct the relationship between the five elements. The herbs are classified under the five elements according to the remedial action of their taste — sweet, sour, bitter, pungent, and salty – and their opposing *yin–yang* qualities of hot and cold. For example, skullcap is a bitter, cold herb that can be used to lower a fever.

Herbs are usually prescribed as a formula of 10–15 dried herbs on the basis of their reputation and record for treating a particular pattern of disharmony. For example, a practitioner might decide to treat a case of infected allergic eczema, which he would diagnose as "damp-heat eczema with fire poison" (*see p.170*), with Gentian Drain the Gallbladder Decoction (*Long Dan Xie Gan Tang*).

The practitioner often adapts a basic formula to match the patient's individual pattern of disharmony. Remedies are usually taken as teas that are prepared in daily doses. They may also be taken as pills, powders, ointments, creams, and lotions.

T'ai chi

This ancient movement therapy is practiced daily by millions of Chinese people. It is sometimes referred to as meditation in motion. T'ai chi is a martial art that emphasizes relaxation, balance, and timing with sequences of slow, graceful movements that improve the flow of *Qi*, calm the mind, and promote self-healing. T'ai chi is a safe and enjoyable form of exercise and can be learned and practiced by people of any age. Research shows that it relaxes the muscles and calms the nervous system, thus improving the function of the body. It also benefits

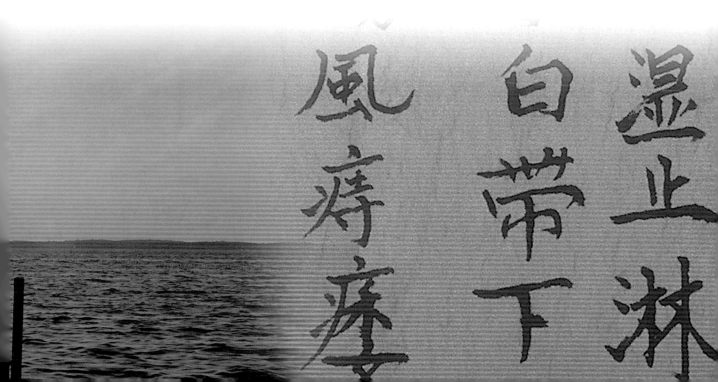

THE FIVE ELEMENTS

Practitioners of Traditional Chinese Medicine have a profound understanding of the relationship between *yin* and *yang* and a practical grasp of the qualities that feature in five-phase theory. The five phases of TCM are fire, earth, metal, water, and wood. These categories represent the qualities of everything in the universe, including the body's Internal Organs, which are more than simply organs as understood by the Western mind. The interplay between these phases gives rise to the unfolding and unceasing changes that are involved in maintaining well-being and restoring balance in our lives. Each phase relates to a *yin* organ and a *yang* organ and is associated with a specific taste, emotion, and season (*see below*). In five-phase theory, one phase supports or inhibits the function of another: fire melts metal, water douses fire, wood breaks through earth, metal lets water condense, water nourishes wood, earth dries up water, metal cuts through wood. In the body, the organs share the same relationships: the Heart (fire) controls the Lungs (metal); the Kidneys (water) control the Heart. The TCM practitioner will use the qualities of the five phases to understand the pattern of disharmony in the body and to restore the balance of the fundamental forces.

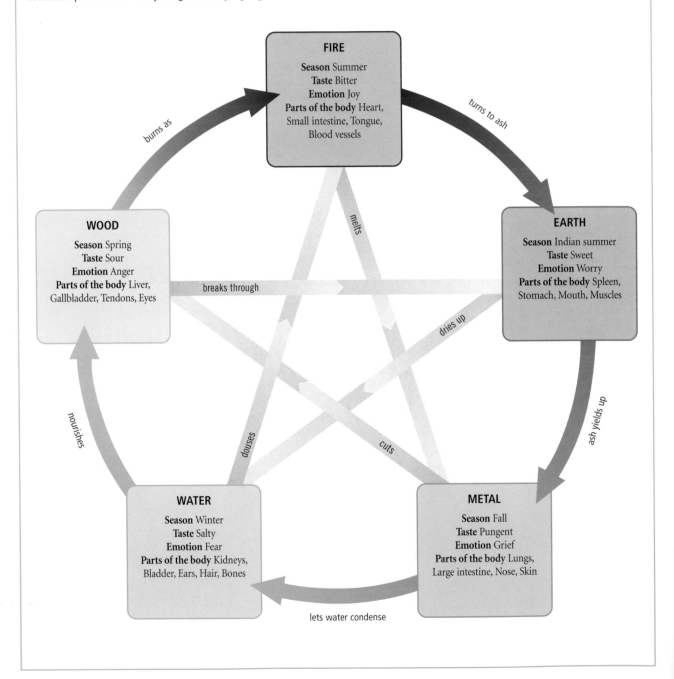

posture, balance, and flexibility, thereby helping people who have arthritis and other musculoskeletal disorders.

Many people with arthritis who have practiced t'ai chi praise its benefits, saying that it helps relieve their pain and stiffness, brings relaxation and lifts their spirits, and increases their flexibility and muscle strength. Studies have shown that t'ai chi can not only improve balance but can also prevent falls. In 1996, a trial in Atlanta, Georgia, found that t'ai chi improved the health of elderly people and another American study in 1989 found that it improved breathing without straining the heart. A recent study indicated possible benefits of immune functions with the regular practice of t'ai chi.

Key Concepts of TCM

Holism means that a person's mind, body, and emotions are seen as a single interacting whole. Ideally, they are in a state of harmony, both internally and in relation to the external environment. Problems in one part of the whole person affect the health of other parts. Holism is one of the key concepts of TCM, which also include *yin* and *yang*, the five elements (*see box, left*), *Qi*, the Internal Organs, the meridians, and the acupuncture points.

Yin and yang

These are the two complementary and fundamental processes of nature of ancient Chinese philosophy. They are qualities that are both opposite and yet at the same time interdependent. Many of the familiar pairs of opposites are described as either *yin* (contraction, cold, water, female, moon, black) or *yang* (expansion, hot, fire, male, sun, white). From the unceasing interplay of *yin* and *yang*, everything grows, develops, and changes.

Yin and *yang* are in a state of continual change and influence everything in the universe, from the very large to the very small. This includes a person's health, which is affected by qualities in the external environment and the harmony of internal energy. Disease-causing (pathogenic) factors can disturb the balance between *yin* and *yang*. For example, a disturbed balance might lead to *yin* conditions that involve hardenings, such as osteoarthritis, or to *yang* conditions that involve inflammations. A TCM practitioner will diagnose the imbalance by assessing the flow of *Qi* with various techniques, such as feeling the pulses in the wrist (*see p.79*), and will then concentrate treatment on restoring the balance.

Qi

Qi is the "vital energy" or "life force" that exists in every living thing. The concept is difficult to explain in Western terms. One way of looking at *Qi* is to say there are three kinds. The first is the *Qi* that is given to a child by its parents at conception — this *Qi* is stored in the kidneys

and contributes to the child's constitution. The second is the *Qi* that we receive from the digestion of food. The third is the *Qi* that we absorb from the air we breathe.

Qi moves between *yin* and *yang*: it can move inward to the center (*yin*) or outward to the surface (*yang*). It governs the functions of the Internal Organs, and circulates via the meridians to every part of the body. Pain, for instance, results from disturbances in this circulation.

Two main categories of *Qi* can bring disharmony — deficiency and stagnation. When *Qi* becomes deficient it might affect the whole person or a single Internal Organ, such as the Kidneys. When it stagnates, *Qi* ceases to flow smoothly through the meridians, leading to aches and pains or a dysfunction of an Organ.

Internal Organs

The Internal Organs are not the same as the Western equivalent although they have the same names, such as liver, kidneys, heart, and spleen. To help avoid confusion, the Chinese ones are written as starting with a capital letter, e.g., Liver, Kidneys, Heart, and Spleen, and Internal Organs.

TCM sees each organ as a complex system that includes not only its anatomical entity and physiological functions, but also recognizes its corresponding emotional and mental function.

Meridians

The meridians are pathways, or channels, in which *Qi* energy circulates throughout the body (*for a diagram of their locations see p.84*). Each meridian is associated with an Internal Organ.

Acupoints

Acupuncture points, also known as acupoints, are specific sites through which the *Qi* reaches the body's surface. An acupuncturist can manipulate the circulating *Qi* via these points to restore health in the relevant organs or meridians.

FINDING A PRACTITIONER

It is essential to find a suitably qualified Chinese herbalist. The National Certification Commission for Acupuncture and Oriental Medicine (*see p.486*) has a list of practitioners online, at www.nccaom.org. Expect the first session to last about an hour and subsequent ones about 30 minutes. You may be given a mixture of herbs to prepare as a tea each day, but herbs may also be prescribed as pills, powders, and ointments.

Do not treat yourself with Chinese herbs unless they are prescribed by your herbalist. Make sure that you give the practitioner full details of any conventional drugs and nutritional supplements you are taking.

If you would like to learn t'ai chi, the T'ai Chi Association (*see p.486*) can help you locate a qualified teacher.

ACUPUNCTURE

PROFESSOR GEORGE LEWITH

Acupuncture is an integral part of Traditional Chinese Medicine (*see p.78*). Traditional Chinese acupuncturists understand patterns of health and illness according to the flow of *Qi* (energy) in the body and apply needles or moxibustion (heated cones or sticks of moxa) to stimulate acupuncture points situated along energy channels called meridians. Acupuncture is becoming an accepted part of clinical health care, particularly for pain management.

History of Acupuncture

"Acupuncture" was coined by Willem Ten Rhyne, a Dutch physician, for the practice he saw on a visit to Japan in the 17th century. It literally means "to puncture with a needle," from the Latin *acus* (needle) and *punctura* (puncture). Acupuncture is a method of stimulating certain points on the body by inserting special needles in order to modify the perception of pain, normalize physiological functions, and treat or prevent disease. Its aim, like the other practices in Traditional Chinese Medicine (*see p.78*), is to restore the balance of *yin* and *yang* in the body and to harmonize the flow of the energy known as *Qi*, which is disrupted in illness.

The *Huang Di Nei Jing* (The Yellow Emperor's Classic of Internal Medicine) is the first record of the teachings that form the foundation of Traditional Chinese Medicine. The book emphasises three of the ideals of Taoist philosophy — balance, harmony, and moderation in all things.

The Chinese practiced acupuncture for several centuries before it reached the rest of the world — it was first practiced in Korea in about 600 AD and soon after in Japan. The West first learned of it in the 17th century when Jesuit missionaries brought European medical practices to China. At this time, Western medicine was still based on the four humors and used purges, leeches, and herbs. However, Western physicians and surgeons had a good knowledge of anatomy, derived from dissection.

Acupuncture reached its zenith during the Ming dynasty (1368–1644), then declined during the Qing dynasty (1644–1911) under Manchu rule and Western influence. During this period, herbal medicine was emphasized and, in 1822, the authorities ordered the closure of the acupuncture–moxibustion department of the Imperial Medical College.

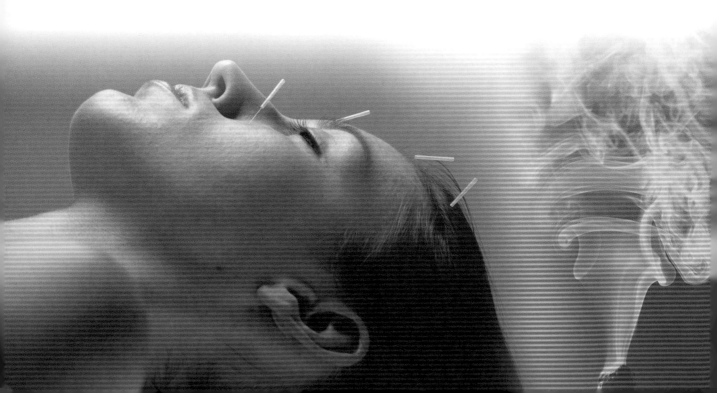

In Europe, acupuncture was widely practiced by the medical profession during the first half of the 19th century, and good results were reported for pain and rheumatism. In 1823, acupuncture was mentioned in the first issue of *The Lancet*. However, it gradually fell into disrepute when practitioners failed to employ it in a selective manner. Having improved their methods, a growing number of Western doctors now practice acupuncture to supplement conventional treatment.

Acupuncture Treatment

There are two main types of acupuncture. In traditional Chinese acupuncture, the acupuncture points are selected in accordance with traditional Chinese theories, such as the individual "pattern of disharmony" (*see p.78*), rather than a Western medical diagnosis. In neuroanatomical acupuncture, certain trigger points (*see p.55*) are needled to treat pain. Although practitioners who use acupuncture make no use of Chinese theories, there is a close correlation between trigger points and acupuncture points for pain.

Modern acupuncture needles are usually made of stainless steel and are single-use, disposable needles. In general, one of the first things a patient will want to know before commencing treatment is "Will it hurt?" In skilled hands, it is not especially painful. It is much less traumatic than an injection because it involves the use of a very small-gauge needle. Moxibustion is often used with acupuncture by the Chinese. This involves burning moxa, the dried leaves of the herb mugwort (*Artemisia vulgaris*), near particular acupuncture points. The heat is believed to help stimulate the acupuncture points and flow of *Qi*.

The Chinese believe that for acupuncture to obtain its maximum effect, a patient should feel a "needling sensation," which involves manipulating the needle after insertion into an acupuncture point. The patient may experience a dull, aching, heavy, numb, sore, distending, or warm sensation around the needle. This is known in Chinese as *De Qi*, and signifies the arrival of *Qi* at the needle. Sometimes, sensations may radiate along the path of a channel (meridian) on which the acupuncture point is situated — the so-called "propagated channel sensation" (PCS). Interestingly, needling trigger points produces the same sort of local sensation, and three-quarters of trigger points are also acupuncture points.

Generally, only a few needles (perhaps 6–10) are inserted during a treatment. They are usually left in place for about 20 minutes before being removed. It is common to experience a degree of relaxation during and following acupuncture. Some patients may experience drowsiness or go to sleep; others say they feel elated and "high" for a short time. These effects may be due to release of endorphins (pain-relieving chemicals produced by the brain).

In general, acute conditions will respond quickly and need few treatments. Chronic disorders respond more slowly and require a more prolonged course of treatment. However, individuals vary quite considerably in their response to acupuncture. Sometimes, immediate relief may be experienced on insertion of a needle, but in other situations three or four sessions may be required before any benefit is noticed at all. Occasionally, patients may find improvement only some weeks after treatment.

Improvement after the first treatment may be temporary and short-lived, but with each treatment a better and more

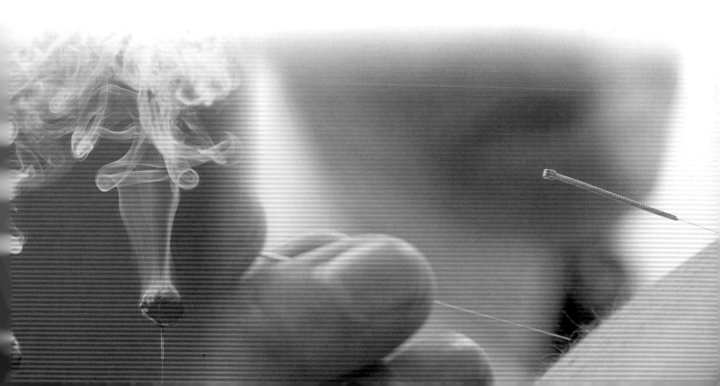

MERIDIANS AND ACUPOINTS

There are 14 meridians in the body. Six are associated with a solid *yin* organ (such as the Liver) and six with a hollow *yang* organ (such as the Lungs). Two more meridians, the Conception and the Governing vessels, control the other 12. *Qi* energy flows along the meridians and is accessible to the acupuncturist via acupoints.

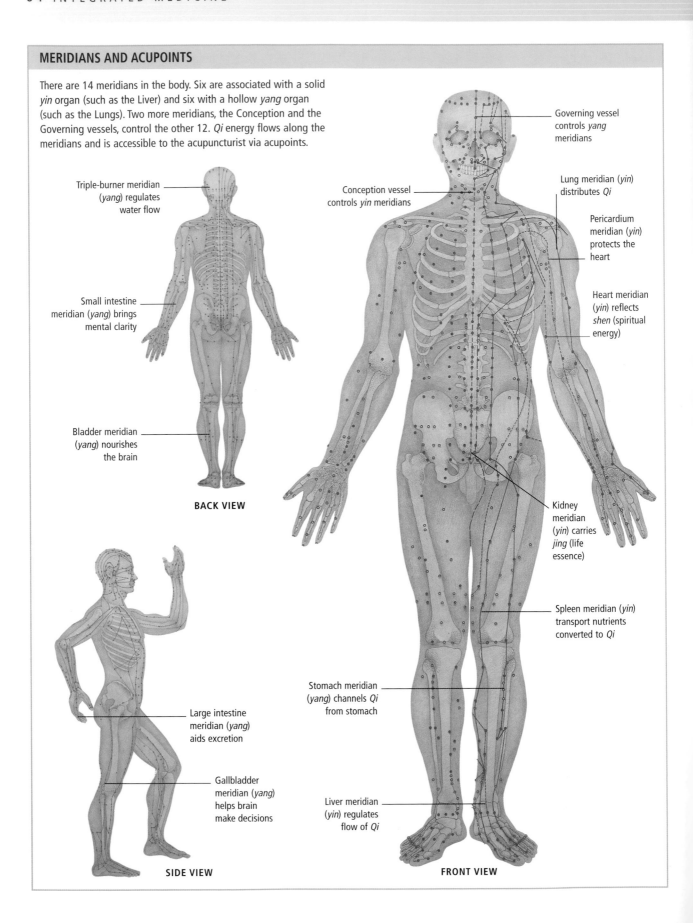

Triple-burner meridian (*yang*) regulates water flow

Small intestine meridian (*yang*) brings mental clarity

Bladder meridian (*yang*) nourishes the brain

BACK VIEW

Large intestine meridian (*yang*) aids excretion

Gallbladder meridian (*yang*) helps brain make decisions

SIDE VIEW

Governing vessel controls *yang* meridians

Conception vessel controls *yin* meridians

Lung meridian (*yin*) distributes *Qi*

Pericardium meridian (*yin*) protects the heart

Heart meridian (*yin*) reflects *shen* (spiritual energy)

Kidney meridian (*yin*) carries *jing* (life essence)

Spleen meridian (*yin*) transport nutrients converted to *Qi*

Stomach meridian (*yang*) channels *Qi* from stomach

Liver meridian (*yin*) regulates flow of *Qi*

FRONT VIEW

prolonged effect should occur. Three or four treatments should be adequate to determine whether a patient will respond. If there is no response after four treatments, then it is unlikely that treatment will be successful.

Most acupuncturists continue to treat patients until they are fully recovered or until there is no further improvement in their condition. A typical course of acupuncture might consist of four to twelve sessions.

Western uses of acupuncture

Traditional Chinese acupuncturists treat a wide range of conditions, from irritable bowel syndrome to asthma. In the West, acupuncture is primarily used for the treatment of pain, particularly neuromuscular pain. The underlying mechanism of how acupuncture works in conventional medical terms is unclear, but its therapeutic effects are probably mediated through the autonomic nervous system, which controls involuntary functions.

Acupuncture treatment for pain works either locally by secretion of neurohormones in the tissue adjacent to the needle, or centrally through nervous pathways mediated by neurotransmitters, such as serotonin (*see p.437*) and norepinephrine. More detailed research reveals these neurophysiological mechanisms.

Effectiveness of Acupuncture

It is difficult to design placebo-controlled trials that test the effectiveness of acupuncture. Researchers involved in clinical trials continue to argue about acupuncture, largely because they tend to look for specific effects compared to a placebo. No appropriate placebo has yet been developed for acupuncture. Two models of sham needles were validated. This adds to the confusion, particularly when comparing so-called "real acupuncture" (acupuncture that needles the correct acupuncture points) with "sham acupuncture" (which does not use actual acupuncture points) — the difference in outcome between the two seems to be much less than might be expected. In other words, it may not matter as much exactly where the practitioner places the needles; the benefit may come from experiencing the whole process of acupuncture. Another major methodological issue is protocolized versus individualized acupuncture.

Evidence for its effectiveness
Positive evidence from clinical trials, based on systematic reviews and meta-analyses of acupuncture trials, supports its use for nausea and vomiting, dental pain, and headaches. There is a growing body of evidence for the effectiveness of acupuncture for treating knee pain that is caused by osteoarthritis. The efficacy of acupuncture treatment in back pain is less clear, with one positive systematic review, one neutral, and one negative review.

Inconclusive evidence exists for the treatment of stroke, asthma, and neck pain, and there is clear negative evidence for the use of acupuncture in weight loss and giving up smoking. However, the effect of acupuncture in smoking cessation trials is similar to that of nicotine patches. Acupuncture is currently used in many pain clinics throughout the US and in primary care both for pain and nonpain-related symptoms.

Needling trigger points
One particularly effective aspect of acupuncture is the practice of needling trigger points (or intramuscular stimulation) in the treatment of pain. Interestingly, the pain referral pattern emanating from a myofascial trigger point often radiates along the pathway of a meridian, and it seems possible that some of the traditional meridian ideas may have developed as a consequence.

Is Acupuncture Safe?

Although serious side effects may occur with acupuncture, they are rare. They include local infection and local tissue damage, such as bruising. Very rarely, serious damage to superficial nerves or internal organs may cause events such as a punctured lung or kidney. The chances of a needle breaking are extremely small, but if one does there may be problems due to the migration of broken or embedded needle fragments.

Two surveys of acupuncture safety, involving 66,000 consultations, demonstrated a very low incidence of minor side effects, but warned against some preventable ones. The transmission by acupuncture needles of infections such as hepatitis B and C is a very real possibility. Unsterilized needles probably caused millions of liver disease cases in China and Japan. It is vitally important to make sure that your practitioner is using disposable needles. It is also essential be diagnosed by a medical doctor before initiating acupuncture treatment, particularly for persistent pain, because acupuncture might mask a disease by reducing pain, breathlessness, and other troublesome symptoms.

FINDING A PRACTITIONER

The National Certification Commission for Acupuncture and Oriental Medicine (www.nccaom.org) and the American Association of Oriental Medicine (www.aaom) have online lists (*see p.486*) of licensed acupunturists. The American Academy of Medical Acupuncture (www.medicalacupuncture.org) lists physicians trained in acupuncture. Commercial services such as www.acufinder.com also list a large number of practitioners, both physicians and licensed acupuncturists. Before you receive acupuncture, make sure that disposable needles are used. Always tell the practitioner if you are pregnant (certain acupuncture points should be avoided).

ENVIRONMENTAL HEALTH

DR DAVID KIEFER

Environmental health examines the impact that the environment makes on human health and disease. The World Health Organization includes physical, chemical, biological, social, and psychosocial factors in their definition of environmental health, and is concerned with both present and future generations. For centuries, scientific research has discovered connections between symptoms of ill health and their possible environmental causes. This knowledge helps doctors treat existing environmental illnesses, and to encourage changes that will help prevent these conditions in the future.

Environmental Hazards

The physical environment is a very important factor in human health. Clean air, sunlight, and clean water are all vital for everyone. Realizing that environmental factors can have serious consequences for human health is not new: the detrimental effects of overcrowding, poor sanitation, infectious diseases, and breathing or ingesting toxins have long been recognized. Environmental health experts use data from animal tests, ecological studies, laboratory tests, and observation of the effects that substances have on humans to assess the risks that different hazards pose. Following is a summary of some of the most potent threats.

Environmental toxins

Toxins can take the form of chemicals, biological agents, radiation (e.g. X-rays or ultraviolet light), or even tobacco smoke, all of which can have negative effects on health. They may enter the body in several ways, including ingestion, inhalation, or from contact with the skin. In some cases toxins can have immediate effects, so the cause of ill health is relatively easy to pinpoint. Some toxins, however, have effects that may become apparent only after many years of low-level exposure.

Many of the chemicals that are now in use in the modern world have not been adequately assessed for their toxicity either to humans or the environment.

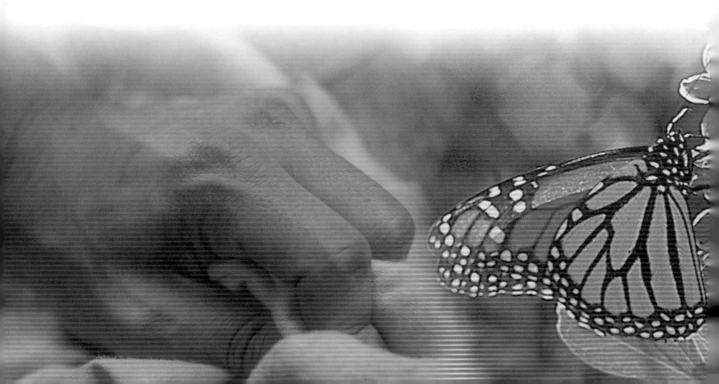

Air pollution

In the past, a few major episodes of stagnant air pollution in large cities resulted in many deaths among people with lung and heart problems. Subsequent investigations led to the identification of many different air pollutants connected to human illness and disease, such as sulfur dioxide, carbon monoxide, nitrogen oxides, polycyclic aromatic hydrocarbons, and ozone. Many of these are produced by the burning of fossil fuels (such as coal, oil, and gasoline) and they constitute the growing problem of "smog" in major cities across the globe, adversely affecting the health of many people. Other airborne pollutants, such as CFCs (*see p.90*), can create distant health problems.

Indoor air pollution is also a problem, whether it results from smoke from tobacco, indoor fires or stoves, or the compounds emitted from modern building materials (including carpets, paint, and walls) used in modern office buildings and homes.

Water contamination

Water supplies can be contaminated with potentially dangerous microbes and chemicals, either from a specific source ("point pollution," e.g. from a factory) or from many scattered sources (e.g. runoff from agricultural fields). Both types of pollution can contaminate lakes, rivers, reservoirs, and other surface waters, and seep into groundwater, contaminating wells and aquifers.

Industrial pollution is responsible for contamination by a wide range of compounds, including volatile organic solvents and heavy metals (especially lead and arsenic).

Lead is a well-researched contaminant. It enters the water supply from old pipes, which are made of lead, or lead has been used as a solder, or it leaches from soil contaminated by the fallout from combusted leaded gasoline.

Microbes from human and animal waste, such as *Cryptosporidium*, and the common gut bacteria *E. coli*, can contaminate water. These can lead to outbreaks of intestinal diseases. Nitrates and pesticides can enter drinking water supplies, mainly from farmland runoff. Nitrates can be harmful to very young babies. In the US, water is treated and pesticide and nitrate levels are usually very low.

Some chemicals are intentionally added to drinking water. Chlorine, which is a common disinfectant, is used to kill pathogens such as *E. coli* from sewage. Trihalomethanes (THMs) are produced when chlorine combines with naturally present organic matter. THMs in drinking water have been linked to higher incidences of miscarriage, but evidence is inconsistent and inconclusive. Chlorine and THMs evaporate easily, so leaving tap water in an open container, preferably in the refrigerator, for a few hours can reduce the chlorine content and improve the taste.

Our bodies need a trace amount of fluoride and it is added to the water supply in some areas for dental health. There have been widely publicized health concerns about fluoride, but little evidence for harm has been published.

Water filters can remove pesticides, nitrates, and chlorine, but the filters must be changed regularly or they become ineffective, and they need to be cleaned regularly. Tap water undergoes a series of mandatory tests, so in most cases it is pure. However, if you are concerned, ask your supplier or have your well water tested.

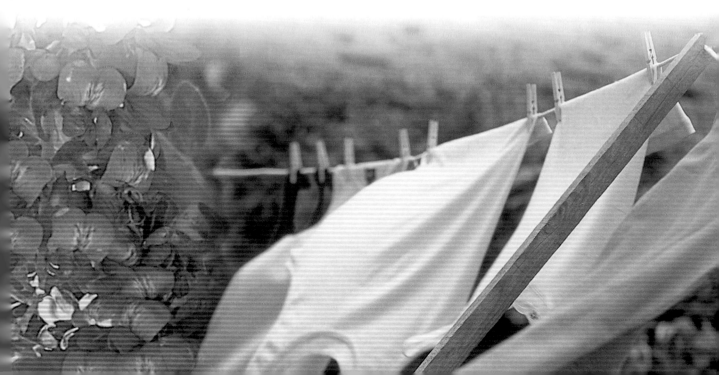

Food contamination

Even healthy foods, such as fruit and vegetables, can be contaminated with potentially harmful chemicals. In agriculture, chemicals are used to reduce pests (pesticides), diseases (fungicides, antimicrobials, and antiparasitics), or weeds (herbicides). They are also used to control the rate of crop growth and ripening (growth regulators). Some crop sprays stay on the surface of the plant, while others (systemic chemicals) are designed to spread throughout the plant. Chemicals can be added after harvesting, to improve the appearance or shelf life of the crop.

Crop chemicals are generally designed to stick to the plant, so that they are not washed off when it rains. This means that a quick rinse under the faucet is not enough to remove them: thorough washing with soap or other detergent is required. Some may also be absorbed into the plant's surface layers, so peeling helps reduce the amount ingested. Systemic chemicals, because they permeate the whole plant, are not removable.

Current pesticide regulations and testing ensure that residues of pesticides in food are extremely low and, in many cases, below the detection limit. However, almost all tests for chemical safety are conducted on individual chemicals, rather than on the cocktail to which we are exposed through our food. There are, however, steps you can take to minimize your exposure to these chemicals. One step is to buy organic foods. By doing this, as well as by reducing your intake of chemical residues, you are also supporting an industry that pollutes the wider environment far less than intensive agriculture does.

Cereal and cereal products

We tend to consume large quantities of cereals (e.g. bread, breakfast cereals, and pasta), so the chemicals that are used to cultivate these plants are particularly important. Intensively-grown wheat, barley, and other cereals are sprayed with a range of chemicals during their growth, including chlormequat, pirimiphos-methyl (an organo-phosphate), glyphosate, and phosphine. The effects of this chemical cocktail on human health has not yet been studied.

On the positive side, chemicals have helped eliminate problems caused by contamination of cereals with poisonous weed seeds and fungal diseases. Ergot, a fungus, used to cause major health problems in Western countries, especially in wet years. Symptoms of poisoning included hallucination, manic depression, gangrene, and abortion, and could lead to a painful convulsive death.

Fruit and vegetables

Potatoes are another staple food that people tend to consume in large quantities. After harvesting, potatoes are usually sprayed with chemicals to keep them from sprouting. Unless you are using organic potatoes, always peel them and avoid eating the skin.

Surface contamination can also be avoided in many fruits. Nonorganic oranges and lemons are treated with waxes and other postharvest chemical sprays to prolong shelf life and add shine. Try to buy organic, unwaxed lemons, especially if you are using the zest (peel). Alternatively, scrub them thoroughly, using warm soapy water.

Buying organic bananas is another good idea. Non-organic bananas often contain residues of pesticides that have been implicated in thyroid disorders in plantation workers. Some chemicals that are applied before shipping to prevent mold are in high quantities at the surface.

Strawberries and other soft fruits are highly susceptible to molds, so fungicides are often used on them. These fruits obviously cannot be scrubbed. Also, high levels of the insecticides acephate and methamidophos have been found in nonorganic peaches and nectarines. Because these chemicals are systemic, they spread through the fruit, so washing will not remove them. Fruit and vegetables produced organically have much lower, or negligible, chemical contamination.

Red meat

Animals can be contaminated with potentially harmful chemicals through their food and medication. If their pastures have been sprayed, or their food is contaminated, the chemicals are absorbed into their bodies. Fat-soluble chemicals, such as dieldrin, DDT, and dioxins are present in small quantities in plants, but they accumulate in animals that eat those plants. When humans eat the animals in turn, the chemicals accumulate in higher concentrations. Meat reared organically is inherently lower in contam-inants since far fewer chemicals are allowed: animals are fed organic foodstuffs and have only minimal medication.

Chicken and eggs

Poultry can be medicated for parasites and disease-causing bacteria, or chemicals can be routinely added to their food. Residues can survive in meat or eggs if the birds are not given enough time to clear the chemicals from their systems.

Low doses of antimicrobial chemicals have been routinely fed to poultry as growth promoters. This has sparked concerns that the practice could lead to drug-resistant bacteria evolving and threatening human health.

Birds reared in high-intensity conditions are likely to need the most chemical treatments to keep them healthy, so try to avoid factory-farmed eggs and meat.

Fish

Through the food they eat, fish are able to absorb chemical pollution from the general environment. Farmed salmon can contain 16 times more PCBs (cancer-causing, dioxin-like chemicals) than wild salmon. This comes mainly from the fishmeal (ground, pelleted fish) on which they are fed. Farmed fish are also likely to be treated with antibiotics and pesticides to control infections and infestations.

HARMFUL CHEMICALS AND THEIR EFFECTS

CHEMICAL	SOURCE AND TOXIC LEVELS	PEOPLE AT RISK AND EFFECTS ON HEALTH
Arsenic	**Source:** natural and manmade, such as wood preservatives and pesticides. **Toxic levels** (for adults of normal body weight): between 300 and 30,000 ppb of inorganic arsenic in food or water can cause adverse health effects. Above 60,000 ppb in food or water can be fatal.	**At risk:** people who (a) breathe in air with sawdust or smoke from arsenic-treated wood; (b) live near contaminated waste sites; or (c) live near rocks with high levels of arsenic. **Health effects:** stomachache, nausea, vomiting and diarrhea, darkening of skin; small corns/warts on torso, palms, or soles.
Benzene	**Source:** natural (volcanoes, forest fires, fossil fuels) and manmade (rubber, pesticides, dyes, drugs, lubricants, etc.). **Toxic levels:** (for adults of normal body weight): between 700 and 3,000 ppm can cause adverse health effects. Exposure to 10,000 to 20,000 ppm for 5 to 10 minutes can be fatal.	**At risk:** people who breathe tobacco smoke, exhausts, industrial emissions, or vapor from glues or paints. **Health effects:** high levels cause dizziness, drowsiness, increased heart rate, vomiting, irritated stomach. Persistent exposure damages bone marrow, disturbs immune system, and may cause leukemia.
Lead	**Source:** natural and manmade (industrial). **Toxic levels:** (for adults of normal body weight): more than 1.5 µg/m3 inhaled on average over 3 months and more than 0.015 mg/L in drinking water may cause adverse health effects.	**At risk:** people who (a) drink water from lead plumbing; (b) work with lead; (c) eat food from lead-contaminated soils. **Health effects:** damage to the central nervous system (especially children's), kidneys. High levels may slow reaction times, weaken joints, cause anemia, lead to miscarriages, and damage sperm production. May be carcinogenic.
Nitrates	**Source:** fertilizer, manure, sewage. **Toxic levels:** (for adults of normal body weight): more than 10 mg/L of nitrate-nitrogen or 45 mg of nitrate in drinking water may have adverse effects.	**At risk:** babies who drink water with high levels of nitrate. **Health effects:** high levels in drinking water can reduce the ability of hemoglobin to carry oxygen, especially in babies up to 6 months old (gut bacteria turn nitrates into toxic nitrites).
Phthalates	**Source:** manmade (plastic softeners, plastic and vinyl toys, solvents, insecticides, wood finishes, cosmetics, personal care products). May be absorbed through skin. **Toxic levels** (for adults of normal body weight): more than 6 ppb in drinking water may cause adverse health effects.	**At risk:** people who (a) eat food stored in plastic wrapping; (b) eat fatty foods, fish, meat, vegetable oils; (c) breathe in certain perfumes, nail polishes, deodorants, hair sprays; (d) drink contaminated water; (e) have excessive mouth contact with plastic (plastic tubing, plastic toys). **Health effects:** gastrointestinal problems, nausea, vertigo. Long-term, potential damage to developing testes and liver, and to developing fetus. May be carcinogenic.
Polycyclic aromatic hydrocarbons (PAHs)	**Source:** natural (volcanoes, forest fires) and manmade (pesticides, dyes, plastics, medicines). **Toxic levels** (for adults of normal body weight): more than a level of 0.015 to 0.03 mg (depending on the PAH) per lb of body weight per day may cause adverse health effects.	**At risk:** people who (a) breathe air from incomplete burning of fossil fuels, waste, or other organic substances; (b) breathe soot, exhaust fumes, contaminated dust; (c) drink contaminated water or milk. **Health effects:** not proven, but animal research suggests PAHs may affect reproductive system, skin, body fluids, and immune system, and may cause cancer.
Polychlorinated biphenyls (PCBs)	**Source:** manmade (pre-1977 manufacture of electrical insulation equipment). **Toxic levels** (for adults of normal body weight) causing adverse health effects vary from 0.5 ppb (drinking water) to 3 ppm (fat of poultry and red meat), and consistently breathing air with more than 0.5 to 1 mg/m3.	**At risk:** people who (a) breathe air from spills and leaks from hazardous waste sites, or from combustion of PCB-containing products; (b) drink contaminated water; (c) eat fish and aquatic mammals in which PCBs accumulate. **Health effects:** animal research suggests large amounts of PCBs may damage the liver, stomach, blood, immune system, and skin (causing acne and rashes). Probably carcinogenic.
	(ppm= parts per million; ppb=parts per billion)	

Wild fish, however, can also be contaminated with harmful environmental chemicals. Some substances, such as PCBs and DDT (a pesticide), which are oil-soluble, accumulate in fat and oil. Oily fish (e.g. mackerel) and predatory fish (e.g. tuna), which are higher up the food chain, are likely to have accumulated more contaminants.

When there is a choice, opt for wild fish, and, if possible, try to be selective about the source of your fish. Those caught in restricted waters, such as the Baltic, are much more likely to be more polluted than those caught in the open Pacific or Atlantic Oceans.

Since contamination levels can be high, women who are pregnant or may become pregnant, or who are breast-feeding, should eat fewer than the one to four portions of oily fish per week that is recommended for others.

Nuclear radiation

Radioactive contamination occurs with nuclear fallout from nuclear reactor accidents, spills at military, research, and commercial facilities, and nuclear weapons testing. All of these sources have exposed workers and the general public to varying doses of radiation. Although the details are being debated by scientists, radiation seems to be related to an increased incidence of cancer beyond what would normally be expected in a population. Some researchers even point out that "there is no threshold level below which radiation exposure is safe."

Global climate change

Environmental change has many far-reaching effects, including changes in patterns of human health problems. The weather affects health not only directly (for example, heatstroke), but also indirectly (for example, warm, wet weather encourages insects such as mosquitoes that may transmit diseases to breed).

Current climate variations offer clues to how long-term climate change might affect health. Every few years, natural changes in ocean temperature affect convection currents (the mass movements of air that form weather systems), creating warmer, more stormy conditions than usual in various parts of the world. During these "El Niño" years higher temperatures in some areas of Peru have been connected to more gastrointestinal diseases, whereas El Niño-related droughts and fires in Indonesia contributed to a worsening of air pollution and a risk in related health conditions such as asthma in southeast Asia. If climate change proceeds as predicted, health effects will be diverse. Some experts predict, for example, that if global warming increases flooding of major rivers and coastal areas, these may release and distribute toxins from agricultural fields, human septic systems, and toxic dumps. Also, some areas of the world may become more susceptible to drought, worsening malnutrition and its resulting health problems.

The ozone hole

It is now widely realized that pollution in one part of the globe can affect people and environments elsewhere. For example, ozone-depleting chlorofluorocarbons (CFCs) produced in industrialized nations may travel thousands of miles and contribute to the "ozone hole" in the Southern Hemisphere. These chemicals, combined with compounds from natural sources such as volcano eruptions, react in the atmosphere to deplete ozone and permit greater amounts of certain types of ultraviolet radiation (UV-A and UV-B) from the sun to reach the earth's surface. Some of these UV rays are very harmful, increasing the occurrence of skin cancer and eye problems, such as cataracts. It is also possible that UV rays may cause a suppression of the immune system. The global dispersal of CFCs is an example of how environmental problems and resulting health effects have become international as well as regional.

Furthermore, human health may also be indirectly affected by changes to the environment resulting from stratospheric ozone depletion. For example, UVB radiation contributes to photochemical smog: it can increase ozone at ground level, aggravating respiratory conditions such as asthma. A potentially more dramatic effect could stem from a decrease in food production due to the effects of stratospheric ozone depletion on certain plants and animals. However, these indirect health effects are less easily measured than direct effects on human health.

Children's health

Children are exposed to a large quantity of different pesticides and toxins through their food and water, at home, in schools, and in gardens and parks. The effects of a toxin on children's behavior, physiology, and physique may be different from its effects on adults. Children have a higher caloric and fluid intake relative to their body weight compared to adults, making low-level contamination of food and water a more significant factor for them. Children also favor certain foods and drinks over others, and this too can contribute to toxic exposure. For example, in the US, toddlers are estimated to drink 16.7 times more apple juice than the average for the population. Thus, any pesticide residues in apple juice would be more significant for toddlers than for other age groups. Also, children are growing and developing in many ways and small, seemingly insignificant exposures may not cause obvious symptoms for many years.

Governments are beginning to recognize these factors and establish recommendations that are specific to children. In the US, the 1996 Food Quality Protection Act dictated that the Environmental Protection Agency must assess the pesticide content of foods and their safety for children. The act also made allowable levels of pesticides lower for infants and children than for adults.

Workplace exposure

Many workplace risks are related to environmental exposures. By understanding the risks in your particular occupation, you can act to lessen or eliminate possible harm, and stay healthy in your career.

A thorough assessment by an environmental or occupational health expert should help you pinpoint hazards. These will be specific to each job, but may include exposures to corrosive substances (acids, alkalis), dusts, fibers (asbestos, fiberglass), gases, heavy metals, agricultural chemicals, plastics (di-isocyanates, phthalates), petrochemicals, physical agents (such as noise, heat, vibration, repetitive lifting), radiation (including electromagnetic, X-rays, and ultraviolet), and solvents.

When you have identified relevant exposures, ensure that you are trained to deal with them, and take all necessary safety precautions. For example, if you are a mechanic you may be exposed to fumes from exhaust, gasoline, and solvents, so you should ensure that your workplace is well ventilated. Or, if you use agricultural chemicals, follow the manufacturer's instructions when mixing or applying them, and wear appropriate protective clothing.

In the office, the compounds emitted from modern building materials and furnishings create indoor air pollution. Some people feel that low-level exposure to these compounds causes sick building syndrome: headache, fatigue, inflammation, and respiratory symptoms. Low-emitting building materials, continuous ventilation, and nontoxic office supplies will reduce these exposures.

HEALTHY HOUSE

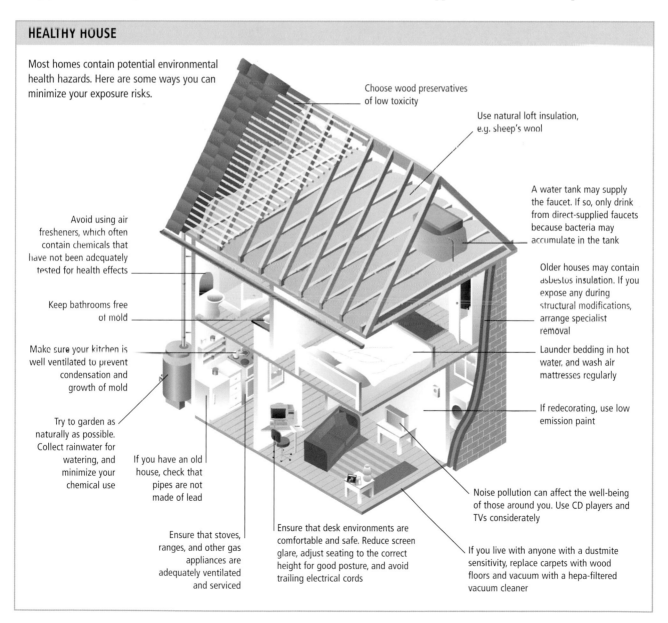

Most homes contain potential environmental health hazards. Here are some ways you can minimize your exposure risks.

Choose wood preservatives of low toxicity

Use natural loft insulation, e.g. sheep's wool

A water tank may supply the faucet. If so, only drink from direct-supplied faucets because bacteria may accumulate in the tank

Avoid using air fresheners, which often contain chemicals that have not been adequately tested for health effects

Older houses may contain asbestos insulation. If you expose any during structural modifications, arrange specialist removal

Keep bathrooms free of mold

Launder bedding in hot water, and wash air mattresses regularly

Make sure your kitchen is well ventilated to prevent condensation and growth of mold

If redecorating, use low emission paint

Try to garden as naturally as possible. Collect rainwater for watering, and minimize your chemical use

If you have an old house, check that pipes are not made of lead

Noise pollution can affect the well-being of those around you. Use CD players and TVs considerately

Ensure that stoves, ranges, and other gas appliances are adequately ventilated and serviced

Ensure that desk environments are comfortable and safe. Reduce screen glare, adjust seating to the correct height for good posture, and avoid trailing electrical cords

If you live with anyone with a dustmite sensitivity, replace carpets with wood floors and vacuum with a hepa-filtered vacuum cleaner

Environmental Health and Cancer Risk

Many factors in the environment are potentially carcinogenic, i.e. are capable of causing changes in body cells that can lead to cancer. Often though, the links have been difficult to study. Epidemiologists (scientists who study the causes and patterns of disease in populations) need large numbers of cases before they can untangle the issues involved. In addition to environmental factors, people's diet, lifestyle, and genetic susceptibility all play a role. This means that environmental factors are rarely the "cause" of cancer. Instead, they can only be described as "risk factors," but 90 percent of cancers can be induced by environmental factors.

Scientists continue to work on current cancer concerns. It is worth noting that research has not shown, to date, that artificial sweeteners and using mobile phones are carcinogenic. There is also no good evidence to link antiperspirant use to breast cancer.

Risk factors

Cancer is essentially a condition where cells keep dividing, out of control. Anything that affects cell division, or that damages the cells' DNA (molecular instructions), is likely to be a risk factor.

Ionizing radiation, of the type given off by X-rays, cosmic radiation from the solar system, and radioactive particles, is known to damage DNA. Many individual chemicals are toxic and directly interfere with cell division. Free radical compounds also increase cancer risk. These are short-lived but very destructive compounds that can damage DNA. One of the main sources of free radicals in the body is oxidation of certain types of fats. Antioxidants such as vitamin C and beta-carotene "mop up" these free radicals, so a diet high in the antioxidant vitamins is especially important (*see p.36*).

Organs and susceptibility

Different parts of the body interact with the environment in different ways. The lungs are vulnerable to airborne contaminants. The link between cigarette smoke and lung cancer is well established. Other breathable carcinogens include asbestos and radioactive particles (dust).

The skin is relatively impermeable to chemicals because of its protective, waterproofing layer. However, skin is exposed to sunlight and the damaging effects of its UV rays. The risk of developing skin cancer is higher for people living or vacationing regularly in an area with strong sunlight. People with fair skin are particularly at risk, since their skin contains less melanin, the pigment that gives skin its color and helps protect it from the sun's rays. Over-use of tanning booths may also contribute to skin cancer.

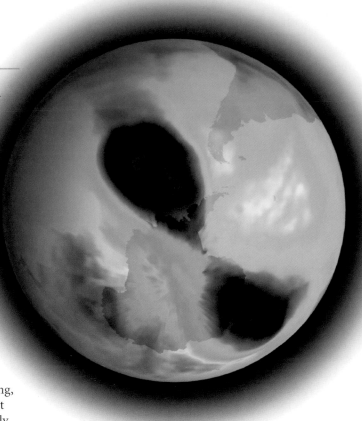

The ozone layer of the upper atmosphere filters the sun's damaging UV rays, but it has thinned over the last few decades. This may be a factor in the rise in skin cancer cases. The thinnest region – the "ozone hole" – is over the Antarctic.

Female breast tissue is naturally very responsive to certain hormones. The hormone estrogen appears to play an important role in the development and progress of breast cancer. Estrogen "mimics" taken either as contraceptive or HRT drugs may slightly increase the risk of breast cancer if used long-term. Many pesticides and other environmental contaminants mimic natural hormones and can potentially affect cell reproduction.

The digestive system is also exposed to environmental contaminants through the food we eat. Some foods are known to be carcinogenic. These include salted, pickled, and smoked foods, charred meat, and meats treated with nitrites, all of which should be eaten in only small amounts or avoided altogether. A very salty diet has been linked to stomach cancer, and a diet low in fiber is thought to be a risk factor for colorectal cancer. Long-term exposure to aflatoxins, chemicals produced by a fungus that can contaminate peanuts and grains, increases the risk of developing liver cancer.

Cancer and genetics

Genes control how our cells deal with toxins and other contaminants and how well our DNA is repaired when it does get damaged. Each of us has a unique combination of genes, which partly explains why some people get cancer when others do not, even if they have been exposed to the same environment. About 10 percent of breast cancer cases, for example, is linked to an abnormal gene. Your doctor can advise on screening programs if you have a relative with cancer and are concerned about genetic links.

Improving Environmental Health

If you suspect that an illness has an environmental health component, an important first step in any diagnosis is to visit an environmental health specialist. He or she will try to discover if you have been exposed to a toxin from food, water, air, building materials, or cleaning supplies and then connect any exposures with your clinical symptoms.

Tests

Tests may provide evidence of certain exposures. For example, a blood test can reveal if you have been exposed to dangerous levels of lead. Blood tests can also detect exposure to elemental mercury (found in dental amalgams, thermometers, and gas meters), whereas urine samples collected over 24 hours are the best way to detect chronic or recent exposures to the other two forms of mercury, methylmercury (found in fish) and inorganic mercury (found in a variety of substances, including industrial pollutants). In many other cases, laboratory tests may be inaccurate, have technical limitations or otherwise fail to help establish a diagnosis.

Treatment strategies

There are many possible treatment strategies for environmental health problems. In general, environmental health experts recommend decreasing exposure to toxins that may be related to health problems and encouraging the excretion or release of toxins from the body.

Decreasing exposure involves awareness of the sources of the problem, and then taking steps to minimize exposure. These might include changing the cleaning products used in the home, or eating organic food where possible.

Detoxification

Some experts recommend taking steps to improve the liver's ability to metabolize and dispose of toxins. This detoxification approach is a strategy employed by many other cultures and traditional healing systems, such as Ayurveda, Traditional Chinese Medicine, and Native American medicine, where it is used as a preventive and treatment option for "periodic cleansing of the body." Liver detoxification may be improved by using liver-toning

herbs, such as milk thistle (*Silybum marianum*), or specific supplements, such as vitamin C, vitamin E, selenium, green tea, and mixed carotenes. To help release toxins from the body, some experts recommend increasing fluid intake to flush certain toxins out through the kidneys. They also recommend increasing fiber intake to facilitate bowel clearance, and sweating by exercising or taking saunas. Other possibilities include bodywork, such as massage, to free toxins from the muscle tissue so that they can then be excreted; homeopathy, to increase the excretion of certain toxins; and colonic irrigation to facilitate bowel excretion of some compounds. However, although these therapies are advocated by some practitioners, they are not yet supported by research or clinical trials.

A strategy example: lead removal

People are exposed to lead in various ways (*see table, p.89*). Most of the adverse effects of lead exposure occur in babies and small children, causing reduced IQ and behavioral difficulties. In adults, low levels of lead exposure may be related to high blood pressure, slow reaction times, anemia, and hearing loss. However, in many cases there are no symptoms.

Governmental and individual efforts have reduced lead exposure in recent decades. These measures have included controlling dust and paint chip residues, using cold water (not hot) for drinking and mixing baby formula milk, and switching to unleaded gasoline to prevent lead from entering the environment.

Time outdoors

Everyone can benefit from being in and interacting with the natural environment, whether gardening, sitting in a park, taking a walk on a beach, or hiking through the mountains. Research has demonstrated some of these benefits, such as improved responses to stress when compared to people restricted to manmade environments. People recovering from surgery do better in hospital rooms with windows, and people are also able to concentrate better after surgery if they are engaged in a restorative nature activity, such as sitting in a park or tending plants. A close association with trees can help improve well-being. And, of course, our parks and other open spaces are common grounds that foster social interactions and contribute to our overall social well-being.

FINDING A PRACTITIONER

When looking for an environmental health expert, make sure that he or she is a member of the American Academy of Environmental Medicine (www.aaem.org); you can find a directory of referable physicians on their Web site. These professionals are physicians or doctors of osteopathy who have passed the core curriculum in environmental medicine. See also p.486 for useful addresses.

MIND–BODY MEDICINE

DR KENNETH R. PELLETIER

Mind–body therapies not only improve overall health but also have a positive and measurable effect on specific conditions and diseases. Two key principles underpin the various therapies. First, the mind can affect the body in positive or harmful ways. Second, whatever you do physically also has an impact on consciousness. A great deal of research reveals that psychological and spiritual practices, such as meditation, relaxation, guided imagery, and biofeedback, can have a useful impact on physical problems, including pain.

The Role of Mind–Body Medicine

Doctors are traditionally sceptical about innovation. When the stethoscope was introduced in 1916, for example, critics were concerned that the unorthodox diagnosis device might distance doctors from their patients. Integrating mind–body medicine fully with other forms of medicine remains a challenge, but of all CAM (complementary and alternative medicine) therapies, mind–body practices are supported by the greatest body of scientific evidence for the greatest number of conditions for the largest number of people. Compared to other CAM therapies, they have also gained the widest acceptance within conventional health-care systems. In fact, mind–body medicine is so widely used by the public and by the medical profession that it may be considered to belong more to conventional than to complementary medicine.

According to the National Center for Complementary and Alternative Medicine (NCCAM) in the US, "Only a subset of mind–body interventions are considered CAM. Many that have a well-documented theoretical basis — for example, patient education and cognitive behavioral approaches — are now considered mainstream." On the other hand, meditation, dance, music and art therapy, and prayer and mental healing are categorized as alternative. NCCAM states that "Many CAM therapies are called holistic, which generally means they consider the whole person, including physical, mental, emotional, and spiritual aspects."

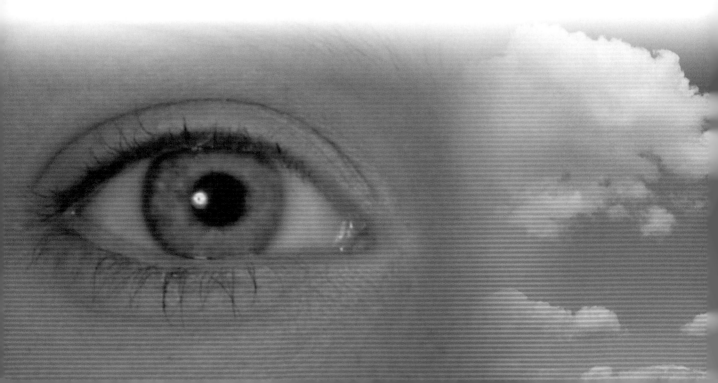

What is mind–body medicine?

In 2001, NCCAM defined mind–body practices as those that employ "a variety of techniques designed to facilitate the mind's capacity to affect bodily function and symptoms." Generally speaking, mind–body practices, which include meditation, relaxation, guided imagery, hypnosis, and biofeedback, produce a beneficial, biologically regenerative, relaxed state, in which the body is more able to heal itself and function optimally. Under the direction of a skilled clinician, these therapies can be used to treat a wide array of medical and psychological conditions. However, they can also be safely used by everyone as "self-care practices" to prevent and reverse the harmful effects of stress and to complement conventional treatments.

Generally, the extensive research into the efficacy of mind–body medicine focuses on major chronic diseases, such as general pain syndromes and insomnia, where a combination of professional therapy and self-care practice is the most effective way of achieving the maximum improvement in health and well-being.

History of Mind–Body Medicine

Mind–body medicine is an ancient concept. Until about 300 years ago, virtually all philosophy and medicine treated the body and mind as an integral whole. Then, in the 18th century, adherents of the Enlightenment introduced a mechanistic and reductionistic scientific model that led to the study of body and mind being separated. The 18th-century paradigm reached its height in the 20th century, when modern scientific medicine helped end the epidemics of infectious diseases, such as smallpox, cholera, and tuberculosis, which had formerly been major causes of mortality. (It should be said, however, that these diseases had already declined due to public health measures, such as improved sanitation, safer water, improved housing, and better nutrition.)

Currently, the diseases that are killing more people in the developed nations worldwide are no longer these infections, but chronic degenerative conditions, such as coronary artery disease, hypertension (high blood pressure), cancer, and diabetes, for which there are no chemical "magic bullets." These diseases are inextricably related to psychological, environmental, and lifestyle factors. Increasingly, stress is recognized as a major causal factor in both the onset of acute diseases and in chronic diseases. Mind–body practices can give people the skills to manage the inevitable stress of life and, therefore, they have an increasingly important role in preventing and reversing the effects of stress and disease.

Asian healing systems

The rise in popularity of mind–body medicine has been stimulated by the introduction of Asian healing methods and systems, such as yoga and Traditional Chinese Medicine, into mainstream Western culture. In the 1970s, Western medical researchers discovered that people who practiced advanced forms of yoga, for example, were able to regulate physical functions that were once considered beyond the reach of conscious control. These include the electrical activity of the brain, the temperature of the body,

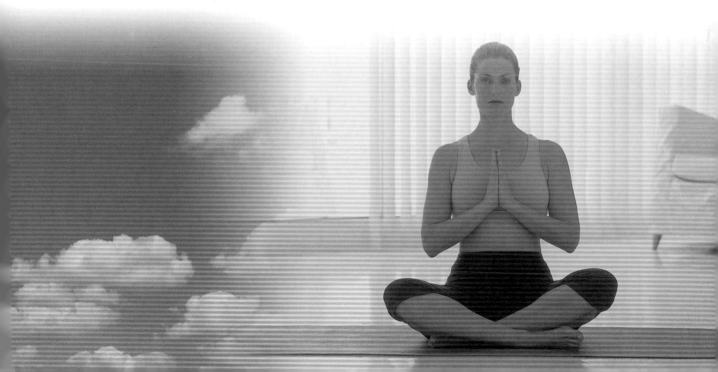

THE INTRICATE MIND–BODY CONNECTION

Mind–body interactions are not rare events but common occurrences in our everyday lives. Often mediated by the activities of nerves and hormones, the effects that one has on the other indicate that they are integrated and part of the same whole. This table lists some of those effects.

EFFECTS OF THE MIND ON THE BODY

Emotions
Emotions such as embarrassment cause physical responses such as blushing.

Stress responses
Stress and anxiety raise the levels of the hormones cortisol and epinephrine in the body. These have a variety of physical effects including:
- changes to the immune system
- increased heart rate
- slowing the digestive system.

Humor
Laughter has been shown to:
- lower blood pressure
- reduce levels of stress hormones
- boost immunity (increasing T-cells and B-cells)
- release endorphins that are natural analgesics and produce a general sense of well-being.

Imagery
We can affect the way our body behaves just by using our imagination. For example, imagine unwrapping a chocolate. Feel the paper crinkling under your fingers, smell the aroma that is released, then imagine the taste and feel of it melting on your tongue. This imagery will no doubt have activated your salivary glands!

Placebo response
Placebos (dummy treatments, such as sugar pills) can be effective in about 30 percent of patients. In other words, believing that the treatment will work can produce positive physiological responses.

EFFECTS OF THE BODY ON THE MIND

Exercise
Exercise has a variety of effects on the brain including:
- improved blood flow to the brain
- release of endorphins, mood enhancers, and analgesics similar to morphine
- alteration of serotonin levels in the brain
- increased production of a chemical called BDNF (Brain-Derived Neurotrophic Factor). This chemical helps neurons (brain cells) grow and connect.

Massage and physical contact
Physical contact with another human (or an animal) can induce feelings of relaxation and well-being.

Massage is a recognized agent for lowering stress.

Sex hormones
Sex hormones (testosterone and estrogen) alter thoughts and behavior.

Posture
Studies have established that if we stand upright, head erect, smile, and breathe deeply, it is impossible to "feel" depressed.

Immune system
Immune molecules known as cytokines can initiate brain actions. Some cytokines help the body recuperate by sending messages to the brain that set off a series of sickness responses, such as fever. The immune molecules also can trigger feelings of sluggishness, sleepiness, and loss of appetite, behaviors that encourage people to rest while they are ill.

Listening
Music can enhance mood and even have analgesic effect by encouraging endorphin release.

Biological sounds, such as a mother's heartbeat, have been used to lower infants' stress. Conversely, noise can increase heart rate, blood pressure, respiration rate, and blood cholesterol levels.

Breathing
By controlling breathing patterns, it is possible to reduce anxiety and stress responses (*see pp. 408 and 414*).

An electroencephalogram (EEG) measures the activity of delta, theta, alpha, and beta brain waves. Delta waves, on the top, are dominant in sleep. Next come theta waves, typical of a person who is drowsy or daydreaming. Alpha waves feature in drowsy adults who are relaxed or meditating. Beta waves are typical when we are focusing on something or actively engaged in a project or discussion.

the heart rate and blood pressure. Incorporating some of these Asian healing systems, researchers have discovered new ways to forestall and heal diseases that have long been considered inevitable consequences of aging.

Reclaiming wholeness

Mind–body medicine recognizes that healing does not necessarily stop when all the physical symptoms of an illness or condition disappear. Healing literally means "to make whole." From this perspective, treating illness can be viewed as an opportunity to reclaim wholeness and restore completeness, even in the face of ongoing disease. However, this can occur only when the mind and body are integrated into a whole, dynamic healing system. It is not simply a question of "mind over matter," but rather that mind matters. The Asian healing systems, such as Traditional Chinese Medicine, have affirmed the power of techniques such as relaxation and meditation and made it clear that a person's inner well-being is crucial to health.

Benefits of Mind–Body Medicine

Essential to all complementary and alternative therapies, but often overlooked, is the notion that the healing process does not work independently of the individual. Rather, it relies on internal changes in an individual's consciousness and behavior — attitude, lifestyle, self-orientation, and environmental awareness are all important. Such a holistic approach demands continuous change from an individual — one has to transform one's psychology and actively engage in the well-being of the mind and body. Since mind–body approaches necessitate such an orientation, they constitute an integral and essential part of all complementary and alternative therapies.

From the perspective of mind–body medicine, the mind, body, and spirit are interrelated, not only with each other but also with the larger social and physical environment. Physical interventions are not solely physical in their effect but also have an impact on consciousness.

Exercise, yoga, meditation, dance, relaxation therapies, visualization, imagery, and manipulative therapies can not only resolve problems in the physical organism but can also create an enhanced psychological and spiritual sense of well-being. Psychological treatments, such as meditation, psychotherapy, or imagery work, can have a demonstrable impact on physical problems, such as pain and high blood pressure, as well as their extensive psychological benefits.

Relieving stress and depression

An ever-growing body of evidence has demonstrated that psychosocial stress is an important factor in many medical conditions, ranging from coronary artery disease and chronic pain to immune problems. Within the confines of our modern environment, mental cues such as anxious thoughts, crowds, work pressures, and traffic jams, are often perceived as threatening and can trigger the fight-or-flight response even though no physical threat is involved. Moreover, psychological stressors may linger and allow the alarm response to persist far beyond its useful time. Powerful hormones released during this stress response have a specific physical impact on the body and can contribute to disease (*see Coping with Stress, p.408*).

Other negative emotions and personality traits have also been found to be associated with the risk of chronic disease. It was once thought that the "Type A" personality, which is marked by highly stressed, time-pressured, and aggressive behavior, was a reliable predictor of mortality from coronary artery disease. Actually, hostility is the Type A factor that seems to be predictive of heart attacks. In 1995, Dr. Murray Mittleman and other researchers at Harvard Medical School in the US reported their analysis of interviews with patients after they had had a heart attack. They reported that the likelihood of having a heart attack was 2.3 times greater within two hours of having an angry outburst than at other times.

Depression is also common in patients with coronary artery disease and is associated with a higher incidence of heart disease and an increased mortality rate following heart attacks. In 1996, a team of researchers led by Dr. Barefoot at Duke University studied mortality statistics for people who had a documented history of heart disease. They discovered that the mortality rate was 78 percent higher in those individuals with moderate to severe depression compared to those who were not depressed. Of course, this depression could have been the result rather than the cause of the physical illness, but clearly the entanglement of mind and body influenced the outcome of the illness.

Among their other benefits, most mind–body therapies create a relaxed state which is the opposite of the arousal characteristic of the stress response. Practicing meditation, relaxation techniques, imagery work, hypnosis, and movement therapies, such as yoga and qi gong, can all produce a beneficial relaxed state.

Techniques from cognitive behavioral therapies (CBT) (*see also Psychological Therapy, p.104*) are also employed in teaching stress management. Individuals learn to recognize stress triggers and respond to them in a different, healthier way by learning a technique called reframing, which allows them to think more positively about the stress-inducing situations they encounter. Through practicing a wide variety of CBT techniques, people learn to master symptoms that had previously been overwhelming. This allows them to build up self-confidence, which then spills over into other aspects of their professional and personal life and enables them to make positive lifestyle changes that go well beyond the alleviation of specific symptoms.

Self-care for good health

Eighty percent of all medical symptoms are self-diagnosed, self-treated, and self-limiting, which means they resolve without the need for formal medical care. Nevertheless, people often need help in learning how to take care of their health (self-care) in order to avoid more serious conditions. Mind–body therapies address the kind of psychosocial issues that need to change before people can successfully implement effective self-care. The therapies provide simple structured steps for individuals to take to benefit their health and well-being. Meditation, for example, helps people relax and become more focused. Consequently, they find it easier to give up smoking, which in turn sets up an upward spiral of health improvement.

In 1993, Dr. McGinnis and Dr. Foege published an article in the *Journal of the American Medical Association* citing a dire yet familiar litany of mortality — in other words, the ten leading causes of death. Their contention was that this list, which included cancer, heart disease, and HIV, belied a more fundamental issue. These are the terminal diseases cited in a pathologist's report or upon autopsy, but the actual causes of death include factors such as tobacco, alcohol, poor diet and inactivity patterns, stress, certain infections, drug use, deadly drug interactions from prescription medications, and so on.

Many of these "causes of death" can be avoided with better self-care practices. Mind–body therapies provide the behavioral basis for individuals to make healthy changes and are thereby the foundation for helpful self-care strategies, such as exercise, good nutritional habits, and more appropriate use of conventional medicines.

Mind–Body Approaches

There are four main mind–body approaches in Western medicine: meditation and relaxation, guided imagery, clinical biofeedback, and hypnosis. In addition, there are a number of other therapies recommended throughout the ailment section of this book. Some therapies overlap. Relaxation and stress-management techniques, in particular, are essential components of all of the therapies. Physiological benefits of relaxing include:

- Decreased levels of epinephrine, sugar, and cholesterol in the blood.
- Reduced blood pressure and less stress on the cardiovascular system.
- Slower breathing with improved lung function and metabolic rate.
- Relaxed muscles, which contain less lactic acid.
- Improved digestion.
- Skin cools down with less activity from the sweat glands.

Meditation and relaxation

Meditation is a long-standing feature of various spiritual and religious traditions. In the secular context, it is a self-directed practice that quiets the mind and relaxes the body, bringing benefits for health and a sense of well-being. The heightened awareness and inner peace that meditation brings can combat stress and anxiety, relieve headaches and fatigue, and help people cope with long-term pain.

During the 1960s, reports reached the West about yogis and practitioners of meditation in India and elsewhere who were able to achieve an extraordinary degree of

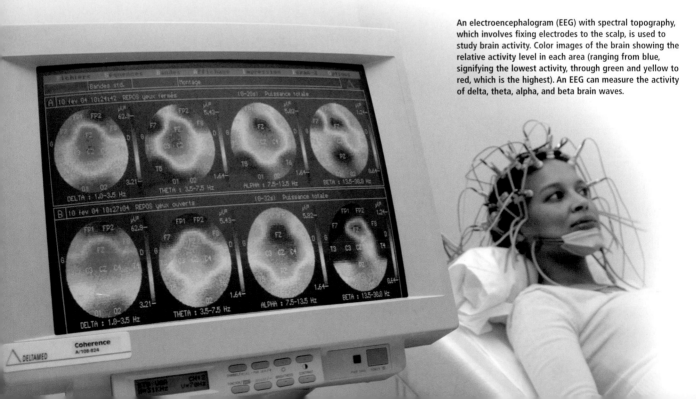

An electroencephalogram (EEG) with spectral topography, which involves fixing electrodes to the scalp, is used to study brain activity. Color images of the brain showing the relative activity level in each area (ranging from blue, signifying the lowest activity, through green and yellow to red, which is the highest). An EEG can measure the activity of delta, theta, alpha, and beta brain waves.

control over supposedly involuntary bodily functions such as breathing, pulse rates, and blood pressure. Studies by myself and my colleagues at medical research centers, including Harvard Medical School, UCLA, Menninger Foundation, and the University of California School of Medicine in San Francisco, substantiated the reports of these remarkable abilities of self-regulation.

While there are major philosophical differences underpinning the hundreds of forms of meditation, at a biological level they have very similar effects on human biochemistry and on the nervous and immune systems. The benefits that research has discovered are based mainly on studies into transcendental meditation, but they can be attributed equally to other types of meditative practice.

Transcendental meditation
One of the most prominent meditation movements in the US in the 1960s was Transcendental Meditation (TM), developed by the Maharashi Mahesh Yogi and popularized by the Beatles. This practice consists of sitting and silently repeating a mantra (a word or a sound) twice a day for 20 minutes, for the stated purpose of achieving "restful alertness" and a state of "unifying capacity."

Studies by Professor Herbert Benson (of the Mind/Body Medical Institute of Harvard Medical School) and others in the late 1960s showed that TM brings about a healthy state of relaxation. An individual in this relaxed state exhibits a decreased responsiveness of the autonomic nervous system, a reduced heart and respiration rate, a decreased output of cortisol released by the adrenal glands, and an increased occurrence of alpha waves, the brainwave frequency associated with a relaxed state. Eventually, Benson developed a generic relaxation method which he termed the "relaxation response" (*see box, right*).

Mindfulness meditation
Among the most commonly used and well-documented forms of meditation in clinical research is "mindfulness" meditation. The art of this Buddhist-based practice is to maintain awareness, in the present moment, of the bodily sensations and flow of thoughts but without passing judgment on them. It differs from concentrative meditation, such as TM, which maintains passive attention on a word, a bodily process (such as breathing), or another stimulus.

Guided imagery

Imagery is a flow of thoughts that embody sensory qualities. It has been used for millennia in every indigenous culture and country of the world as part of shamanic healing practices. As a mind–body therapy, it enlists an individual's imagination in evoking one or more of the senses, usually sound, vision, warmth, and movement. In modern clinical settings the therapist generally guides the individual's creation of images. Individuals may also employ imagery

---

RELAXATION

Practice the following steps for 10–20 minutes every day (but not within two hours of eating a meal) to help ease tension and relieve stress.

- Find a comfortable position, sit quietly, and close your eyes.
- Starting at your feet, relax your muscles. Work your way up your legs, torso, hands, arms, neck, face, and head, relaxing the muscles as you go. Keep all the muscles relaxed.
- Inhale through your nose and focus on your breathing. As you exhale, silently say "ONE" in your mind. Continue breathing consciously but naturally for 10–20 minutes. Thoughts will try to distract you — just repeat "ONE" as you exhale and continue your breathing.
- To finish, sit quietly for a few minutes — at first with closed eyes and then with them open.

---

on their own without any instruction or supervision from health practitioners. Sometimes spontaneous imagery in sleep or daydreaming episodes can provide profound personal insights and can be the basis for creativity and scientific discoveries.

Imagery is often incorrectly referred to as visualization, but it can equally entail imagining smell, touch, hearing, taste, proprioception (the unconscious perception of movement and spatial orientation), and motion.

Many mind–body therapies contain a spontaneous and/or a "guided" imagery component. Guided imagery is purely psychological and can occur with or without a physically quiet state. Biofeedback, desensitization, and aversion techniques, hypnosis, autogenic training, gestalt therapy, Jacobson's progressive relaxation, neurolinguistic programming (NLP), and rational emotive behavior therapy (REBT) include guided imagery in their approach.

Meditation that involves focusing on a mantra, imagined sound, or object of contemplation also uses imagery, as do relaxation techniques that include sensory instructions. Imagery is also related to hypnosis in that they both elicit similar states of consciousness and have similar uses in practice. In fact, research has discovered that there is a correlation between the ability to imagine and the capacity to enter into an altered or hypnotic state.

Imagery for better health
Imagery may be used early on in a therapy session to help the practitioner arrive at a diagnosis. A person may be asked to describe his or her condition or problem in sensory terms. Often, the resulting description can provide a basis for the kinds of therapeutic treatments that are chosen and give a significant insight into the person's subjective experience of his or her condition. Imagery is also a powerful aid in achieving insight and perspective into a person's health and in making contact with emotions.

EXERCISES FOR IMAGERY AND AUTOSUGGESTION

Imagery can help you relax and deal with pain or other problems by imagining positive images and desired outcomes. Here are some suggestions for images:
- Imagine your symptoms as a slowly melting block of ice.
- Picture the affected part of your body working perfectly.
- To induce serenity, try a "focused daydream." Imagine walking up a sunlit path alongside a waterfall, or picture a stormy sea that slowly quiets down as you sail into port.

Practice the following up to three times a day:
- Choose an image or desired outcome that you wish to visualize.
- Find a quiet place and either lie down or sit comfortably so that your whole body can relax and you can let your mind go.
- Inhale and exhale slowly through your nose until you relax.
- Concentrate on your chosen image for as long as you can. Focus on every detail. What can you hear? How do you feel?

You can learn to hypnotize yourself safely and effectively with the following autosuggestion technique. Make sure you are clear about the purpose of the self-hypnosis — for example, to ease your asthma, be less anxious, or become more confident — and be prepared to practice it every day.

- Sit or lie in a comfortable position, close your eyes and relax your whole body.
- Count from ten to zero and imagine yourself walking down a flight of stairs or along a clearly defined woodland path.
- Repeat words that positively summarize what you want to achieve, such as "the pain is going away." Alternatively, listen to a recording of the words.
- When you have finished, count from zero to ten as you walk up the flight of stairs or return along the path.
- Rest for a minute with your eyes closed.

One way of doing this is to use imagery in a receptive mode, in which the person has an imaginary dialogue with an image that represents his or her symptoms or illness, and the image communicates information about the meaning of sensations and symptoms.

Imagery work can also be used by therapists to put patients in touch with an "inner advisor" who helps them achieve insight into their medical problems.

Mental rehearsal

In a technique called mental or psychological rehearsal, imagery is used to help the person prepare for medical procedures, such as invasive diagnostics or surgery. The technique can help relieve pain and anxiety and prevent side effects from procedures, such as chemotherapy, which may be aggravated by intense emotional reactions. When imagery is used in this way, the patient is generally guided by a therapist into a relaxed state and then led through a series of images in which the treatment and the recovery process are described in sensory terms, along with the desired outcome.

Patients may be encouraged to create their own system of images involving the healing process, or they may be guided through a series of images to relax, divert their attention, or diminish sympathetic nervous system arousal. Preparatory imagery work can help patients experience less pain following surgery. It can encourage them to relax the muscles around the incision site as well as hasten the return of bowel function and prevent excessive blood loss by redirecting blood flow to other parts of the body. Mental rehearsal imagery also helps patients deal with anxiety-producing diagnostic procedures, such as MRI scans, which can make some people feel claustrophobic because they have to spend time inside a scanner.

Research with mental rehearsal has yielded highly positive and often dramatic results, which include: reduced pain and anxiety, shorter hospital stays, less need for medication, and a reduction in the number and intensity of side-effects from treatment. Mental rehearsal is also used regularly to help prepare mothers-to-be for natural childbirth.

Clinical biofeedback

Clinical biofeedback is a training technique in which people learn to consciously regulate bodily functions, such as heart rate or blood pressure, that are not normally accessible to voluntary control. It applies to any process that measures and reports back information about the system that the individual is attempting to control, with the goal of improving or eliminating a symptom or illness.

Biofeedback dates back to the late 1930s, when Dr. O. Hobart Mowrer invented an alarm that could be triggered by urine as a way to train children to stop bed-wetting. In 1961, noted psychologist Dr. Neal Miller from Yale University explored the unorthodox hypothesis that responses of the autonomic nervous system, such as heart rate and bowel movement, could be conditioned. He conducted a series of groundbreaking experiments that demonstrated how control of autonomic processes could be learned through biofeedback techniques.

In the early 1960s, Dr. Joe Kaniya of the University of California School of Medicine in San Francisco, Dr. Barbara Brown at the Veterans Administration Hospital in Sepulveda, California, and Dr. Elmer and Dr. Alyce Green at the Menninger Foundation, Kansas, used biofeedback devices to monitor and record self-regulatory feats of yogis. It was through these remarkable experiments that biofeedback began to attract wider attention.

Measurements and devices

Most commonly, clinical biofeedback is a feature of several measurements and devices. Electrocardiographs (ECGs), for example, reveal the electrical activity of the heartbeat (*see Angina, p.249*) and echocardiographs provide ultrasound scans of the heart muscle. Electroencephalographs (EEGs) provide feedback on electrical brainwave activity and electromyographs (EMGs) monitor muscle tension via visual or auditory signals. Skin temperature gauges measure the heat generated at the surface of the skin and galvanic skin response (GSR) sensors detect the electrical conductivity of the skin, which increases when the skin sweats because of stress.

In a typical biofeedback session, people are connected to biofeedback devices and then use breathing, muscle relaxation, and other techniques to help them relax. The machines transmit signals when this is achieved. In this way, people learn to relax at will and and achieve their desired outcome, such as reducing blood pressure, relieving headaches, and coping with asthma. It takes practice, but soon people can attain a slow but even heartbeat, plenty of alpha brainwaves, low-level muscle activity, and a warm skin with little activity in the sweat glands.

With the development of increasingly sophisticated monitoring devices and computerized, multiple-channel instrumentation, new possibilities have been opened up for clinical biofeedback training. For example, sensors can monitor and feed back the activity of the rectal sphincter and the muscles controlling the bladder to help people who are incontinent. Esophageal motility can be monitored to provide feedback on the muscles of the esophagus since esophageal spasms are very painful and can be self-regulated through hypnosis and/or clinical biofeedback. Other instruments can monitor gastrointestinal functions and stomach acidity.

Hypnosis and hypnotherapy

In the late 18th century, the practice of the power of suggestion was introduced to medicine by the French physician Dr. Franz Anton Mesmer under the name of Mesmerism. He attributed the effects of hypnosis to the presence of a universal fluid that produced disease when it was out of balance in the body. After his ideas were discredited, the name was changed to hypnosis (from the Greek word *hypnos*, meaning sleep). Dr. James Esdaile, an English surgeon stationed in India, performed surgery using hypnotic anesthesia. In the late 19th century, hypnosis became popular when Sigmund Freud used it in his early psychiatric practice.

A hypnotherapist guides an individual from ordinary consciousnesses into a state of focused concentration, in which the individual is highly responsive to suggestion. Hypnotherapy, as the practice of hypnosis has come to be called, was recognized as a valid medical treatment by the American Medical Association in 1958 and by the British Medical Association in 1955.

Today, the American Society of Clinical Hypnosis (ASCH) is the main professional organization in the US, with more than 4,000 members who must be licensed health professionals and have achieved a minimum of 20 hours of training in hypnotherapy. There are between 3,000–6,000 other practitioners of hypnotherapy, including nurses, social workers, and lay therapists.

In the UK, there are about 300 qualified hypnotherapists registered with the UK Council for Psychotherapy (UKCP), with a larger number registered with other organizations, such as the General Hypnotherapy Register and the National Council for Hypnotherapy (NCH).

Benefits of hypnosis

Physiologically, the hypnotic state, which does not necessarily involve a trance, is similar to other forms of deep relaxation, with reduced sympathetic nervous system activity, decreased blood pressure, slowed heart rate, and increased activity of the alpha and theta brainwaves. Compared to guided imagery, self-hypnosis is much more purely physical and can occur without the use of any imagery — guided or otherwise.

Hypnosis has come to be viewed as a way of gaining access to deep levels of the mind in order to bring about changes in behavior or alterations in psychological states. Hypnotherapy often uses imagery to modify feelings of pain, anxiety, and fear, or to introduce suggestions regarding the behavior required to achieve therapeutic goals. Once out of the hypnotic state, the subject is expected to practice these new behaviors.

How hypnosis works

Doctors, psychotherapists, dentists, and other health-care providers use hypnotherapy to treat a wide variety of medical and psychological problems. Methods of hypnotic induction and specific suggestions and imagery are tailored to meet the needs of the individual client. It can be used as a form of analgesia in surgery, to control allergies, reduce stress, and produce changes in behavior for better health; for example, it can help people to quit smoking.

Hypnotherapy can be employed either by itself or in conjunction with other forms of treatment. When used in the treatment of chronic illness, hypnosis can help alleviate anxiety, decrease the need for medication, and make medical procedures more comfortable. In 1989, one study showed that hypnosis could increase pain tolerance by 113 percent among highly hypnotizable subjects when compared to a control group.

When employed by qualified practitioners (*see above*), hypnosis is very safe, but it is a powerful technique that must be used with caution. Consequently, individuals who have a history of serious psychiatric problems are not appropriate candidates for hypnotherapy.

Hypnotizability

Individuals vary greatly in their "hypnotizability" — their susceptibility to hypnosis. According to a 1983 World Health Organization estimate, 90 percent of people can be hypnotized and 20–30 percent are susceptible enough to enter the deep state that makes them ideally responsive to hypnotic suggestion. Most people can learn to hypnotize themselves, either from a book with audio tapes or from a hypnotherapist, with a technique called autosuggestion. You may be able to use this self-hypnosis to relieve pain, boost self-confidence, and ease an attack of asthma.

Experimental evidence suggests that elderly people are less susceptible to hypnosis, and hence they may not make as good candidates for hypnotherapy as younger subjects. A 1972 study tested susceptibility to hypnosis among different age groups and produced evidence that confirmed that hypnotizability decreases with age. Other factors that may influence hypnotizability include a compromised autonomic nervous system, which is also characteristic of some elderly people. Many studies of hypnosis have been based on research with students and other young people, which may make the results inapplicable to the elderly.

Other mind–body techniques

In addition to the four main approaches described above, a number of other mind–body therapies are suggested in this book. Movement therapies (*see p.62*) such as yoga and t'ai chi have mind–body components and there is also an overlap between mind–body therapies and psychological techniques (*see p.104*).

Autogenic training (AT)

This is a series of six mental exercises that switch off the body's stress responses and encourage calmness in the mind and relaxation in both involuntary and voluntary muscles. The name is derived from Greek and means "generated from within." Devised by German neurologist and psychiatrist Dr. Johannes Schultz in Berlin in the 1920s, AT is normally taught by a practitioner in eight weekly sessions that last for 90 minutes each. AT can help various ailments, from stress and anxiety to high blood pressure and eczema. The length of treatment does not seem to affect clinical outcome.

Gestalt therapy

In this technique, which is also used in humanistic psychotherapy (*see Psychological Therapy, p.104*), a practitioner helps the client gain self-awareness of habitual thoughts, feelings, and actions, and express any thoughts and emotions that may be repressed. The name derives from German and means "organized whole." Developed by German psychoanalyst Fritz Perls in the 1960s, gestalt therapy sessions are held weekly, either on a one-to-one basis or in groups, and may involve recalling a dream and role playing.

Eye-movement desensitization and reprocessing (EMDR)

This information-processing therapy is a technique that integrates elements of various psychotherapies, such as cognitive behavioral therapy, psychodynamic therapy, experiential therapy, and interpersonal psychotherapy (*see p.107, and Post-Traumatic Stress disorder, p.422*). EMDR was discovered by American psychologist Francine Shapiro in 1987 and has proved useful in treating traumatic disorders, such as PTSD, phobias, and anxiety.

Meditation helps bring thoughts under control and relieve any stress you may be feeling. Regular practice can lower the breathing and heart rate and induce a sense of calm.

During EMDR treatment, patients move their eyes from side to side while simultaneously discussing their anxieties with the therapist. The eye movement is thought to help the brain process painful thoughts. Sessions are held on a one-to-one basis and vary in duration according to an individual's needs.

Jacobson's progressive relaxation

American physiologist Edmund Jacobson developed his relaxation method in the 1930s. It involves systematically tensing and relaxing every major muscle group in their body (*see box on Relaxation, p.99*).

Neurolinguistic programming (NLP)

Developed in the 1970s by American psychotherapists John Grinder and Richard Bandler, this technique combines cognitive behavioral therapy with elements of humanistic psychotherapy (*see Psychological Therapy, p.104*) and hypnotherapy. An NLP practitioner helps a person consciously reprogram their patterns of speech and body language with the aim of improving their communication skills and bringing about personal change. Sessions may be held weekly on a one-to-one basis and vary according to an individual's needs.

Psychoeducation

By using books, brochures, illustrations, videos, and/or audio tapes the patient can literally be educated on the specific nature of their condition to give them a sense of greater mastery and control through better understanding. This can be an important method of providing advice and information about a person's psychological or behavioral problems. Psychoeducation benefits the person and his or her family so that they are better informed about the kinds of treatment that are required and better prepared for the treatment itself. The technique has proved useful for people with cancer, eating disorders, ADHD, and depression.

Rational emotive behavior therapy (REBT)

This cognitive behavioral technique is designed to replace the irrational thinking behind negative emotions with more positive and flexible patterns of thought to help people attain their goals. Developed by American psychoanalyst Albert Ellis in 1955, it is useful for anxiety, stammering, depression, and addictions. Generally, REBT sessions lasting up to an hour may take place once a week, with homework assignments designed to help patients learn skills faster.

Visualization

More correctly known as imagery (*see Guided Imagery, p.99*), visualization encourages people to imagine positive images and desired outcomes in order to help them change negative attitudes and overcome various ailments, such as stress, pain, anxieties, and phobias, and to cope with chronic illnesses, such as cancer.

Summary of Research Evidence

Dr. John A. Astin of the Complementary Medicine Program at the California Pacific Medical Center, San Francisco, has conducted one of the best designed overviews of the applications of mind–body medicine. He writes "There is now considerable evidence that an array of mind–body therapies can be used as effective adjuncts to conventional medical treatment for a number of common clinical conditions." Astin's 2002 review underscores the fact that mind–body therapies can be readily integrated into the treatment of many conditions, often combining self-care practice with clinical care.

Moderate to strong evidence

Extensive randomized controlled trials (*see p.23*) and/or systematic reviews (critical statistical analysis of previously published research) reveal that there is moderate to strong evidence of the clinical efficacy of mind–body therapies for the following 11 conditions: coronary artery disease (*see p.252*); high blood pressure (*see p.244*); insomnia (*see p.448*); general pain syndromes (*see Persistent Pain, p.144*); low back pain (*see p.268*); headaches (*see p.114*); fibromyalgia (*see p.298*); arthritis self-care (*see p.289* and *p.293*); living with cancer (*see p.464*); incontinence; and recovery from surgery.

Mind–body therapies are at least as good as, if not better than, many common conventional treatments. Given their relative simplicity, low cost, and absence of side effects, the findings are particularly significant.

Positive efficacy

Most current randomized controlled trials indicate that mind–body therapies are useful for the following conditions: allergies (*see p.456*); asthma (*see p.205*); chronic obstructive pulmonary disease; dermatological disorders (*see Skin, p.156*); diabetes (*see p.314*); living with HIV (*see p.470*); irritable bowel syndrome (*see p.222*); peptic ulcers (*see p.219*); post-stroke rehabilitation (*see p.148*); pregnancy and labor (*see p.358*); and tinnitus (*see p.188*).

FINDING A PRACTITIONER

Many practitioners work in the field of mind–body medicine, so before arranging a consultation make sure they are qualified and registered. Contact the relevant professional organization for details and lists of practitioners in your area (*see Useful Addresses, p.486*). Some psychologists practice hypnosis — your doctor may be able to refer you. Classes for meditation and other self-help mind–body skills are widely available — check your local listings for details.

PSYCHOLOGICAL THERAPY

DR. ADRIAN HEMMINGS

Psychological therapy focuses on the talking therapies, which are grouped together into five general approaches. Qualified practitioners provide a formal and professional relationship within which a person can usefully explore difficult, and often painful, emotions and experiences. These may include feelings of anxiety, depression, trauma, or perhaps the loss of meaning in life. It is a process that seeks to help the person gain an increased capacity for choice, thereby becoming more autonomous and self-determined.

Psychological health

The health of the human mind (*psyche*) is much more difficult to establish than the well-being of the body. How we deal with people and the world around us says a lot about our ability to cope with the ups and downs of life, but whether it exposes the secret world of unconscious motivations is another matter.

In general, a healthy mind implies being content with yourself. For healthy people, on the whole, life has meaning and fulfillment. They have friends and family to whom they can express thoughts and emotions. They do not fear change and are always ready to learn. Amid the stresses and strains of everyday life they are able to enjoy themselves. A healthy mind is one that can deal with both positive and negative events, from getting married to a death in the family. It is normal to feel frustration as well as happiness, or anger as well as joy. It is how people deal with the stresses and the intensity of feelings that is important. This depends on an innate ability (nature) as well as the psychological responses learned during the growing up process (nurture).

Psychological problems and their causes

There are many signs of psychological problems. There may be a marked personality change or simply an inability to cope. Some people may have strange, grandiose, or obsessive ideas. A prolonged period of depression and apathy, as well as marked changes in eating or sleeping patterns, may also be indications of psychological

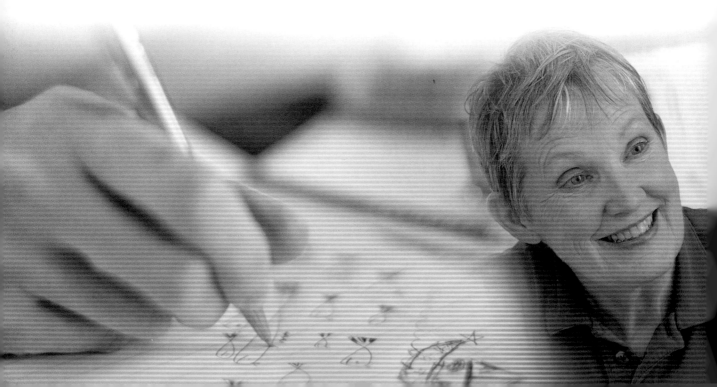

problems. Thinking or talking about suicide, extreme emotional highs and lows, and the abuse of alcohol or drugs are signs of psychological difficulties, as are excessive outbursts of anger, hostility, or violent behavior.

Psychological problems have various origins, which can be placed in a number of categories. An individual's life history is an important factor in the development of psychological problems. It is when people are young that they develop their basic assumptions of others and themselves, as well as their strategies for coping with life. These strategies need continual updating — a strategy that may have been appropriate at the age of five is no longer useful at the age of 40. Sometimes people cling to outmoded and detrimental strategies that then lead to difficulties in current relationships and eventually to psychological and emotional distress.

Some people have a genetic propensity to psychological problems. This could be due to the way in which their brain is formed or because they easily produce excess stress hormones, making them more likely to be susceptible to stressful life events. Physical ill-health can affect a person's psychological well-being, too. Seriously ill people may become depressed or anxious. This in turn can affect their physical health, slowing their recovery and possibly making them more depressed — and so the cycle continues.

Situational factors can negatively influence psychological well-being — for example, living in a socially deprived area with frequent vandalism and drug abuse. Trauma, such as a car accident or physical attack, or even the witnessing of a traumatic event, can produce adverse reactions that can lead to post-traumatic stress. Loss and bereavement, while a natural part of life, can also affect people's psychological health and while all societies have rituals in place to facilitate the grieving process, some people find it very difficult to come to terms with their loss.

Cultural factors can affect the person's sense of identity and belonging and can have a direct effect on an individual's sense of psychological well-being. For example, people from immigrant populations encounter more psychosocial problems than those in the dominant culture.

Each category can produce psychological problems on its own, but it is usually when there are two or more factors that psychological "dis-ease" takes hold. For instance, if someone has had a very difficult early life, he or she may respond more negatively to a traumatic event than someone who has had a stable, loving childhood. However, people's reactions are unpredictable. Someone with a difficult early life, for example, may have learned at an early age to cope with trauma and therefore manage better than the person with a stable background who has not encountered any traumatic events.

The beginnings of psychoanalysis

Many identify the birth of talking therapies as we know them with Sigmund Freud and his mentor Josef Breuer. When Breuer hypnotized a woman with symptoms that included paralysis, blackouts, and an aversion to water, she revisited her childhood memories and became distressed. The experience had a profound cathartic effect, causing many of her symptoms to disappear. Such cases inspired Freud to introduce the concept of the unconscious where, he believed, the motives for our emotions, thoughts, and actions lie buried. He developed psychoanalysis to allow

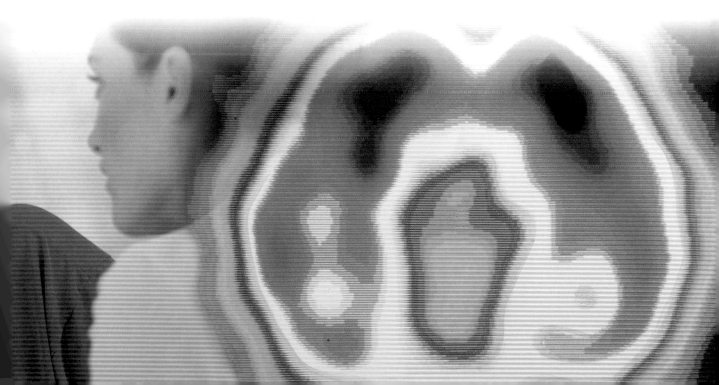

THE FIVE APPROACHES OF PSYCHOLOGICAL THERAPIES

Talking therapies can be broadly grouped into five categories, depending on the approach adopted.	APPROACH	DESCRIPTION	EXAMPLES	CONDITIONS
	Psychoanalytical and psychodynamic	A therapist listens to your experiences and explores links between present emotions and actions and past events, particularly those in your childhood.	Jungian analytic therapy Psychodynamic therapy	Personality disorders Depression Eating disorders
	Cognitive behavioral	This combines concepts and techniques from cognitive (thinking) and behavior therapies. The therapist listens to your experiences and offers insights into your negative thoughts, beliefs, and behaviors, and then encourages you to explore and practice a new way of thinking or behaving.	Cognitive-behavioral therapy (CBT) Systemic desensitization Behavioral therapy 12-step program for addiction	Post-traumatic stress disorder Depressive disorders Anxiety disorders and phobias Eating disorders Schizrenia Addiction Chronic fatigue
	Systemic	A systemic therapist explores relationships by treating them as systems,. For example, in a family system one person's behavior provokes reactions in others. Systemic approaches are most often used with couples and families or other groups, but can be used by individuals.	Family therapy	Eating disorders in adolescents (involving a whole family)
	Humanistic	Counselors often use a humanistic approach. By exploring and understanding your experiences in an accepting and non-judgmental atmosphere, the therapist can help increase your awareness of your problems and your potential for finding solutions.	Client-centered therapy (a form of counseling, although counselors can use many different approaches)	Help adjusting to life events, illnesses, disabilities, or losses
	Interpersonal	In-depth exploration of how people relate to others, and ways of changing the pattern of those relationships.	Interpersonal group therapy	Relationship difficulties Depressive disorders Eating disorders Addiction

his patients to talk freely so that they could reveal their buried motives and be released from their psychological crisis. One of his pupils, Carl Jung, believed that people share a collective unconscious and that individuals had a "shadow" side, which they repressed. He evolved his own version of psychoanalysis to help individuals integrate this shadow side into their lives and thereby find their true self.

The five approaches

Since the time of Freud and Jung, the talking therapies have developed considerably. About 400 recognizable types can be grouped into five approaches that differ mainly in their emphasis rather than in fundamental assumptions.

Psychoanalytic and psychodynamic approach

These therapies originate in the ideas of Freud and include Jungian analytic therapy and psychodynamic therapy, which is used for depression, post-traumatic stress disorder, and eating disorders. The therapist listens to the person's account of his or her experiences and explores the connections between what the person is thinking, doing,

and feeling in both the present and the past, particularly in childhood. Thoughts, emotions, and feelings that were repressed earlier in life emerge into consciousness and may cause problems, such as conflicts, anguish, or anxiety.

Analyzing the person's dreams, creative experiences, and relationships with others is crucial. The key to the process of psychoanalysis is "transference," by which the person transfers feelings onto the therapist as a means of exposing, identifying, and resolving them.

This approach often takes a long time (several sessions a week for one to seven years). However, adapted techniques can shorten this to about 10 weeks when there is a specific problem such as a bereavement. Psychoanalysis can be carried out individually or in groups.

Cognitive behavioral approach

Clinical psychologists developed this approach in the 1960s by combining features from behavioral and cognitive therapy. Behavior therapy, which is based on the work of Ivan Pavlov and B. F. Skinner, uses reward and punishment as a way of "reconditioning" behavior. Cognitive therapy, developed by psychotherapist Aaron T. Beck, relies on the power of a person's mind to identify and transform his or her negative mental processes (cognition) into more positive powers of self-perception.

Cognitive behavioral therapies (CBTs) focus on the "how" rather than the "why" of problems. At first, the therapist helps people become more aware of problematic thoughts and habits, and then initiates a plan whereby the person is encouraged to think of new ways of behaving and to record the thoughts and feelings inspired by them.

CBTs can prove particularly useful for depression and anxiety. Individual therapies include gradual exposure therapy for phobias and obsessive–compulsive disorder (OCD); systematic desensitization for phobias; behavioral therapy for insomnia; ritual prevention for OCD; and brief therapy for depression. CBTs for post-traumatic stress disorder include anxiety management, stress inoculation therapy, systematic desensitization, and eye movement desensitisation and reprocessing (EMDR, *see p.424*).

Systemic approach

In the 1940s, systems theory was developed to explain the way phenomena were organized, by focusing on the arrangement and relationship of the parts as they belonged to the whole. Systemic psychological therapies developed when systems theory was considered in tandem with the feedback mechanisms of cybernetics and the family studies of social anthropology. The systemic approach focuses on a human system, such as a family, team, or community, in which people live or work together. The family therapist examines how members of a family relate to and communicate with each other, and how the family as a whole maintains itself and what, for them, constitutes "normality." If, for instance, a family member behaves uncharacteristically, the other members are likely to change their behavior in order to keep things as "normal" as possible (known as maintaining homeostasis). Therapists may then actively help the family resolve their problems. Systemic approaches are usually short term and carried out with groups, such as families or couples, but they can also be used as a way of understanding an individual.

Experiential or humanistic approaches

These approaches from the 1950s and 1960s are rooted in the work of Abraham Maslow and others, and in the philosophies of humanism, existentialism, and phenomenology. Humanists believe moral values come from human nature and experience. Existentialists believe that, because of our desire to be rational in an irrational universe, the individual defines everything in his or her own world. Phenomenologists believe in the primacy of perception; to them, the human mind needs to relearn the way it engages with immediate experience.

These approaches include gestalt therapy, client-centered therapy, person-centered psychosynthesis, transactional analysis, psychodrama, primal therapy, and rebirthing.

Their emphasis is on the experience of the person living in an environment that is often hostile and dehumanizing. The therapist encourages the person to become more aware of the immediate experience and to notice how he or she has adapted to their environment. The person may then be facilitated to risk becoming more authentic and "real." Experiental and humanistic therapies are carried out with individuals, couples, and groups.

Interpersonal approach (ITP)

ITP was developed in the 1980s by Gerald Kerman and Myrna Weissman from the ideas of Harry Sullivan, as a way of treating depression. The approaches have been adapted for use with various problems, such as bulimia and substance abuse. ITP is highly structured and focuses on the problems that arise between people in a work, social, family, or marital environment. The therapist encourages people to examine how they relate to others and to look at ways of changing their "relational style." It involves identifying why breakdowns in communication and unreasonable expectations take place. ITP is short term: individuals attend 12–16 sessions that last an hour and take place weekly.

Do psychological therapies work?

Talking therapies can help people cope better with depression, anxieties, eating disorders, relationship problems, substance abuse and behavioral dependency, psychotic illness, sexual dysfunction, sexual abuse, bereavement, irritable bowel syndrome, asthma, chronic pain, and long-term illnesses such as cancer and HIV. Thousands of research studies support the use of talking therapies. Meta-analyses (statistical overviews of independent studies) have shown that people who have participated in a talking therapy are 80 percent more likely to recover than those who did not. Some studies have compared the effectiveness of different pyschological approaches but not enough research has been done in this area. When reading about diseases in this book, bear in mind that where one talking therapy is suggested as effective for an ailment, it may simply mean that others have not yet been researched for that condition.

FINDING A PRACTITIONER

Membership in a recognized organization and a list of qualifications may not be a guarantee of good practice, but it does provide some safeguards. Check if a therapist is an accredited member of an organization such as the National Mental Health Association (*see p.486*). At the first session, ask the therapist to explain about confidentiality, payment, and how many sessions you are likely to need.

Diseases &

Disorders

GENERAL ADVICE & PRECAUTIONS

The 110 conditions that appear in this book have been selected because they respond best to an integrated, holistic approach to treatment that combines complementary therapies with conventional medical practice. The objective of the book is to provide readers with an overview of each condition — what it is, why it occurs, who is most likely to be affected — and a unique summary of the best treatments for these conditions. The text for each treatment has been written by a leading practitioner in the field (see Contributors, p.5). The juxtaposition of these varied approaches demonstrate how, in many cases, complementary and conventional medicine can work in tandem to alleviate symptoms, improve well-being, and, in some cases, provide a cure.

ESSENTIAL COMPONENTS

Information is organized for each condition in a standard way. Each ailment has a number of essential components. These include lists, boxes, and bulleted compilations of practical advice to which you can turn for help or immediate relief.

Symptoms, factors, and triggers
The symptoms of a condition, and the reasons it may have arisen, are listed on the left-hand side of each opening page. Predisposing factors make the condition more likely. Triggers are known to cause the condition.

Caution boxes warn you of side effects, alert you to potential interactions between treatments, provide advice on when some treatments are not appropriate, and tell when you should consult a practitioner.

WHAT ARE THE SYMPTOMS?

Symptoms usually begin 1–3 weeks following infection and may include:
- A mild fever, headache, or flulike symptoms
- Rash that appears as crops of small red spots. The spots become itchy and fluid-filled, then dry out and form scabs
- Discomfort in the mouth if spots develop there
- Possible complications include bacterial infections of the rash

WHY MIGHT MY CHILD HAVE THIS?

PREDISPOSING FACTORS
- Weakened immune system

TREATMENT PLAN

PRIMARY TREATMENTS
- Give fluids and acetaminophen (see *Helping Your Child, right*)
- Antiviral drugs (in some cases, e.g., where immunity is compromised by other illnesses or drugs)

BACKUP TREATMENTS
- Antibiotics (if a secondary infection occurs)
- Nutritional therapy
- Rhus toxicodendron and other homeopathic medicines

For an explanation of how treatments are rated, see p.111.

CHICKENPOX

Chickenpox, also known as varicella, is a contagious viral illness that is common in children. It is caused by the varicella zoster virus and results in a characteristic rash of fluid-filled spots that are usually widespread over the body. Chickenpox is usually mild in children, but symptoms tend to be more severe in young babies, adolescents, and adults. The main aim of treatment is to fight the virus and enhance the function of the immune system.

WHY DOES IT OCCUR?

The varicella zoster virus that causes chickenpox is transmitted through airborne droplets contained in the coughs and sneezes of infected people. It can also be transmitted by direct contact with the rash of spots and blisters.

Once the rash appears, the tiny red spots quickly turn into itchy, fluid-filled blisters. These dry out within 24 hours and form scabs. Several crops of spots can appear.

Someone with chickenpox is infectious from about two days before the rash appears until the last spots have formed scabs, usually 10–14 days after the onset of the rash.

COMPLICATIONS Bacterial infection of the blisters caused by scratching the itchy rash is the most common complication of chickenpox. Newborn babies and people with weakened immune systems (such as those who are undergoing chemotherapy) are likely to have more serious varicella infections and may also develop other complications, such as pneumonia.

THE RELATIONSHIP OF CHICKENPOX TO SHINGLES People who have had chickenpox are then immune to the disease and cannot catch it again. However, the virus remains dormant in nerve cells and may be reactivated later in life, causing shingles (see p.165). People who have not had chickenpox can catch it from someone with the shingles rash and not via coughs and sneezes. However, it is not possible to develop shingles without having first had chickenpox, even if it was only a very mild episode a long time ago.

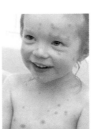
The chickenpox rash first affects the skin on the body, then spreads to the face and limbs. The spots become itchy, fluid-filled blisters that dry out and then form scabs.

HELPING YOUR CHILD

PRIMARY TREATMENT For a child with a mild infection who does not need to see a doctor, try the following measures:
- Let your child rest.
- Reduce the fever by dabbing the skin with a cool washcloth. Encourage your child to drink plenty of cool fluids to prevent dehydration. Thirst is often

IMPORTANT

Pregnant women who develop chickenpox, or who are exposed to the infection for the first time, should see their doctor.

absent and dehydration is a real danger, especially for babies. Offering a lot of small sips is usually best, especially when nausea is a problem. A plastic medicine dropper that holds a few fluid ounces is useful.
- To relieve discomfort, give acetaminophen to children over three months (do not give aspirin to children under the age of 12 years because of the risk of Reye syndrome).
- Give your child a warm-water bath that contains either a handful of bicarbonate of soda or two cups of powdered oatmeal to soothe itching.
- Use cotton to gently dab calamine lotion onto the spots to relieve itching. Alternatively, apply a gel of chickweed (*Stellaria media*) and/or a paste made from slippery elm (*Ulmus fulva*) powder, baking soda, and water to the spots.
- Keep your child's fingernails short and try to prevent him or her from scratching the spots and blisters to prevent skin infections. Babies may need to wear mittens to keep them from scratching.

TREATMENTS IN DETAIL

Conventional Medicine

If your child is healthy, the infection is likely to be mild and will not need treatment. The child will normally recover fully between 10–14 days after the onset of the first crop of the chickenpox rash. Simply focus on relieving the itching and preventing your child from scratching the blisters (see *Helping Your Child, p.400*). Permanent scars may result from blisters that are scratched and become infected.

PRIMARY TREATMENT Babies or individuals with reduced immunity, such as those who are undergoing chemotherapy or who are HIV-positive, should see a doctor at once regarding possible treatment with antiviral drugs.

Chickenpox does not usually require any treatment, although antiviral drugs, such as acyclovir, may be considered for adults. Antiviral drugs may limit the effects of the varicella infection but they need to be administered in the early stages of the disease if they are to be of help.

Antibiotics are needed if a secondary bacterial infection of the rash occurs.

IMMUNIZATION Doctors in the US have introduced a program of chickenpox immunization as a routine measure for children between 12–18 months, with catch-up immunizations offered for children 13–18 years old who have not been previously vaccinated.

CAUTION

Antiviral drugs have potential side effects; ask your doctor to explain these to you.

Nutritional Therapy

PRIMARY TREATMENT VITAMIN C AND ZINC SUPPLEMENTS may help boost the immune system, which can encourage healing and speed recovery.

Give 500–1,000mg of vitamin C per day, divided into three or four doses, together with 10mg of zinc, once or twice a day for 1-2 weeks. (This dosage of zinc is safe for children aged two years or more.) Taking zinc supplements over a long period can deplete the body of copper, so give your child 1mg of copper for each 15mg of zinc.

VITAMIN A SUPPLEMENTS Studies show that the chickenpox infection causes a lowering of vitamin A levels in children. Giving 3,000–5,000 IU of vitamin A every day for 10 days from the start of infection seems to help children with chickenpox. If given at the very start of the infection, vitamin A supplementation can help shorten the illness. Moreover, it may also help complications, such as pneumonia, conjunctivitis, and gastroenteritis.

MULTIVITAMIN/MINERAL SUPPLEMENT In 2001, a study revealed that a daily multivitamin and mineral formulation made children much less likely to contract chickenpox when there was an outbreak at school. A multivitamin and mineral supplement are believed to help boost a child's immune defenses.

CAUTION

Consult your doctor before giving zinc or vitamin C with antibiotics (see p.46).

Homeopathy

Chickenpox is usually a mild disease in young children, settling without complications, but it can be a severe illness in people with a suppressed immune system (which occurs, for example, as a side effect of certain drugs).

RHUS TOXICODENDRON The classical homeopathic treatment for chickenpox is *Rhus toxicodendron*. This medicine is frequently helpful, particularly if the rash is very itchy, with small blisters. Give your child two pills of the 6C strength, 4 times a day until the rash heals (see p.77).

> Chickenpox can be extremely dangerous in women who are pregnant

BELLADONNA AND ACONITE *Belladonna* and *Aconite* may help in the early stages of the infection, when there is fever and the child is generally unwell. *Aconite* is likely to help if the child feels both chilly and frightened. *Belladonna* is appropriate if the child feels hot and flushed.

PULSATILLA may help with children who are miserable, clingy, and tearful with the illness. They may have a fever, but are strangely not thirsty. *Antimonium tartaricum* has a reputation for helping when the skin rash is slow to subside.

PREVENTION PLAN

The following may help prevent your children from catching chickenpox:
- Stay away from people infected with chickenpox or shingles
- Give them a daily multivitamin and mineral supplement
- Make sure they are immunized against varicella

Treatment Plan lists treatments in order of priority, helping you make more informed choices. Primary treatments should be the first line of treatment in all cases. For an explanation of ratings, see p.111.

Important boxes highlight safety information regarding a condition, including special situations when it is essential that you see your doctor or go to the hospital.

Prevention Plan appears at the end of ailments for which preventive measures may be effective. It lists simple things you can do yourself to help prevent a condition.

General Precautions

- Always consult your doctor for a diagnosis — do not try to diagnose an illness or condition yourself.
- See a doctor immediately if you have any of the red flag symptoms listed below.
- See your doctor if there is no improvement in a condition within two weeks (48 hours for children under five years old).
- Do not stop taking prescribed medicine without consulting your doctor first.
- Tell your doctor about any complementary therapies you are using, and tell a complementary practitioner about any conventional treatment you are receiving.
- If you have a diagnosed medical condition, check with your doctor before using any complementary treatments.
- If you do not do exercise regularly, check with your doctor before starting a new exercise program. This is especially important if you have heart disease or back pain, or if you are pregnant.
- If you pregnant, breast-feeding, or trying to conceive, do not take any over-the-counter medicines or any herbal medicines without consulting your doctor.

Specific Precautions

Conventional Medicine
- Tell your doctor (or pharmacist if you are buying over-the-counter medicines) of all the other medicines and complementary remedies you are taking.
- Only take medicines that are prescribed for you and complete the full course.
- Seek medical help if you develop unexpected side-effects.
- Do not keep medicines beyond their expiration dates.

Nutritional Therapy
- Do not take more than the recommended dose. Excessive doses of vitamins and minerals may have toxic side effects.
- Some nutritional supplements interact with conventional drugs. See p.46 before taking a nutritional supplement.
- Do not exceed the recommended dosage without consulting a doctor or dietician.
- Check with your doctor before giving supplements to children under 12.
- During pregnancy, limit your intake of supplements that contain vitamin A. If you are in doubt, consult with your doctor.

Western and Chinese Herbal Medicine
- See p.69 before taking a herb. Some interact with drugs and supplements.
- Some herbs are not recommended for people with certain medical conditions; be aware of each herb's contraindications.
- Do not take herbal with conventional medicines before consulting your doctor.
- Do not give herbal remedies to children under 12 without consulting a health-care practitioner trained in herbal medicine.
- Do not take herbs during pregnancy, while breast-feeding, or while trying to conceive without a healthcare practitioner knowledgable in herbal medicine.
- Seek medical advice before taking herbal medicines if you have ever had hepatitis or another liver disease.
- Always seek professional advice if you do not recover as soon as expected when taking a herbal remedy.

Bodywork Therapies and Massage
- Inform your practitioner of your medical condition. This is especially important if you are pregnant or have osteoporosis, a fracture, cancer, or circulatory problems.

Acupuncture
- Make sure that your practitioner is qualified and uses disposable needles.
- Tell your practitioner if you are pregnant or if you have hepatitis B or C or HIV/AIDS.

Mind–Body Therapies
- If you have severe depression, psychosis, or epilepsy, you may be disturbed by hypnosis or hypnotherapy. Ask your doctor or psychiatrist before using these therapies.

How Treatments are Rated

Throughout this section, treatments are divided into three categories to help readers decide on their treatment path. Primary treatments are those that a reader should definitely try first. In many cases there is good scientific evidence from randomized controlled trials and meta-analyses (*see* p.480) to support their use. In all cases they are recommended by the authors of this book, who are doctors and complementary practitioners with extensive knowledge of treatments for these conditions.

Backup treatments have some positive evidence to support their use. Treatments in the third category are worth considering because they have a history of traditional use or there is some practitioner experience to suggest they may work.

This is an evidence-based book and the authors have cited references for all the treatments described. The scientific evidence for the primary treatments is listed on p.494. All the other references for treatments are listed on the DK website. Go to www.dk.com/newmedicine.

RED FLAG SYMPTOMS

You should see a doctor immediately if you experience any of the following symptoms or if you have any other symptoms that concern you:

- Chest pain or shortness of breath. If you have pain in the chest, arms, jaw, or throat, call 911 or your local EMS.
- Unexplained dizziness
- Persistent hoarseness, cough, sore throat
- Difficulty swallowing
- Persistent abdominal pain or indigestion
- Coughing up blood
- Persistent weight loss or fatigue
- A mole that has changed shape, size, or color, or itches or bleeds
- A sore that does not heal, or unexplained swellings under the skin

- Change in bowel or bladder habits
- Passing blood in the stools or urine
- Vaginal bleeding between menstrual periods, after sex, or following menopause, or any unusual vaginal discharge
- Thickening or lump in a breast; discharge or bleeding from a nipple; change in shape or size of a breast
- Swelling or lump in a testis; change in shape or size of a testis; total and persistent failure to get an erection
- Severe headaches; persistent one-sided headaches; visual disturbance
- Frequent and persistent back pain
- Unexplained leg pain and swelling
- Unexplained fever

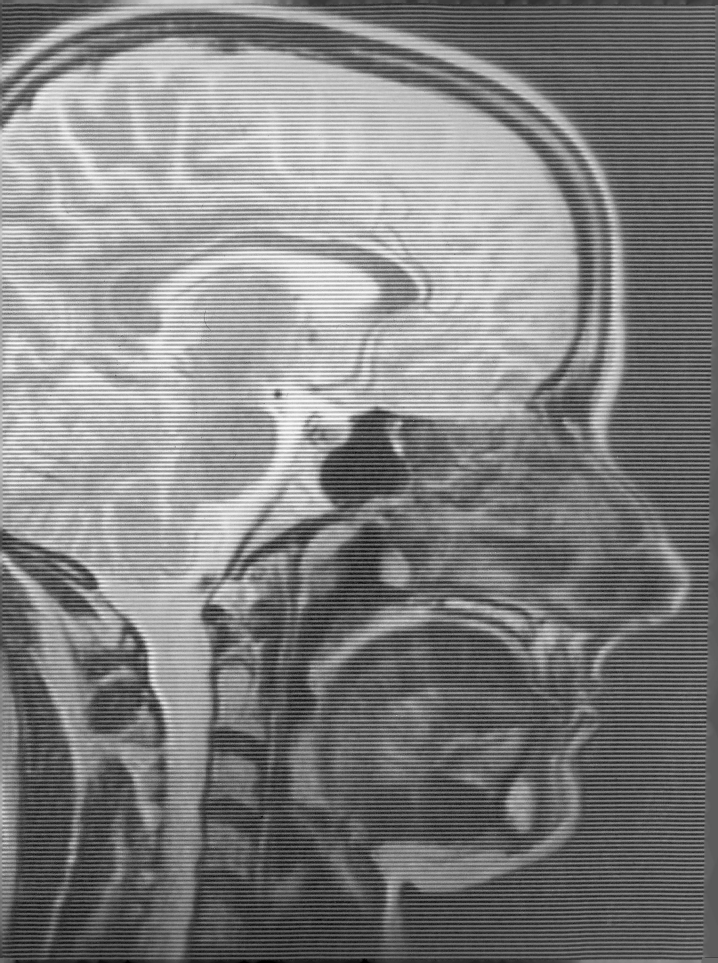

Brain & Nervous System

The mysterious brain and the nerves that network through the body coordinate the way we think, feel, and sense. Integrated medicine treats the whole person — body and mind. Nutritional and herbal medicines support the nervous system and drugs and complementary therapies work well in tandem for disorders ranging from stroke to migraine.

HEADACHES

Most people have at least one headache every year, making this a very common complaint. The majority of headaches last only a few hours, but some can last for days or even weeks. They have a variety of causes, most of which are not serious. Analgesics and other drugs are used for immediate relief. Eating regularly and making dietary changes might also be helpful in preventing recurrences. Depending on the cause, postural rehabilitation, manipulation techniques, dental treatment, biofeedback training, and relaxation therapy could also be appropriate.

WHAT ARE THE SYMPTOMS?

- Pain that may involve the entire head or only one area, such as the temples or the area above the eyes

WHY MIGHT I HAVE THIS?

PREDISPOSING FACTORS

- Tense neck muscles or temperomandibular jaw dysfunction
- Vision problems
- Depression
- Food sensitivities
- Low magnesium levels
- Prolonged use of analgesics
- Noisy, stuffy environment
- Poor posture
- Polluted environments

TRIGGERS

- Stress
- Caffeine withdrawal
- Alcohol use
- Low blood-sugar levels
- Dehydration

WHY DOES IT OCCUR?

TENSION A variety of factors may cause headaches, but the majority are brought on by tension in the neck or scalp muscles. The trapezius muscle, which runs from the middle of the back to the shoulders and base of the neck, is one of the strongest muscles in the body. When it contracts, it causes the muscles of the neck to contract as well, and the resulting "pull" or tension at the base of the skull can generate a tension headache, along with constriction of other muscles of the head and face. Recurrent tension headaches often affect people with depression or those under prolonged stress. Tension headaches are often worse in noise and hot, stuffy environments.

OTHER CAUSES There may be various other triggers for headaches. Sinusitis, a cold, or a viral infection can cause headaches. Alcohol, low blood-sugar levels, mild dehydration, food sensitivities, too much caffeine or caffeine withdrawal, and low levels of magnesium in the diet are thought to contribute. A history of head trauma can also cause chronic headaches. Prolonged use of strong analgesics can cause rebound headaches. Occasionally, high blood pressure can be a cause.

Poor posture, trigger points (sensitive areas in muscles), joint restrictions in the neck and upper back, and stress can contribute to headaches. Problems with the temporomandibular joint that connects the jaw to the skull, as well as dental problems or whiplash injuries, can also result in headaches. In some cases, vision problems may be a cause. You should have your prescription for glasses or contact lenses checked if you have recurrent headaches.

IMPORTANT

See a doctor if you have an unusual, severe, one-sided, or persistent headache, especially if it is accompanied by scalp tenderness, a stiff neck, nausea, fever, sensitivity to light, a rash that does not fade when pressed, or drowsiness. These symptoms could indicate more serious causes of headache.

TREATMENT PLAN

PRIMARY TREATMENTS

- Rest, analgesics, and other self-help measures (*see Immediate Relief, opposite*)
- Blood-sugar stabilizing diet
- Food elimination diet
- Increased water intake
- Avoid caffeine
- Magnesium supplements
- Relaxation training and biofeedback

BACKUP TREATMENTS

- Fish oil supplements
- Homeopathy
- Western and Chinese herbalism
- Alexander technique (if poor posture is a factor)
- Environmental health measures
- Chiropractic and osteopathy
- Acupuncture
- Mind–body therapies

For an explanation of how treatments are rated, see p.111.

Headaches may occasionally have a serious cause, such as giant-cell arteritis (*see below*), meningitis, a brain tumor, an aneurysm, or a subarachnoid hemorrhage.

CLUSTER HEADACHES A cluster headache is similar to a migraine in that it often affects one side of the head only and the pain is usually severe. However, they last for only an hour or so, and attacks tend to come in groups, with headache-free periods in between.

GIANT-CELL ARTERITIS A headache and tenderness over the scalp or temple may occur as a result of giant-cell arteritis (also known as temporal arteritis), a serious condition that particularly affects women and older people and is caused by inflammation of blood vessels in the head. The cause is unknown, but it may be due to an autoimmune reaction in which the immune system attacks the arteries. Immediate treatment with corticosteroids is required to prevent sudden blindness.

HEADACHES IN CHILDREN In children, short-lived headaches are usually caused by a viral infection. Some school-age children suffer from recurrent tension headaches, which may start in the afternoon and last less than 24 hours. These may be related to stress or to eye disease.

IMMEDIATE RELIEF

- Take an analgesic (for example, ibuprofen or acetaminophen) with plenty of water; for NSAIDs, take pill after food.
- Splash cold water on your face and lie down for 30 minutes. Applying an ice pack to the back of your neck may help.
- Practice deep breathing and try to rest.
- Using your fingertips, massage around your neck, the base of your skull, and over your scalp. Focus extra attention on any particular areas of tenderness that you discover.

TREATMENTS IN DETAIL

Conventional Medicine

PRIMARY TREATMENT If your headache is unusual or very severe, the doctor will do a physical examination and may arrange for you to have various tests, such as a CT or an MRI scan, in order to exclude an underlying cause. However, in most cases no tests will be needed. He or she may recommend ways of dealing with underlying stress and may prescribe analgesics such as acetaminophen or ibuprofen. However, it is often helpful to stop taking analgesics entirely because overuse of these drugs can contribute to

> The majority of people who experience recurrent cluster headaches are male

persistent headaches. Low doses of antidepressants may be helpful in some chronic cases; many controlled trials have found that different kinds of antidepressants had a beneficial effect on headaches.

CAUTION

Drugs for headaches can cause a range of possible side effects; ask your doctor to explain these to you.

Nutritional Therapy

PRIMARY TREATMENT **BLOOD-SUGAR STABILIZING DIET** One factor that is common in nonmigraine headaches is low blood-sugar levels. People who are prone to headaches when they skip a meal are most at risk. Taking steps to stabilize your blood-sugar levels and reduce the effects of stress are often very effective in combating headaches that are associated with low blood-sugar levels (*for more details, see p.42*).

PRIMARY TREATMENT **INCREASED WATER INTAKE** A common and often overlooked cause of headaches is dehydration. The tissues that surround the brain are composed mostly of water. When these tissues lose fluid, they shrink, and this can give rise to pain and irritation. Many people find that just drinking about a quart (1 liter) of water a day can lead to a substantial reduction in the frequency and/or severity of their headaches.

PRIMARY TREATMENT **AVOIDING CAFFEINE WITHDRAWAL** People who regularly drink coffee, tea, or other caffeinated drinks normally find that stopping caffeine can lead to a headache for a day or two, after which headaches are reduced or stop altogether. The most immediate way to stop a caffeine-withdrawal headache is by drinking a caffeinated beverage. Alternatively, you could permanently eliminate all forms of caffeine-containing foodstuffs from your diet, including coffee, tea, chocolate, cocoa, and caffeinated soft drinks. Beverages that are naturally caffeine free — for example, herb and fruit teas as well as coffee substitutes that are based on barley or chicory — are good alternatives to caffeinated drinks.

PRIMARY TREATMENT **MAGNESIUM SUPPLEMENTS** Studies are mixed on whether magnesium helps headaches; some studies have found a benefit, while others have not. You could try taking 300–500mg daily, divided into two or three doses. Too much magnesium can cause diarrhea; if this happens, reduce the dose.

CAUTION

Consult your doctor before taking magnesium and fish oils because they can interfere with other medication (*for more information, see p.46*)

FISH OILS The effectiveness of fish oils, at a dose of approximately 800mg EPA and 500mg DHA per day, to prevent migraine headaches and treat headaches that have already started was examined. A study showed that teenagers who took fish-oil supplements for two months had fewer headaches that resolved more quickly. However, neither result was significantly different from the headaches experienced by those who received placebo.

ASPARTAME Some people report that consuming food or drinks with aspartame, an artificial sweetener, causes headaches. An experiment in which aspartame was given to people who believed that they were sensitive provided evidence supporting this effect.

Homeopathy

Homeopathic treatment of headaches is controversial, and some clinical trials have been negative. A review found that three out of four randomized placebo-controlled trials of homeopathy treatments for migraine or other headaches found no benefit of homeopathy. It is difficult to generalize about homeopathic treatment of headaches and which remedy might be best because it very much depends on the individual. For best results, visit a reliable practitioner rather than trying to self-treat.

NATRUM MURIATICUM, a remedy made from salt, is probably the most commonly used homeopathic medicine for chronic headaches, although many others may be appropriate. It is usually prescribed on "constitutional" grounds (treating the person, not the disease, *see p.73*), for people who are conscientious and controlled. They may be quite depressed, but hide it well, and do not like to discuss their own feelings, although they may be very sympa-

thetic to the problems of others. They may also crave salty, food. Take two 30C pills of *Natrum mur.* once or twice a week.

NUX VOMICA, which is derived from the southeast Asian poison-nut tree, is a homeopathic remedy that is used to treat "sick headaches." It is therefore suitable for treating headaches accompanied by nausea or by actual vomiting. These headaches are normally at their worst first thing in the morning and may be triggered by overindulgence the night before.

Western Herbal Medicine

Calming herbs, such as chamomile (*Matricaria recutita*), valerian (*Valeriana officinalis*), lavender (*Lavandula officinalis*), and lemon balm (*Melissa officinalis*), help reduce the stress that contributes to tension headaches. Applying diluted essential oils of rosemary (*Rosmarinus officinalis*), lavender, or mint (*Mentha* spp.) to the temples when a headache threatens can be very helpful. Essential oils can be diluted with almond

oil, olive oil, or any vegetable oil. Use 3–5 drops of essential oil per teaspoon of carrier oil, being careful that the oils do not get into your eyes. Follow this by sipping a cup of chamomile or lemon balm tea.

HERBAL OILS rubbed into tense muscles in the head and neck may be relaxing and effective in treating tension headaches. Topically applied peppermint oil (10 percent peppermint oil in ethanol) was more effective than placebo and as effective as 1,000 millegrams of acetaminophen for tension headaches. The oil was spread across the forehead and temples every 15 minutes for 45 minutes. Another study found that a similar preparation relaxed the muscle over the temple. Eucalyptus oil was also tested in this study but it was shown to be no more effective than the placebo.

> **CAUTION**
>
> See p.69 before taking an herbal remedy. If you are taking a prescribed medication, consult an herbal medicine expert first.

TRIGGER POINTS AND HEADACHE

Tension headaches may be partly due to areas of sensitized tissue in the muscles of the jaw, neck, and shoulders, known as trigger points (*see p.55*). These sensitive areas often develop from habitual

tightening of the muscles when a person is under stress. Trigger points may be responsible for causing pain not only at the site where they have developed, but also in tissue some distance away ("referred pain"). It is possible

to release the trigger points (*see Osteopathy and Chiropractic, p.118*). This, together with regular relaxation exercises, can help to reduce both the duration and frequency of tension headaches.

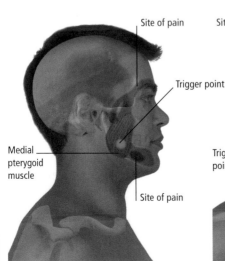

A trigger point in the jaw muscle can cause pain in both the jaw and above the eye.

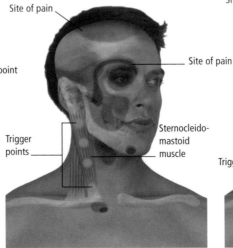

Trigger points in the neck may cause pain at the back of the head and around the eyes.

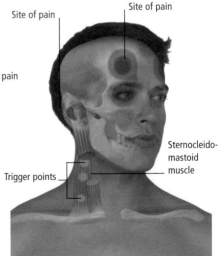

Forehead pain may be due to trigger points in the sternocleidomastoid muscle.

Chinese Herbal Medicine

In Traditional Chinese Medicine, headaches are differentiated by their location, external symptoms, and internal imbalances of energy, both of excess and deficiency. A common type of headache is said to be a result of "Liver Yang Rising," associated with irritability and anger. Another common type is "Kidney Yin Deficiency," associated with mental and physical overexertion. The Four Substances decoction is used to treat "blood-deficient" headache, which usually affects women, and "blood stasis" headache, marked by chronic unremitting episodes and sometimes associated with a head injury. There are many other types of headaches and, therefore, a diagnosis by a qualified practitioner is essential.

> **CAUTION**
>
> Self-medication with Chinese herbal medicine is inadvisable for headaches. Consult a qualified Chinese herbalist.

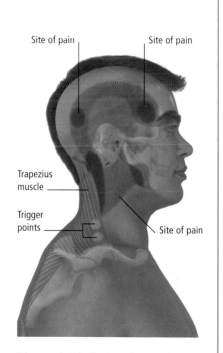

Site of pain

Site of pain

Trapezius muscle

Trigger points

Site of pain

Trigger points in the trapezius muscle may cause pain in both the neck and temple.

Environmental Health

Some believe that environmental chemicals may injure the nervous system, resulting in symptoms such as headaches. For example, some claim that the myriad symptoms (including headaches) in Gulf War syndrome represent injury to the nervous system. There are many possible causes for this, including exposure to chemical warfare, pesticides, extremes of heat and cold, dust, and smoke from oil-well fires. However, other studies have found no association between resulting symptoms and such exposures or even combat time in the Persian Gulf.

EVERYDAY HAZARDS Loud noises, strong light, and altitude changes can cause headaches in some people. The weather can be a culprit: some people may experience a worsening of their headaches in thunderstorms or humid conditions, a phenomenon that has been borne out in scientific studies. Other individuals may develop symptoms from the use of hand-held mobile phones, with symptoms worsening with longer use.

LEAD AND GASOLINE High blood-lead levels, such as those found in people who live close to and downwind from lead smelters, are related to increased headaches. Headaches may also result from exposure to gasoline fumes and other environmental toxicants (such as benzene, sulfur dioxide, and photoionizable dust) in the air around service stations, a particular problem for people who work at those sites.

SICK-BUILDING SYNDROME It is thought that a group of symptoms, including headaches, fatigue, inflammation, and respiratory symptoms, could be the result of low-level exposure to compounds such as chemicals in new carpets in inadequately ventilated buildings.

Carbon monoxide, which is a by-product of the combustion of fossil fuels, can build up in poorly ventilated rooms near cars, furnaces, air-conditioning systems, and gas stoves. It can be very dangerous because it is odorless and is therefore not easily detected. It can build up to the point where it can cause serious central nervous system toxicity and, eventually, death. You can reduce your exposure by using low-emitting

building materials and nontoxic office supplies, continuous ventilation, and by storing all chemicals.

AVOIDING FOOD ADDITIVES Monosodium glutamate (MSG), a flavor-enhancing substance that is often found in Chinese food, potato chips, processed foods, and seasonings, is known to cause headaches in some people. If you think you might be sensitive to food additives, you should read the ingredient labels on foods, and make a point of avoiding anything that contains MSG.

MERCURY Leaching of mercury from dental amalgam fillings is often mentioned as a cause for a variety of health problems, including headaches, but this is doubted by many researchers. Most mercury toxicity occurs as a result of occupational exposure (mining, ore smelting, and in dental offices) or from eating tainted fish.

Acupuncture and Acupressure

Several studies of acupuncture as a treatment for tension headaches show a benefit. A study of electroacupuncture found that it was superior to sham acupuncture (the use of acupuncture needles but not in trigger points to conduct controlled experiments) for decreasing headache frequency, duration, and pain. A review of controlled trials of acupuncture for recurrent headaches indicated that acupuncture has a role in the treatment of this type of headache. Economic analysis of the cost-effectiveness of acupuncture was also found to be favorable.

To treat headaches successfully, a series of acupuncture treatments is usually needed. The exact treatment and its duration depends on the individual's symptoms. Applying pressure to the LI4 (He Ju) point in the hollow between the thumb and index finger can provide temporary relief.

Bodywork and Movement Therapies

The many different causes of headaches require different approaches to treatment. Some approaches focus on posture, some on neck restrictions, some on trigger points (sensitive areas in muscles; see p.55), and others on imbalances affecting the jaw (see also p.280).

ALEXANDER TECHNIQUE Spending a great deal of time standing or sitting with your head thrust forward, in a slouched posture, puts a great deal of stress on the muscles and joints of the upper back and neck, which may lead to formation of trigger points, nerve irritation, and headaches. The Alexander technique aims to correct such "patterns of misuse." It takes time and you need an Alexander teacher to guide you through the procedure. What feels uncomfortable at first (such as holding the head correctly) gradually becomes comfortable, and starts to "feel right."

Teachers of the Alexander Technique have perfected a gradual rehabilitation program, which should ideally be accompanied by treatment (and self-treatment) aimed at stretching and releasing tight muscles and joints and at toning and balancing the body as a whole.

CRANIAL OSTEOPATHY AND DENTISTRY Osteopaths and dentists believe that jaw misalignment can cause headaches. Cranial osteopaths and dentists apply techniques to ease the stresses in the jaw area that may cause headaches, either by working on correcting possible misalignment of the upper and lower teeth or by encouraging better function of the jaw itself. However, a comprehensive review of controlled studies found that occlusal adjustment was not effective treatment for headaches and other symptoms caused by temperomandibular disorders.

OSTEOPATHY AND CHIROPRACTIC Some injuries to the neck, particularly whiplash (caused by a sudden, extreme "whipping" movement of the head and neck; *see p.268*), can cause long-term tissue irritation that leads to chronic headaches. Chiropractors and osteopaths manipulate restricted joints of the neck or use soft-tissue techniques to encourage greater freedom of movement and ease possible nerve irritations. This approach can reduce the incidence of chronic headaches.

A review of randomized controlled trials of spinal manipulation as a treatment for chronic headaches found spinal adjustment as effective as the antidepressant amitriptyline for preventing episodes of tension headaches or migraines.

Some headaches may result from activation of trigger points in muscles and there is evidence that deactivating these trigger points reduces the incidence of headaches. The headaches that are most improved by trigger-point treatment are those that are accompanied by tenderness of the muscles that attach to the head (*See also Migraine, p.119*).

Mind–Body Therapies

STRESS AND HEADACHES Numerous scientific studies have shown a strong link between stress and both tension and migraine headaches. A study of young

> ## About 3 percent of people experience a tension-type headache on most days

adults who experienced regular tension headaches found that feeling under stress and not functioning well emotionally were both predictive of greater frequency and intensity as well as longer duration of headache symptoms.

Another study found that stress associated with negative life events, such as divorce, was related to how often people experienced headaches. In fact, when people who have regular headaches are asked about the most common precipitating factors, stress and tension are almost universally cited. Finally, a national survey of people in Taiwan found a strong link between job stress and incidence of a number of health-related problems, including headache and musculoskeletal discomfort.

PRIMARY TREATMENT **BIOFEEDBACK, RELAXATION TRAINING** and other specific psychological skills can help relax tense muscles that lead to headaches and counteract the negative effects of pain caused by excessive muscle tension. A comprehensive review of studies that examined nondrug approaches to recurrent tension headaches found that relaxation training and biofeedback, as well as a combination of the two, yielded nearly a 50 percent reduction in headaches.

A review of psychological treatments for pain in children found that relaxation and cognitive behavioral therapy reduce the severity and duration of headaches in children and adolescents.

Biofeedback therapy, if used to treat tension headaches, usually involves electromyographic (EMG) biofeedback. Electrodes are attached to muscles in the forehead and temple region. The electrodes monitor tension in the muscles, which is translated into an audio or visual signal. For example, a beeping signal may become faster when a muscle is contracted, and slower when a muscle is relaxed. Learning to slow down the beeping means that the person is learning to relax the muscles that contribute to tension headaches. Once the person can reliably relax the specific muscles, machines are no longer needed. The technique can be used at any time, anywhere, with no further cost after the training is completed. Some people learn the technique in only a few sessions, while others require 10 or 20 sessions.

The aim of relaxation techniques is usually to achieve generalized relaxation rather than specific muscles. Techniques vary; one involves tensing and then releasing the tension in groups of muscles in succession, with the aim of eventually being able to relax all of the major muscle groups at once. Different forms of relaxation techiques are taught in meditation or yoga classes.

Evidence has shown that home-based psychological approaches, such as relaxation exercises, are as effective as clinic-based treatments. If you have regular headaches and your doctor has excluded a serious cause, try simple relaxation exercises or meditation for 20 minutes a day (*for details, see p.98*).

PREVENTION PLAN

- Eat regular meals to ensure stable blood-sugar levels
- Drink plenty of fluids, especially water
- Limit your intake of caffeine and alcohol
- Do relaxation exercises if you feel tense
- Reserve time for yourself on a daily basis

MIGRAINE

Migraine is characterized by recurrent headaches that are often accompanied by visual disturbances, nausea, and vomiting. A migraine can last for several days and may be may be preceded by a period of feeling irritable, known as the prodrome. A tendency to migraines sometimes runs in families, suggesting that genetic factors may play a role. Treatment involves a range of measures, such as dietary changes, massage, and relaxation, as well as medication to treat an attack and to prevent further attacks from occurring.

WHY DOES IT OCCUR?

The cause of migraine is unknown but various factors may be involved. Certain foods play a role in triggering migraines in many people. Low blood-sugar levels, low levels of magnesium in the diet, female hormones, and stress also seem to be contributory factors. Some people develop migraine type headaches in response to vigorous exercise, possibly due to the increase in blood pressure and blood flow. Trigger points, which are sensitive points in the muscles (*see p.55*), and nerve irritation in the head and neck are also thought by some specialists to cause severe migraine-like headaches.

TYPES OF MIGRAINE There are two main types of migraine as well as many other, less common types. The first is a classical migraine, in which the headache occurs on one side of the head and is preceded or accompanied by an "aura." This may involve a range of phenomena, including visual disturbances, tingling and/or numbness in various parts of the body, and feelings of restlessness or depression. The cause of the aura is not fully understood. The second main type is known as a common migraine, in which there is no aura preceding the headache, which usually involves both sides of the head. Some

IMPORTANT

See your doctor if a headache comes on after vigorous exercise; is accompanied by fever, stiff neck, drowsiness, or a rash; if the headache follows a head injury; or if self-help remedies do not bring relief after three days.

TREATMENT PLAN

PRIMARY TREATMENTS

- Rest and other self-help measures (*see Self-Help, p.120*)
- Over-the-counter analgesics and antinausea drugs
- Triptan and other drugs (for severe attacks)
- Feverfew and other Western herbs
- Magnesium supplements
- Food elimination diet
- Blood-sugar stabilizing diet
- Neck manipulation and massage

BACKUP TREATMENTS

- Nutritional therapy
- Bodywork therapies
- Relaxation training
- Acupuncture

WORTH CONSIDERING

- Homeopathy
- Chinese herbal medicine
- Environmental health measures

For an explanation of how treatments are rated, see p.111.

people experience a "visual" migraine, in which they have blurred vision or other visual disturbances but no headache. Others, especially children, may have an "abdominal" migraine, in which the symptoms include recurrent episodes of abdominal pain or vomiting, and the one-sided headaches and nausea typical of the condition in adults may not occur. Migraine is a significant cause of headache in children, particularly girls, and by the age of 15 about 1 in 20 children has experienced a migraine attack.

Some people have migraines once a year while others may have attacks as often as once or twice a month. Attacks may last a few hours or several days. Sometimes sleep will end an attack.

SELF-HELP

- Take analgesics and other medication as prescribed.
- Splash your face with cold water or put a cold compress or an ice pack on your forehead and the back of your neck.
- Rest in a dark room away from noise.
- Drink plenty of water to avoid becoming dehydrated.
- Massage your temples and neck with a few drops of lavender, rosemary, or peppermint essential oil, diluted in a little vegetable oil.
- Sip a cup of peppermint tea or ginger tea to help relieve any nausea associated with migraine.

TREATMENTS IN DETAIL

Conventional Medicine

Your doctor will diagnose the condition from a description of the symptoms. He or she will be able to give you advice about lifestyle changes and prescribe drugs if necessary. Your doctor will also be able to help you identify and avoid migraine triggers, with the aim of reducing the number and severity of attacks.

PRIMARY TREATMENT **OVER-THE-COUNTER DRUGS** Analgesics may be helpful when an attack occurs. It may be necessary to experiment to find the common drug that works best for you; aspirin, ibuprofen, or other nonsteroidal anti-inflammatory drugs (NSAIDs) may be very useful.

PRIMARY TREATMENT **PRESCRIPTION DRUGS** Your doctor may prescribe triptans, such as sumatriptan, which are often helpful in relieving more severe migraine attacks. They work by narrowing the blood vessels that supply the brain. In addition to being available as pills that are taken orally, these drugs may be given by either injection or nasal spray. If your migraines occur frequently, there are also various drugs

> Around 20 percent of people have migraines in both developed and undeveloped countries

available that may be prescribed for use on a daily basis — for example, the beta-blocker propranolol and the antidepressant amitriptyline. Some of the anticonvulsant medications, especially sodium valproate, are also an effective treatment for migraine. These medications can prevent migraines as well as lessening their severity when they do occur, but it may take a month or two for the maximum effect of the drugs to be realized.

CAUTION

Drugs for migraine can cause a range of possible side effects; ask your doctor to explain these to you.

Nutritional Therapy

PRIMARY TREATMENT **FOOD ELIMINATION DIET** Food sensitivity is a major cause of migraine according to a number of studies. Certain foods known to trigger migraine include cheese, chocolate, citrus fruits, monosodium glutamate (MSG), aspartame, ice cream, milk, and eggs, as well as alcohol, especially red wine and beer. Caffeine withdrawal may also be a trigger for migraine. However, research has suggested that the most common trigger food of migraine is actually wheat.

People with such sensitivities can be treated with food elimination diets. In one study of 60 people on a five-day elimination diet, which was limited to pears, spring water, and lamb, the participants reported a very significant improvement in

their symptoms after eliminating on average 10 foods to which they were sensitive. (*For more details about food elimination diets, see p.39.*)

PRIMARY TREATMENT **BLOOD-SUGAR STABILIZING DIET** Migraine can sometimes be triggered if the level of sugar in the blood becomes too low — a condition known as hypoglycemia. This may explain why some people are prone to a migraine attack if they miss a meal. To ensure a stable blood-sugar level, avoid long periods without food: eat regular meals with healthy snacks, such as fresh fruit and nuts, in between. In general, base your diet on unprocessed foods, such as fresh fruits and vegetables and meat and fish. Choose whole-grain starches, such as whole-wheat bread and brown rice, which are broken down more slowly by the body than their white counterparts. This type of diet gives a steady release of glucose and helps prevent blood-sugar levels from fluctuating (*see also p.42*).

PRIMARY TREATMENT **MAGNESIUM SUPPLEMENTS** Migraine has been related to low magnesium levels and magnesium deficiency, which increase the risk of spasm in the arteries. Some studies of magnesium supplementation have shown a benefit. Another study, however, found no effect of magnesium supplements for migraines.

Magnesium supplements may be particularly helpful for women who suffer from premenstrual migraines. One study found that 360mg of magnesium a day for the last half of the menstrual cycle, decreased menstrual migraines. Compared with placebo, magnesium reduced pain and the number of days that women experienced headaches. If you have regular migraines, try taking 200mg of magnesium twice a day. However, too much magnesium can cause diarrhea; if this occurs, try reducing the dose.

FISH OIL Two studies found that fish oil was no more effective than placebo for preventing migraines. Those treated with fish oil did have fewer headaches, but so did those treated with placebo. Another study tested 6g omega-3 fatty acids daily for 4 months. Although the fish-oil group had one fewer migraine during the study than the placebo group, there was no difference in headaches experienced during the last month of treatment.

> **CAUTION**
>
> Consult your doctor before taking magnesium and fish oils because they can interfere with other medication (*for more information see p.46*).

5-HYDROXYTRYPTOPHAN (5-HT) has been tested in a study and found to be as effective as methysergide, a medication popular for treating migraines at the time of the study. 5-hydroxytryptophan is related to tryptophan, which is no longer available in the US because of its link with a serious condition called eosinophilia myalgia syndrome. Although this syndrome was most likely caused by a contaminant in tryptophan that was made by a specific manufacturer, it is not clear whether this same sort of contamination could also affect 5-HT. This supplement is available over the counter, but caution would dictate avoiding it.

RIBOFLAVIN High doses of riboflavin, a B vitamin, have been found to be effective for reducing the frequency of migraines. A randomized controlled trial found that 400mg riboflavin a day, given for four months, was significantly better than placebo for reducing the frequency of attacks and days with headaches. Although this dose is more than 300 times higher than the recommended daily allowance of riboflavin, this vitamin has not been associated with serious adverse effects. In the trial above, one patient taking riboflavin reported diarrhea, and another reported increased urination.

AVOIDING FOOD ADDITIVES Certain chemicals and food additives can cause migraines. Some of the most common of these are nitrates (preservatives that are added to preserved meats), and monosodium glutamate (MSG), which is naturally present in mushrooms, kelp, and scallops, but is also added to Chinese restaurant food and snack foods.

ASPARTAME, an artificial sweetener that is found in many products from soft drinks to chewing gum, may cause migraines. Interestingly, aspartame may have been involved in continuing headaches because there is antimigraine medication with aspartame added to it. If you are prone to migraines it is worth checking the ingredients listed on packaging and trying to avoid medications that contain aspartame.

Homeopathy

The evidence on homeopathy and migraine is rather confusing — there are some positive results, some negative results, and some equivocal results. The differences may be accounted for by different types of patients, different types of homeopathic prescribing, and different ways of measuring outcomes. However, an Italian research group led by Gennaro Muscari-Tomaioli found that homeopathy had very positive results on the quality of life of people with migraines. The usual medicines given were *Natrum muriaticum*, *Staphysagria*, *Lycopodium*, *Lachesis*, and *Nux vomica*. All were prescribed at least partly on a "whole person" basis (*see p.73*).

NATRUM MURIATICUM is suggested for severe headaches with visual problems that tend to be worse in the sun. The affected person may also have streaming eyes. It is one of the medicines prescribed for "weekend migraine," which typically comes on when the patient takes time to relax.

STAPHYSAGRIA may be used for headaches brought on by anger or indignation, especially if these feelings are not expressed. Affected people may also have styes.

LYCOPODIUM is often appropriate when the headache is right-sided or moves from right to left. These migraines tend to be worse in late afternoon and are often associated with bloating and gas.

LACHESIS is given for headaches that are usually left-sided and worse in the morning. In women they occur before periods or as menopause approaches.

OTHER REMEDIES *Kalium bichromicum* is suggested if there is an aura preceding the headache by several hours. There may also be sinusitis. *Spigelia* is often used to treat left-sided headaches which affect the eye and which are also sometimes accompanied by palpitations.

Western Herbal Medicine

For best results you should visit a healthcare practitioner who is knowledgable about herbal remedies. He or she can assess your symptoms and prescribe an appropriate herb or mixture of herbs to take. The most popular herb for preventing migraines is feverfew.

PRIMARY TREATMENT **FEVERFEW** (*Tanacetum parthenium*), a member of the chrysanthemum family, has been studied for preventing migraine. Some migraine sufferers grow feverfew and eat a leaf or two every day, or eat a leaf every hour or two when they are getting an attack. No studies have examined the effectiveness of feverfew for treating migraines but several studies have looked at feverfew for preventing attacks. A review found that four of six randomized, double-blind, placebo-controlled trials of feverfew showed a benefit of the herb for preventing migraine. Another recent study looked at a special CO_2 extract and found that it only helped prevent migraines in people who suffer from headaches at least four times a month. In some people, this herb can cause mouth ulcers even when taken as capsules. It is available in pill form or as a tincture.

BUTTERBUR An extract of butterbur called Petadolex reduced migraine frequency in a controlled trial and fewer people in the butterbur group had to use medicines to treat their migraines than those who were in the placebo group. Butterbur contains pyrrolizidine alkaloids, toxic compounds that are harmful to the liver; therefore, only extracts from which these compounds have been removed should be used.

PREMENSTRUAL MIGRAINES For the pain of premenstrual migraines, some herbalists use Chaste tree berry (*Vitex agnus-castus*), motherwort (*Leonarus cardiaca*), *dong guai* (*Angelica sinensis*), and black cohosh (*Actaea racemosa*).

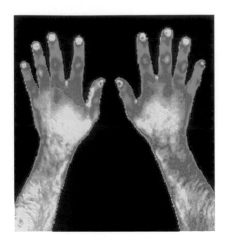

During a migraine, blood flow to the body's extremities is reduced. This thermogram reveals decreased heat in the hands and fingers, which show up as green and blue.

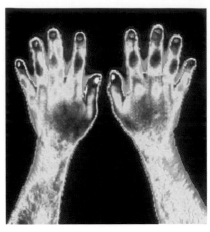

After the person has used thermal biofeedback, the hands are much warmer. This technique can help relieve migraine by encouraging blood to flow to the hands and away from the head.

RELAXING TENSE MUSCLES Very tense, tight shoulder and neck muscles can be eased by taking cramp bark (*Viburnum* sp.) and chamomile (*Matricaria recituta*) and by gentle massaging such tense areas with essential oils — for example, lavender (*Lavendula officinalis*), rosemary (*Rosmarinus officinalis*), cinnamon (*Cinnamomum cassia*), and orange — diluted in almond oil. Massaging the neck and temples with a few drops of diluted essential oils of rosemary, lavender, or mint (*Mentha* spp.) as soon as a migraine threatens can be helpful as well.

> **CAUTION**
>
> See p. 69 before taking a herbal remedy and, if you are taking prescribed medication, consult an herbal medicine expert first.

Chinese Herbal Medicine

No clinical trials of traditional Chinese Medicine (TCM) in the treatment of migraine have been performed.

WIND INVASION If you feel under the weather, practitioners of traditional Chinese Herbal Medicine believe you may indeed have been invaded by adverse climatic factors. Wind is seen as a particularly disrupting influence, unsettling *qi* (vital force) and blood flow to the head. Wind may invade together with cold, damp, or heat. "Wind-cold" headaches are often treated with Ligusticum-Tea Blended Powder (Chuan Qiong ChaTiao Wan), a formula that contains green tea, while "wind-heat" headache is treated with Chrysanthemum Tea Adjusted Powder. It is interesting that chrysanthemum, j*u hua* (*Chrysanthemum morifolium*), one of the main Chinese remedies for headache, is a relative of feverfew used by Western herbalists for the same purpose.

ENERGY IMBALANCES In TCM, the liver provides *qi* (vital force) to enable the smooth flow of blood and nutrients to the brain. Its function is easily disrupted by stress, anger, worry, and tension. This disordered *qi* flow, described as "liver *yang* and internal wind rising," brings on a painful, throbbing headache, typically affecting one side of the head — a characteristic migraine presentation. The classical prescription is Gastrodia Uncaria Decoction (Tian Ma Gou Teng Yin).

> **CAUTION**
>
> Self-medication with Chinese herbal medicine is not advisable for migraine. Consult a qualified Chinese herbalist.

Environmental Health

Environmental factors that may increase the occurrence of migraine headaches include exposure to strong light, changes in the weather, for example humidity and thunderstorms, and being at a high altitude, as well as more local factors such as exposure to solvents and pesticides.

Acupuncture and Acupressure

Migraine has frequently been treated with acupuncture and there are a number of quality studies in this area. However, many look simply at headache in general and do not necessarily differentiate "classical" migraine from regular headaches alone.

Studies have looked at using a traditional Chinese approach to the diagnosis and treatment of migraine, as well as more Westernized techniques involving the use of tender trigger points in the head and neck. A number of these studies, particularly those published in the early 1980s, have been of poor quality, but on balance there is much more evidence to show that acupuncture will be of benefit in treating migraines than reports that it has no effect. The majority of studies suggest that the frequency and intensity of migraine can be helped with acupuncture, and that acupuncture can be used to prevent migraine attacks.

Acupuncture reatment can be based on either a traditional Chinese approach or a Western approach and usually needs to be given initially on a weekly basis. Generally, six to eight treatments are required, with the frequency of treatment related to frequency of attacks.

A study of 401 people with chronic headaches, predominantly migraine, showed that acupuncture (up to 12 treatments for three months) offered substantial benefits compared to routine conventional treatment. Headaches were reduced not only at the conclusion of the study but a year later as well. Acupuncture treatment also reduced medication use.

Acupressure may also be an effective treatment; applying pressure to the LI4 (He Ju) point in the hollow between the thumb and index finger can provide temporary relief from migraine.

Bodywork Therapies

Despite having many of the same symptoms as true migraine (such as nausea), many one-sided headaches may not be migraines at all but arise instead from nerve irritation, or trigger-point activity, in the neck. It is also not uncommon for people to experience both migraines and severe headaches that derive from nerve irritation in the neck. A recent study of patients with neck injuries reported that 35 percent experienced headaches deriving from their necks, while another 11 percent had both neck-related headaches and migraines.

PRIMARY TREATMENT **NECK MANIPULATION AND MASSAGE** Osteopaths and chiropractors believe that your headache, whether diagnosed as migraine or not, may be helped by treatment of the neck muscles and joints. This might involve mobilization or manipulation of restricted joints, release of excessive tension in muscles of the region, or deactivation of trigger points. Chiropractic or osteopathic spinal or neck adjustment may be helpful for migraines.

A controlled trial of neck manipulative therapy found that 14 sessions over eight weeks reduced scores on a headache index (a combination of headache frequency and severity); the effect was similar to that of the antidepressant amitriptyline. Manipulative therapy appeared to have a more lasting effect than amitriptyline after treatments were stopped. Another study that compared spinal manipulative therapy (up to 16 times over eight weeks) with a sham therapy found that the treated group had fewer headaches and used less medication but that there were no differences in headache severity between the two groups.

Massage releases muscle tension and helps restore normal blood flow to the blood vessels in the neck, scalp, and face. It also has a wider therapeutic effect, helping relieve stress and tension. A 1998 study evaluated the potential benefits of massage in treatment of migraine. The results after five weeks were that a group of people receiving massage therapy for their migraines reported a greater number of headache-free days, a reduced need for migraine medication, more hours of sleep, and less interrupted sleep.

PEMF (pulsing electromagnetic fields) A Cochrane review identified two trials of pulsing electromagnetic fields that found a benefit for migraine but concluded that evidence was weaker for this therapy than for neck manipulative therapy.

DEACTIVATION OF TRIGGER POINTS Migraines are often associated with trigger points (sensitive areas in the muscles) in the neck and facial muscles. It is very simple to prove the connection for yourself. If you have a particular pattern of headache, gently feel around in the muscles of the neck and face for tender areas (trigger points). Once you locate them, press them firmly, one at a time, for 10 seconds or so, until you identify points that reproduce or exaggerate the headache pain pattern you usually have. If you find such active trigger points, they should be treated by a suitable practitioner, such as an osteopath, a chiropractor, physical therapist, massage therapist, neuromuscular therapist, or an acupuncturist.

Mind–Body Therapies

Many studies have shown a link between stress and both tension and migraine headaches. Emotional factors such as anxiety seem to influence physiological factors that can trigger migraines.

RELAXATION TRAINING AND BIOFEEDBACK, as well as a combination of the two, yielded nearly a 50 percent reduction in headaches in a review of the literature examining nondrug treatments for recurrent migraines. Moreover, home-based relaxation was as effective at reducing headaches as treatment in a clinic. The consensus panel of the United States Headache Consortium concluded there is strong evidence for the effectiveness of psychological therapies, including relaxation, biofeedback, and cognitive behavioral therapy, in the prevention of migraines. If you have regular migraine headaches, experiment with a program of relaxation exercises or meditate for 20 minutes each day (*for relaxation and meditation sequences, see p.99 and 100*).

THERMAL BIOFEEDBACK has been shown to be particularly valuable in preventing migraine. Visualization is used to get blood to flow to the body's periphery and away from the brain, which seems to prevent the full onset of a migraine (*see p.100*).

The best time to do thermal biofeedback is during the early onset or "aura." The technique, which must be learned in a clinic, involves placing a temperature sensor, called a thermistor, on the fingers. When a migraine begins, temperatures in the fingers can fall from their usual range of the 90°s F (mid-30°s C) to the 80°s F (low 30°s C) or even lower. When a patient can see these lowered temperatures on the thermistor, he or she uses general relaxation and/or visual imagery (such as imagining the warm sun shining on the hands) to help the hands warm up. By watching the tiny changes registered on the thermistor, the patient can learn which relaxation techniques and/or visual images are most useful for raising the temperature.

In addition to being a preventive technique, even during a migraine attack, the use of thermal biofeedback can occasionally alleviate the severity and/or duration of the migraine. However, medications that constrict excessive blood flow to the brain are still the first line of treatment.

> Peak prevalence for migraine is from 30 to 39. After the age of 50 they are less common

PREVENTION PLAN

- Keep a diary of your migraines so that you can determine when they occur and what are the likely triggers. Make a note of factors such as foods eaten, changes in the weather, sleep patterns, and stress levels

- Avoid any foods or situations that seem to bring on attacks

- Take propranolol or any other medication that is prescribed by your doctor for prevention

- Eat regular meals and try to get enough sleep at night

- If stress is a trigger, do relaxation exercises regularly (*see p.99*)

NEURALGIA

Episodes of severe pain in the area supplied by a nerve is known as neuralgia. In one common type, trigeminal neuralgia, a severe, stabbing pain is felt around the side of the face and the cheek — areas supplied by the trigeminal nerve. Postherpetic neuralgia is persistent pain in an area previously affected by shingles (*see p.165*). Neuralgia may also occur in the suboccipital region, which is at the back of the head, or in an arm or a leg if a nerve is affected by a prolapsed disk. A variety of treatments bring relief, including medications and bodywork therapy.

WHAT ARE THE SYMPTOMS?

- Pain that may involve any part of the body, depending on the cause
- In postherpetic neuralgia, burning and continuous pain in the area previously affected by shingles
- In trigeminal and suboccipital neuralgia, intense, stabbing pain in attacks lasting from a few seconds to a few minutes

WHY MIGHT I HAVE THIS?

PREDISPOSING FACTORS

- Shingles
- Heavy dental work
- Head or back injury
- Aspartame (an artificial sweetner), in trigeminal neuralgia
- Caffeine, in trigeminal neuralgia

TRIGGERS

For trigeminal neuralgia

- Eating, talking, brushing the teeth, and washing the face.
- Touching certain areas on the face (known as trigger points)

WHY DOES IT OCCUR?

The pain of neuralgia is caused by damage to a nerve. Various factors can cause it, including prolonged pressure on or injury to the nerve, as may happen due to a prolapsed disk (*see p.274*). Infection, such as with the herpes zoster virus in shingles (*see p.165*), may also cause postherpetic neuralgia in the area that is affected. Facial surgery or heavy dental work, such as having a tooth extracted or root canal treatment, may also cause neuralgia.

However, in many cases the cause of neuralgia is not known. For example, doctors are usually not able to identify a cause for trigeminal neuralgia or glossopharyngeal neuralgia (in which there is severe, stabbing pain at the back of the tongue and in the back of the throat).

Trigeminal neuralgia is more common in women and in people who have multiple sclerosis (*see p.140*). In rare cases, trigeminal neuralgia may be found to be caused by compression of the trigeminal nerve by a tumor or an enlarged blood vessel.

WHAT SETS OFF THE PAIN? Some people with established neuralgia find that exposure to cold triggers attacks. In some instances, only very slight disturbance to an affected area is enough to bring on stabbing pain. In trigeminal neuralgia, for example, facial movements such as smiling or frowning may be sufficient to set off an attack. In postherpetic neuralgia, merely touching the skin may bring on the pain, while sometimes attacks can occur spontaneously, without a trigger.

IMPORTANT

See your doctor if you experience symptoms of neuralgia. In rare cases there may be a serious underlying cause.

TREATMENT PLAN

PRIMARY TREATMENTS

For postherpetic neuralgia:

- Drugs and anesthetic creams for pain relief

For trigeminal neuralgia:

- Carbamazepine (and other antiepileptics) for pain relief
- Acupuncture

BACKUP TREATMENTS

- Avoid aspartame and caffeine

- Vitamin B supplements
- Capsaicin cream

WORTH CONSIDERING

- Homeopathy
- Osteopathy, chiropractic,and cranial manipulation
- Relaxation and biofeedback
- Surgery (if trigeminal neuralgia persists)

For an explanation of how treatments are rated, see p.111.

TRIGEMINAL NEURALGIA

One of the most common types of neuralgia affects the trigeminal nerve. This nerve transmits sensation from some areas of the face to the brain. It is also involved in controlling the muscles that move the jaw to chew. Damage to the trigeminal nerve may cause bursts of stabbing pain that are felt anywhere along the path of the three branches of the nerve on a single side of the face. The cause is often not known. Attacks of trigeminal neuralgia may be brought on by chewing or certain facial movements, or by touching areas of the face.

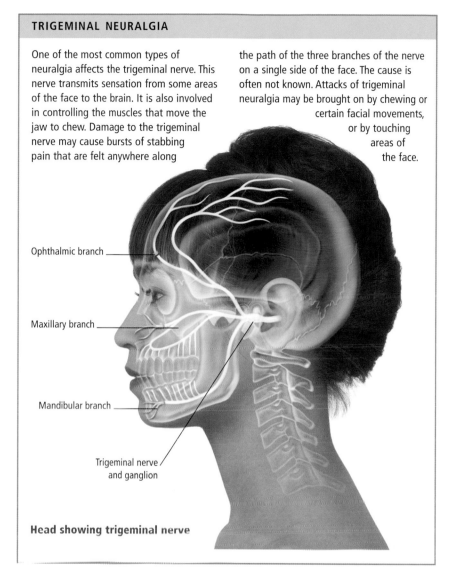

Ophthalmic branch

Maxillary branch

Mandibular branch

Trigeminal nerve and ganglion

Head showing trigeminal nerve

CAUTION

Drugs for neuralgia can cause a range of possible side effects; ask your doctor to explain these to you.

SURGERY may be considered if the symptoms of trigeminal neuralgia persist. Options include heat treatment to destroy the trigeminal nerve or microsurgery to cut it. Both procedures will cause permanent numbness on the affected side of the face. If a tumor or enlarged blood vessel is found to be the cause, surgery may be recommended to remove it.

Nutritional Therapy

ELIMINATING ASPARTAME, an artificial sweetener widely found in soft drinks and processed food, from your diet may help if you have trigeminal neuralgia. A component of aspartame, the alcohol methanol, is known to be toxic to the nerves.

CAFFEINE Avoiding caffeine, which is found in cola, chocolate, and even in some analgesics — as well as in coffee — may help if you have trigeminal neuralgia. In a case study, a woman had complete relief from her symptoms of trigeminal neuralgia after adopting a caffeine-free diet. It is possible that caffeine may trigger trigeminal neuralgia because it has a nerve-stimulating action.

B VITAMIN SUPPLEMENTS seem to be helpful in treating neuralgia. A German study showed that symptoms of neuralgia improved when patients took a B-vitamin preparation. If you have neuralgia, take a daily high-potency multi-B vitamin supplement containing at least 25mg of the major B vitamins (B_1, B_2, B_3, B_5, and B_6).

CAUTION

Ask your doctor before taking vitamin B supplements. These may interfere with the action of certain drugs. See p.46.

Homeopathy

ACONITUM NAPELLUS AND ARSENICUM ALBUM A number of homeopathic medicines may be helpful for neuralgia. *Aconitum napellus* often helps with acute

TREATMENTS IN DETAIL

Conventional Medicine

The doctor will probably be able diagnose neuralgia from the symptoms. He or she may also evaluate other possible causes of the pain. In some cases, neuralgia may be cured spontaneously. In other cases, treating any underlying cause (such as a prolapsed disk) helps relieve the pain.

PRIMARY TREATMENT **ANTIVIRAL DRUGS** (such as acyclovir) reduce the likelihood of persistent postherpetic neuralgia developing if they are started early in attacks of shingles (*see p.165*), and can also shorten the shingles attack itself. Other treatments for postherpetic neuralgia include topical preparations containing anesthetics that can be applied directly to the affected area to help relieve the pain.

PRIMARY TREATMENT **TRICYCLIC ANTIDEPRESSANTS** such as amitriptyline or nortriptyline help relieve pain caused by postherpetic neuralgia, but it is not understood why these drugs are effective.

GABAPENTIN, an antiepileptic drug, can help relieve the pain of trigeminal neuralgia. Other antiepileptic drugs may be effective in some cases. As with tricyclic antidepressants, it is not known why antiepileptic drugs relieve neuralgia. It may be that both types of drugs alter the transmission of nerve impulses, but this has not been shown.

attacks of the pain, especially if the condition is triggered by exposure to cold and particularly to dry, cold wind. In people who respond to it, the pain may alternate with a sensation of tingling or swelling and the person is usually anxious and restless during the attack.

Aconitum napellus and *Arsenicum album* patients are both anxious and restless during the attack, and the pain is made worse by cold. However, *Arsenicum album* is deeper acting and more likely to help with the underlying condition. People who respond to it are often very organized and "uptight"; they feel the cold greatly and often have dry, flaky skin. The neuralgic pain itself is usually described as of burning character and is relieved by heat.

OTHER REMEDIES *Agaricus muscaris* (made from the Fly agaric toadstool) may help when the pain is described as being like "icy needles." People who respond to it may have twitching or a facial tic, sometimes with very itchy chilblains. *Spigelia antihelmica* is one of the most important medicines for trigeminal neuralgia, especially when it is left-sided. Those whom it helps have pain that affects the eye and may be associated with palpitations.

Kalmia latifolia is associated with similar symptoms to those of *Spigelia antihelmica*, but usually on the right side. *Hypericum perforatum* may be helpful if the neuralgia came on following an injury.

Western Herbal Medicine

PRIMARY TREATMENT **CAPSAICIN** cream, derived from chili peppers (*Capsicum* spp.), 0.025% or 0.075%, may be useful for the pain of postherpetic neuralgia (*see also p.129*). It should be rubbed on the site only when the skin is unbroken. The pain will worsen for a day or two until the cream starts working, so keep using it as directed.

Acupuncture

PRIMARY TREATMENT Neuralgia is often an important component of chronic pain, and acupuncture, as well as related techniques such as transcutaneous electrical nerve stimulation (TENS), are frequently used in pain clinics to treat a variety of chronic pain syndromes. Acupuncture has a bearing on a number of pain mechanisms. It can affect the nerve transmission of pain and stimulate the production of chemicals in the body that act naturally to relieve pain (for example, endorphins and encephalins). (*See also Chronic Pain, p.144.*) Acupuncture appears to be an effective treatment for many neuralgias. One acupuncture technique, percutaneous electrical nerve stimulation (PENS), developed by Dr. William Craig, has been effective in treating nerve pain that has been caused by diabetes. The evidence for its wide use is unfortunately lacking, largely because there are so few clinical trials in this area.

TREATMENT The acupuncturist should, in general, try to avoid placing needles in the painful area. Usually needles will need to be placed in other parts of the body, or possibly the ear. Treatment should be given once or twice a week initially, but if after six to eight treatments there is no obvious benefit, then acupuncture is unlikely to be helpful. Frequently, neuralgia is an indication of some underlying imbalance that may be amenable to acupuncture. If initial treatment with acupuncture is successful, regular treatment, on a monthly basis, is likely to be recommended.

Bodywork Therapies

OSTEOPATHY OR CHIROPRACTIC may be able to relieve the frequency and intensity of trigeminal or suboccipital neuralgia when it is associated with restrictions of the facial or cranial joints.

Research at the University of Florida College of Dentistry suggests that 5 to 10 percent of patients may experience secondary trigeminal neuralgia after facial surgery, and 1 to 5 percent of patients may experience secondary trigeminal neuralgia after dental extractions. If the area was injured or subjected to heavy dental work before the onset of symptoms, there may be a mechanical factor in the nerve irritation that manipulation might relieve.

Research has also shown that trigeminal neuralgia can originate from damage to the upper spinal cord and neck area. Trauma to the head and neck, such as concussion or whiplash, may result in injury to nerve pathways. The trauma may trigger facial pain immediately or develop over months or years.

CRANIAL MANIPULATION (also known as cranial osteopathy, craniosacral technique, or sacro-occipital technique) is the specialized application of very mild forces to areas of the head. This therapy is designed to restore normal freedom of the extremely small degrees of movement that are possible at the various sutures (fixed joints in the skull) and other joints of the skull and between the facial bones. Cranial manipulation may help relieve the pain of neuralgia affecting the face and back of the head.

TRIGGER POINTS (tender points in the muscles; *see p.55*) either in the face itself or in the muscles at the front and side of the neck can produce pain that is so similar to that of trigeminal neuralgia that it can be easily confused with it.

Trigger points can be deactivated by acupuncture as well as by the manual pressure and stretching techniques that are used by osteopaths, massage therapists (particularly those with a neuromuscular therapy training), and some physical therapists and chiropractors.

Mind–Body Therapies

RELAXATION EXERCISES AND BIOFEEDBACK may be worth considering, using either electromyographic (EMG) biofeedback (*see p.101*) or muscle tension techniques. (*See also Chronic Pain, p.144.*) For some people, stress may be a factor in their neuralgia, and taking steps to reduce the incidence of stress and finding more time for relaxation may help. (*For relaxation and meditation sequences, see p.99.*)

PREVENTION PLAN

- If you develop shingles, see your doctor promptly so that antiviral drugs can be started
- If you have shingles, get plenty of rest in order to recuperate fully
- Avoid triggers such as exposure to cold weather
- Avoid caffeinated beverages and aspartame if you are prone to trigeminal neuralgia

NEUROPATHY

The peripheral nerves originate from the spinal cord and branch out to supply the body. Any disorder of these nerves is known as neuropathy. The cranial nerves, which extend from the brain to supply the head and neck, may be affected and cause facial palsy. Nerves supplying internal organs may also be affected. Neuropathies cause a range of symptoms and may be acute and short-lived or long-term. Drugs, dietary supplements, and bodywork therapies may be used to treat the underlying cause and to relieve symptoms.

WHAT ARE THE SYMPTOMS?

SENSORY NEUROPATHIES

- Tingling, pain (which may feel like an electric shock), or burning and numbness in the hands, feet, and limbs

MOTOR NERVE NEUROPATHIES

- Muscle weakness and wasting and eventually impaired mobility in some cases

AUTONOMIC NEUROPATHIES

- Fainting, diarrhea, or occasionally constipation, inability to urinate, erectile dysfunction, and an irregular heartbeat

WHY MIGHT I HAVE THIS?

PREDISPOSING FACTORS

- Exposure to toxic substances
- Alcohol abuse
- Some cancers
- Overuse of power tools that cause vibration

TRIGGERS

- Diabetes mellitus
- Vitamin deficiencies
- Infection
- Certain drugs
- Cancer
- Injury or compression of a nerve
- Inflammation of blood vessels supplying a nerve

IMPORTANT

See a doctor if you develop the symptoms of neuropathy. In some cases neuropathy may have a serious underlying cause.

WHY DOES IT OCCUR?

While some causes of neuropathy seem to damage the nerve cells directly, others harm the outer layer (the myelin sheath) of the nerves. Sometimes both are damaged. In all cases, the normal passage of signals along the peripheral nerves is disrupted, leading to the symptoms of neuropathy (see diagram p.128).

Depending on the particular nerve or nerves affected, neuropathy may affect sensation (sensory neuropathy), movement (motor neuropathy), or autonomic functions, such as bladder control (autonomic neuropathy). Neuropathy affecting the neck is known as cervical radiculopathy; when it affects the lower back it is known as lumbar radiculopathy. If the facial nerve is affected, facial palsy may result. Bell's palsy is a type of facial palsy that causes weakness or paralysis of the muscles on one side of the face.

In a mononeuropathy, one nerve is affected and the symptoms are restricted to the area supplied by that nerve. Damage to a single nerve may be due to injury or compression. For instance, carpal tunnel syndrome (see p.152) is caused by compression of the median nerve that supplies the hand. When many nerves are affected, the symptoms are more widespread; this condition is called polyneuropathy.

COMMON CAUSES The most common cause of neuropathy in developed countries is diabetes mellitus (see p.314). If diabetes is poorly controlled, high blood glucose levels may damage the peripheral nerves and the blood vessels supplying them. Deficiencies in certain B vitamins and other nutrients may also cause neuropathy. The most common cause worldwide is Hansen's disease (leprosy); infection with other viruses, such as HIV (see p.470), may also cause neuropathy.

Neuropathy may develop if the blood vessels that supply the nerves become inflamed, as occurs in polyarteritis nodosa. Some cancers can cause neuropathy. Certain drugs and toxic substances can damage nerves, as can vibration resulting from overuse of power tools. Sometimes the cause of a neuropathy is unknown.

TREATMENT PLAN

PRIMARY TREATMENTS

- Treatment of underlying cause

BACK-UP TREATMENTS

- Vitamin B_{12} injections and vitamin B_6
- Capsaicin (for diabetic neuropathy)
- Environmental health measures
- Acupuncture

WORTH CONSIDERING

- Bodywork therapies and yoga
- Evening primrose oil (for diabetic neuropathy)

For an explanation of how treatments are rated, see p.111.

SELF-HELP

The following measures can help you manage diabetic neuropathy:

- Check your feet every day for signs of injury, which you may not be able to feel due to nerve damage. See your

doctor immediately if you notice any changes.
- Make sure that nothing in your shoes can injure or irritate your feet, such as ill-fitting linings or soles.
- Use a moisturizer if the skin on your feet is dry and/or thin.
- Limit your caffeine intake. Caffeine may make the pain of neuropathy worse.
- Get regular exercise.
- Massage your hands and feet every day.

TREATMENTS IN DETAIL

Conventional Medicine

Your doctor will probably diagnose neuropathy from your symptoms. He or she may do a physical examination and arrange for other tests, such as electromyography and nerve conduction tests, to find out more. Further tests may be done to look for an underlying cause, for example, a blood test to measure blood sugar levels.

PRIMARY TREATMENT **TREATING AN UNDERLYING CAUSE** when possible is the first approach. If alcohol abuse is a cause, vitamin B₁ supplements will be recommended. Corticosteroids may be given for polyarteritis nodosa.

Nutritional Therapy

VITAMIN B₁₂ (methylcobalamin) may accelerate recovery from Bell's palsy. In one study, 60 people with Bell's palsy were given standard steroid therapy, standard steroid therapy plus methylcobalamin, or methylcobalamin alone. The group given methylcobalamin alone recovered most quickly. The time required for complete recovery of facial nerve function was significantly shorter in the methylcobalamin and methylcobalamin plus steroid groups (average of about two weeks) than in the steroid group (average of about nine weeks). The dose of methylcobalamin used in the study was 500mcg. It was injected intramuscularly, three times a week for at least eight weeks or until recovery was complete. People considering vitamin B₁₂ injections for facial palsy should consult their doctor.

Vitamin B₁₂ (cobalamin) treatment may also be useful in treating other forms of neuropathy. Deficiency of cobalamin can

produce a number of neurologic problems, including neuropathy in the nerves in the limbs and in the optic nerve, and these always need thorough investigation. If you have a neuropathy and vitamin B₁₂ deficiency is suspected, medical investigation is always needed.

VITAMIN B₆ (pyroxidine) may also be useful. People with diabetic neuropathy may have an underlying vitamin B₆ deficiency. In one study, people with diabetic neuropathy took supplements of 150mg of pyridoxine per day. Most people in the study experienced some initial relief of pain and abnormal sensation within approximately 10 days. Improvement continued throughout the experimental period with lessening or a disappearance of symptoms. After the experimental period, 70 percent of patients asked to continue taking B₆ supplements. Within three weeks of stopping pyridoxine therapy, the remaining 30 percent of patients had a recurrence of their diabetic neuropathy symptoms. If you have diabetic neuropathy, try taking 50mg of B₆, two or three times a day

CAUTION

Vitamin B may reduce the effectiveness of certain drugs: ask your doctor for advice (*see also p.46*). High doses of vitamin B₆ (over 500mg per day, or 150mg per day for some people) can cause neuropathy.

ALPHA-LINOLENIC ACID (ALA), an antioxidant sold as a dietary supplement, has been used to treat diabetic neuropathy. Clinical trials have mainly examined intravenous use; a large, controlled trial that looked at a combination of intravenous and oral alpha-lipoic acid found no improvement of symptoms, but the treatment helped prevent deterioration of nerve function.

GAMMA-LINOLENIC ACID (GLA) is an essential fatty acid in the omega-6 series, formed in the body from linoleic acid (provided by vegetable oils). People with diabetes generally have a reduced ability to convert dietary linoleic acid in the diet to GLA. The lack of GLA and the molecules it converts to in the body may play a role in the development of neuropathy.

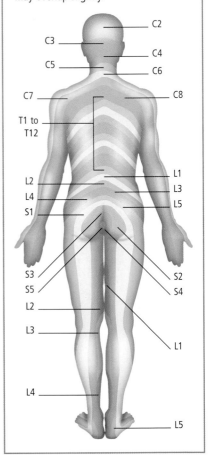

NERVES AND DERMATOMES

The spinal nerves branch out from the spinal cord and supply different areas of the body. The areas of the surface of the skin supplied by specific spinal nerves are known as dermatomes. The dermatomes in the trunk are all horizontal, while the dermatomes in the limbs are vertical. Dermatomes are named according to the spinal nerves that supply them — "C" stands for cervical (neck region), "T" indicates the thoracic (chest region), "L" stands for lumbar (low back and parts of thighs and legs), and "S" refers to sacral (parts of thighs and legs, buttocks, genital areas, and feet). Areas of sensation may overlap slightly.

GLA supplements have been noted to bring about improvements in diabetic neuropathy. In one trial, GLA supplementation at a dose of 480mg per day for a year was shown to reverse existing diabetic neuropathy. Evening primrose oil contains GLA and has been found to help alleviate the symptoms of diabetic neuropathy. If you have diabetic neuropathy, try taking 4–6g of evening primrose oil a day.

Western Herbal Medicine

CAPSAICIN CREAM Capsaicin is the active ingredient in chili peppers (*Capsicum* spp.), making them irritating to the tongue and skin. When used in a cream to treat diabetic neuropathy, capsaicin appears to deplete the chemical messengers that send signals through the peripheral nerves, lessening the sensation of pain despite the fact that the cause is still present. Several trials suggest that capsaicin cream is an effective and safe way to treat diabetic neuropathy.

Creams, gels, and roll-on preparations containing capsaicin are available in strengths ranging from 0.025% to 0.075%. It is probably best to begin using capsaicin cream at the lowest strength and progress to stronger concentrations if necessary. Some people experience a burning sensation and redness at the site where the cream is applied, but this generally lessens with repeated applications. Capsaicin cream should not be applied more than four times a day, and it may take up to four weeks for maximum benefit to be seen.

> **CAUTION**
>
> Keep all medications containing capsaicin away from the eyes and the mucous membranes. Do not apply the cream immediately after bathing or showering. Wash your hands very carefully after each application.

Acupuncture

Acupuncture appears to provide pain relief in some cases of neuropathy. It affects some of the pain mechanisms, such as the transmission of pain by nerves, and encourages the production of certain chemicals, such as endorphins and encephalins, that inhibit pain. Acupuncture can also deactivate trigger points (tender areas in muscles) that may arise due to a neuropathy. The evidence for acupuncture to treat neuropathy is limited and few clinical trials are available. The main disadvantage in using acupuncture to treat degenerative neurological conditions is that treatment may need to be

repeated frequently. Acupuncture treatment for neuropathy should be given on a weekly basis and abandoned if no effect is seen after six to eight sessions.

Environmental Health

An environmental health expert may be able to help detect the cause of a neuropathy. Environmental causes include compounds toxic to the nerves, certain medications (including some of the chemotherapeutic agents used to treat cancer), and mechanical injury resulting in compression of a nerve. Even simple pressure on nerves, such as prolonged use of crutches or sitting in the same position for a long time, can cause it, as can therapeutic drugs, workplace chemicals, and environmental pollutants.

Exposure to heavy metals such as lead, mercury, arsenic, and mercury has well-documented neurological effects. Nerve degeneration can be associated with chronic cocaine or stimulant abuse; recreational drugs can induce both neurological and psychiatric impact.

EXTREME COLD AND VIRUSES There are two possible causes of the specific neuropathy known as Bell's palsy, which affects the facial nerve. In some people, exposure to extreme cold temperatures can lead to symptoms of Bell's palsy. In others, a viral cause occurs with exposure to anything that lowers the activity or effectiveness of our immune systems. This weakening of the immune system allows latent viruses to become activated and inflict certain nerve cells, as with the case of trichloroethylene and the herpes simplex virus.

Bodywork Therapies

TRIGGER POINT DEACTIVATION Some forms of neuropathy activate trigger points that aggravate the symptoms. An acupuncturist or osteopath, a physical therapist, massage therapist, or chiropractor may be able to deactivate any trigger points. This can be helpful in addition to whatever else is done to treat the neuropathy itself.

CRANIAL MANIPULATION aimed at restoring normal movement to the joints of the face and skull may, in some cases, be effective in relieving Bell's palsy.

Neuropathic symptoms elsewhere in the body that are specifically caused by nerve entrapment or compression can often be eased or relieved by specialized physical therapy methods involving very precise, carefully performed stretching and mobilization techniques. Among the most common neuropathies that can be improved using these methods are carpal tunnel syndrome (*see p.152*) and the ulnar tunnel neuropathy (affecting the elbow).

OSTEOPATHY AND CHIROPRACTIC When neuropathy results from spinal nerve compression, possibly involving disk damage, osteopathic and chiropractic manipulation may effectively ease the pain that can result from the nerve compression or irritation. However, manipulation in the presence of a prolapsed disk requires expert skills; be sure that your practitioner has experience in dealing with prolapsed disks.

MASSAGE Regular massage of the hands and feet can help maintain circulation in diabetic neuropathy and prevent complications, such as ulceration, that result from poor blood flow to the extremities. Massage appears to work whether self-administered or done by another person.

Yoga

Certain neuropathic conditions involving nerve entrapment, such as carpal tunnel syndrome (*see p.152*), have been treated using yoga stretching techniques. For peripheral neuropathy, yoga may help relax tense muscles, lessen pain, and make it easier for individuals to cope with their condition. Yoga is also a good form of exercise for people with diabetic retinopathy because it tends to be gentle and is unlikely to cause damage to tissues.

> **PREVENTION PLAN**
>
> **The following may help prevent the development of neuropathy:**
> - Avoid environmental hazards
> - Take a vitamin B-complex supplement
> - If you have diabetes mellitus, keep your blood-sugar levels well controlled

MEMORY IMPAIRMENT

A certain degree of memory impairment is a normal consequence of aging. The decline may begin as early as the mid-30s and be noticeable by the mid-40s. It usually has a gradual onset and mainly affects short-term memory. Lack of regular mental stimulation, which can occur when a person retires, may contribute to the condition. Treatment for poor memory might involve drugs if there is an underlying cause, dietary changes, vitamin supplements, physical exercise, and psychological techniques to improve memory recall.

WHAT ARE THE SYMPTOMS?

- Inability to recall short-term events
- Inability to remember short-term information

WHY MIGHT I HAVE THIS?

PREDISPOSING FACTORS

- Normal aging and lack of mental stimulation
- Free radical damage
- Raised homocysteine levels
- Underlying physical or psychological disorder
- Certain drugs, such as antiepiltleptic drugs and mood stabilizers

TRIGGERS

- Fatigue

TREATMENT PLAN

PRIMARY TREATMENTS

- Drugs to treat any underlying condition (e.g., hypothyroidism)
- Ginkgo biloba
- Memory tasks

BACKUP TREATMENTS

- Oily fish
- Antioxidants and B vitamins

WORTH CONSIDERING

- Homeopathy
- Acupuncture
- Exercise
- Breathing techniques

For an explanation of how treatments are rated, see p.111.

WHY DOES IT OCCUR?

NORMAL AGING Some degree of memory impairment can be expected with age. As a person grows older, the ability to learn gradually declines, although life experience increases and the intellectual faculties continue to develop. By 50 to 70 years of age, short-term memory and the ability to concentrate become reduced. By 90, the brain has lost up to 10 percent of its tissue.

BRAIN DISORDERS Memory impairment may occur as a result of various brain disorders. It may be caused by dementia (*see p.133*), or it may follow a head injury, in which case memory may return to normal after a few weeks. An underlying physical illness, such as hypothyroidism (*see p.319*), or a psychological condition, such as severe depression (*see p.436*), or anxiety (*see p.414*) may contribute to poor memory. Certain drugs, including antiepileptics and mood stabilizers, can also cause memory loss.

OTHER FACTORS Low levels of essential fatty acids and vitamin E in the diet and raised levels of homocysteine in the body have been linked with poor memory. It may also be caused by a deficiency of vitamin B, or pernicious anemia, or even lack of mental stimulation. Respiratory alkalosis, in which the blood is too alkaline due to rapid deep breathing, may contribute to poor short-term memory by creating an oxygen deficit in the brain.

IMPORTANT

See your doctor if memory impairment is causing concern or interfering with daily life.

TREATMENTS IN DETAIL

Conventional Medicine

The doctor will assess memory and brain functions. If memory impairment is considered to be worse than expected for a person's age, tests (such as thyroid function tests and CT or MRI scanning of the brain) may be performed to rule out an underlying condition.

PRIMARY TREATMENT **UNDERLYING CAUSE** Treatment of memory loss is aimed at treating the underlying cause wherever possible. For example, hypothyroidism is treated by thyroid hormone supplements and depression may be relieved by antidepressant drugs.

Nutritional Therapy

Brain tissue is rich in healthy essential fats known as long-chain polyunsaturated fatty acids (PUFAs). In recent years, a lot of scientific attention has been focused on the role in brain function of the omega-3 PUFAs, such as eicosapentaenoic acid (EPA) and docosahexaenoic acid (DHA).

Some people have a tendency to low blood sugar. Their concentration and memory may deteriorate whenever blood-sugar levels dip too low. (*For information on stabilizing blood sugar, see p.42.*)

OILY FISH EPA and DHA are found in abundance in oily fish (such as salmon, trout, tuna, mackerel, herring, and sardines), and studies suggest that high fish consumption helps reduce the risk of brain function decline. Two Dutch observational studies found that those who ate a lot of

MIND MAPPING

Mind mapping brings the creative thinking and visual areas of the brain into play to help jog memory recall. To start a mind map, write down in the centre of some paper a main theme, for example "holiday". From the central word, draw a line or arrow and jot down items to be remembered such as "passport". Use another line for tasks to be done before you leave, such as "empty fridge". Your map can be as elaborate or simple as you like. Below are some tips to guide you.

DRAW YOUR MAP	KEEP IT SIMPLE	THINK VISUALLY
• Write the map's theme in the center and work outward. • Group related items together. • Use colored pens for different sections. • Look for relationships and use arrows or lines to link related ideas. • Leave some space to add more ideas later. • Try capital letters to make key words stand out clearly.	• Just have key words or images — not sentences. • Write down words as they occur. • Allow ideas to flow. • If you can't think what to add in one area, move on to another.	• Illustrate with doodles, shapes, or little pictures. They create a visual relationship with the idea that helps you remember things later. • Try an image at the center of the map — this is particularly effective. • Use colors to highlight key tasks or to group related items. • Enjoy the task — creativity aids memory.

fish had about half the risk of developing dementia compared to those who ate little or no fish. No clinical studies of fish or fish oil and memory impairment have been done in humans, but supplements of EPA and DHA have been shown to improve memory in animals. Including at least two portions of oily fish in the diet per week might be useful in maintaining memory. Taking daily supplements of concentrated fish oils at a dose of 2g per day may also help preserve memory in the long term.

ANTIOXIDANTS The mental decline that occurs with aging may be related to damaging molecules known as free radicals. Free radicals are quenched in the body by antioxidant substances, such as beta-carotene and vitamins C and E. There is some evidence that increasing intakes of antioxidant nutrients might help maintain mental sharpness. One study found that people who consumed 2.1mg (3,500 IU) of beta-carotene per day were half as likely to experience cognitive impairment, disorientation, or have difficulty solving problems compared to those taking 0.9mg (1500 IU) or less per day. Another study found that higher levels of vitamin C and beta-carotene in the body were associated with better memory. Citrus and kiwi fruits, strawberries, broccoli, cabbage, and brussels sprouts are especially rich in vitamin C, while deep green and yellow-orange vegetables (e.g. carrots, spinach, and sweet potatoes) are all good sources of beta-carotene. It would be reasonable to supplement the diet with 5,000–10,000 IU of beta-carotene and 1g of vitamin C daily to see if it helps memory.

The antioxidant vitamin E has also been related to memory. In one study, people with the lowest vitamin E levels were almost three times worse at remembering than those with the highest levels. Other studies also show that high vitamin E levels are associated with good brain function.

Good sources of vitamin E include nuts and seeds. In addition, supplementing with vitamin E at a dose of 400–800 IU per day may be helpful.

FOLIC ACID AND OTHER B VITAMINS Another link between nutrition and brain function concerns the amino acid homocysteine. Raised levels of homocysteine have been linked to chronic diseases such as heart disease and osteoporosis. Research also shows a relationship between raised homocysteine levels and reduced mental performance. Folic acid (which is a B vitamin), vitamin B_{12}, and vitamin B_6 have all been found to help reduce homocysteine levels in the body.

Interestingly, studies have found people with low folic acid levels have impaired memory function compared to people with normal folic acid levels. Folic acid is found in green leafy vegetables, and liver, avocado, bananas, and fish are rich in vitamin B_6. Foods that contain vitamin B_{12} include meat, fish, and eggs.

You may also want to take a supplement. A study into the effects of supplements on women found that taking 750mcg of folic acid, 15mcg of vitamin B_{12}, and 75mg of vitamin B_6 each day for 35 days had a significant positive effect on some measures of memory performance in comparison to a placebo, which had no effect. Taking a vitamin B-complex supplement each day may also help memory.

> **CAUTION**
> Vitamin B_6 may react with certain drugs, including anticonvulsants such as phenytoin. Ask your doctor for advice.

Homeopathy

A number of homeopathic medicines may help with memory. (*For dosages, see p.77.*)

BARYTA CARBONICA AND LYCOPODIUM are the most important for age-related memory problems. *Baryta carbonica* is effective where there are arteriosclerosis (hardening of the arteries), memory problems, and mental slowness. The person affected may become timid and childish and have offensive foot odor. Symptoms may be worse in cold, damp weather and affected people may get recurrent colds with neck glands that become very hard and swollen. *Baryta carbonica* may also be helpful for younger people who experience memory problems after illnesses, especially infectious mononucleosis.

People who respond to *Lycopodium* are often serious intellectual people who may have held responsible jobs. These people become depressed and reclusive because they lose self-confidence over their memory problems. These people often have stomach trouble, with gas and bloating, and have a sweet tooth.

PHOSPHORIC ACID is another medicine that may be helpful for younger people, especially when they experience the effects of intellectual and emotional stress combined — for instance, the stress of exams combined with relationship difficulties. They appear depressed, apathetic, and slow to answer questions.

ANACARDIUM ORIENTALE is sometimes helpful if there is sudden memory loss, as happens when a name or an idea suddenly goes out of someone's head. Affected people may also have sudden, violent tempers.

Western Herbal Medicine

GINKGO (*Ginkgo biloba*) Research on ginkgo for memory impairment that is associated with age has had conflicting results, with some studies showing benefit and other research not showing a benefit.

> **CAUTION**
>
> See p.69 before taking a herbal remedy and, if you are taking prescribed medication, consult an herbal medicine expert first.

Acupuncture

If memory impairment is considered as part of a traditional Chinese diagnosis, then regular acupuncture treatment may improve overall balance and function including memory, either through a traditional Chinese approach or through the more Westernized explanation of improved cerebral circulation. Although there are no controlled trials suggesting that acupuncture improves memory, there are a number of anecdotal suggestions that it may help. Usually, treatments on a weekly basis are required to obtain a sustained improvement. If the underlying cause of memory impairment is a disease such as Alzheimer's, treatment such as acupuncture might slow down the development of dementia. Although studies in rats showed a possible role for acupuncture in memory impairment, no clinical trials have been performed. It is known that acupuncture is not effective at curing the underlying cause of the memory loss, but can only relieve the memory loss itself, to some degree in some people. The individual's memory capacity should be tested before the start of treatment and after six to eight weekly sessions have been completed. If no progress is made, acupuncture should be abandoned.

Exercise and Breathing

Respiratory alkalosis (*see p.57*) may cause short-term memory loss and an inability to "stay focused." The condition prevents red blood cells from releasing oxygen efficiently, which increases the oxygen deficit in the brain, known as the Bohr effect. The solution is to increase the efficiency of delivery of oxygenated blood to the brain and aid the release of oxygen to body tissues.

EXERCISE is one of the most obvious and beneficial ways to improve delivery of oxygenated blood to the brain. Researchers have also found that there is a clear link between high blood-sugar levels and reduced volume of the hippocampus, a structure within the brain that is concerned with memory and learning. People whose blood-sugar regulation is impaired commonly perform more poorly than normal in memory tests. Since weight loss and exercise can both normalize blood-sugar levels, it seems obvious that a healthy lifestyle that includes regular exercise can help improve your memory.

In important research on the relationship between exercise and memory, it was discovered that people with the respiratory condition chronic obstructive pulmonary disease (COPD) demonstrated instant improvement in their thinking processes and memory immediately after 20 minutes of riding a stationary bicycle, at a rate that reached their peak performance level. The assessment after exercise evaluated verbal processing, attention span, short-term memory, and motor skills. The results indicate an improved ability on the part of each participant to process and retain information than he or she could before exercise. These people, because of their diseased lungs, had been forced to adopt a breathing pattern that led to excessive carbon dioxide exhalation. This resulted in an oxygen deficit in the brain, which the exercise helped reverse. The research shows the potential for improving short-term memory loss by stimulating circulation through even modest amounts of exercise.

BREATHING TECHNIQUES Slowing your breathing rate and improving your abdominal breathing also improve the efficiency of delivery of oxygenated blood around the body. (*For details, see p.62.*)

Mind–Body Therapies

Memory impairment is a common aspect of aging. However, along with physical trauma, it can be associated with a number of other psychological problems, such as anxiety (*see p.414*) and depression (*see p.436*). Post-traumatic stress (*see p.422*) may also affect memory in that traumatic memories intrude into everyday life.

PRIMARY TREATMENT **MEMORY TASKS** Dementia (*p.133*) is probably the most common cause of memory impairment and recently some talking therapy techniques have been developed to help address the memory loss aspect. (*See also box, p.131.*) In spaced retrieval (SR), a patient is given a memory task at increasingly extended intervals, which helps the person recall how to remember. A number of studies have supported this method of working. Cueing hierarchy, in which a correct sequence of words must be remembered, is another method and has been compared directly with SR. In studies both treatments were effective, although more goals were attained using SR.

> **PREVENTION PLAN**
>
> - Take ginkgo biloba supplements
> - Practice memory techniques
> - Exercise regularly
> - Follow a healthy diet

DEMENTIA

Memory loss, personality changes, and a decline in intellectual ability characterize dementia. The condition is more common in people over the age of 65, and genetic factors may play a part in some types. An essential first step is an assessment to identify and treat any underlying disorders. Although the condition usually cannot be cured, a range of treatments might help control the symptoms, including drugs, dietary methods, massage, music therapy, and relaxation training.

WHAT ARE THE SYMPTOMS?

- Impaired memory, especially regarding recent events
- Loss of intellect that affects reasoning and understanding
- Difficulty holding a conversation
- Reduced vocabulary
- Emotional outbursts and agitation
- Physical wandering
- Neglect of personal hygiene

WHY MIGHT I HAVE THIS?

PREDISPOSING FACTORS

- Risk factors for stroke, including high blood pressure, smoking, and diabetes mellitus
- Long-term alcohol abuse
- Raised homocysteine levels
- Advanced age
- Genetics (in some types)

IMPORTANT

Anyone suspected of having dementia should have a thorough medical assessment. Elderly people with severe depression may seem to have dementia because the conditions share some symptoms, such as forgetfulness.

WHY DOES IT OCCUR?

The underlying abnormality in dementia is degeneration of the brain tissue, but the exact cause of the condition is often not known. Alzheimer's disease is probably the best known and most common type of dementia, but there are many others, including multi-infarct dementia, Pick's disease, and Lewy body disease.

In Alzheimer's disease, cells in some areas of the brain are destroyed, while other cells become less responsive to neurotransmitters (chemicals that transmit messages in the brain). Chemical changes in the brain are thought to play a role in the condition, with a decline in levels of acetylcholine and other neurotransmitters. Abnormal tissues and deposits of abnormal protein also appear in the brains of people with Alzheimer's disease.

Dementia sometimes results from an underlying cause, such as damage to the brain from interruption to its blood supply by recurrent small strokes (known as multi-infarct dementia). Other possible causes include long-term alcohol abuse, hypothyroidism (see p.319), and HIV infection (see p.170). It may develop after a heart attack or a brain injury and some types of dementia may have genetic factors involved.

Recent research has shown that people who have had a stroke (see p.148) are at a high risk of developing dementia. Dementia that develops after stroke begins as an Alzheimer's-type condition, but later takes on the characteristics of vascular dementia.

Alzheimer's disease usually develops gradually, while multi-infarct dementia tends to develop more rapidly. People with dementia often do not realize that there is anything wrong with them, which can make the condition even more distressing for friends and family. In the initial stages, however, they may be aware of what is happening, which can cause depression. Caregivers for people with dementia often need support themselves.

TREATMENT PLAN

PRIMARY TREATMENTS
- Treatment of any underlying cause
- Donepezil and galantamine (for mild to moderate Alzheimer's disease)
- Emotional and practical support

BACKUP TREATMENTS
- Drugs for symptoms (such as agitation)
- Dietary changes
- Antioxidant vitamins
- Western herbal medicine

WORTH CONSIDERING
- Environmental health measures
- Contact with nature (for its calming effect)
- Exercise
- Bodywork therapies
- Acupuncture
- Mind–body therapies

For an explanation of how treatments are rated, see p.111.

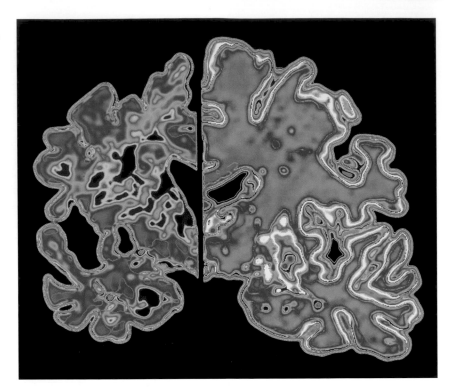

This color-enhanced scan of an Alzheimer's disease brain *(left)* and a normal brain *(right)* shows how the Alzheimer's brain is considerably shrunken and the surface is more deeply folded than the normal brain.

TREATMENTS IN DETAIL

Conventional Medicine

PRIMARY TREATMENT The doctor will do a careful medical history of the person affected and will often speak with a close relative or friend as well to get additional information. He may also refer the person affected for cognitive testing to assess intellectual function, and may arrange other tests, such as blood tests to check thyroid gland function. Where possible, the doctor will aim to treat the underlying cause. Sometimes side effects of certain drugs or severe depression can mimic dementia.

PRIMARY TREATMENT **DRUGS** are now available for treating some people with mild to moderate Alzheimer's disease. Examples include donepezil, tacrine, and galantamine (which was originally isolated from daffodil bulbs). There is some evidence to suggest that they may slow the disease or sometimes even improve intellectual ability. Regular assessments are performed to monitor any change. A drug is likely to be stopped if there is no response. Drugs such as sedatives may also be prescribed to treat other symptoms of dementia, such as agitation.

CAUTION

Drugs for dementia have a range of possible side effects; ask your doctor to explain these to you.

PRIMARY TREATMENT **SUPPORT** A person with dementia usually needs assistance with day-to-day living and may at some point require full-time care in a nursing home. In the later stages of dementia, behavioral and psychiatric symptoms can be the worst aspect of the disease for caregivers. Learning behavioral techniques can be essential in helping control patients.

People who care for someone with dementia in the home usually find the task very demanding and stressful and are often in need of support themselves. The doctor can put caregivers in touch with organizations and support groups who can offer them both practical and emotional support. Respite care, where the caregiver is able to have some time off or go on vacation, can often be arranged. (*See also Useful Addresses, p.486.*)

PRIMARY TREATMENT **EXERCISE** Physical activity may help prevent dementia; one study found that men and women over 65 who exercised regularly had about half the risk of Alzeimer's disease or other types of dementia as people who did not. Exercise may also help relieve depression in patients with Alzheimer's disease. Intellectual stimulation may also help protect against dementia.

Nutritional Therapy

DIETARY CHANGES Oily fish (e.g. salmon, trout, tuna, mackerel, herring) and foods such as flaxseed oil contain omega-3 fatty acids. Eating fish regularly may reduce the risk of dementia.

In addition, studies show that the levels of DHA are generally lower in the brains and blood plasma of Alzheimer's patients than in those of normal elderly individuals. Individuals wishing to stave off Alzheimer's disease and dementia may do well to consume a diet high in omega-3 fatty acids, for example by eating two portions of oily fish a week.

Monounsaturated fats, found in extra-virgin olive oil, avocados, and nuts, have also been found to slow brain function decline. Eating plenty of these foods may help maintain brain function.

ANTIOXIDANTS Some scientists have been looking at the role that damaging molecules called free radicals play in Alzheimer's disease. Free radicals damage cell membranes (including nerve cells) and are quenched in the body by antioxidants. It is thought that brain function may be protected if antioxidant intake is increased.

Vitamin E (an important antioxidant nutrient) at a dose of 2000 IU per day has been shown to help protect against Alzheimer's disease, and to extend the time that people with Alzheimer's disease are able to care for themselves. Studies have found that supplements of vitamins C and E and high dietary intakes of these nutrients are associated with a reduced risk of dementia and Alzheimer's disease.

Another antioxidant, beta-carotene, may also be helpful in preventing cognitive decline. In a study of more than 5,000 individuals aged 55 to 95, it was found that those consuming 2.1mg (3,500 IU) of the antioxidant beta-carotene per day were half as likely to suffer cognitive impairment, or disorientation, and have difficulty

called phosphatidylcholine, which our bodies can synthesize and is contained in all our cells. Dietary sources include eggs, soybeans, and meat. Many studies of lecithin for treating dementia have been performed, but the results do not show a

inflammation within it, the net effect being to stabilize and strengthen nervous system function. Most research on ginkgo extract has been done on a standardized extract, EGb761, which is sold under several different brand names, including Ginkgold and Ginkgoba. Many studies of ginkgo extract have been performed, and some have found a benefit for mental function and mood. In the studies with positive results, cognitive activity, including memory and recall, is stimulated; other research has not found a benefit. Clinical research has shown that ginkgo is most effective in mitigating mild to moderate dementia, but there are indications that it can also slow deterioration in severe dementia. The usual dose is 40mg of standardized ginkgo extract, 2–3 times a day. If it is taken at the recommended dose, side effects are rare.

> An estimated 18 million people worldwide have dementia. By 2025 that number will double

in problem-solving compared to those who took 0.9 mg (1,500 IU) or more per day. Taking 5,000–10,000 IU of beta-carotene, 600–800 IU of vitamin E, and 1–2g of vitamin C per day may provide some protection from the onset of dementia in the long term.

VITAMIN B High levels of the blood chemical homocysteine have also been found in people with Alzheimer's disease. The authors of one study concluded that an increased plasma homocysteine level is a strong independent risk factor for the development of dementia and Alzheimer's disease. A raised homocysteine level (determined by a blood test) can often be successfully treated with supplements of vitamin B_6 (at least 10mg per day), vitamin B_{12} (at least 50mcg per day), and folic acid (at least 400mcg per day). In the light of current research, it is quite likely that taking a daily B-complex supplement may help preserve brain function in the long run. Nutritional approaches are worth trying in dementia regardless of its cause, whether it is caused by multiple small strokes or Alzheimer's disease.

ACETYL-L-CARNITINE can increase the production of the brain neurotransmitter acetylcholine. Although early studies suggested that acetyl-L-carnitine was helpful for dementia, more recent, larger studies have not shown a benefit of this therapy on mental or social function. Acetyl-L-carnitine is fairly safe but can antagonize thyroid hormone; therefore, people with thyroid problems should avoid it. The normal dose of acetyl-l-carnitine is 500–1,000mg, three times a day.

LECITHIN, which is made commercially from soybeans, is rich in a phospholipid

clear benefit. However, lecithin is harmless. The usual dose for dementia is 1/2–1oz (15–30g) three times daily; if pure phosphatidylcholine is being used, the dose is 1–2 teaspoons (5–10g) three times daily.

VINPOCETINE is a synthetic form of a substance found in lesser periwinkle (*Vinca minor*). It is sold in the US as a dietary supplement. Several studies that looked at short-term use of vinpocetine found a benefit, but more definite studies should be done. Vinpocetine appears to be safe.

Western Herbal Medicine

Several herbal medicines may be useful in the prevention and treatment of dementia, in particular, Alzheimer's disease. People who are seeking to treat dementia with herbal medicine should consult a healthcare practitioner knowledgable about herbal medicines, who will prescribe herbs that enhance cerebral blood flow and promote anti-inflammatory and antioxidant activity within the brain.

Anxiety and depression are commonly associated with dementia, so uplifting and relaxing herbs such as lemon balm (*Melissa officinalis*) and St. John's wort (*Hypericum perforatum*) may be suggested. You may also want to consider massaging tense neck and shoulder muscles with lavender (*Lavandula* spp.) oil.

GINKGO (*Ginkgo biloba*) and members of the mint family, such as sage and rosemary, are among the best-known herbal treatments for dementia. Ginkgo is the herb of choice in treating dementia, having been the subject of extensive laboratory and clinical research. Gingko extracts improve circulation to the brain and inhibits

SAGE (*Salvia officinalis*) Substances from sage inhibit the enzyme acetylcholinesterose; several drugs that are used to treat dementia have the same effect. A short-term (four-month) study showed a benefit of treatment with sage extract on the mental function of Alzheimer's patients. However, sage contains thujone, a potentially toxic compound; therefore, it cannot be recommended for longer term use.

AROMATHERAPY The fragrance of some herbs may help soothe patients with dementia. A small study found no effect of inhaling essential oils of lavender, sweet orange, or tea tree, but a larger study found that applying lotion scented with essential oil of lemon balm (*Melissa officinalis*) was more effective for reducing agitation than the lotion alone.

> **CAUTION**
>
> See p.69 before taking a herbal remedy and, if you are taking prescribed medication, consult an herbal medicine expert first.

Environmental Health

There are many chemicals that could damage neurons and lead to dementia, although definitive proof is often lacking.

ENVIRONMENTAL HAZARDS People in occupations that could expose them to electromagnetic fields (radio and television stations, power plants, airports, electrical plants, or telephone repair) could be at increased risk of developing dementia.

An elevated level of aluminum in your drinking water is associated with an increased risk of dementia and Alzheimer's disease. Chronic solvent exposure may lead to memory problems. However, one study did not find an association between Alzheimer's disease and exposure to solvents, although this may be due to the difficulty in characterizing and measuring exposure to solvents. The true nature of these exposures and the risk that they pose for the development of dementia are still speculative and will need further study.

PROTECTION There may be a significant amount of individual variation with respect to susceptibility to environmental chemicals that may lead to dementia. It is possible that the mechanism for damage from these compounds is through free-radical formation (*see Nutrititional Therapy, p.134*); if further research confirms this, then free-radical scavengers (antioxidants) such as vitamin E may be useful in prevention and treatment.

CONTACT WITH NATURE may have a beneficial influence on people with dementia. A study has shown that people with progressive Alzheimer's disease who live in nursing homes without gardens tend to become more aggressive than people with the condition who have access to the outdoors.

Acupuncture

There is preliminary evidence showing that acupuncture may be helpful for treatment of Alzheimer's disease. It is believed to induce the proliferation and differentiation of neural hippocampal stem cells.

Bodywork Therapies

Dementia is often accompanied by outbursts of agitated behavior, sometimes verbal and sometimes involving physical violence. This behavior can be extremely upsetting and disturbing to the patients' families and other caregivers. Research studies have shown that body massage, hand massage, and/or peaceful background music can play an important role in reducing the incidence of agitated behavior in people with dementia.

MASSAGE AND MUSIC In a study comparing the effects of ten minutes of soothing music with ten minutes of calming hand massage, it was found that both methods reduced nonaggressive agitated behavior for at least an hour afterward, but neither method had any effect on the aggressive behavior sometimes associated with the

> Only a small number of dementia cases are thought to be due to genetic factors

later stages of Alzheimer's disease. The music used in this type of research had a slow tempo, soft dynamic levels, and repetitive themes; care was taken to avoid recognizable melodies that might evoke emotional responses.

Back massage too can be a soothing influence: in one study people with dementia in a nursing home were given back massage and displays of agitated behavior reduced in frequency, although verbal agitation was unaffected.

Mind–Body Therapies

RELAXATION TRAINING A relaxation session may temporarily help relieve symptoms. A study of the effects of relaxation on dementia investigated the effectiveness of intensive relaxation training in people ranging in age from 52 to 93 years old who had been diagnosed with either Alzheimer's disease or multi-infarct dementia. The results demonstrated that relaxation training may be an effective aid in the management of behavioral problems such as forgetfulness and disorientation in elderly patients who have dementia. Music therapy may also be instrumental in relaxation (*see Bodywork Therapies, left*).

COGNITIVE STIMULATION THERAPY A recent study showed that cognitive stimulation therapy (CST) appears to improve both cognitive function and the quality of life in people who have various forms of dementia. This technique involves having people with dementia do various cognitive "tasks" that are related to real-world events and people. In the randomized controlled study, 115 older people with dementia took part in

a CST program that ran twice weekly for 45 minutes at a time. Sessions began with a physical warmup activity, followed by activities that encouraged the processing of information rather than a simple recall of facts. The topics that were included in the CST sessions involved money, current events, famous faces, and word games. None of the participants in the program took medication for their dementia. At the end of the 14-week trial period, the group who had attended the CST sessions demonstrated significant improvement in cognitive skills as well as basic quality of life over the control group, who had had no treatment. However, the authors concluded CST sessions would need to be ongoing and on at least a weekly basis for the improvements to be maintained.

REMINISCENCE THERAPY is a psychological technique that helps people who are suffering from dementia recall events in their lives, using videos, objects, photographs, and music from their past. Reminiscence therapy may assist dementia patients in regaining a sense of self.

PREVENTION PLAN

- Eat oily fish twice a week and take antioxidant supplements

- Take supplements of ginkgo and vitamins C, E, and B complex daily

- Have blood pressure and homocysteine levels checked regularly (these may be risk factors for dementia)

- Exercise

- Read, learn new skills, and maintain social networks and existing hobbies to keep the mind active

- Practice visual memory techniques (*see above*)

- Avoid factors that provoke stress and anxiety as much as possible

DIZZINESS AND VERTIGO

The term dizziness is commonly used to describe various symptoms, from mild light-headedness to vertigo, a more specific term that describes a false sensation of moving or rotating. Both may be accompanied by nausea and vomiting. Dizziness may result from various causes, including panic attacks or anemia. Vertigo may result from disturbance to the organs of balance in the inner ear, or from other causes. There are no well-established natural treatments for vertigo, but dietary changes, breathing exercises, and chiropractic might bring relief.

WHAT ARE THE SYMPTOMS?

- A sensation of moving or rotating
- Nausea
- Vomiting

WHY MIGHT I HAVE THIS?

PREDISPOSING FACTORS

- Labyrinthitis
- Benign positional vertigo
- Ménière's disease
- Head or neck injury
- Stroke
- Medications
- Autonomic dysfunction
- Anemia
- Standing for long periods
- Arthritis in neck joints
- Multiple sclerosis
- Tumor

TRIGGERS

- Inner ear infection
- Hyperventilation
- Fatigue
- Dehydration
- Excessive alcohol consumption

TREATMENT PLAN

PRIMARY TREATMENTS

- Immediate Relief measures *(see right)*
- Antihistamines; adjusting medication

BACKUP TREATMENTS

- Blood-sugar stabilizing diet
- Epley procedure (for benign positional vertigo)
- Chiropractic or osteopathy

WORTH CONSIDERING

- Homeopathy
- Craniosacral therapy/cranial osteopathy
- Breathing retraining
- Mind–body therapies

For an explanation of how treatments are rated, see p.111.

WHY DOES IT OCCUR?

Mild dizziness may be caused by many different factors, including panic attacks, anemia, fatigue, shallow breathing, low blood-sugar levels, or drinking too much alcohol. It may also occur after long periods of standing still. Very often, the cause of dizziness cannot be found.

Vertigo is due to problems with the nerve that connects the inner ear to the brain, or to problems in the areas of the brain that are concerned with balance. Another cause of vertigo is an inflammation of the inner ear that affects the organs of balance (labyrinthitis). This type of vertigo usually comes on rapidly. It may last for up to two months but tends to disappear without treatment.

Benign positional vertigo, which often arises due to a buildup of calcium debris in the semicircular canals in the inner ear, is a common cause of episodes of vertigo that are triggered by moving the head. These episodes are normally short-lived, typically lasting for less than one minute.

Recurrent vertigo may result from the inner ear disorder Ménière's disease, in which the pressure in the inner ear is intermittently raised. Any type of vertigo may be accompanied by nausea and vomiting.

Arthritis in the joints of the neck can sometimes cause recurrent episodes of vertigo and, in rare cases, vertigo may be a feature of multiple sclerosis *(see p.140)*. Other rare causes of dizziness and vertigo include a tumor affecting the nerve that connects the inner ear to the brain, a stroke, or a head or neck injury. These serious conditions may cause other symptoms affecting speech, vision, or movement and require immediate medical attention.

IMMEDIATE RELIEF

During an attack, lie still and avoid any sudden movements.
- Press the pericardium 6 (P6) point for 5 to 10 minutes. This point lies about two of your own thumb-widths above the front wrist crease, in line with your ring finger. You can also buy special wrist straps ("sea-bands") designed to help motion and morning sickness; they put pressure on these points. Ask for them at your local pharmacy.

IMPORTANT

If your dizziness or vertigo is accompanied by problems with your speech, vision, or mobility, seek medical help immediately.

TREATMENTS IN DETAIL

Conventional Medicine

Your doctor will do an examination that focuses on the functioning of your ears, eyes, and nervous system, and may also arrange tests in order to check the vestibular apparatus (structures of the inner ear). Investigations, such as blood tests and CT scanning, may be done to look for underlying disorders of the dizziness or vertigo, which will be treated where possible.

EPLEY PROCEDURE If you have benign positional vertigo, your doctor may recommend that you do the Epley procedure. This is a series of head movements that help reposition any calcium debris that has become loose in the semicircular canals in the inner ear *(see box, pp.138, 139)*.

PRIMARY TREATMENT **ANTIHISTAMINES**, such as meclizine, may help reduce vertigo and any associated nausea. Antihistamines can cause drowsiness.

Nutritional Therapy

BLOOD-SUGAR STABILIZING DIET Dizziness or vertigo can sometimes be symptoms of blood-sugar fluctuation; dizziness is often associated with low blood-sugar levels (*see p.42*).

Homeopathy

Many remedies may be suitable for dizziness and vertigo. You will need to visit a homeopath as the choice of remedy is dictated by your constitution and symptoms (*see p.73*). Some of the more commonly prescribed remedies are as follows:

VERTIGO HEEL is a complex homeopathic medicine that has been shown to be equally effective as one of the leading conventional treatments for treating Ménières disease. *Vertigo Heel* contains *Conium, Cocculus indicus, Petroleum,* and *Ambra grisea.*

MENIERE'S DISEASE AND LABYRINTHITIS *Chininum sulphuricum* is one of the homeopathic medicines that is most frequently prescribed and is often helpful for symptoms of Ménière's disease, such as dizziness with ringing in the ears and deafness. *Tabacum* may be helpful for treating labyrinthitis, symptoms of which include severe dizziness, nausea, vomiting, and cold sweats. *Gelsemium* may also be useful in treating this condition when the nausea is less severe but the patient feels weak and tremulous. *Theridion* is rarely used in general; however, it is helpful for vertigo that is associated with the rare symptom of extreme sensitivity to noise, which seems to go right through the patient.

VERTIGO IN OLDER PEOPLE *Conium, Baryta carbonicum,* and *Phosphorus* are the homeopathic medicines often indicated for older people who have vertigo associated with circulatory problems. *Conium* is appropriate for people who find that their vertigo is worse while they are lying down or move their head, even very limited movement. *Baryta carbonicum* is suggested when vertigo is associated with difficulty in thinking and poor memory. There may also be hard, swollen glands, particularly in the neck, and cold feet.

Phosphorus will generally be prescribed on "whole person" grounds, where the symptoms include great fatigue that is only temporarily improved by rest. Other symptoms include easy bruising and, in general, easy bleeding (for example, nosebleeds). Phosphorus may also be indicated in cases where there is anxiety with phobias and excessive sensitivity, not only to the physical surroundings but also to the human environment, associated with emotional changeability.

Acupuncture

Acupuncture has been used as a treatment for dizziness and vertigo, particularly if the dizziness is associated with problems in the neck. There have been case reports but, unfortunately, no good clinical trials have been performed to test the efficacy of acupuncture for this condition.

Bodywork Therapies

EASING SPINAL RESTRICTIONS A chiropractor or osteopath may be able to ease underlying spinal restrictions. Dizziness that derives from neck problems is characterized by feelings of unsteadiness when either walking or standing, and is usually made worse by turning the neck. Causes include restriction of circulation, nerve irritation, or the brain receiving contradictory messages from the tiny nerve structures about the position different parts of the body are in and the movements taking place.

Ménière's disease, which involves dizziness, may sometimes be the result of irritation of nerves in the neck. An uncontrolled study of 235 people with symptoms

---

THE EPLEY PROCEDURE

The Epley procedure, which is used to treat benign positional vertigo, was developed by Dr. John Epley to reposition calcium debris in the inner ear, which can cause vertigo. Tiny calcium crystals, known as canaliths, are usually attached to the base of the semicircular canals in the inner ear. These crystals may become detached, for unknown reasons, and move through the canals, causing a sensation of dizziness when the head moves. The Epley procedure repositions the canaliths back to the base of the canals. Shown here is a modified version for self-help use.

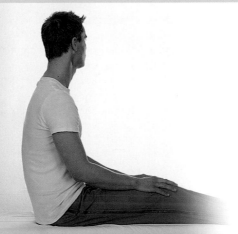

1. Sit on the edge of a bed. Turn your head to the side on which nystagmus (involuntary eye movement) has occurred.

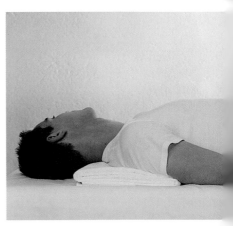

2. Keeping your head turned, lower yourself backward until you are lying on the bed. This can sometimes trigger the nystagmus.

of dizziness following neck injuries found that almost half of them were able to create their symptoms by keeping their head still, while they turned their body, thereby producing rotation of the neck. Nearly all of the 112 patients in the study were found to have specific restrictions between the vertebrae of the neck, primarily in the part located just underneath the skull where it joins the upper neck. After an average of 18 treatments, 101 of these people were symptom-free and an additional six patients had much reduced levels of dizziness. Out of the original control group, only five were unchanged.

CHIROPRACTIC If the dizziness begins after a neck injury (such as might result from a fall or a traffic accident), try consulting either an osteopath or a chiropractor. Good results have been achieved using chiropractic manipulation with large numbers of people whose vertigo started after a neck injury such as whiplash. Chiropractic treatment can also help relieve the dizziness that is caused by chronic tension in the neck.

CRANIOSACRAL THERAPY AND CRANIAL OSTEOPATHY practitioners maintain that their gentle manipulation of the head and neck achieves good results in many cases of vertigo; however, there are no research studies to back these claims.

Breathing Retraining

Rapid and shallow upper-chest breathing (hyperventilation), which is commonly triggered by stress or anxiety, typically results in the elimination of too much carbon dioxide from the body. This can cause the blood to become too alkaline, which in turn causes the smooth muscle layer around the blood vessels to contract, causing dizziness.

Another result of this increased alkalinity of the blood is the Bohr effect, in which the red blood cells that carry oxygen to the brain as well as to other body tissues release oxygen less readily than usual. This combination of a reduced blood supply and poor oxygen release can starve the brain of oxygen, leading to dizziness and other symptoms.

Breathing-pattern disorders that lead to this situation can usually be improved or corrected by breathing rehabilitation, which involves slow, diaphragmatic (yoga-type) breathing methods (*see p.62*), as well as correction of restrictions that may have developed over time in overused and stressed muscles and joints. These restrictions tend to reinforce any abnormal breathing pattern that has developed, and it is important to treat both the stressed muscle and joint problems and the abnormal breathing patterns to alleviate the dizziness.

Mind–Body Therapies

Vertigo can be difficult to treat because of the often subjective nature of dizziness, the frequent failure of medications to alleviate the symptoms, and the psychological factors that may complicate the condition. However, relaxation techniques can be useful in combating underlying stress, and they may also help people who are prone to panic attacks, of which dizziness is a common component.

Dizziness is not uncommon after a traffic accident, especially if the incident was frightening or involved loss of consciousness. If your dizziness began after an accident or any other traumatic experience, you should consider trying psychological treatments as well as bodywork, because the mind as well as the body reacts to sudden, shocking events.

PREVENTION PLAN

If you are prone to dizziness:

- Avoid triggers as much as possible
- Eat regular meals
- Do regular yoga or diaphragmatic breathing exercises
- Avoid standing still for long periods

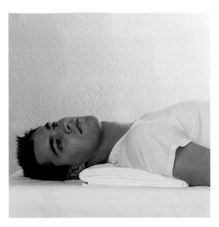

3. After waiting for 30 seconds, turn your head carefully and slowly to the opposite side (your "good" side). Wait another 30 seconds.

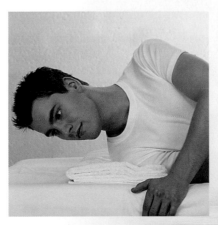

4. Keeping your head very still, use your arms to lever yourself up slowly from the bed into a sitting position.

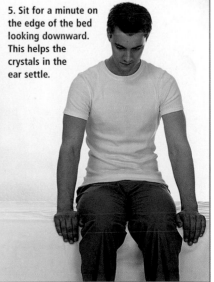

5. Sit for a minute on the edge of the bed looking downward. This helps the crystals in the ear settle.

MULTIPLE SCLEROSIS

In multiple sclerosis (MS), nerves in the brain and the spinal cord are progressively damaged, causing a range of symptoms that can affect feeling, movement, bodily functions, and balance. Symptoms and their severity differ from person to person. Multiple sclerosis is more common in the Northern Hemisphere and tends to develop between early adulthood and middle age. Although there is no cure, treatment might include drugs to ease symptoms and improve functioning, as well as dietary changes, acupuncture, and homeopathy.

WHAT ARE THE SYMPTOMS?

The symptoms of MS vary according to which parts of the brain and spinal cord are affected and may include:

- Blurred vision
- Numbness or tingling anywhere in the body
- Fatigue, which may be persistent
- Weakness and a feeling of heaviness in the limbs
- Coordination and balance problems, including vertigo (a sensation of moving or rotating)
- Slurred speech
- Stiff movement of the limbs (spasticity)
- Tremor

WHY MIGHT I HAVE THIS?

PREDISPOSING FACTORS

- Having a close relative with MS
- Diet high in saturated fat
- Smoking

WHY DOES IT OCCUR?

Many nerves in the brain and spinal cord have a sheath of fatty material called myelin, which acts as insulation. In MS, small areas of myelin are damaged, leaving holes in the sheath (demyelination). Nerve impulses are not conducted normally, causing a wide range of symptoms that affect sensation, movement, body functions, and balance. Eventually, the damaged areas of myelin are replaced by scar tissue. Evidence suggests that MS is an autoimmune disorder, in which the body's immune system produces antibodies against its own tissues, in this case the brain and the spinal cord.

It is thought that MS may be triggered by factors such as a viral infection in childhood in genetically susceptible people. There is also evidence that development of MS may be related to certain dietary fats, but no trigger has been identified.

IMPORTANT

If you think you may have MS, consult a doctor without delay.

There are two types of MS. In the more common type, "relapsing-remitting" MS, symptoms may be intermittent, lasting for days or weeks and alternating with months or even years with no symptoms (remission). In the other type, "secondary progressive" MS, chronic symptoms become progressively worse. Relapsing-remitting MS may become secondary progressive over time.

Symptoms may occur singly early on in the disorder and together as it progresses. Depression is common and memory may be affected. Bladder problems may develop and men may have problems achieving an erection. Eventually there may be painful muscle spasms and poor mobility.

TREATMENT PLAN

PRIMARY TREATMENTS

- Corticosteroids, interferon-beta, immunosuppressants (*see Drugs to Treat Relapses, p.141*)
- The Swank diet

BACKUP TREATMENTS

- Drugs for fatigue, depression, and other symptoms
- Physical therapy
- Emotional support
- Omega-3 fatty acids

- Nutritional supplements

WORTH CONSIDERING

- Homeopathy
- Environmental health measures
- Acupuncture
- Tai chi
- Bodywork therapies
- Cognitive behavioral therapy

For an explanation of how treatments are rated, see p.111.

DAMAGE TO NERVES IN MULTIPLE SCLEROSIS

Nerve cells, or neurons, originate, transmit, and receive nerve impulses. In addition to having nuclei and other features common to all cells, neurons have special projections. Some are called dendrites, and others are known as nerve fibers (or axons). These fibers link the neuron to other neurons or cells and carry nerve signals, often forming long communication chains in the body. Some nerve fibers are covered in a fatty substance called myelin, which helps speed up the transmission of nerve impulses. If this myelin is damaged, as occurs in MS, nerve impulses along the fiber are slowed or stopped.

In MS areas of demyelination develop. Nerve impulses are not conducted normally across nerve fibers, leading to symptoms such as blurred vision and poor balance.

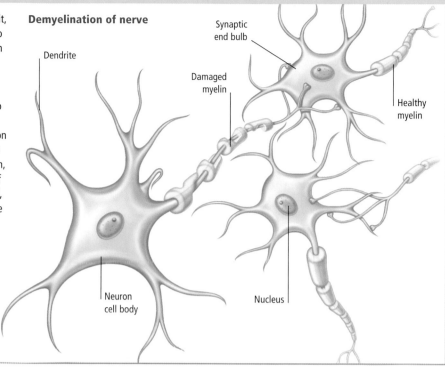

Demyelination of nerve

Dendrite

Synaptic end bulb

Damaged myelin

Healthy myelin

Neuron cell body

Nucleus

TREATMENTS IN DETAIL

Conventional Medicine

The doctor will arrange for tests, such as magnetic resonance imaging (MRI) of the brain and spinal cord to look for areas of demyelination. Drug treatments for MS can be divided into two main groups: those that aim to reduce either the severity or the frequency of relapses in relapsing-remitting MS, and those that aim to relieve specific symptoms. Research is in progress into the use of cannabinoids to relieve certain MS symptoms, for example, spasticity and tremor.

PRIMARY TREATMENT | **DRUGS TO TREAT RELAPSES** Intravenous or oral corticosteroids may be given as short courses to reduce the severity of symptoms during relapses. These drugs reduce inflammation, which has a role in demyelination. Short courses of corticosteroids should not cause any significant or long-term side effects. Interferon beta, which is given by injection, may be prescribed in some cases and may reduce the number of relapses, as may immunosuppressants, such as azathioprine, and other drugs including glatiramer

acetate, which is also given by injection. Mitoxantrone, which is a chemotherapeutic drug, may be prescribed to treat worsening relapsing-remitting as well as secondary progressive MS. For progressive disease, immunosuppressants are emphasized; glatiramer is not effective at this stage of the disease.

DRUGS FOR SYMPTOMS Many different medications are available to treat the symptoms of MS. For example, the drug amantadine may help with fatigue, while antidepressants may be recommended to treat depression. Anticonvulsants can help treat paroxysmal symptoms such as spasms or seizures. Drugs that act on the muscles of the bladder, such as oxybutinin, may help relieve bladder symptoms; but self-catheterization may be necessary to help the bladder empty completely. Treatments for erectile dysfunction include sildenafil. Muscle spasms may be relieved by muscle relaxant drugs, such as baclofen.

> **CAUTION**
>
> Drugs for multiple sclerosis can cause a range of possible side effects; ask your doctor to explain these to you.

PHYSICAL THERAPY may be recommended in order to improve muscle strength and mobility and help relieve muscle spasms if they occur. If movement is affected, occupational therapists can offer advice on the many aids that are available, and can also advise on other measures to help with everyday living — for example, how to adapt cooking, sleeping, and bathing facilities to maintain a high degree of independence.

EMOTIONAL SUPPORT is extremely important for people with MS and their families in the long term. An affected individual's health-care team will help provide this, and there are support groups and organizations that can also offer both practical and emotional assistance (*see p.486*).

Nutritional Therapy

OMEGA-3 FATTY ACIDS, such as those found in oily fish, appear to be protective. This type of fat may be important through its modulation of the inflammatory and immune processes. Inflammation in the blood vessels of the brain may be an underlying feature of multiple sclerosis. The omega-3 fatty acids EPA and DHA, which are found in abundance in oily fish, can be made into anti-inflammatory chemicals by the body. By contrast, arachidonic acid, which is an omega-6 fatty acid found in foods such as red meat, eggs, liver, and kidneys, can be made into chemicals that have an inflammatory effect. One study found that people who eat more red meat, which is rich in arachidonic acid, have higher rates of MS. If you have MS, you may wish to eat more oily fish and less red meat. Some people with MS have been found to be deficient in the omega-3 fatty acids EPA and DHA. Fish oil supplements, which are rich in EPA and DHA, may be useful for people with MS. If you have MS, you may wish to take about 350mg per day of EPA and 250mg per day of DHA. Taking 1–2g concentrated fish oils each day will provide good levels of EPA and DHA.

PRIMARY TREATMENT **THE SWANK DIET** There is some evidence that the sooner the Swank diet is started, the less risk there is of significant disability. Dr. Roy Swank studied the effect of a low-fat diet in 150 patients with MS between 1949 and 1984. The diet restricted saturated fat to 20g per day and eliminated partially hydrogenated fats, such as margarine and many processed fats. People were given healthy fats in the form of cod-liver oil (5g per day) and vegetable oils (10–40g per day). Compared to untreated individuals, those who adhered strictly to this regime deteriorated less. The treated group also enjoyed much better overall survival, with about 70 percent surviving over the study period compared to about 20 percent in the untreated group. Consult a nutritionist (*see p. 47*) for further information.

NUTRITIONAL SUPPLEMENTS There is evidence to suggest that calcium, magnesium, selenium, vitamin D, vitamin E, vitamin B_{12}, and other B vitamins may be important in MS. A daily multivitamin may also help; it certainly won't hurt.

Homeopathy

There has not been any scientific research on homeopathic treatment of MS, but a number of case reports show improvement in symptoms or, apparently, in the underlying disease. Since the condition is so variable, individualized treatment from a trained practitioner is required (*see p.73*) and the condition is not suitable for self-help or self treatment.

PHOSPHORUS may be helpful in MS, especially if blurred vision or vertigo are problems. People who respond to this remedy usually feel very tired and may catnap. They may also have numbness or altered sensation, particularly burning sensations in the hands, feet, and elsewhere. They are often thirsty, especially for cold drinks, and may also crave salty foods. They tend to be nervous and oversensitive.

SILICEA AND NATRUM MURIATICUM are other constitutional medicines (i.e., they match the person' constitutional type, *see p.73*) that may help. *Silicea* patients typically are thin, pale, and chilly but have sweaty, cold hands and feet. A very characteristic feature of these people is weak nails, often with lengthwise ridging. Affected people often say that their nails became weak and their hair thinner and finer around the time they fell ill. They seem to pick up infections easily and are slow to recover. Mentally they are timid, although they may be stubborn and push themselves to exhaustion if they have decided to do something.

In people who respond to *Natrum muriaticum*, it is not uncommon to find that the problem seems to have been triggered by mental stress, for instance, an unhappy relationship or bereavement, but it is very typical of these patients that they try to avoid discussing their inner feelings.

MEDICINES TO RELIEVE SYMPTOMS *Nux vomica* or *Ignatia* may be useful for the painful spasms, usually in the legs, that may occur in MS and are sometimes triggered by quite trivial stimuli or even have no apparent stimulus. The person who responds to *Nux vomica* tends to be bad-tempered and often has indigestion. The *Ignatia* patient is nervous, sometimes to the point of being hysterical. *Equisetum* may help with bladder control, *Gelsemium* with double vision and tremor and *Conium* with vertigo.

Environmental Health

GEOGRAPHICAL DISTRIBUTION The view that the environment has a bearing on MS is supported by population studies showing that the disease occurs in clusters. The geographical distribution of MS is not random. Cases of the disease increase as latitude increases (in both directions), even in ethnically homogeneous countries. The northern portion of the US, northern and central Europe, and New Zealand are among the high-risk regions for the development of the disease. When people move from an area of low MS risk to an area of high risk, they become at high risk of MS. So, it is likely that something in the environment, perhaps combined with a genetic predisposition, causes MS.

Environmental triggers proposed for MS are many and include viral infections, smoking, injuries, lack of sunshine, heavy metals, anesthesia, psychological stress, organic solvents, and artificial sweeteners.

The farther you live from the equator (in either direction), the greater your risk of having MS

However, it has so far been impossible to assign specific causes to a disease that has so many different presentations and has a genetic component as well. In the absence of carefully controlled studies, we are left with epidemiological studies and some specific avoidance advice.

INFECTIONS There is strong evidence that viral infections act as triggers for MS flare-ups. People with MS are twice as likely to experience an acute flare-up following an upper respiratory infection, and this risk is more than threefold in people who have a high level of antibodies to viruses in their bloodstream. Bacterial infections may also play a role in causing relapses in MS. If you have MS you should avoid such exposure as much as possible. This means avoiding crowded, confined places during outbreaks of flu and respiratory disease. Most importantly, wash your hands frequently and avoid touching your face.

SMOKING Smoking has been associated with a transient worsening of MS symptoms and if you have MS you should not smoke. Many studies show a strong association between smoking and the development of MS. There are no studies examining a role of second-hand smoke in MS, but if you have the condition, it would be wise to avoid all exposure to smoke.

CHEMICAL SOLVENTS Exposure to certain chemical solvents has been proposed as a trigger for MS, but the evidence is controversial. There have been over a dozen studies in the past decade that have suggested a relationship between solvents and the development of MS, but many occupational exposure studies have not shown any MS clusters in occupations that involve high exposure to organic solvents, such as painters, printers, and carpenters.

HEAVY METALS Exposure to heavy metals, such as mercury, seems to play a role in the development of the disease, according to studies into MS clusters. Some researchers believe that exposure to heavy metals in the soil is responsible for the geographic variation in MS cases. This has been used as an argument to link mercury in amalgam dental fillings with MS, a theory that has not been supported by any meaningful research. It is not necessary to remove fillings, but it may help to have your drinking water tested and install a purifying system if the heavy metal content is high (this is especially important if you use water from a well). Limit or avoid tuna, shark, and swordfish (which often contain high levels of methylmercury), gelatin (which may contain lead), and some calcium supplements (which, like gelatin, may contain lead from bones).

PESTICIDES AND HERBICIDES Many compounds used in pesticides and herbicides can be toxic to the nervous system. Do not use these chemicals in your garden or walk where they have recently been applied.

SUN EXPOSURE Exposure to sunlight has been examined in relation to MS ever since the geographical distribution was noticed. In people with MS, it seems that higher sun exposure is linked to a decreased risk of death. Some researchers feel that this protective effect of sunlight is due to increases in vitamin D production, since sunlight is necessary for the body to make vitamin D. People with MS who have higher levels of vitamin D have fewer MS lesions on MRI scans. Studies on animals with MS-like diseases also show improvements with vitamin D treatments.

> Sclerosis means scars. In MS, scars in the brain and on nerve fibers interrupt nerve transmission

If you have MS, try taking a daily vitamin D supplement and go out in the sun every day. However, limit your sun exposure to 15–20 minutes daily (without sunscreen) to protect against skin cancer.

Chinese Herbal Medicine

Some of the herbs used in traditional folk medicine may make a difference in MS. In a double-blind study, 100 MS patients received an Tibetan herbal formula known as Adoprin. Half of the patients who received this formula experienced overall improvement in addition to increased muscle strength and improved bladder function.

Acupuncture

There is no evidence that acupuncture will alter the course or severity of MS. However, neuralgia-like pain (see p.124) is common in MS, and acupuncture can provide pain relief. As with all degenerative neurological conditions, acupuncture may only work for a short time, and treatment may need to be repeated frequently.

Bodywork and Movement Therapies

MASSAGE has been shown in several small research studies to be helpful in treating aspects of MS. In one study, patients who were massaged had significantly improved levels of self-esteem and better body-image and social functioning, although the neurological symptoms had not improved. In another study, massage appeared to improve well-being and mood and reduce tension and fatigue.

REFLEXOLOGY is recommended on the basis of some randomized controlled trials. In one study, over 70 people with MS were divided into two groups, one receiving reflexology and the other just massage of the calf. The reflexology group showed significant improvement in muscle and bladder control. In another study, 14 people with MS received a one-hour reflexology treatment every week, while 12 people acted as a control group. The results after 18 weeks revealed that those patients in the treatment group experienced some improvements in 45 percent of their symptoms.

YOGA A randomized controlled trial of six months of yoga or exercise found that both were effective in reducing fatigue, although neither improved cognitive function.

TAI CHI The gentle flowing movements of tai chi can help control MS symptoms. When a group of people with MS did tai chi, symptoms such as depression, problems with balance and walking, muscle spasms, and bladder control all improved.

Mind–Body Therapies

COGNITIVE BEHAVIORAL TECHNIQUES show promise in the treatment of MS. Stress is known to make MS symptoms worse. For example, a study of patients with relapsing-remitting MS found that stressful events unconnected with the disease doubled their chance of having a flare-up. Relaxation or meditation exercises may help (see p.99), but cognitive behavioral methods may be even more effective; ask your caregiver if this method might work for you. In a small 2002 study, MS patients using a cognitive behavioral program in order to improve their coping skills developed fewer MS-related brain lesions.

CHRONIC PAIN

Acute (sudden) pain is the body's warning signal that something specific is wrong. Chronic (persistent) pain is defined as pain lasting for six months or longer. It may be the result of chronic inflammation, as occurs in some kinds of arthritis, or nerve damage. However, chronic pain may also derive from a complex problem involving both mind and body, when the nervous system begins to generate pain signals even though no underlying physical cause is involved. Mind–body therapies are important to treatment, along with analgesics and acupuncture.

WHAT ARE THE SYMPTOMS?

- Long-term pain anywhere in the body

WHY MIGHT I HAVE THIS?

PREDISPOSING FACTORS

- An infection, injury, or other cause, even if it has healed
- Being depressed (states of mind and other mind-body issues can affect perception of pain)

WHY DOES IT OCCUR?

The sensation of pain can stem from injury, infection, and many other causes. Some of the most common causes of pain include injuries, rheumatoid arthritis (*see p.293*), osteoarthritis (*see p.289*), back problems (*see p.268*), and neuralgia (*see p.124*). Sometimes pain is perceived in the wrong area of the body. In angina, for example, pain signals from the heart travel up the sensory nerves of the spinal cord together with signals from the left arm. The brain becomes confused and senses pain in an unexpected part of the body (the left arm, neck, or jaw).

PERSISTENT PAIN AND GATE CONTROL In some cases it is not possible to identify an underlying cause for chronic pain and there is often no clear explanation for why some pain persists even after the disease or condition that triggered it has healed. However, persistent pain syndromes are very real and incapacitating, and often have a devastating effect on work and relationships. Persistent pain affects up to 30 percent of people and is increasingly being viewed as a disorder in its own right rather than just as a symptom of an underlying cause.

According to the "gate control" theory, nerve impulses traveling from the body via the spinal cord to pain receptors in the brain can be influenced by nerve cells in the spinal cord that behave like gates. By shutting or opening these "gates," the brain is able either to magnify or to reduce pain signals. Chemicals called endorphins are the body's natural analgesics. They work

TREATMENT PLAN

PRIMARY TREATMENTS

- Treatment of underlying cause where possible
- Analgesics (for short-term use)
- Other drugs to relieve pain, such as NSAIDs
- Physical treatments, e.g. TENS
- Psychological treatments, e.g. counseling

BACKUP TREATMENTS

- Corticosteroid injections for joint pain
- Opioid drugs for intractable pain
- Nerve blocks for severe pain
- Antidepressants

WORTH CONSIDERING

- Fish oil supplements
- Tryptophan
- Acupuncture
- Bodywork and movement therapies
- Exercise
- Meditation
- Cognitive behavioral therapy

For an explanation of how treatments are rated, see p.111.

by stimulating receptors located in the brain, spinal cord, and nerve endings, where they block pain impulses. How wide the pain gates open and how much pain information reaches the brain depends partly on the quantity of endorphins that are circulating in the body.

TOLERANCE of pain varies, partly as a result of an individual's psychological state. This is because emotional states modify the levels of endorphins in the body. The effect of psychological state on perception of pain explains why athletes who are injured in competition are often able to continue, and how soldiers are sometimes able to fight on in the heat of battle despite devastating injury. Pain is perceived as being worse or more intense by people when they are depressed and less intense when they are distracted by something that they find enjoyable.

How someone interprets pain and any ideas that he or she may have about it and its consequences affect his or her pain tolerance. Past experiences and associations with pain, in addition to general life stresses, also play a part in the perception and tolerance of pain.

VICIOUS CYCLE People who suffer from chronic pain tend to immobilize themselves because of their fear that any exercise will be intensely painful. Instead, if they did exercise they would discover that it releases pain-killing endorphins, thereby lessening their pain and, consequently, their sense of fear and depression.

Lack of physical activity also weakens and shortens muscles and causes them to become tense, creating muscle spasms and, as a result, more pain. This pain-tension cycle can cause deepening depression, helplessness, and lower pain tolerance. Breathing pattern disorders may also occur as a reaction to pain. These patterns can further contribute to the vicious cycles of tension that serve either to worsen or to perpetuate the pain.

HYPERSENSITIVITY Continual pain can make a pain pathway more sensitive to pain impulses, long after the original cause of the pain has been healed. Psychological states are known to directly affect the body: for example, in one experiment, just thinking about painful experiences led to tensed

USING TENS FOR PAIN RELIEF

Transcutaneous electrical nerve stimulation (TENS) is a technique that is used to help relieve pain. The TENS unit produces minute electrical impulses that pass into the body via electrode pads attached to the skin. The pulses are supposed to interrupt the pathways along which pain signals travel and prevent them from reaching the brain, where they are registered as pain. Here a TENS unit is being used on the knee. TENS is frequently used to relieve pain during labor.

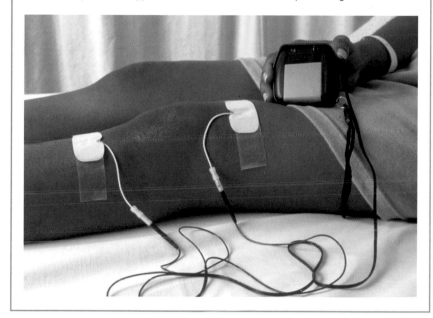

back muscles in people who complained of chronic back pain. By expecting the worst when a migraine begins, people who have regular migraines may tighten muscles and restrict blood flow, making the migraine attack longer and more severe.

SELF-HELP

The following measures may help reduce pain and improve well-being:
- Keep a diary to record episodes of pain in order to identify factors that make it better or worse.
- Avoid becoming tired and get adequate rest each day.
- Do regular aerobic exercise such as walking, swimming, or tennis, as well as yoga or stretching to prevent muscles from becoming stiff.
- Do meditation or relaxation exercises (*see p.98*) every day.
- Make time for friends and family as well as for enjoyable hobbies and activities that distract you and lift your mood.
- Take fish-oil supplements (*see p.146*).
- Have regular relaxing massages.

TREATMENTS IN DETAIL
Conventional Medicine

PRIMARY TREATMENT **TREATING AN UNDERLYING CAUSE** Your doctor will order tests to be performed to look for an underlying cause of persistent pain, which will be treated wherever possible. Various measures may be helpful in treating persistent pain and there is ongoing research into potential new treatments. For example, research shows that cannabis may relieve muscle pain in multiple sclerosis, although prescribing it remains a controversial issue in most countries. You may also be referred to a local pain specialist or to a multidisciplinary pain clinic, if one is located in your area. In these specialized hospitals, experts in pain management can help reduce your pain levels and maximize normal function and well-being.

PRIMARY TREATMENT **PAIN-RELIEVING DRUGS** Various pain-relieving drugs are available, ranging from mild analgesics to powerful opiate drugs. Nonsteroidal anti-inflammatory drugs (NSAIDs) are also helpful in some cases, such as in joint pain caused by inflammation.

Some drugs relieve certain types of pain in addition to their primary action. These drugs include tricyclic antidepressants such as amitriptyline, and anticonvulsants, which may be used to treat chronic pain.

INJECTIONS AND NERVE BLOCKS Corticosteroid injections into joints may help relieve pain in certain joint diseases, such as osteoarthritis. Nerve blocks are another option for certain types of chronic pain. For example, epidurals, in which a local anesthetic is injected into the space around the membranes enveloping the spinal cord, may offer temporary relief for back pain. Very severe pain arising from surgery or serious injury may be treated with injections of opioids. These drugs are usually not prescribed for long-term use due to their addictive properties. However, morphine and other opiates are an appropriate treatment for cancer pain and some other chronic pain syndromes.

> **CAUTION**
>
> Drugs for chronic pain can cause a range of possible side effects; ask your doctor to explain them to you.

PRIMARY TREATMENT | PHYSICAL TREAMENTS A variety of physical treatments are available to help relieve pain, including acupuncture, massage, and ultrasound therapy. In transcutaneous electrical nerve stimulation (TENS), electrical impulses are relayed from a portable impulse generator to electrodes stuck to the skin in the painful area. They are usually left in place for about 30 minutes. TENS treatment may relieve persistent pain, such as chronic back pain, for several hours.

PRIMARY TREATMENT | PSYCHOLOGICAL HELP Pain is stressful, and your doctor may suggest counseling to help you cope. Cognitive behavioral therapy may be especially useful (*see p.147*). In addition there are organizations (*see p.486*) that can offer emotional support and practical day-to-day advice. Antidepressants may be prescribed for the depression that often accompanies persistent pain.

Nutritional Therapy

FISH-OIL SUPPLEMENTS Pain associated with inflammation may be helped by supplementing your regular diet with omega-3 fatty acids. Excessive consumption of omega-6 polyunsaturated fatty acids (found in vegetable oils and fast foods) and a relative lack of omega-3 fatty acids (found in oily fish) seems to promote inflammation and pain.

Supplementation with omega-3 fatty acids has been demonstrated in studies to reduce inflammatory processes and pain in the body. Omega-3 fatty acids can be found in some nuts (such as walnuts) and seeds, and in oily fish such as salmon, mackerel, trout, and sardines. Including these foods in the diet may help you control the pain. Taking 1–3g of fish oil each day is likely to help persistent pain also.

TRYPTOPHAN The amino acid tryptophan is required for the release of the substance beta-endorphin, which is one of the body's natural pain-relieving compounds. Tryptophan is also needed for the production of serotonin, a brain chemical that may reduce the tendency to sense pain. Supplementing the diet with foods containing tryptophan may change the pain threshold so that pain is not sensed as readily. Tryptophan exists naturally in certain foods,

including meat, tofu, almonds, peanuts, and pumpkin and sesame seeds. Tryptophan supplements are not available in the US, however, because batches of tryptophan were associated with a serious disease called eosinophilia-myalgia syndrome, first reported in New Mexico in 1989. Although 5-hydroxytryptophan (5-HTP), a substance that tryptophan is converted into before it is made into serotonin, is available, it is not clear whether or not it is actually safer than tryptophan.

Acupuncture

Acupuncture is often used by multidisciplinary pain teams to treat unexplained pain and appears to be an effective treatment. It seems to work by stimulating the release of endorphins and "closing pain gates" by stimulating nerve fibers that block pain. It may also be helpful in relieving the anxiety and depression that accompanies long-term pain. Clinical trials are mixed; since persistent pain is not in itself a diagnosis, it is almost impossible for clinical trials to provide evidence in this area. Almost all acupuncture techniques have been used at some point to treat persistent pain and there is no real evidence to suggest which are best. Persist with treatment over a month or two to see if pain relief can be obtained.

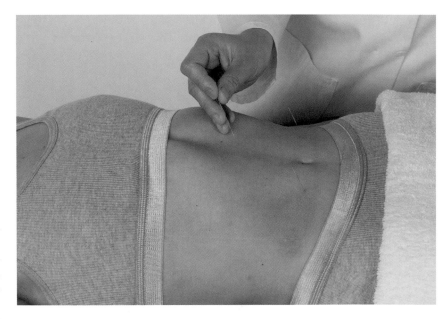

Acupuncture has been effective in some cases for treating unexplained chronic pain. Fine needles are inserted (here on the Kidney meridian) to stimulate nerve fibers.

Five out of six people with chronic pain take analgesics, but 70 percent still have pain

Bodywork and Movement Therapies

MANIPULATION THERAPIES Easing pain that arises from the central nervous system may require surgical or other interventions, such as nerve blocks (injections, *see p.146*), that aim to interrupt the transmission of pain messages. This is especially true if the pain is extreme and/or longstanding. Although there are no clinical studies, postural therapies such as Feldenkrais and the Alexander technique can teach chronic pain patients to sit, stand, and move around in ways that avoid aggravating pain.

However, if the persistent pain stems from a peripheral source, such as the nerves in an arm or leg, some manual therapies (such as neuromuscular therapy or osteopathic soft-tissue manipulation) may be able to alter the mechanism giving rise to the pain through manipulation, soft-tissue treatment, or a combination of both of these treatments. Practitioners can also help patients reduce their general sensitivity to pain through teaching them certain breathing rehabilitiation and relaxation methods.

MASSAGE When it is accompanied by other therapies, massage can be useful in reducing pain through relaxation.

DEACTIVATION OF TRIGGER POINTS The researchers Wall and Melzack have shown that, whatever other factors are involved, all chronic pain involves trigger points in muscles.. They are a factor in the continuing painful state and may even be the primary cause of the pain. Trigger points (particularly sensitive areas in the muscles, *see p.55*) can be eliminated by various means, including soft-tissue manipulation, local anesthetic injection, and acupuncture. Percutaneous electrical nerve stimulation (PENS) is an acupuncture technique that has been found to be successful. Releasing trigger points allows the circulation to be restored to tense muscles.

HYDROTHERAPY can be both relaxing and invigorating, helping improve the circulation. There are a number of forms of hydrotherapy, from exercising in heated swimming pools to applying cold compresses to the painful area. Therapy using water, particularly supervised exercises in thermal or mineral water, known as balneotherapy, has been studied as a means of relieving general chronic pain. It can significantly help relieve pain and improve general functioning. The hydrostatic force of the water is thought to bring about pain relief, possibly by taking stress off the affected joint, relaxation, or other factors.

Exercise

Pain can make people reluctant to exercise but this should be resisted because lack of activity weakens, tenses, and shortens muscles, which in turn can create more pain. It is easy to fall into the vicious circle of avoiding exercise and thereby inadvertently increasing the level of pain. Doing gentle exercise each day, such as walking, cycling, or swimming, as your condition allows, helps promote the release of endorphins, improve sleep, relieve depression, and reduce the perception of pain. Start slowly and remember to work within your limitations. A doctor or physical therapist may be able to advise you on suitable activities. In addition to aerobic forms of exercise, gentle yoga or stretching at home also may be therapeutic. Breathing exercises may be helpful in relieving chronic back pain.

Mind–Body Therapies

A 1994 study showed that there is a strong link between someone's "control belief" and their experience of pain. This means that the more you believe that you can influence or control your symptoms, the less pain you are likely to experience. Specifically, the higher your belief in your ability to control the pain level, the lower the level of pain you will tend to experience. These and a body of other findings

provide very strong support for using psychological approaches to control chronic pain that is not cancer-related.

MINDFULNESS MEDITATION An uncontrolled study of "mindfulness" meditation (*see p.99*) was undertaken by Dr. Jon Kabat-Zinn and his colleagues at the University of Massachusetts School of Medicine. Patients with chronic pain were trained in this form of meditation as part of a 10-week stress-reduction and relaxation program. People in the study found that using this technique they could ignore "present-moment pain." They also found that their other symptoms, such as depression and negative body image, improved. At the same time, use of pain-relieving drugs decreased and activity levels and feelings of self-esteem increased.

Most improvements were maintained for up to 15 months after the initial training and many participants continued the meditation practice as a daily routine.

OTHER PSYCHOLOGICAL THERAPIES A major 1999 review looked at the effectiveness of psychological therapies in the treatment of persistent chronic pain. Psychological treatments, such as cognitive behavioral therapy, were associated with significant physical and psychological improvement in people who participated in the studies. The review concluded that active psychological treatments that are based on the principle of behavioral therapy are very effective in managing persistent chronic pain.

If you are experiencing chronic pain (whatever the cause), you could try spending 20 minutes every day doing either relaxation exercises or meditation (*see p.98*). You could also explore the possibility of learning biofeedback techniques (*see p.100*) or of having cognitive behavioral therapy, either of which can help you develop a sense of control over the painful condition.

PREVENTION PLAN

See your doctor if you have chronic pain. Many people put off having treatment for their condition but that can make the problem worse.

STROKE

Damage to the brain caused by an interruption of its blood supply is known as a stroke. It may occur due to a blockage or a leak in one of the arteries that supply the brain. Stroke is more common over the age of 70 and affects more men than women. Smoking and a diet high in saturated fat are risk factors for stroke, as are high blood pressure and diabetes. Rehabilitation and prevention of further strokes might incorporate various approaches including dietary and lifestyle changes, drugs, and speech, occupational, and physical therapy.

WHAT ARE THE SYMPTOMS?

Symptoms often develop rapidly over a matter of seconds or minutes. The exact symptoms depend on the area of the brain that is affected, but may include:

- Weakness or inability to move on one side of the body
- Numbness on one side of the body
- Tremor and clumsiness
- Blurred vision or loss of vision in one eye
- Very severe headache, possibly at the back of the head
- Difficulty in speaking or understanding what is said
- Vomiting, loss of balance, and vertigo (feeling of dizziness)
- Unconsciousness

WHY MIGHT I HAVE THIS?

PREDISPOSING FACTORS

- High blood pressure
- Smoking
- Over 70 years old
- Sedentary lifestyle
- Obesity
- Diet high in saturated fat
- Raised homocysteine levels
- Atrial fibrillation
- Diabetes

WHY DOES IT OCCUR?

Most strokes are due either to cerebral thrombosis, in which a blood clot forms in an artery in the brain, or to cerebral embolism, when a fragment of a blood clot that has formed elsewhere travels to the brain. Blood clots are more likely to form in arteries damaged by atherosclerosis, a condition in which fatty deposits build up in the lining of the arteries. In this sense, the disease is generally similar in cause to coronary artery disease (*see p.252*).

About 10 percent of strokes result from cerebral hemorrhage, which occurs when an artery in the brain ruptures, leaking blood into the brain tissue. In some cases, the underlying cause is an aneurysm, a tiny bulge in the blood vessel.

Strokes that are caused by a cerebral hemorrhage tend to be more serious and are often accompanied by a very severe headache. Bleeding strokes are more common in those taking warfarin or another antocoagulant drug. Hemorrhagic strokes

IMPORTANT

If someone develops any of the symptoms of a stroke (*see left*), call an ambulance immediately.

are more likely than other types of strokes to result in loss of consciousness and to be life-threatening, but both bleeding and hemorrhagic strokes can be fatal.

In most cases strokes come on without warning. Symptoms that disappear in 24 hours are due to transient ischemic attacks (TIA), which are a neurologic warning sign of susceptibility to a future stroke. TIAs usually result from spasm in narrowed blood vessels.

The aftereffects of a stroke vary greatly in their severity (*see box, p.151*). About a third of strokes result in death, and about a third result in eventual full recovery. About a third of people survive with deficits including mild, temporary symptoms and localized muscle weakness, to permanent

TREATMENT PLAN

PRIMARY TREATMENTS

- Giving up smoking (*see Self-Help, p.149*)
- Treatment of underlying cause, e.g. high blood pressure
- Aspirin, anticoagulants, and other drugs
- Carotid endarterectomy and other surgery
- Rehabilitation
- Treadmill walking

BACKUP TREATMENTS

- Nutritional therapy
- Physical therapy

WORTH CONSIDERING

- Acupuncture
- EMG biofeedback

For an explanation of how treatments are rated, see p.111.

This X-ray shows an aneurysm (balloonlike swelling) in the carotid artery. If an aneurysm in the brain ruptures, cerebral hemorrhage and stroke result.

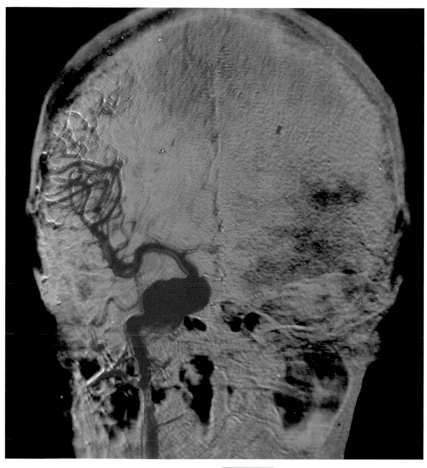

disability, loss of speech, and changes in cognition. Some people who have had a stroke develop dementia (see p.133). Most treatment aims to prevent further strokes since anyone who has had a stroke is at high risk for another one.

SELF-HELP

If you have had a stroke:
- Do not smoke.
- Eat a diet rich in fruit, vegetables, and oily fish and low in fat (see p.44).
- Exercise on a regular basis.
- Watch your weight.
- If you have high blood pressure, follow your doctor's advice on how to reduce it and take any medication correctly.

TREATMENTS IN DETAIL

Conventional Medicine

ASSESSMENT Anyone who is suspected of having a stroke should be taken to the hospital as soon as possible. A doctor will carry out a thorough examination in order to assess the symptoms, identify any risk factors (such as high blood pressure), and look for possible sources of emboli (fragments of blood clots) that may have caused the stroke.

The doctor may arrange for various tests, including CT scanning or MRI, which will show the site and extent of the damage in addition to revealing whether the stroke resulted from a blockage or a hemorrhage. Carotid doppler scanning, in which an ultrasound probe is moved over the path of an artery to assess the blood flow through it, may be used to look for narrowing of the carotid arteries. An EKG may be done in order to evaluate the heart rhythm, and an echocardiogram may be performed to evaluate the motion of the heart muscle.

TREATMENT will involve identifying and treating any underlying conditions that caused the stroke, such as high blood pressure. Other possible measures depend on whether the stroke was caused by a blockage

or a hemorrhage. Clot strokes are treated with thrombolytic (clot-busting) drugs, such as alteplase, which are administered intravenously or by injection. If you smoke, your doctor will advise you to stop. You will also be advised to change your diet to include less fat and more fresh fruit and vegetables (see p.44).

PRIMARY TREATMENT **ASPIRIN AND OTHER DRUGS** If the stroke resulted from a blockage, you may be prescribed a high dose of aspirin for several days. This has been shown to improve chances of recovery and reduce the risk of death. High-dose aspirin treatment will be followed by low-dose aspirin taken daily. Long-term low-dose aspirin has been shown to reduce the risk of a further stroke by making the platelets less likely to clump together, which occurs when clots form. Anticoagulants, which reduce the clotting tendency of the blood, are routinely prescribed. Cholesterol-lowering drugs are important in anyone with elevated cholesterol.

CAUTION

Drugs for stroke can cause a range of possible side effects; ask your doctor to explain these to you.

PRIMARY TREATMENT **CAROTID ENDARTERECTOMY** If the carotid arteries in the neck are found to be greatly narrowed, carotid endarterectomy may be performed. In this procedure, material that is causing the narrowing is removed from the lining of the arteries. Risks include the small possibility of causing a further stroke.

PRIMARY TREATMENT **SURGERY** If the stroke resulted from a hemorrhage, urgent surgery may be performed to remove the clot formed by the leaked blood. In certain cases, where aneurysms are present, it may be possible to clip off the aneurysm to prevent further leakage of blood.

REHABILITATION is a key part of treatment for stroke. It may involve physical therapy (*see also right*) and speech and language therapy, depending on the disability experienced. If your disability is ongoing, occupational therapists can advise you on special utensils, walking aids, and other items that help with everyday living. There are also a number of organizations that can provide both practical and emotional support for people who have had a stroke and their caregivers. Talk to your health-care provider or see p.486.

Nutritional Therapy

DIET In general, the best diet for stroke prevention is one rich in fruits, vegetables, nuts, seeds, and oily fish, and low in fast and processed foods and other sources of salt and saturated fat. Fruit and vegetables seem to be particularly important because they are rich in potassium, which helps lower blood pressure and may help reduce stroke risk. Interestingly, low potassium levels (hypokalemia) have been found to be common after a stroke, and may be associated with a poorer recovery.

Flavonoids, which are also found in fruit and vegetables, are associated with a lower risk of stroke. In one study, people with the highest levels of quercetin, a flavonoid, had a 71 percent lower risk of stroke. If you want to protect yourself from stroke, try to eat at least five portions of fruit and vegetables daily.

Studies have found that people who eat fish regularly tend to be at less risk of stroke than those who do not eat fish. The protective effect seems to be due to the omega-3 fatty acids that fish contains. To reduce your risk of stroke, eat at least two portions of fish a week, especially oily fish (such as salmon, mackerel, trout, and sardines), which are especially high in omega-3 fatty acids.

SUPPLEMENTS There is some evidence that supplementation with vitamins, minerals, protein, and calories may improve general nutrition and health and reduce mortality in stroke patients. Together with a healthy diet, a multivitamin and mineral supplement may help improve the outcome in individuals who have had a stroke. One study found that people who had high blood levels of vitamin C had a 41 percent lower risk of having a stroke. Taking 1g of vitamin C per day, in addition to a multivitamin supplement, may help prevent stroke.

Some studies show that moderately raised homocysteine levels may be a risk factor for stroke. Raised homocysteine levels are associated with a low dietary intake of folic acid, vitamin B_6, and vitamin B_{12}. Taking a daily vitamin B-complex supplement in addition to a daily multivitamin may help you reduce your risk of stroke.

See p.44 for more information on nutritional approaches that may help not only in the prevention but also in the treatment of a stroke.

Acupuncture

The Chinese tend to use acupuncture, given daily, for treating stroke and head injury. There are some quite specific techniques that are claimed to help accelerate the recovery from a stroke. Because acupuncture is said to work by enhancing the local blood circulation around the injured area of brain, treatment should not be started for a week or two after the stroke occurred in order to avoid further bleeding.

RESULTS OF TRIALS The several rigorous clinical trials looking at the use of specific acupuncture points in the treatment of stroke show that acupuncture appears to be safe but does not appear to have a specific effect in aiding stroke recovery. The first clinical trials, which suggested that it might be very effective, were small and not well designed. The more recent clinical trials leave no doubt that, while acupuncture may have some effect on improving spasticity and enhancing individual independence, it does not accelerate stroke recovery. Anecdotal evidence suggested that acupuncture may be more effective if combined with hyperbaric therapy.

If acupuncture is to be considered following a stroke, at least 10–15 treatments are needed, and they should be given over a month or so before deciding whether this treatment is effective.

Bodywork and Movement Therapies

It is well established that early treatment of a stroke, using tactics such as exercise and movement in order to ensure that an optimal supply of oxygen is delivered to the brain and tissues, reduces long-term neurological damage and decisively improves survival chances.

PRIMARY TREATMENT **PHYSICAL THERAPY AND OTHER TECHNIQUES** Recovery from the effects of a stroke depends, to a large extent, on efficient and effective rehabilitation strategies, based on physical therapy, occupational therapy, and in some cases, speech therapy. A recent review concluded that therapy-based rehabilitation services (physical therapy, occupational therapy, and speech therapy), when they were targeted at stroke patients who were living at home, appeared to improve their independence in the personal activities involved in daily living.

One study looked at patients who still had difficulty with normal functions such as walking a year after a stroke had occurred. The results of this study showed that in such cases rehabilitation treatment could lead to significant, although clinically small, improvements in the patients' mobility and walking. However, these improvements are not usually sustained after treatment ends, and the rehabilitation treatment was found to have no lasting effect on the patients' daily activity, social activity, anxiety, depression, and their number of falls, nor on the emotional stress of their caregivers.

PRIMARY TREATMENT **TREADMILL WALKING** Recent studies have demonstrated that walking on a treadmill, with the patient's body weight partially supported on the arms of the equipment, is among the most effective ways of regaining the ability to walk independently after a stroke. This method of physical therapy gives patients who cannot walk alone the

Some people who have had a stroke go on to develop dementia

AFTEREFFECTS OF STROKE

The aftereffects of stroke depend on what caused the stroke, its severity, and the location in the brain where it occurred. Different areas of the brain are responsible for different functions and abilities in the body. The right side (or hemisphere) of the brain is responsible for controlling the left side of the body, and vice versa. A stroke may also affect the brain stem, which is located at the base of the brain and is responsible for the control of many of the body's vital functions, such as breathing and heart beat.

STROKES IN THE RIGHT SIDE OF THE BRAIN MAY CAUSE:	STROKES IN THE LEFT SIDE OF THE BRAIN MAY CAUSE:	STROKES AFFECTING THE BRAIN STEM MAY CAUSE:
• Weakness or paralysis on the left side of the body • Denial that weakness or paralysis has occurred ("left neglect") • Visual problems, especially with the left visual field • Problems with spatial awareness, such as depth perception • Difficulty recognizing or locating body parts • Difficulty reading maps or finding clothing or other items • Problems with memory • Changes in behavior, including lack of concern about problems, impulsiveness, inappropriate actions, and depression	• Weakness or paralysis in the right side of the body • Difficulties with speech and comprehension • Visual problems, especially with the right visual field • Problems with mathematics and with organizing and reasoning • Behavioral changes, including cautiousness, inability to make decisions and depression • Problems with reading and writing • Difficulty in assimilating new information • Problems with memory	• Problems with breathing and heart functions • Trouble controlling body temperature • Problems with balance and coordination • Weakness or paralysis affecting the entire body • Difficulties chewing, speaking, and swallowing • Problems with vision • Coma

opportunity for repetitive practice, encouraging them to walk more symmetrically with less muscle spasm and better cardiovascular efficiency when compared to walking on the floor. Several controlled trials that have looked at survivors of acute strokes have shown that treadmill training is at least as effective as other physical therapy approaches.

ROBOT-ASSISTED MOVEMENT Results of trials demonstrated that using a robot to assist the shoulder and elbow movements of people who had had a stroke helped them recover both faster and more fully when compared with conventional rehabilitation that involved exercising, occupational therapy, and physical therapy. By six months after the stroke, however, there was no effective difference between the patients who had been treated conventionally and those who had received robotic assistance.

CHINESE TECHNIQUES In China, acupressure, acupuncture (see p.150), and Tuina (TCM manipulation and massage) is commonly used to treat the aftereffects of strokes and to encourage rehabilitation. These methods are most effective when they are used as part of an intensive rehabilitation program. Tai chi has also been used to increase muscle strength.

Mind–Body Therapies

EMG BIOFEEDBACK can be an effective way of learning to regain control of weakened muscles. You may be taught electromyographic (EMG), or muscle activity, biofeedback. This involves using special instruments to measure the electrical activity of the muscles, and then learning to increase this activity through various techniques. EMG biofeedback treatment has also been used specifically for walking rehabilitation, but the results of trials are controversial. However, a recent study concluded that EMG biofeedback increases muscle strength and improves walking in patients with impaired function on one side and foot-drop after a stroke. Another study showed that it is superior to conventional physical therapy alone for improving ankle muscle strength in people having rehabilitation following a stroke.

PREVENTION PLAN

- Do not smoke
- Eat a healthy diet low in saturated fat with two portions of oily fish weekly
- Do regular gentle exercise
- Lose excess weight
- Treat high blood pressure and high cholesterol levels if necessary

CARPAL TUNNEL SYNDROME

In carpal tunnel syndrome, the median nerve, which supplies certain parts of the hand, is compressed where it passes through the narrow space (the carpal tunnel) formed by the bones of the wrist and the strong band of tissue that overlies them. The compression causes painful tingling in the hand, wrist, and forearm, which is often worse at night and first thing in the morning, or after strenuous exercise. A combination of yoga stretches, anti-inflammatory drugs, nutritional supplements, and other therapies all help bring relief.

WHAT ARE THE SYMPTOMS?

Initial symptoms may include:

- Burning or tingling sensation in the hand
- Pain in the hand that may extend up the forearm

As the condition progresses, further symptoms may develop, including:

- Numbness of the hand
- Weakening of the grip
- Wasting and weakness in some muscles in the hand, especially at the base of the thumb

WHY MIGHT I HAVE THIS?

PREDISPOSING FACTORS

- Repetitive hand movements, e.g., using a keyboard
- Pregnancy
- Obesity
- Low thyroid function (hypothyroidism)
- Diabetes mellitus (*see p.314*)
- Oral contraceptives
- Kidney failure
- Blood disorders

TREATMENT PLAN

PRIMARY TREATMENTS

- Splinting the wrist at night
- Corticosteroids
- Osteopathic manipulation
- *Namaste* pose and other yoga exercises

BACKUP TREATMENTS

- Vitamins and bromelain
- Surgery (in severe cases)

WORTH CONSIDERING

- Homeopathy
- Acupuncture

For an explanation of how treatments are rated, see p.111.

WHY DOES IT OCCUR?

The underlying cause of the nerve compression that causes carpal tunnel syndrome may not be identifiable. However, in some cases the soft tissues inside the carpal tunnel swell, putting pressure on the median nerve. This swelling may be associated with fluid retention in pregnancy or with obesity.

Sometimes the carpal tunnel becomes narrowed because of a joint disorder, such as rheumatoid arthritis, or a wrist fracture. Repetitive hand movements, such as typing on a keyboard or playing a musical instrument, may cause inflammation of the tendons in the wrist and may also affect the median nerve.

In women, taking oral contraceptives may sometimes be a factor in developing the condition. Carpal tunnel syndrome is more common in people between the ages of 40 and 60 and tends to affect people who have diabetes mellitus (*see p.314*) or hypothyroidism (*see p.319*).

Symptoms typically affect the area supplied by the median nerve: the thumb, the first and middle fingers, the inside of the third finger, and the palm of the hand. Both hands are often affected. The symptoms of carpal tunnel syndrome may be worse at night, and pain may be severe enough to disturb sleep.

IMPORTANT

Consult a doctor if you think you may have carpal tunnel syndrome.

TREATMENTS IN DETAIL

Conventional Medicine

The doctor will usually be able to diagnose carpal tunnel syndrome from your symptoms alone. He or she will examine your hands and wrists and may tap the inside of your wrists to check whether you experience a tingling sensation. Nerve conduction tests may be done to confirm the diagnosis in severe cases.

If the condition develops in pregnancy, it will probably clear up after the birth. In other cases, treating the cause, if it is identified, usually relieves symptoms. If carpal tunnel syndrome is linked to repetitive hand movements, avoid the repetitive actions that cause the symptoms.

PRIMARY TREATMENT **SPLINTING** Your doctor may advise splinting the wrist at night to give you some relief.

PRIMARY TREATMENT **CORTICOSTEROIDS** An injection in the affected wrist or a short course of oral corticosteroids may be prescribed. These drugs, which work by reducing inflammation, have been found to bring a period of relief.

SURGERY may be necessary to relieve the pressure on the nerve if symptoms are persistent and severe. This may either involve traditional ("open") surgery or endoscopic ("keyhole") surgery, in which smaller incisions are made. Both procedures carry a small risk of complications, such as temporary numbness and wound infections.

YOGA STRETCH FOR THE WRIST

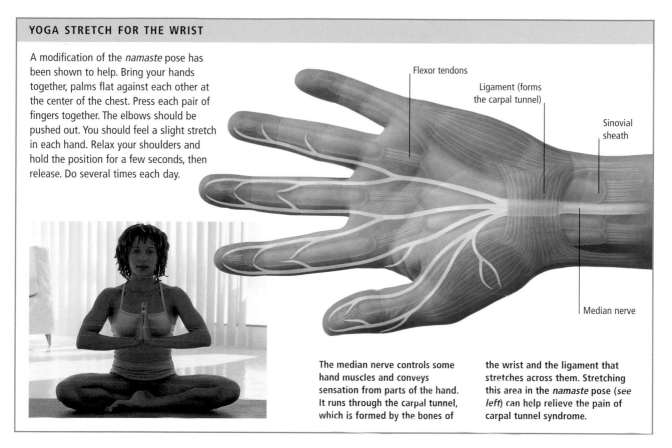

A modification of the *namaste* pose has been shown to help. Bring your hands together, palms flat against each other at the center of the chest. Press each pair of fingers together. The elbows should be pushed out. You should feel a slight stretch in each hand. Relax your shoulders and hold the position for a few seconds, then release. Do several times each day.

Flexor tendons

Ligament (forms the carpal tunnel)

Sinovial sheath

Median nerve

The median nerve controls some hand muscles and conveys sensation from parts of the hand. It runs through the carpal tunnel, which is formed by the bones of the wrist and the ligament that stretches across them. Stretching this area in the *namaste* pose (*see left*) can help relieve the pain of carpal tunnel syndrome.

Nutritional Therapy

VITAMIN SUPPLEMENTS Vitamin B_6 has been found to be very effective in treating carpal tunnel syndrome in some studies but not in others. Vitamin B_6 reduces inflammation in soft tissues and is needed for normal function of nerve cells. Vitamin B_2 can also be effective and the effectiveness is further improved when vitamins B_2 and B_6 are taken together. Try taking 100mg of each one every day for three months. Thereafter, a good B-complex supplement should be sufficient.

CAUTION

Consult your doctor before taking vitamin B6 which can interacts with certain drugs; high doses may cause neuropathy. (*See also p.46.*)

BROMELAIN The pineapple extract bromelain is naturally anti-inflammatory and may be useful in treating carpal tunnel syndrome, especially when taken with vitamin B_6. The recommended dose is 500mg of bromelain three times a day on an empty stomach.

Homeopathy

Ruta graveolens and *Hypericum perforatum* may be used to treat carpal tunnel syndrome. People who respond to *Ruta* have wrists that are weak, stiff, and achy in the morning, but symptoms ease as the day goes on. People who respond to *Hypericum* have severe, usually shooting pain. The problem may be brought on by injury to the median nerve. *Arnica* is effective at reducing postoperative pain.

Acupuncture

The pain and discomfort of carpal tunnel syndrome can often be helped by a few treatments of local acupuncture and it is always worth trying prior to surgery. Sometimes electrical stimulation is required around the wrist, but frequently acupuncture needles alone will provide immediate and sustained relief. This is particularly likely if the condition is recent or triggered by a transitory event, such as pregnancy.

You will know whether acupuncture is likely to be effective for this condition after four or five weekly sessions.

Bodywork Therapies

PRIMARY TREATMENT **OSTEOPATHIC MANIPULATION** methods have been used successfully to treat carpal tunnel syndrome. Myofascial release (a type of stretching) improved carpal tunnel symptoms in a small preliminary trial. Participants' pain, numbness, and weakness decreased.

Yoga

PRIMARY TREATMENT **NAMASTE POSE** In one study, people who suffered from carpal tunnel syndrome did a series of modified yoga postures for the arms daily, holding each of the postures for 30 seconds. (*see above*). After eight weeks, participants in this study reported less pain and said their grip was significantly better.

PREVENTION PLAN

If you work in a job that involves repetitive hand movements, use a wrist support and take regular breaks

MOTION SICKNESS

Almost everyone experiences motion sickness at some time, but the condition is especially common in children. The condition may be caused by road, sea, or air travel, or by amusement park rides. Once the motion stops, the symptoms usually subside soon afterward. Motion sickness can be treated with drugs, but acupressure, acupuncture, avoiding certain foods before travel, and autogenic training exercises can also bring relief.

WHAT ARE THE SYMPTOMS?

- Nausea
- Vomiting
- Headache
- Sweating
- Pallor
- Fatigue and lethargy

WHY MIGHT I HAVE THIS?

PREDISPOSING FACTORS

- Eating salty or fatty foods before traveling
- Trigger point activity in neck muscles
- Anxiety

TRIGGERS

- Fumes from traffic
- Reading or doing close work while traveling, especially in cars or buses

TREATMENT PLAN

PRIMARY TREATMENTS

- Pressing pericardium 6 point on wrist and other self-help measures
- Motion sickness drugs or patches

BACKUP TRATMENTS

- Avoiding certain foods
- Ginger and peppermint
- Homeopathy

WORTH CONSIDERING

- Trigger-point deactivation
- Breathing retraining
- Autogenic training
- Relaxation exercises

For an explanation of how treatments are rated, see p.111.

WHY DOES IT OCCUR?

Motion sickness occurs because of a conflict between the messages the brain receives from the eyes and the messages it receives from the organs of balance (the vestibular apparatus), which are located in the inner ear. For example, if you are traveling in a car, the inner ear senses the motion, but if you are looking at the interior of the car or are focusing on a book in front of you, your eyes may perceive the car as stationary. The conflicting messages the brain receives may bring on nausea or vomiting. The same conflict causes motion sickness from traveling in a plane or boat.

The body's sense of balance can also be disturbed by sensitive areas ("trigger points") in the neck muscles, as well as by restrictions in the joints of the neck, and this is thought by some practitioners to contribute to motion sickness. Psychological factors, such as anxiety about the journey or stress, can also contribute to motion sickness. Some people are sensitive to engine fumes and this can also bring on feelings of nausea.

SELF-HELP

- Firmly press the pericardium 6 (P6) point for 5 to 10 minutes (*see box, below*). You can purchase wrist straps ("seabands") that put pressure on these points at your pharmacy.
- Look at the horizon while traveling.
- Open a window, if possible.
- Avoid eating salty or high-fat foods or dairy products before travel.
- Take ginger or peppermint before and during travel.

THE PERICARDIUM 6 POINT

Feelings of nausea can often be relieved by pressing the pericardium 6 point on the wrist. This point is used in acupuncture, but can also be effective when pressed. To find this point, measure two of your own thumb-widths above the first crease in your wrist as you go up your arm. Then find a point in line with your middle finger on that hand. Press this point firmly, until it hurts just slightly, for five to 10 minutes. You can repeat the procedure on the other wrist. This method can be used as often as necessary to relieve nausea, and is also safe for children to use.

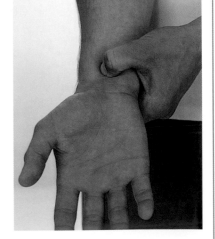

Pressing the pericardium 6 point for nausea

Conventional Medicine

PRIMARY TREATMENT **MOTION-SICKNESS DRUGS** Various treatments may help relieve motion sickness; some can be bought over the counter. Antihistamines, such as meclizine, taken before the trip, may help prevent nausea. Although generally used to treat allergic conditions, they also reduce the vomiting reflex in the brain. Some oral drugs can safely be given to children age 4 years and over.

Prescription skin patches containing scopalamine are helpful in preventing nausea in some people. They have a prolonged action but need to be applied several hours before travel. They should not be used on children under the age of 10 years.

> **CAUTION**
>
> Drugs for motion sickness may cause drowsiness and blurred vision; do not take them if you will be driving or operating machinery.

Nutritional Therapy

FOODS TO AVOID Eating foods that are high in sodium, such as preserved meats, corn chips, potato chips, and salted nuts, correlates significantly with increased airsickness (a form of motion sickness). Consumption of foods high in protein, such as milk products, cheese, and preserved meat, has also been related to an increased risk of airsickness. Avoid these foods for several hours before traveling.

GINGER AND PEPPERMINT Ginger (*Zinziber officinalis*) is a very good treatment for nausea or vomiting, whether from morning sickness in pregnancy or motion sickness. There are research trials that show a benefit with ginger. If you like the taste of ginger, eat some candied ginger or ginger-flavored candies (available at Asian markets), or make a tea out of fresh ginger root. If you don't like the taste, try powdered ginger in capsules (1,000mg 30 minutes before you travel, then 500–1,000mg every two hours while in transit). Peppermint (*Mentha x piperita*) is also a traditional nausea remedy. Try eating peppermint candy before and during a trip. Alternatively, you can either make a tea from peppermint and drink it before you travel or place one drop of peppermint essential oil under your tongue whenever you feel nauseated.

Homeopathy

Homeopathic treatments are frequently used for motion sickness.

COCCULUS (made from the plant *Anamirta cocculus*, the Indian cockle) is among the several homeopathic medicines that may be appropriate. A number of other homeopathic medicines may be used as well. In practice, it is best to use a homeopathic complex, which contains several different homeopathic medicines. A number of such complexes are available, all of which include *Cocculus*. These include Travella (containing homeopathic *Apomorph, Staphysagria, Cocculus, Theridion, Petroleum, Tabacum,* and *Nux vomica*) available in the UK and Cocculine, available in the US, France, Canada, and elsewhere, with a similar composition.

It is best to start treatment the day before travel, with two tablets, three times on the day before, and an additional dose just before leaving.

Acupressure

Acupuncture to points on the front of each forearm, just above the wrists (the P6 points), has been shown by some researchers to have an antinausea and antidizziness effect. Similar benefits are claimed for acupressure, whether the nausea is caused by motion, medication (such as chemotherapy or an anesthetic), or pregnancy. Treatment should be given ideally just before the journey and, if necessary, some acupressure should be applied during the journey if symptoms persist (*see photograph, p.154*).

Bodywork Therapies

TRIGGER-POINT DEACTIVATION Trigger points are sensitive areas in muscles that usually cause pain or discomfort where they are situated as well as in areas some distance away. Trigger points, particularly in the muscles that run from just behind the ear to the breastbone, can produce symptoms of dizziness and/or motion sickness. Trigger points can be deactivated either by acupuncture or by the manual pressure and stretching techniques that are used by osteopaths, massage therapists (particularly those with neuromuscular therapy training), and some physical therapists and chiropractors.

Breathing Retraining

It may be that motion sickness is made worse by the anxiety and tension that accompany it. Therefore symptoms may be reduced if the body is relaxed and the breathing pattern is allowed to calm down. Clinical experience suggests that people who learn to relax their neck and shoulders and breathe deeply with the diaphragm rather than using the upper chest can tolerate motion better. (*See Mind–Body Therapies, below, and p.62 for more information.*)

Mind–Body Therapies

AUTOGENIC TRAINING is a series of six silent verbal exercises that help people relax at will. It may be possible to control motion sickness using autogenic relaxation techniques, especially if anxiety and tension contribute to the condition.

A study compared the effectiveness of intramuscular injections of promethazine and the autogenic-feedback training exercise (AFTE) as treatments for motion sickness. People prone to the condition underwent a rotating-chair test. Motion-sickness tolerance was significantly greater after four hours of AFTE than 25mg or 50mg doses of promethazine. The AFTE group reported fewer or no symptoms at higher rotational speeds than people in the control or promethazine groups. Although it was a small study, the positive results suggest that psychological techniques may help overcoming motion sickness. Try relaxation techniques (*see p.99*) before your trip, and as you travel.

> **PREVENTION PLAN**
>
> Do breathing and relaxation exercises before you travel. Avoid salty and high-fat foods. Bring ginger or peppermint candy.

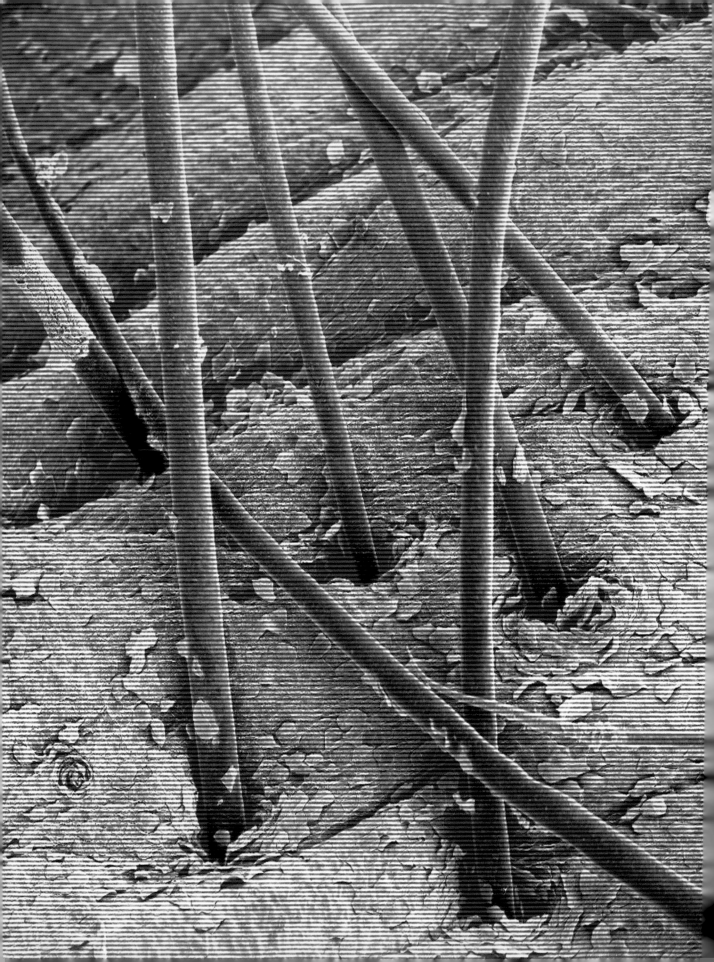

Skin

The skin is the body's largest organ and its first line of defense. Skin ailments are often best resolved using integrated treatment, which can regulate internal imbalances. While treatments usually rely on creams, ointments, and oral drugs, nutritional supplements, homeopathy, herbal remedies, and mind–body therapies can all help.

ACNE

Acne is a rash that usually appears on the face but may also affect other areas, especially the upper back, the middle of the chest, the shoulders, and the neck. The most common form is acne vulgaris, which is the familiar rash that afflicts many teenagers. Regular washing with acne soaps may help prevent bacterial buildup. Depending on the severity, acne may be treated with topical creams, oral antibiotics, or isotretinoin. Acne may also respond to tea tree oil. Rosacea, which causes an acne-type rash on the face, may affect middle-aged women.

WHAT ARE THE SYMPTOMS?

- Small blackheads
- Small, firm whiteheads
- Red pimples, sometimes with pus-filled tips
- Painful, large, firm, red lumps
- Tender lumps without obvious heads (cysts)

WHY MIGHT I HAVE THIS?

PREDISPOSING FACTORS

- Hormonal changes associated with puberty
- Certain drugs, such as corticosteroids
- Genetic factors

WHY DOES IT OCCUR?

Acne vulgaris is more common and more severe in males than females, and is triggered by changes in hormones, such as androgens, associated with puberty. The condition may first appear as early as the age of 10, It usually subsides after adolescence, but can occasionally persist after the age of 30. There may also be genetic factors, since acne vulgaris sometimes runs in families. The condition can cause great psychological distress and often arises during the period when teenagers are most self-conscious about their appearance.

Acne vulgaris is caused by the overproduction of an oily substance called sebum, which is secreted by the sebaceous glands in the skin. Sebum normally drains into the hair follicles and flows out through the follicle openings on the skin surface, lubricating the skin and keeping it supple.

However, in acne vulgaris excess sebum is produced, usually as a result of oversensitivity to androgens (male sex hormones) that are present in both boys and girls at puberty. The excess sebum can block the follicles and harden into tiny plugs. In some acne cases, the follicles may become blocked with keratin, a protein that is produced by skin cells. Bacteria collect and multiply in the blocked follicles, releasing free fatty acids from the sebum. The release of the free fatty acids may be a major factor in the development of acne lesions because they attract the body's inflammatory mechanism.

Less common forms of the condition include occupational acne, which may result from exposure to certain industrial oils; and drug-induced acne, which may be caused by various prescribed drugs, such as corticosteroids. In this case, your doctor

TREATMENT PLAN

PRIMARY TREATMENTS
- Benzoyl peroxide cream (*see Self-Help, p.159*)
- Topical keratolytics
- Topical antibiotics and retinoids

BACKUP TREATMENTS
- Oral antibiotics and retinoids (severe acne)
- Oral contraceptives (for some women)
- Wholefood diet
- Antioxidants
- Fish-oil supplements

- Detoxifying and other diets
- Zinc
- Vitamin B$_6$ (for acne before a period)
- Western and Chinese herbal medicine

WORTH CONSIDERING
- Homeopathy
- Trigger-point deactivation
- Hydrotherapy
- Mind–body therapies

For an explanation of how treatments are rated, see p.111.

may change your prescription. Babies may experience a temporary acne due to exposure to maternal hormones.

In rosacea, the rash that develops on the center of the face, consisting of red pimples with white and yellow heads, resembles acne, but it often causes a stinging, burning, or itching sensation. The cause is unknown, but there may be a genetic factor because it often runs in families. The rash may be triggered by eating a spicy meal, drinking alcohol, or going into a hot room. Rosacea primarily affects women between the ages of 30 and 55.

SELF-HELP

- Wash twice a day with warm water and a mild cleanser, but do not scrub your skin too vigorously.
- Do not pick the pimples; this may make the condition worse and may even result in scarring.
- Apply benzoyl peroxide cream to your acne every day.
- If you have occupational acne, keep your clothes clean.

TREATMENTS IN DETAIL

Conventional Medicine

After making a diagnosis, your doctor may, depending on the severity of your symptoms, recommend antibiotics and other drugs in the form of creams as well as preparations to be taken orally. You may also be referred to a dermatologist.

PRIMARY TREATMENT **TOPICAL KERATOLYTICS,** such as salicylic acid, help relieve mild acne. Your doctor may prescribe a cream containing these, and they are also available over the counter. They help break down the oily plugs that block the opening to the sebaceous gland hair follicle and loosen the dead or hardened cells on the surface of the skin. As a result, the trapped sebum can flow out, reducing the chances of bacterial infection.

PRIMARY TREATMENT **TOPICAL ANTIBIOTICS AND RETINOIDS** can help acne that is mild to moderately severe. Your doctor may prescribe creams or ointments containing these. Retinoids work by reducing sebum production.

DEVELOPMENT OF ACNE VULGARIS

Sebaceous glands around the hair follicles produce sebum (an oily substance) to lubricate hair growth and waterproof the surface of the skin. Sometimes too much sebum is produced during puberty in both sexes due to male hormones (androgens). The excess sebum becomes mixed with dead skin cells, clogging the follicle opening and encouraging bacteria to breed. The result is inflammation and acne.

Four stages of acne

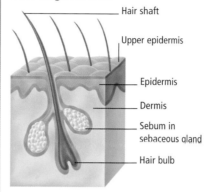

1 HEALTHY SKIN
The sebaceous glands sit in the dermis layer of the skin where they produce the right amount of sebum to lubricate the hair shaft and waterproof the epidermis.

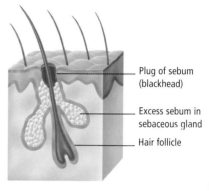

2 BLACKHEAD
A surge in production of sebum blocks the pore. The plug of sebum, bacteria, and skin debris reacts with oxygen in the air and turns black (blackhead or "open comedo").

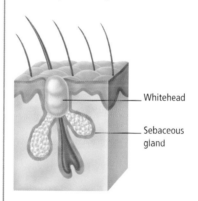

3 WHITEHEAD
Sometimes the plug of sebum does not break through the skin, when it is known as a whitehead or "closed comedo." As it grows larger, it presses on the hair follicle.

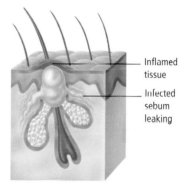

4 INFECTED FOLLICLE AND ACNE
Sebum and the bacteria that feed on it leak from the growing whitehead into the dermis. The surrounding skin tissue and the hair follicle become inflamed (acne).

CAUTION

Most topical creams can cause a burning sensation or skin irritation. Topical retinoids in particular can cause an initial "flare." Sunlight may exacerbate irritation.

ORAL ANTIBIOTICS AND RETOINOIDS If your acne is moderate to severe, your doctor may prescribe an oral antibiotic, such as tetracycline, which you take for 3–4 months; longer use should be avoided, because it results in bacteria becoming resistant to the antibiotics. For severe acne, dermatologists may prescribe a course of retinoids, such as isotretinoin, which is usually taken for four months. Over 90 percent of patients respond to this therapy. Many people are cured by a single course of retinoids, but in some cases, a second course may be prescribed.

CERTAIN COMBINED ORAL CONTRACEP-TIVES reduce male hormone (androgen) levels and have been shown to reduce the

Eating plenty of antioxidant fruit and vegetables is important. Regular intake of carrot juice, for example, can provide beta-carotene, an antioxidant and precursor to vitamin A, which helps control acne. Supplements can help, too: in one study, taking 200mcg of selenium together with 20 IU of vitamin E each day helped reduce acne symptoms.

FISH OIL SUPPLEMENTS can also help reduce the inflammation that may be associated with acne. This inflammation may be linked to excessive amounts of omega-6

VITAMIN B$_6$ can help some women whose acne flares up before a menstrual period. Some female acne sufferers have high levels of male hormones (androgens). Women with premenstrual acne may benefit from taking a 50mg vitamin B$_6$ supplement a day. In a few cases, high-dose B vitamin supplementation has made acne worse. B$_6$ and B$_{12}$ have been associed with acne flares.

Homeopathy

Homeopathy is often used to treat acne and the evidence suggests it responds well. For the best effect, treatment needs to be tailored to the individual by a skilled practitioner. If one is unavailable, you can use a homeopathic complex consisting of several of the medicines indicated below. The following therapies are recommended by homeopaths, but no clinical trials support their use.

SULFUR AND SILICEA Two of the most commonly indicated medicines are *Sulphur* and *Silicea*. Rashes that respond to *Sulphur* are typically very itchy, particularly in the heat. *Sulphur* constitutional types are usually extroverted, untidy, and may be opinionated or garrulous. They tend to be hot-blooded, needing fewer clothes than most people. In particular, their feet may be hot and smelly.

Acne that responds to *Silicea* features pustules that never seem to discharge: they sit under the skin for weeks without bursting, but often forming cysts. *Silicea* people are usually chilly and feel cold, even in a warm room. They tend to be pale and thin, with fine hair and weak, ridged nails. Their hands and feet are cold and clammy.

OTHER REMEDIES *Kalium bromatum* is recommended when the pimples are often itchy. Individuals complain of poor sleep, frequently disturbed by bad dreams. They may be mentally slow, finding it hard to remember and think.

Calcarea sulphurica is suitable if there are large yellow pustules that are slow to

---

> ## The sebaceous glands are active before birth in both of the sexes

severity of acne in some women. All formulations of oral contraceptives appear to be equally effective but may need to be taken for at least six months.

Nutritional Therapy

WHOLE-FOOD DIET Evidence is emerging that the prevalence of acne in developed countries is related to a glut of foods high in refined sugars and starches. These tend to cause the body to secrete copious quantities of insulin, which seem to increase the levels of the male hormones that may be at the root of many acne cases. Cutting back on refined and processed carbohydrates is an important step in clearing acne.

PRIMARY TREATMENT **DETOXIFICATION AND OTHER DIETS** In natural medicine, acne is viewed as a problem of excess toxicity. Clinical experience shows that detoxification can be effective in reducing acne and in improving the condition of the skin. A common factor in acne is an overgrowth of yeast organisms and food sensitivity also appears to be a common underlying theme in acne. See p.40 for diets to address these problems.

ANTIOXIDANTS There is evidence to suggests acne is an inflammatory condition in which free radicals play a role. Antioxidants can help to reduce the inflammation by neutralizing the damaging free radicals.

fatty acids (found in vegetable oils), accompanied by a relative lack of omega-3 fatty acids (found in oily fish). There is some evidence that many people with acne are deficient in the essential fatty acids.

You may be able to control your acne by cutting down on margarine and vegetable oils and eating more oily fish (such as salmon, mackerel, and trout), walnuts, and flaxseeds.

You may also reduce the inflammation associated with acne by taking essential fatty acids, such as gamma linolenic acid (GLA). These are derived from evening primrose (*Oenothera biennis*), borage (*Borage officinalis*), or blackcurrant (*Ribes nigrum*) oil, as well as from fish oil.

PRIMARY TREATMENT **ZINC** Three studies found that zinc therapy can be effective for people with acne. In one study, zinc 30mg for three months successfully reduced lesions in 31 percent of those treated; minocycline, however, reduced lesions in twice as many patients. A topical cream containing chloroxylenol and zinc oxide was as effective as a preparation of 59 percent benzoyl peroxide. Zinc is available in food sources, such as pumpkin seeds, or supplements. Take 30mg of zinc three times a day for 3–4 months and then reduce the dose to 25mg once a day. Taking zinc for a long period can deplete the body of copper, so take 1mg of copper for each 15mg of zinc.

heal and may be itchy. Acne spots that respond to *Hepar sulphuris calcareum* are very sensitive or painful as they develop.

Pulsatilla is particularly (but by no means exclusively) helpful for girls when crops of pimples develop in the week before a menstrual period. It is prescribed mostly on constitutional grounds (*see p.73*). *Pulsatilla* types are mild-tempered or sweet-natured. They lack assertion and are indecisive. Although they easily feel cold, they like fresh air (provided they are well wrapped up) and hate stuffy atmospheres.

Western Herbal Medicine

Herbs are highly effective in controlling excess sebum production and combating the bacteria that proliferate in the plugged outlet at the base of hair follicles. A combination of internal and external treatment brings the best results.

INTERNAL TREATMENTS A daily dose of chasteberry (*Vitex agnus-castus*) may help to control surges of the hormones (especially at puberty) that increase the size of sebaceous glands and the production of sebum. Sage (*Salvia officinalis*), motherwort (*Leonurus cardiaca*), and red clover (*Trifolium pratense*) may also help reduce surplus sebum by modulating hormone levels. Regular cups of green tea (*Camellia sinensis*) may adjust the overproduction of male and other hormones and serve as an anti-inflammatory.

Extracts of poke root (*Phytolacca decandra*), a herb restricted to professional use, seem to cut down the flow of sebum and restrict bacterial proliferation. Burdock (*Arctium lappa*) root and leaf also combats bacteria and reduces inflammation.

An overloaded bowel is a frequent cause of acne. Rhubarb (*Rheum palmatum*) root eliminates toxic wastes and reduces bacterial inflammation. It is laxative, so take it only for a short time. Oregon grape root (*Mahonia aquifolium*) can significantly reduce acne eruptions, while the bitters in artichoke (*Cynara scolymus*) leaf stimulate the liver and production of bile.

EXTERNAL TREATMENTS may help unblock sebaceous glands and kill off bacteria that lead to inflammation of the skin. Try tea tree (*Melaleuca alternifolia*) oil gel, which in clinical trials was as effective as

An Ancient Egyptian remedy for acne featured ostrich egg, olive oil, bile, flour, and milk

benzoyl peroxide and with fewer side effects, although perhaps slower to act.

Washes of astringent herbs, such as rose (*Rosa gallica*), witch hazel (*Hamamelis virginiana*), burnet (*Sanguisorba officinalis*) root, elderflower (*Sambucus nigra*), or cold Earl Grey tea, are recommended by herbalists. Applying fresh lemon juice and/or live yogurt to your skin can also help, especially after a chamomile (*Matricaria recutita*), steam bath has opened up the sebaceous glands. Allow the steam made from chamomile tea to rise over your face.

You can apply a paste of oatmeal, green tea (*Camellia sinensis*), chamomile (*Matricaria recutita*), and calendula (*Calendula officinalis*). Pounded burdock (*Arctium lappa*) leaves mixed with an aqueous cream may calm inflammation and fresh aloe vera gel is good for oily skin. Another topical remedy is an equal mix of cucumber and beet juice, but it can stain the skin.

> **CAUTION**
>
> See p.69 before taking a herbal remedy and, if you are taking a prescribed medication, consult an herbal medicine expert first.

Chinese Herbal Medicine

In Traditional Chinese Medicine (TCM), acne is classified into four types based on the infection, toxicity, inflammation, and stress that contribute to it. Research has not yet backed up the TCM approach. A formulation of *Angelica dahurica*, *Coptis chinensis*, and *Glycyrrhiza glabra* may be helpful for prevention and treatment. Consult a trained practitioner before using TCM herbs (*see p.81*). Self-medication is not recommended due to reports of kidney or liver failure in patients using TCM.

> **CAUTION**
>
> Do not take Chinese herbal remedies with prescribed drugs for acne without first consulting a health care practitioner.

Bodywork Therapies

HYDROTHERAPY, such as the regular use of a facial sauna, can act as a preventive measure. It helps reduce the chances of follicle blockage. A facial sauna that is made from fresh peppermint (*Mentha piperita*), parsley (*Petroselinum crispum*), and lemon (*Citrus limonum*) is especially good for deep cleansing as well as invigorating the skin.

Combine peppermint (*Mentha piperita*), lavender (*Lavandula angustifolia*), yarrow (*Achillea millefolium*), and rosemary (*Rosmarinus officinalis*) for a refreshing facial sauna for particulary oily skin.

> **CAUTION**
>
> Do not take an Epsom salts bath if you are elderly or frail.

Mind-Body Therapies

Acne can have a major emotional impact, especially on self-conscious teenagers, and some practitioners believe that stress can make it worse. In a research study, a combination of biofeedback, visualization, relaxation, and breathing was effective in reducing stress. If you are stressed, try diaphragmatic breathing (*see p.62*) for 10 minutes a day. If your acne causes depression or difficulties in relationships and emotional life, your doctor may suggest psychotherapy to help restore your self-confidence and self-esteem.

> **PREVENTION PLAN**
>
> These may be helpful in preventing acne over the long term:
>
> - Adequate zinc intake
> - Face saunas
> - Hydrotherapy

HERPES SIMPLEX

Herpes simplex is a highly contagious skin infection, which especially affects the mucous membranes of the mouth and genitals. The two viruses responsible cause lesions that are frequently very uncomfortable, especially during the first outbreak. Many carriers of herpes don't know that they are infected. Although there is no cure, antiviral creams and pills reduce the severity and duration of attacks. Boosting the immune system and keeping stress to a minimum using relaxation techniques may reduce the chances of a further outbreak.

WHAT ARE THE SYMPTOMS?

For herpes simplex type 1 (HSV1):

- At first, either no symptoms or painful mouth ulcers
- Cold sores may develop, preceded by tingling in the affected area

For herpes simplex type 2 (HSV2):

- Painful blisters and ulcers in the genital area or lower back — the first episode may be accompanied by a fever, flulike symptoms, and painful urination
- Recurrences are often preceded by tingling in the affected area

WHY MIGHT I HAVE THIS?

PREDISPOSING FACTORS

- Lowered immunity
- Stress
- Poor sleep
- Sunlight
- Menstruation
- Intimate contact with an infected person (kissing, oral sex, genital sex, anal sex)

TREATMENT PLAN

PRIMARY TREATMENTS

- Topical antiviral creams
- Oral antiviral drugs
- Lysine supplements

BACKUP TREATMENTS

- Low-arginine diet
- Homeopathy
- Western and Chinese herbal medicine
- Mind–body therapies

WORTH CONSIDERING

- Various supplements
- Zinc sulfate solution

For an explanation of how treatments are rated, see p.111.

WHY DOES IT OCCUR?

Two closely-related viruses are responsible for causing herpes. Herpes simplex type 1 (HSV1) is more common and generally infects the oral area, whereas herpes simplex type 2 (HSV2) usually infects the seminal area. Although HSV2 has more social stigma attached to it, the two viruses are very similar. Both may cause outbreaks on the lips, mouth, or genital area, and are easily transferred between the genital area and the mouth and throat during oral sex. Only one third of those infected with either virus experience major symptoms.

Neither HSV1 nor HSV2 are major health threats, although a few serious ailments may occur. Herpes that has spread to the eye may cause blindness and, very rarely, herpes may spread to the brain. Pregnant women who have herpes should consult their doctor. If the mother experiences an outbreak of genital herpes during labor, a cesarean section may be necessary to avoid transferring the virus to the baby.

Approximately two-thirds of those with herpes never experience outward signs of the infection and may unknowingly transmit herpes to a sexual partner. However, the chances of this happening are very small — between 4 and 10 percent. When lesions are present, herpes is easily transferred by direct contact. Carriers of the herpes virus are infectious from when symptoms of an outbreak are first experienced until skin is completely healed.

Either herpes virus may be shed before lesions occur, and some people shed virus between attacks. People who have developed antibodies after contracting HSV1 or HSV2 may have some immunity to the other form.

IMPORTANT

See your doctor immediately if you develop a cold sore in or near the eye.

Both types of herpes virus remain dormant in the nerves for life. The exact triggers that cause a herpes outbreak are unknown but when the immune system is weakened, the viruses can be easily reactivated. In some people, an outbreak begins with a tingling feeling or itching in the genital area, or pain in the buttocks or down the leg. Ulcers and blisters may form, causing viruses to be shed. Stress, poor sleep, sunlight, and menstruation can also cause the viruses to reactivate.

ORAL HERPES Over half of all Americans are infected with oral herpes, usually caused by HSV1, during childhood through contact with infected saliva. The initial infection is often symptomless, although painful mouth ulcers sometimes occur. Afterward, the virus lies dormant, most commonly in the trigeminal nerve ganglia near the temple region of the head. During an outbreak, it migrates down the nerve, causing a fresh outbreak of cold sores mainly on the lips. The face and, rarely, the eyes may also be affected.

GENITAL HERPES, usually caused by HSV2, affects 1 in 5 adults and adolescents in the US. The virus can be caught via touching, kissing, or unprotected sex. After the initial attack, this virus retreats to the sacral ganglion, a nerve structure near the base of the spine, from where it may later be reactivated, causing a recurrence of lesions in the genital area or buttocks.

- Place a cold, wet, used tea bag over the affected area as soon as the tingling or painful sensation begins.
- For genital herpes, try sitting in a salt-water or warm bath.

Conventional Medicine

Visit your doctor for individualized treatment options. Herpes is often difficult to diagnose — even when test results are negative, a person may still have the virus.

PRIMARY TREATMENT **TOPICAL ANTIVIRAL CREAMS** contain antiviral drugs, which include acyclovir and penciclovir. These creams are only effective during an initial attack, when they may shorten symptoms by one day.

PRIMARY TREATMENT **ORAL ANTIVIRAL DRUGS** may be prescribed by your doctor to treat attacks of both types of herpes simplex. If you have frequent genital herpes attacks, or have impaired immunity, a doctor may prescribe oral antiviral drugs, such as

acyclovir, to prevent infection from becoming severe. A five-day course of daily oral antivirals, such as acyclovir, famcyclovir, or valacyclovir, needs to start at the first sign of an outbreak. Ask your doctor for a prescription ahead of time so that you can carry a supply of pills with you. These drugs can abort an attack if used early enough.

> **CAUTION**
>
> Antiviral drugs may cause side effects; ask your doctor to explain these to you.

Nutritional Therapy

A LOW-ARGININE DIET may be recommended to help fight the herpes viruses, which need the amino acid arginine to reproduce. Arginine is found in nuts, especially peanuts and cashews, chocolate, and grains. However, no evidence from studies in humans supports this theory.

LYSINE is an amino acid that inhibits the growth of herpes simplex in the laboratory. Although lysine is used in the synthesis of carnitine and, therefore, is important to the transport of fatty acids,

clinical trials of lysine supplements have found it ineffective in preventing outbreaks, rate of healing, or the severity of blisters.

A COMBINATION OF VITAMIN C AND BIOFLAVONOIDS has been used to treat herpes. Take 200mg of vitamin C and 200mg of bioflavonoids 3–5 times a day at the first sign of an attack. Applying vitamin C cream 3 times a day to blisters may also help reduce their severity.

VITAMIN E spread on the skin from a soft gelatin capsule has been used to provide topical relief for herpes blisters. Soak a small piece of tissue in the contents of a vitamin E capsule and apply to the lesions. Apply for 15 minutes, twice a day.

> **CAUTION**
>
> Consult your doctor before taking vitamin E or vitamin C with warfarin, or before taking vitamin C with antibiotics (*see p.46*).

ZINC SULFATE Zinc solutions or creams have been used to treat herpes. A solution of zinc sulfate (0.01–0.025 percent zinc), applied as a compress for 10 minutes each day, has been recommended; however, no controlled trials of this treatment have been performed.

Homeopathy

RHUS TOXICODENDRON is the most commonly used homeopathic medicine for acute attacks of both types of herpes. It is specifically suggested for patients whose itching and pain are relieved by the application of heat.

No clinical trials have been done of homeopathy for herpes. However, other remedies commonly used include *Croton tiglium* for genital herpes, *Natrum muriaticum* for cold sores on the lips, and *Causticum* for the rare occurrence of cold sores in the nose. *Sepia* may be the most effective for recurrent herpes, especially in women. *Agaricus muscarius* and *Arsenicum album* are used for postherpetic neuralgia.

Western Herbal Medicine

LEMON BALM (*Melissa officinalis*) leaves or extracts have been used topically to treat herpes. However, two controlled trials

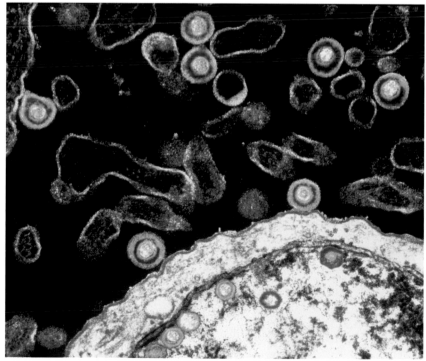

A human cell is under attack from a number of herpes viruses. After each virus enters the cell, its genetic material (yellow) emerges from the protein coat (blue) and reproduces itself.

found little to no benefit for lemon balm extracts. A controlled, year-long study of *Echinaceae purpurea* plant or root extract found no benefit in preventing herpes recurrences.

RHUBARB ROOT One Chinese study has demonstrated that, even in low doses, an ethanol extract of rhubarb (*Rheum officinale*) root can inhibit the spread of the herpes simplex virus that causes cold sores.

> ## Approximately 1 in 5 people infected with genital herpes have only one attack

In addition, it may prevent infection from occuring in the first place.

Rhubarb root was one of four herbs identified by Chinese researchers as having significant inhibitory effect on the herpes virus. The others were the tree peony (*Paeonia suffruticosa*), chinaberry (*Melia toosendan*), and yellow mountain laurel (*Sophora flavescens*).

Other research has confirmed that a sage (*Salvia officinalis*) and rhubarb root cream, applied to the lips, proved as effective as topical acyclovir cream.

PROPOLIS, a resinous material from poplar and conifer buds used by bees to seal their hives, is active against the herpes virus. One study found that a propolis ointment was more effective than acyclovir or placebo for treating genital herpes.

OTHER HERBS Other well-known herbs have shown anti-HSV activity. In clinical studies, topical glycyrrhetentic acid (found in licorice) encouraged herpes blisters to heal and reduced the pain associated with a cold sore outbreak.

Tea tree (*Melaleuca alternifolia*) oil and eucalyptus (*Eucalyptus globulus*) oil show individual antiviral activity against HSV in the laboratory. Siberian ginseng (*Eleutheroccus senticosus*) is also useful. Regular use of creams containing concentrated and dried leaf extract of lemon balm (*Melissa officinalis*) has been studied. The treatment does not appear to be highly effective, but is harmless.

Soothing herbs, such as chickweed (*Stellaria media*) and chamomile (*Matricaria recutita*), applied as creams or gels, or cold chamomile tea bags may provide relief.

TRADITIONAL TREATMENTS Some traditional treatments have yet to be researched. One is the tea bag (*see Immediate Relief, p.163*), which may be effective because of its tannin content. Some herbalists specifically recommend Earl Grey tea bags, which contain bergamot oil. Applying either goldenseal (*Hydrastis canadensis*) powder mixed into live yogurt or fresh grapefruit juice to an outbreak is also said to be effective. Some herbalists advocate the use of aloe vera (*Aloe vera*) gel, while others recommend taking flaxseed oil because the omega-3 oils that it contains can decrease inflammation.

> **CAUTION**
>
> See p.69 before taking an herbal remedy and, if you are taking a prescribed medication, consult a health-care professional first.

Chinese Herbal Medicine

TCM doctors see HSV1 and HSV2 infections as typical "damp–heat" toxins. An acute attack is treated with Gentian Drain the Gallbladder Decoction (*Long Dan Xie Gan Tang*), with a few changes made for legal and safety reasons. For example, akebia (*Akebia trifoliata*) is replaced with phellodendron (*Phellodendron amurense*) bark, yellow mountain laurel (*Sophora flavescens*) root, dyer's woad (*Isatis tinctoria*) leaf, and rhubarb (*Rheum officinale*) root. A paste prepared from natural indigo (*Indigofera suffructicosa* or *Isatis tinctoria*) powder known as *Qing Dai San* can be applied to the cold sores.

> **CAUTION**
>
> See p.69 before taking a Chinese herbal remedy and if you are taking a prescribed medication consult a Chinese herbalist first.

Mind–Body Therapies

The regular practice of a mind–body technique along with lifestyle changes, such as stress reduction and regular exercise, may be effective in controlling the severity and/or frequency of herpes outbreaks.

RELAXATION TECHNIQUES Studies suggest that stress, anxiety, worry, and depression can all make a recurrence of oral or genital herpes more likely. The social stigma of genital herpes enhances a sense of isolation and guilt. If you have either type of herpes, regularly practicing techniques such as progressive muscle relaxation, hypnosis, abdominal breathing, and meditation can all help counter stress by slowing down the heart and respiration rates. In a 2002 study, participants who were prone to genital herpes were taught self-hypnosis over six weeks. Results showed that their herpes attacks were almost halved. Another study suggested that cognitive restructuring, a form of cognitive behavior therapy (CBT) that focuses on changing a person's attitude toward a chronic illness, may also help.

STRESS MANAGEMENT In 1997, research revealed that when a group of men with genital herpes practiced stress management techniques, the frequency of their herpes attacks was significantly reduced. The men also reported less depression, anxiety, and distress. Those who practiced relaxation the most consistently had significantly greater improvement in mood. In 2000, another study revealed that a 10-week period of stress management lowered stress levels, decreased the negative impact on the immune system, and showed an improvement in symptoms.

> **PREVENTION PLAN**
>
> **These may help prevent further attacks:**
>
> - A long course of an oral antiviral drug
> - Daily multivitamin and mineral supplement
> - Regular relaxation and exercise

SHINGLES

The same virus that causes chickenpox (*see p.400*) may later cause herpes zoster, or shingles, a blistering rash overlying a nerve. The herpes zoster virus lies dormant in the body but can be reactivated. Pain or discomfort, known as postherpetic neuralgia, may persist in the affected area for months or years after the rash has disappeared. Treatment involves analgesics and antiviral drugs, with additional measures to treat the postherpetic neuralgia.

WHAT ARE THE SYMPTOMS?

- Initial tingling or pain in the affected area
- Tiny, painful blisters appear in one area and on one side of the body — usually on the chest, abdomen, or face — and later crust over
- Fatigue
- Fever
- Headache
- Pain and discomfort, known as postherpetic neuralgia, may continue for months or years

WHY MIGHT I HAVE THIS?

TRIGGERS

- Stress
- Illness
- Age
- Chemotherapy
- Chronic corticosteroid use

TREATMENT PLAN

PRIMARY TREATMENTS

- Antiviral drugs
- Pain relief
- Antibiotics, if secondary infection occurs

BACKUP TREATMENTS

- Proteolytic enzymes
- Vitamin E
- Acupuncture
- Homeopathy
- Capsaicin cream
- Mind–body therapies

For an explanation of how treatments are rated, see p.111.

WHY DOES IT OCCUR?

Varicella virus initially causes chickenpox and then remains dormant for the rest of the individual's life in the dorsal root ganglia, which are nerve structures near the spine (*see p.166*). Stress or an illness may reactivate the virus to cause shingles. Varicella can be spread by direct contact with a blister. A person who has not had chickenpox can catch the virus from someone with shingles.

Chickenpox rarely recurs, but shingles tends to be a recurrent condition mainly affecting people aged between 50 and 70 years. People who have weakened or depleted immune systems, such as those with AIDS (*see p.470*) or cancer patients undergoing chemotherapy (*see p.464*), are especially susceptible to shingles. In older people, there may be prolonged pain (postherpetic neuralgia, *see p.124*).

TREATMENTS IN DETAIL

Conventional Medicine

Your doctor will be able to diagnose shingles from the appearance of the rash and from other symptoms, such as fatigue, fever, and tingling in the affected area.

IMPORTANT

- Consult your doctor at once if you have the symptoms of shingles.
- Consult your doctor if you are pregnant and have been exposed to chickenpox.
- See your doctor immediately if the rash of shingles affects your face. If a nerve that supplies the eye is affected, it may cause inflammation and scarring of the cornea.

PRIMARY TREATMENT **ORAL DRUGS,** such as the antiviral drug acyclovir, may be given for a week and may help shorten attacks if the medication is started early enough. You will need antibiotics if the blisters become infected. Studies have shown that antiviral drugs and tricyclic antidepressants such as amitriptyline can reduce the likelihood of persistent postherpetic neuralgia.

PRIMARY TREATMENT **PAIN RELIEF** Analgesics can help relieve the pain and discomfort of postherpetic neuralgia. Alternatively, your doctor may prescribe a topical preparation containing anesthetic drugs, which can be applied to the affected area. These drugs are not used while the rash is present.

A treatment known as transcutaneous electrical nerve stimulation (TENS) may also bring relief from the pain. A small device that can be used at home relays tiny electrical impulses (usually for about 30 minutes) to electrodes on the skin in the painful area. The impulses stop the pain signals from reaching the brain.

CAUTION

Antiviral drugs can cause side effects; ask your doctor to explain these to you.

Do not use a TENS device if you have a pacemaker. Do not place the electrodes near your eyes or the front of your neck.

Nutritional Therapy

PROTEOLYTIC ENZYMES There is some evidence to suggest that taking a combination of the proteolytic (protein-digesting) enzymes — chymotrypsin, papain, and

SHINGLES RASH

The shingles rash caused by the herpes zoster virus usually affects the skin of the chest, abdomen, or face. More rarely, the rash may appear on a shoulder or on the scalp. It is common for the rash to occur on only one side of the body because the virus becomes activated on one of the branches of the 12 pairs of dorsal nerves. After lying dormant in the dorsal root ganglion of a spinal nerve, the virus may be activated by stress or an illness. In a shingles attack, blisters appear on the skin along the path of the nerve. The rash may follow a line from the back to the front of the ribs.

The highlighted areas show the potential path of the shingles rash on the skin of the back as if the two nerves were infected.

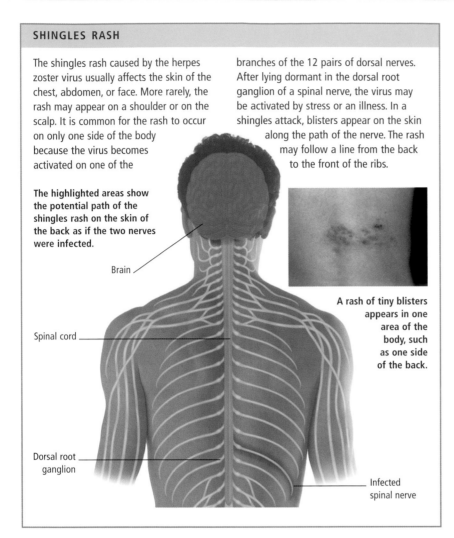

Brain

Spinal cord

Dorsal root ganglion

Infected spinal nerve

A rash of tiny blisters appears in one area of the body, such as one side of the back.

trypsin (administered orally) — may help accelerate the healing of shingles. These enzymes are thought to be involved in decreasing the body's inflammatory response to the virus. Research also shows that oral proteolytic enzymes may help reduce the likelihood of developing postherpetic neuralgia.

In one study, administering 120mg trypsin, 40mg chymotrypsin, and 320mg papain five times a day reduced both the blisters and the pain as effectively as acyclovir. The recommended dose is 500mg of a proteolytic enzyme preparation, which should be taken several times a day while symptoms persist.

VITAMIN E A study in 1976 found that vitamin E in a daily dose of 1200–1600 IU helped alleviate postherpetic neuralgia associated with shingles. However, it can take six months or more to see real benefit.

Acupuncture

In Traditional Chinese Medicine, acupuncture is widely used to treat acute shingles, usually within 48–72 hours of the illness developing. Acupuncture does not help once the neuralgia has become established.

Acupuncture for shingles should be provided in the first few days, on a daily or every other day basis, and gradually discontinued as the rash settles.

Homeopathy

RHUS TOXICODENDRON OR RANUNCULUS BULBOSUS *Rhus toxicodendron* is the most commonly indicated medicine for acute shingles attacks. It is particularly suitable if there are small, intensely itchy blisters, often on a dusky-red background, and if the itching and pain are often relieved by hot applications. *Ranunculus*

bulbosus can be very helpful for shingles, especially if it affects the chest, with severe burning or shooting pain.

AGARICUS MUSCARIUS OR ARSENICUM ALBUM may sometimes help people with postherpetic neuralgia. In those who respond to *Agaricus muscarius*, the pains are reported to be like "icy needles"; the patient may also suffer from tics or twitching. *Arsenicum album* is associated with a burning pain that is relieved by heat. The skin is dry and flaky, while the patient is extremely anxious, tense, and chilly.

Western Herbal Medicine

CAPSAICIN CREAM The pain that may occur after shingles, called postherpetic neuralgia, can be treated with capsaicin, made from chili pepper (*Capsicum* spp.). It is available in an over-the-counter cream in two concentrations (use the 0.075 percent, not the 0.025). You can rub it onto the affected area several times a day but wash your hands after applying. It may cause a burning sensation that usually goes away after several applications. Two studies have shown a benefit from this treatment.

Mind–Body Therapies

You can combat the psychological factors associated with postherpetic neuralgia, such as stress and anxiety, with mind–body techniques, including progressive muscle relaxation, biofeedback, meditation, or abdominal breathing. These techniques lower your heart and respiration rates, and calm your body and mind. Reducing stress may boost your immune response to the virus and help prevent reactivation. One controlled study of T'ai Chi found that taking three classes a week for 15 weeks boosted immune activity against the varicella zoster virus in the elderly.

PREVENTION PLAN

These may help improve immunity and prevent further attacks:

- A diet rich in antioxidants
- Daily B-vitamin supplements

ECZEMA

Eczema, also known as atopic dermatitis, is a chronic condition in which patches of skin become red, inflamed, and itchy. Affected areas may be covered in small, fluid-filled blisters, thickened and red, or crusted or cracked. Eczema commonly affects skin creases, like the insides of elbows or the back of knees. The rash of contact dermatitis may result from irritation or from an allergic reaction. Eczema usually cannot be cured; the aim of treatment is to control symptoms with topical creams, diets, probiotics, avoiding environmental triggers, and taking herbal remedies. Relaxation and breathing retraining may help.

WHAT ARE THE SYMPTOMS?

- Redness and swelling of the skin
- Small, fluid-filled blisters
- Itching, especially at night
- Dry, scaly, and cracked skin
- Thickened skin in long-standing eczema

WHY MIGHT I HAVE THIS?

PREDISPOSING FACTORS

For atopic eczema:

- Genetic tendency
- Fatty acid deficiency
- Stress and anxiety
- Depression
- Biotin deficiency
- Vitamin B$_{12}$ deficiency
- Zinc deficiency
- High histamine levels in the blood

TRIGGERS

For atopic eczema:

- Strong detergents, soaps, dog or cat fur, wearing wool, dust mites
- Food sensitivities
- Dry skin

For contact dermatitis:

- Nickel, rubber

WHY DOES IT OCCUR?

We are witnessing a significant increase in atopic eczema, the most common type of eczema, and environmental factors play a part. Centrally heated houses, dust mites in pillows and carpets, and animal dander from pets may all trigger or worsen eczema in susceptible individuals. However, there are also many other factors (*see left*) — some, such as detergents, are irritants rather than triggers. Eczema tends to recur intermittently throughout life. Each type of eczema may be triggered by different factors.

TYPES OF ECZEMA Atopic eczema may first appear in infancy and continue to flare up throughout adolescence and adulthood. The cause is unknown, but this type of eczema often appears in people with an inherited disposition to other allergic conditions, including asthma and hay fever. Flare-ups in adults may be linked to stress, a change in the temperature, or as an allergic reaction to certain foods, but often has no obvious trigger.

The mechanism underlying eczema is not fully understood. In people with atopic eczema, it seems as though the immune system reacts to an otherwise harmless substance, such as dust, as if it were dangerous. It is thought that inflammatory cells are stimulated to destroy the "allergen," but if too many are activated, the skin becomes red, swollen, and itchy.

In contact dermatitis and other types of eczema, the skin is irritated and there may be an allergic response. Contact dermatitis is a form of eczema that can occur at any age and develops after touching something to which you are sensitive. Poison ivy rash is a classic example, and most people are

TREATMENT PLAN

PRIMARY TREATMENTS

- Emollient creams and topical treatments
- Food-exclusion diet
- Essential fatty acids
- Homeopathy
- Avoidance of environmental irritants

BACKUP TREATMENTS

- Oral corticosteroids and immunosuppressants (for severe eczema)
- Ultraviolet phototherapy

- Probiotics (particularly for children)
- Western and Chinese herbal medicine
- Mind–body therapies

WORTH CONSIDERING

- Breathing retraining
- Zinc, biotin, and vitamin B
- Anti-*Candida* diet

For an explanation of how treatments are rated, see p.111.

easily sensitized. But substances such as nickel, rubber, or cinnamon flavoring, which don't cause a rash in most people, will cause contact dermatitis in some.

Nummular, or discoid eczema, causes itchy, coin-shaped patches on the arms and legs. Affected areas may ooze and become scaly or blistered. It is more common in men. The cause is not known, but it may be related to allergy.

Asteotic eczema, characterized by a scaly rash that is random and cracked, is most common in elderly people. It is caused by dry skin that occurs with aging or as a result of exposure to dry, cold air.

Dishidrotic eczema affects thick-skinned areas, such as the fingers, palms, and soles. The many itchy blisters may joint to form large, oozing areas. that thicken and crack.

IMPORTANT

If you have eczema symptoms, consult your doctor for a diagnosis.

SELF-HELP

- Avoid contact with known irritants and keep notes to find out which factors, whether foods, dust, or stress could be triggering your attacks.
- Use emollient soothing creams frequently and liberally.
- Get rid of dust mites; vacuum bedrooms daily and encase mattresses and quilts in microfiber covers.
- Wear smooth fabrics (does not have to be cotton).
- Do not scratch the affected areas; try tapping the itchy areas instead.
- Expose the affected area to sunlight for ten minutes several times weekly.
- Spread *Calendula* cream on the eczema patches. (However, homeopathic *Calendula* cream may contain lanolin, so you should not use this if you are sensitive to lanolin.)
- Wear gloves when doing housework to protect your hands from detergents and cleaning materials.
- Use hypoallergenic bathwater oil to help moisturize the skin.
- Place 1 lb (500g) of oatmeal in a gauze, cotton, or cheesecloth bag. Hang it under a running hot-water faucet as you

PATCH TESTING FOR CONTACT DERMATITIS

Patch testing of the skin helps determine which substances cause an allergic reaction. Tiny amounts of the substances are placed on small disks, which are stuck to an inert tape and placed on a person's back. After about two days, the disks are removed to reveal either red patches (positive reactions) or no changes (negative reactions). In some cases, the reaction may be delayed.

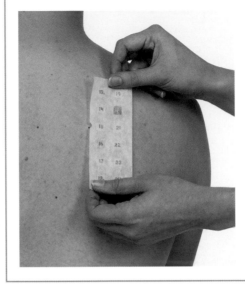

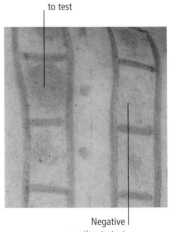

Positive reaction to test

Negative reaction to test

fill a bath. The bathwater should be at body temperature (not too hot). Let the bag float in the bath and use it to gently pat areas of particular irritation. Stay in the water for 20 minutes and then pat yourself dry afterward; don't rub. Comercially made oatmeal bath powders are also available and can be purchased over the counter at a pharmacy.

TREATMENTS IN DETAIL

Conventional Medicine

Your doctor will usually be able to diagnose eczema from the symptoms alone, and may be able to distinguish the type from an examination and a discussion about the possible irritants.

For contact dermatitis, the most important thing is to identify what you are sensitive to, whether fragrance, detergent, hand lotion, cosmetics, topical medication, metals (especially nickel and platinum), or animal hair. The location of your contact dermatitis may help determine the cause. People with contact dermatitis may need patch testing (*see above*), in which trigger substances are applied to areas of skin to see if there is a positive reaction.

PRIMARY TREATMENT **EMOLLIENTS AND TOPICAL TREATMENTS** are your doctor's first option for controlling symptoms of eczema. Emollients help keep the skin moist (hydrated). Topical corticosteroid creams, which reduce inflammation, can help relieve eczema symptoms. If corticosteroid creams are used intermittently and at the right strength for the body area being treated, they are unlikely to cause thinning of the skin or other side effects. Antihistamines are sometimes prescribed. Soap substitutes, such as water-based cream, can also be useful.

If you have developed contact dermatitis, your doctor will determine the cause, if possible, and will advise you to avoid the irritant wherever possible. He or she will treat the condition like atopic eczema, recommending that you take measures such as protecting your hands with emollient creams or gloves.

ORAL DRUGS may be prescribed for people who have very severe atopic eczema. These include corticosteroids, cyclosporine, and azathioprine. Corticosteroids reduce the inflammation, while cyclosporine and azathioprine are immunosuppressants, working by reducing the immune response, are very potent and can have serious side effects. Oral or topical antibiotics may be prescribed if the eczema becomes infected. Some antihistamines may relieve the itching and to be taken at night for their sedating properties .

ULTRAVIOLET PHOTOTHERAPY (UVA) may also be needed in severe cases of eczema in order to reduce the skin inflammation (*see Psoriasis, p.172*).

> **CAUTION**
>
> Oral drugs and ultraviolet phototherapy have a range of possible side effects; ask your doctor to explain these to you.

Nutritional Therapy

PRIMARY TREATMENT **A FOOD-EXCLUSION DIET** is often recommended by complementary practitioners (*See Identifying and Treating Food Sensitivity, p.39*). Most scientific studies, however, show that people do not benefit from elimination diets in treating eczema.

PRIMARY TREATMENT **ESSENTIAL FATTY ACIDS** are needed for keeping the skin healthy. Research suggested that people with eczema may be unable to process these acids normally. Evening primrose oil, which contains omega-6 fatty acids, used to be recommended, but the most recent research shows that it does not help. Although the largest study of fish oil was negative, some studies seem to show that fish oils can reduce the overall severity of symptoms and the scaling and itching of atopic eczema. Take 1.8g of omega-3 fatty acids each day for 1–3 months as a trial. This dose is the equivalent of 3–4g of fish oil, which is the same amount that you would get if you chose to consume a portion of oily fish every day.

Hemp and flaxseed oils are rich sources of essential fatty acids. Take 1–2 tablespoons of oil a day for one month (doses should be reduced for children, in proportion to their weight). It can also be used in ointments to control dry, atopic eczema.

PROBIOTICS contain healthy gut bacteria that may help infants and young children who have atopic eczema. Research has shown that the large intestines of infants with atopic eczema may have a disturbed balance of beneficial and potentially harmful bacteria. Giving probiotics (*Bifidobacterium lactic Bb-12* and *Lactobacillus GG*) in formula milk to infants while they are being weaned can be beneficial in reducing the extent and severity of atopic eczema. Evidence seems to suggest that probiotics benefit the immune system and may also decrease leakage of food allergens (foods that initiate immune reactions) across the gut wall, which can be one element in atopic eczema in early childhood. There is some good news, however, for mothers who are at risk of having a child with eczema (i.e., women who already have a child with eczema, suffer from eczema themselves, have a first-degree relative who has eczema, or whose partner has allergies). Evidence suggests that if you take probiotics during pregnancy and then feed your child probiotics after birth, he or she is less likely to develop eczema.

ANTIOXIDANTS A study that tested vitamin E, selenium, or the combination of the two, found no benefit over placebo in treating eczema.

ZINC OR BIOTIN SUPPLEMENTS may benefit some people with eczema. The clinical research so far fails to identify who is likely to respond to these supplements, but they could be worth trying for a month.

VITAMIN B$_{12}$ SUPPLEMENTS Evidence suggests that eczema and dermatitis may be made worse by a deficiency in vitamin B$_{12}$. It has been known for over 50 years that vitamin B$_{12}$ supplements may help alleviate the symptoms of dermatitis. Since studies suggest that a deficiency of other B vitamins, such as riboflavin, may also be involved in exacerbating eczema, try taking a high-potency vitamin B complex each day for a month. In addition, applying vitamin B$_6$ cream can help control seborrheic eczema in some children.

> **CAUTION**
>
> Consult your doctor before taking fish oil with warfarin (*see p.46*). Do not give high-dose nutritional supplements to children without proper advice.

Homeopathy

Each of the various types of eczema respond well to homeopathic remedies. Although there are only a few clinical trials for evaluating the homeopathic treatment of eczema (the same is also true for conventional treatments), homeopaths consistently report very good results.

PRIMARY TREATMENT Eczema is an ailment that illustrates one of the principles of homeopathy: three different medicines (*Arsenicum album, Graphites,* and *Sulphur*) will help in most cases, but a homeopath must choose the correct remedy for the individual (*see p. 73*).

ARSENICUM ALBUM AND SULPHUR People who respond to these two remedies have similar characteristic skin symptoms — they experience intensely itchy rashes that burn after scratching. However, the types of people who respond to these two medicines are markedly different. The typical person who responds to *Arsenicum album* is tidy, fastidious, tends to be anxious, and feels the cold excessively.

On the other hand, people who respond to *Sulphur* are often untidy and tend to be extroverts who relish a good argument. In addition, they are often warm blooded (they feel heat) with hot feet.

GRAPHITES In *Graphites* cases of eczema, the rash tends to crack and ooze a clear or yellowish, sticky liquid when scratched. It often affects particular areas, such as behind the ears or on the nipples; in women, the eczema may become worse before menstruation. (*See also Locals, mentals, and generals, p.76.*)

TAKING REMEDIES Start each of the above treatments by taking two pills of the 6C strength, twice daily. Beware of "aggravations," in which you experience temporary flare-ups of the symptoms, followed by improvement. Aggravations are quite common in the homeopathic treatment of skin conditions and are considered a positive sign because they indicate that you are reacting to the medicine. If you develop an aggravation, stop treatment and do not take any more of the remedy until the aggravation has fully settled. This may take up to 2–3 weeks.

Western Herbal Medicine

External treatments play a role in controlling the symptoms of eczema, but effective herbal healing of eczema usually requires internal treatment as well. The best way to take the herbs for this condition is in an infusion or a decoction, not as a tincture.

BORAGE SEED OIL, applied to childrens' seborrheic dermatitis (cradle cap), can lead to considerable improvement within 3–4 weeks. Borage (*Borago officinalis*) is also known as starflower. Rub ten drops of borage seed oil into the affected region twice a day for a month. Repeat as necessary. Studies are mixed on internal use.

OTHER EXTERNAL TREATMENTS When washing yourself, try using oatmeal sealed in old pantyhose instead of soap (*see Self-Help, p.168*). If you are having a bath, run the hot water through a bag of oatmeal. To control the symptoms of atopic eczema apply an ointment with hemp oil to the skin.

Try a paste of slippery elm (*Ulmus fulva*) powder and oatmeal mixed with chamomile (*Matricaria recutita*), elderflower (*Sambucus nigra*) tea, and distilled witch hazel (*Hamamelis virginiana*). An ointment prepared from nettle (*Urtica dioica*) juice may bring relief, too, although it is not commonly available in the US.

Compresses of chickweed (*Stellaria media*) or cold cucumber are soothing. The healing astringent action of a compress prepared from the leaves of walnut (*Juglans regia*) can bring relief to weeping lesions, as can a compress of oak (*Quercus robur*) bark tea, which is rich in tannins. Witch hazel (*Hamamelis virginiana*) also soothes inflamed skin. Licorice (*Glycyrriza*

glabra) paste mixed with a drop or two of chamomile (*Matricaria recutita*) or peppermint (*Mentha piperita*) oil applied externally may also reduce the inflammation and itch. Licorice has a mild steroidal-like effect and an active principle within the plant, glycyrrhetinic acid, applied in an ointment to eczematous rashes displayed an improvement similar to the effect of cortisone. One study tested chamomile cream for eczema and did not find a benefit, while two others suggest that topical chamomile creams may work as well as topical hydrocortisone.

INTERNAL TREATMENTS Western herbalists advise patients to drink infusions and decoctions made with blood-cooling herbs to calm inflamed skin. These include nettle (*Urtica dioica*), heartsease (*Viola tricolor*), figwort (*Scrophularia nodosa*), red clover (*Trifolium pratense*), burdock (*Arctium lappa*) root and leaf, and yellow dock (*Rumex crispus*) root.

Teas made from elderflower (*Sambucus nigra*), lindenflower (*Tilea cordata*), and Rooibosch (*Aspalathus linearis*) can help reduce itching. Weeping eczema may respond to the antibacterial action of Oregon grape root (*Mahonia aquifolium*), fumitory (*Fumaria officinalis*), dandelion (*Taraxacum officinale*) root, and golden seal (*Hydrastis canadensis*). Inulin, found in dandelion and burdock (*Arctium lappa*) root, may increase the resistance of the immune system and reduce histamine release.

Chinese Herbal Medicine

Eczema is known in Traditional Chinese Medicine (TCM) as *Si Wan Feng*, in which "dampness" plays an important part.

Clinical control trials in the 1990s of a standard formula of ten herbs for the treatment of dry atopic eczema showed significant effects in both adults and children. Approximately half of the children who took part continued to benefit from the formula a year later. Two-thirds of studies have shown positive results with normal liver function. Later trials of TCM herbs for eczema have not confirmed the original good results.

TYPES OF ECZEMA There are a number of typical presentations, one of which is damp–heat eczema with "fire poison" (i.e. a bacterial infection). The skin is very red with raised, red papules, vesicles (small, fluid-filled blisters), and pustules (pus-filled spots) that may weep. Treatment is likely to be based on Gentian Drain the Gallbladder Decoction (*Long Dan Xie Gan Tang*) but omitting *Mu Tong*, which is illegal in the US.

Acute eczema that corresponds to widespread, dry, atopic eczema is "heat in the blood with resulting wind" (i.e. disrupted *Qi* flow) but little or no dampness. There is no weeping from the inflamed skin. TCM doctors may treat this by modifying a combination of three classical treatments that cool the blood and correct *Qi* flow.

In chronic attacks of eczema that are repeated over a period of months or years, a pattern may develop that is caused by blood deficiency. Affected skin is dry, rough, thickened, and very itchy. The patient is chronically fatigued and suffers from dry, thinning hair and ridged nails that break easily. The correct strategy is to nourish the blood, clear the heat and correct *Qi* flow. A typical prescription is a variation of Chinese Angelica Decoction (*Dang Gui Yin Zi*).

EXTERNAL TREATMENTS Skullcap (*Scutellaria laterifolia*) root, phellodendron (*Phellodendron amurense*) bark, and sophora (*Sophora flavescens*) root can be combined to make a soothing wash for inflamed skin. A paste, wash, or ointment that contains burnet (*Sanguisorba officinalis*) root can calm irritated skin.

The incidence of eczema has increased threefold in the last 30 years

Environmental Health

Allergic contact dermatitis and irritant contact dermatitis are the most common skin problems caused by exposure to environmental agents.

PRIMARY TREATMENT **AVOIDING IRRITANTS** Common agents known to cause contact dermatitis are acids, alkalis, solvents, and other highly irritant chemicals. They are found in everyday products, such as deodorants, hair products, antistatic compounds, antiseptics, disinfectants, alcohols, soaps, cleaners, detergents, softeners, fiberglass, solvents, gasoline, paraffin, paint, adhesives, lacquers, degreasing agents, pesticides, and latex. Ultraviolet radiation may also cause contact dermatitis.

Skin irritation may result from a specific product or a specific ingredient in a group of products. For example, an irritant contact dermatitis may be caused by compounds in personal hygiene products, the chlorine-containing compounds in cleaning products, or the organohalogen substances present in some pesticides.

Most environmental agents can cause dermatitis in one of two ways. They can either act as "sensitizers" by dissolving the protective oily layer on the skin, impairing its barrier function and sensitizing it to other chemicals and irritants that would otherwise not pose a problem. Alternatively, environmental agents can act as "irritants" directly.

PERSONAL HISTORY It is important to identify and avoid the chemicals that trigger eczema. Ask an environmental health expert to help identify which chemicals you have been exposed to and to match potential exposures to your particular skin problem. This involves an analysis of your specific circumstances, such as your work or home environment and even the weather, to determine when your symptoms are either better or worse. You will need to answer various questions, such as "Do you live or work near any hazardous chemical facilities?" and "Does anyone around you have similar symptoms?"

NONTOXIC ALTERNATIVES Try to use low-emitting building materials, continuous ventilation, and nontoxic office and cleaning supplies. Carefully store the chemicals in your home or office. For a trial period,

> ## More than 15 million people in the US suffer from eczema symptoms

limit contact with known irritants, such as latex, antiseptics, and detergents, and avoid prolonged exposure to the sun without proper protection.

If you find that you are sensitive to a particular substance, look for an alternative. For example, you can replace products that are made from latex, which are ubiquitous in both industry and health-care, with those made from nitrile. Many stores now stock environmentally friendly, natural, organic, or nontoxic versions of common household and garden products, such as pesticides.

Breathing Retraining

Diaphragmatic, yoga-type breathing exercises help retrain breathing. People who habitually breathe with only their upper chest expire excessive amounts of carbon dioxide. This makes the blood more alkaline and increases allergic responses, which may make eczema worse.

Breathing retraining is a simple exercise that focuses on the diaphragm and breaks the habit of upper-chest breathing (see p.57). It is based on yoga and, if practiced for at least a three-month period, has been shown to change breathing habits, especially when it is coupled with massage and other types of bodywork that release and relax the chest and upper back.

Mind–Body Therapies

People who have eczema may become anxious, stressed, and, if the condition affects the face or other visible areas of skin, markedly depressed. Stress may precipitate and make eczema worse in vulnerable individuals.

A 1995 study provided evidence that mind–body therapies, such as biofeedback, autogenic training, and hypnotherapy, may all help treat the psychological components of atopic dermatitis and manage the symptoms, particularly if given in tandem with medical treatment. Group psychotherapy,

as a supplement to a regular medical regime, can help, too.

BIOFEEDBACK When combined with progressive relaxation at home, biofeedback can help reduce the severity of eczema and the irritation associated with the disorder. Research shows that mind–body relaxation, when it is combined with guided imagery, may be more effective than relaxation alone in lowering the anxiety levels and itchy sensations of atopic eczema.

AUTOGENIC TRAINING As a way of managing the stress and anxiety associated with eczema, autogenic training has been shown to be comparable with other mind–body therapies, such as biofeedback and techniques that are focused more exclusively on muscular relaxation. It is a series of six mental exercises that changes body chemistry to encourage relaxation. It regulates unwanted tension in both involuntary muscles, such as those in the blood vessels, and voluntary muscles, such as those in the back. However, there are no studies showing that this therapy can alleviate eczema symptoms.

HYPNOTHERAPY can control itching. After inducing a state of profound relaxation, a practitioner will aim to plant positive suggestions in the subconscious mind to help relieve anxiety and reduce the desire to scratch the skin. An unblinded study of hypnosis feedback found a benefit for skin damage but not for redness.

PREVENTION PLAN

These strategies may all help if you are prone to eczema:

- Avoidance of irritant chemicals
- Healthy diet
- Relaxation

WHAT ARE THE SYMPTOMS?

For plaque psoriasis:
- Patches of thickened, red, scaly, silvery skin, usually on the knees, elbows, lower back, and scalp, and sometimes on old scars
- Intermittent itchiness or soreness of the affected areas
- Discolored nails with small pits

For guttate psoriasis:
- Coin-shaped, pink patches of scaly skin, about 0.4in (1cm) across, mainly on the back and chest
- Intermittent itchiness of the affected areas

For pustular psoriasis:
- Small fluid-filled blisters on a red base, mainly on the palms of the hands and the soles of the feet
- Gradual replacement of blisters by brown spots or small, scaly patches
- In the severe form, many blisters usually develop quickly, together with a fever

For inverse psoriasis:
- Large, clearly defined, red areas in the folds of skin. The rash often affects the groin, the armpits, and the skin under the breasts

WHY MIGHT I HAVE THIS?

PREDISPOSING FACTORS
- Genetic factors
- HIV infection

TRIGGERS
- Excessive alcohol intake
- Drugs, e.g. some antimalarials and, rarely, beta-blockers
- Food sensitivity
- Stress or anxiety

PSORIASIS

Psoriasis is an inflammatory disorder that can affect many areas of the body at once, and it may be associated with arthritis. The most common of the four types is plaque psoriasis, but all forms involve reddening and thickening of the skin. Treatment combines skin preparations with a nutritional regime that incorporates foods that are rich in omega-3 fatty acids, fresh fruit and vegetables, and supplements of selenium or vitamin E. Oral drugs, such as immunosuppressants, are reserved for severe cases that do not respond to other treatments.

WHY DOES IT OCCUR?

In psoriasis, new skin cells are produced at a much faster rate than dead cells are shed, so an excess of skin cells accumulates to form thickened patches. The cause of psoriasis is not known, but episodes may be triggered by local trauma, excessive alcohol, food sensitivity, irritation, sunburn, infection, injury, stress, and anxiety. Certain medications, such as antimalarials, beta blockers, and antidepressants, can trigger psoriasis. The condition often runs in families — approximately 1 in 3 people with psoriasis has a close relative with the condition. About 10 percent of people who have a form of psoriasis eventually develop a psoriatic arthritis.

TYPES OF PSORIASIS Of the four types, only plaque psoriasis (also known as psoriasis vulgaris), which may develop at any age and is the most common type of psoriasis, is usually a lifelong disorder.

Guttate psoriasis, which affects mainly children and adolescents, often develops about two weeks after a bacterial throat infection. This type usually clears up

TREATMENT PLAN

PRIMARY TREATMENTS
- Topical treatments
- Sarsaparilla
- Homeopathic *Calendula* cream (for immediate relief)

BACKUP TREATMENTS
- UV phototherapy (for severe psoriasis)
- Oral drugs (for severe psoriasis)
- Food-exclusion
- Omega-3 fatty acids and dietary changes
- Homeopathy (*see also Immediate Relief, p.173*)
- Western and Chinese herbal medicine
- Mind–body therapies

WORTH CONSIDERING
- Acupuncture

For an explanation of how treatments are rated, see p.111.

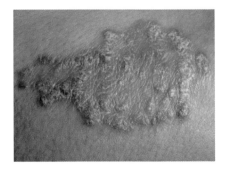

The elbow is one of the common locations for the characteristic patches of thickened skin. Other sites where plaque psoriasis develops include the scalp, knees and forearms.

IMPORTANT

See your doctor if you experience symptoms of psoriasis. In rare cases, there may be a serious underlying cause.

spontaneously after 4–7months, but it may recur or plaque psoriasis may develop.

A rare type, pustular psoriasis, may become life-threatening if the severe form occurs, affecting the entire body, because dehydration, kidney failure, and severe infections may develop.

Inverse psoriasis, in which large, moist, red areas develop in skin folds rather than over widespread body areas, mainly affects elderly people. This form of psoriasis usually clears up without treatment. Some people are affected by more than one type of psoriasis.

IMMEDIATE RELIEF

Apply homeopathic *Calendula* (marigold) cream freely to psoriasis patches (avoid if you are allergic to lanolin).

TREATMENTS IN DETAIL

Conventional Medicine

Your doctor will be able to diagnose which type of psoriasis you have from the appearance of the skin patches.

Since plaque psoriasis cannot be cured completely, doctors try to control the symptoms and will usually start by prescribing creams to apply to the skin.

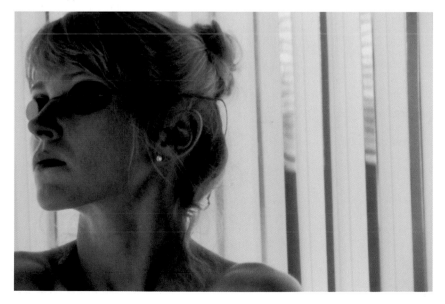

PUVA phototherapy involves regular exposure to ultraviolet light under hospital supervision. It is believed to help people with psoriasis by slowing down the rate of skin cell division.

Guttate and plaque psoriasis are usually treated with topical medications and, sometimes, with ultraviolet light therapies. Pustular psoriasis that is restricted to the hands and feet may be treated with very strong topical steroids or PUVA light therapy (*see below*).

Severe pustular psoriasis requires urgent hospital admission for monitoring, with drugs and supportive measures provided. Inverse psoriasis can often be controlled by mild topical steroids.

PRIMARY TREATMENT **TOPICAL TREATMENTS** Emollient creams and lotions can help bring relief by hydrating (moistening) and softening the skin. There are various other topical treatments, all of which are usually applied to the psoriasis patches once or twice a day. Some should not to be used by pregnant women but your doctor will advise you on this and any other potential side effects.

Corticosteroid creams of a mild to moderate strength may provide short-term relief by reducing inflammation. Purified coal tar, widely available in the form of bath products, ointments, and pastes, also helps relieve inflammation by increasing the skin's sensitivity to sunlight.

Calcipotriene, which is derived from vitamin D, can be used either as an ointment and cream or as a preparation to be applied to the scalp but not to the face. Its action appears to decrease the production of the skin cells involved in the process of skin thickening and patch formation.

Calcipotriene cream can help by slowing down the rate at which skin cells divide. Make sure you wash it off within an hour of applying it. Tazarotene, which is a retinoid drug derived from vitamin A, is a gel you can spread on the affected areas. It is not yet known how this drug works.

PUVA AND UVB PHOTOTHERAPY reduce skin inflammation. They involve treatment with the two different types of ultraviolet light (UVA and UVB) and are sometimes combined with topical treatments.

In PUVA (psoralen ultraviolet A) phototherapy, patients take a psoralen drug, such as methoxsalen, that makes the skin more sensitive to the effects of the light. The drug enhances the treatment with long-wave ultraviolet light (UVA), which is delivered by special lamps in hospitals. The use of PUVA is carefully regulated.

UVB phototherapy involves supervised and regulated exposure to sunlight or to the radiation from ultraviolet B lamps.

ORAL DRUGS may be needed if plaque psoriasis is so severe that it does not respond adequately to topical treatments. Oral drugs, which are prescribed by a doctor, are much more potent and have many more side effects than topical preparations. The oral drugs include: acitretin, a retinoid drug that may start to have an effect after 2–4 weeks; cyclosporine, an immunosuppressant; and methotrexate, also an immunosuppressant, usually taken just once a week.

CAUTION

Topical treatments, oral drugs, and phototherapy all have potential side effects; ask your doctor to explain them to you.

Nutritional Therapy

A FOOD-EXCLUSION DIET may help some people, since some practitioners believe that some cases may be linked to food sensitivity (*see p.39*). One study reported that eliminating gluten — found in wheat, barley, and rye — improved psoriasis in some people.

OMEGA-3 AND OMEGA-6 FATTY ACIDS Eating less foods containing the unhealthy omega-6 fatty acids and more foods containing the healthy omega-3 fatty acids (*see p.34*) may help people with psoriasis, who tend to have elevated levels of a fat known as arachidonic acid in their blood. It seems to encourage inflammation in the body, leading some scientists to believe that it may be an important underlying factor in psoriasis.

In the body, arachidonic acid can be formed from omega-6 fatty acids — found in many margarines, vegetable oils, processed foods, fast foods, and baked goods, such as muffins, cakes, and cookies. Foods that are rich in arachidonic acid include dairy products and red meat.

Supplementing your diet with omega-3 fatty acids, which have anti-inflammatory effects in the body, may help relieve psoriasis. In one study, taking 10g of fish oil daily improved the skin patches of psoriasis.

Psoriasis affects 6.4 million Americans

Patients had less itching, scaling, and redness, and the affected area had diminished in size compared to those of the people taking the placebo.

Omega-3 fatty acids are found in some nuts and seeds, especially walnuts and flaxseeds, and oily fish, such as mackerel, salmon, and sardines. People with psoriasis may benefit from regular inclusion of these foods in their diet or with a daily supplement of 5–10g of concentrated fish oil.

FISH OIL It is unclear whether fish oil helps psoriasis. Most controlled studies that tested the effect of oral fish oil on psoriasis found a benefit, but a few trials have found no benefit. Several studies that tested intravenous infusions of omega-3 lipid emulsion found the treatment more effective than omega-6 lipid infusions for severe plaque psoriasis and guttate psoriasis; however, this treatment is not available in the US. A combination of fish oil and evening primrose oil has been tested for psoriasis and psoriatic arthritis; the treatment was ineffective. For those who do not like the odor of fish oil, deodorized preparations are available. Another good alternative is flaxseed oil, which has three times as much omega-3 fatty acids as omega-6 fatty acids.

One interesting study tested oily fish consumption against white fish consumption in patients with plaque psoriasis. Oily fish (salmon, sardines, mackerel, herring) is much higher in fish oil than white fish. Each patient ate about 6oz (170g) of one type of fish daily for six weeks, then switched. A small but significant improvement was noted during the periods when patients ate oily fish.

Three studies have found a benefit of oral fish oil (1.8–12g polyunsaturated fatty acids daily) for psoriasis; one study found no benefit. Topical fish oil preparations have also been tested; one trial found a benefit over placebo for relieving scaling but not itching. Another found no benefit. There is no harm in eating more fish or trying fish oil supplements; try taking 3–5g fish oil daily. Other research reports that intravenous infusions of a fish-oil emulsion can help ameliorate the symptoms of chronic plaque psoriasis.

FRESH FRUIT AND VEGETABLES Clinical experience indicates that people with psoriasis often benefit from a diet rich in fruit and vegetables. These foods are full of many different nutrients, especially vitamin C and beta-carotene, which have antioxidant properties, combat free radicals, and may thereby help quell inflammation.

SELENIUM Although selenium is sometimes recommended to treat psoriasis, a randomized trial found no benefit for a selenium preparation (selenomethionine 200 mcg/day for four weeks).

Homeopathy

Homeopaths believe that many patients with psoriasis benefit from homeopathic treatment, although in the majority of cases the problem does not clear up completely. Treatment needs to be prescribed on an individual basis. Among the most important medicines are: *Arsenicum album, Arsenicum iodatum, Graphites, Sulphur, Lycopodium,* and *Sepia.*

ARSENICUMS The two *Arsenicums* are usually used for guttate psoriasis in which plaques tend to be small, rounded, and flaky. *Arsenicum album* may also be very helpful in pustular psoriasis. The rash is often very itchy and burns after scratching.

With *Arsenicum album,* the itching is relieved by heat. *Arsenicum iodatum* has less of these features, but patients frequently have severe hay fever and other allergies particularly affecting the eyes.

OTHER REMEDIES *Graphites* may be an appropriate remedy for use in cases of inverse psoriasis and in psoriasis that is unusually distributed around the body — for instance, in the fold behind the ears, where the eruption cracks and may ooze clear colorless or yellow fluid.

The psoriasis that responds to *Sulfur* is usually the plaque type: intensely itchy and often the rash is red and raw because of scratching. Heat makes the itching worse (for instance, in bed). The patient is generally hot-blooded, often with hot feet, kicking off shoes at every opportunity, and sticking his or her feet out of bed at night. *Sulphur* types are hot, scruffy, usually extroverted, and untidy or flamboyant.

The psoriasis in people who respond to *Lycopodium* and *Sepia* is not very specific. Homeopaths prescribe these medicines mostly according to the person's mental and general features (*see Constitutional medicines and polychrests, pp.74–5*); they see psoriasis as an internal disease that is manifested on the skin.

Western Herbal Medicine

Creams made from aloe leaf extracts or Oregon grape root may be helpful. Oregon Grape (*Mahonia aquafolium*) root cream, applied topically, had a beneficial effect on psoriasis in one study. Other herbs that are used to treat various forms of psoriasis include sarsaparilla (*Smilax ornata*) and red clover (*Trifolium pratense*). The little research that has been done on sarsaparilla supports its traditional use in treating psoriasis. In a controlled study of 92 patients, sarsaparilla significantly improved the psoriasis of 62 percent and achieved complete clearance in 18 percent of the subjects. Its anti-inflammatory properties make it useful for combating the arthritis that sometimes affects people with psoriasis.

Ten percent of adults with psoriasis may have developed it before the age of 10

ALOE A controlled trial of an aloe leaf extract (0.5%), applied three times daily for five out of seven days a week for a month at a time, found that the treatment was very effective, compared with placebo. Aloe leaf is different from aloe gel, which occurs inside the leaf.

CAPSAICIN The substance in chili peppers (*Capsicum* spp.) that provides the hot sensation, capsaicin is available in over-the-counter creams to treat arthritis and other conditions. Capsaicin cream appears to be helpful in psoriasis. A controlled trial tested capsaicin 0.025% cream applied four times daily for six weeks in patients with pruritic (itchy) psoriasis. Compared to placebo, capsaicin cream improved itching significantly. Overall evaluation scores improved as well. Some patients reported a burning sensation when they first used the cream; usually this sensation went away after a few uses. It is very important to wash your hands after using capsaicin cream, and not to touch your eyes or mouth before thoroughly washing the cream off. Roll-on applicators are available and are a convenient alternative.

COMFREY Herbalists have also used topical preparations containing comfrey (*Symphytum officinale*) to treat psoriasis patches. Although these are harmless when used on closed skin, comfrey should not be taken internally.

DETOXIFICATION HERBS Herbalists may recommend herbs because of their ability to clean out or soothe the bowel, such as sarsaparilla. Although many herbalists believe that bowel "detoxification" can help relieve psoriasis and other skin conditions, there is no evidence that supports this theory. Herbs that are used to "detoxify" or heal the bowel include burdock, aloe vera gel, flaxseed, and psyllium seed or husk.

OIL OF WINTERGREEN in topical preparations should probably be avoided by those with psoriasis. Psoriatic skin absorbs the oil more easily than does normal skin, and toxicity from the salicylates in wintergreen can result.

> **CAUTION**
>
> See p.69 before taking a herbal remedy, and if you are taking a prescribed medication, consult an herbal medicine expert first.

Chinese Herbal Medicine

Chinese herbal medicine categorizes psoriasis in ways that may be unfamiliar to Western doctors. For example, acutely progressive psoriasis, marked by widespread, distinct and raised red patches, is seen as caused by heat in the blood. The main prescription for this is based on the Sarsaparilla and Sophora Decoction (*Tu Hai Yin*), which contains herbs for cooling the blood.

The TCM herbalist will also generally advise those with psoriasis to avoid alcohol, spicy food, shellfish, and "hot" meats, such as lamb and beef.

Self-medication is not recommended due to reports of kidney or liver failure in patients using TCM.

> **CAUTION**
>
> Do not take Chinese herbal remedies without first consulting an expert in traditional Chinese medicine (TCM).

Acupuncture

No trials indicate that acupuncture is effective for psoriasis. In one controlled trial in which 56 patients were treated with traditional diagnosis and therapy over three months, the control group fared better than those receiving acupuncture. If acupuncture is to have an effect, then the treatment will need to be prolonged. Weekly treatment for eight to ten weeks would be reasonable.

Mind–Body Therapies

STRESS MANAGEMENT People with psoriasis may experience significant psychological stress and distress, which appear to aggravate the the course of the disease. If you have psoriasis, yoga or a relaxation therapy, such as diaphragmatic breathing (*see p.62*), may be helpful to reduce stress.

Preliminary studies suggest that psychological therapies may be effective in the management of psoriasis. One study indicated that people with psoriasis benefited from a six-week course of an integrated, multidisciplinary, stress management approach, called the Psoriasis Syndrome Management Program (PSMP). Participants experienced a greater reduction in the clinical severity of psoriasis symptoms as well as a reduced incidence in anxiety, depression, psoriasis-related stress, and disability. Moreover, the reductions were sustained for six months.

MINDFULNESS MEDITATION is one of the most innovative approaches to treating psoriasis. Research suggests that a brief session of this Buddhist-based practice, which maintains awareness in the present moment of body sensations and thoughts without passing judgment on them (*see p.99*), can be beneficial in the treatment of psoriasis. Listening to an audiotape during UVA phototherapy or photochemotherapy (PUVA) (*see p.173*), can reduce the stress that is experienced by individuals with psoriasis while increasing the rate at which the psoriatic patches heal. One study combined the mind–body techniques of meditation and guided imagery to help 18 people with psoriasis of the scalp. Results showed that meditating may be clinically effective for some patients in reducing their patches of psoriasis, but that guided imagery made no significant impact on their symptoms. Overall, meditation can be regarded as a useful treatment for some patients with psoriasis.

> **PREVENTION PLAN**
>
> **These may help prevent psoriasis outbreaks:**
>
> - Whole-food diets with plenty of fruit, vegetables, and oily fish.
> - Regular relaxation and meditation.

URTICARIA

Also known as hives, urticaria is an intensely itchy rash that may affect the entire body or just one area. It is often part of an allergic reaction and consists of red, raised areas and, sometimes, fluid-filled white lumps. The swellings develop rapidly over a few minutes and last for several minutes to several hours. Urticaria may occur with angioedema or anaphylaxis, both of which require urgent medical attention. The condition can be treated with oral antihistamines. In some cases, a food exclusion diet, eliminating certain problem foods, may help.

WHY DOES IT OCCUR?

Urticaria may be part of an allergic reaction, when skin cells release histamine and other substances that cause local inflammation. The itchy red rash that results may affect a small area of skin or it may erupt over the entire body.

The reaction may follow exposure to a particular substance, such as ingestion of a drug or food, such as nuts or strawberries. Urticaria can also follow an insect sting or bite, or contact with a plant, such as nettles. In some cases, no cause can be found. A tendency to develop urticaria may run in families.

A rash that lasts longer than six weeks (chronical urticaria) occurs in about a third of cases. "Physical urticaria" results when the skin temperature is raised, as in a hot bath or shower and exercise, or during an emotional response, such as anger or stress. Even sunlight or contact with water may trigger the rash. Some people with chronic urticaria have dermatographism, in which even light scratching of the skin will cause the rash.

ANGIOEDEMA Urticaria may occur with angioedema, when a part of the body (often around the eyes, lips, and hands) suddenly swells. Occasionally, the mucous lining of the mouth, tongue, and throat may suddenly swell, too. This can seriously affect the ability to talk, breathe, and swallow and is a medical emergency.

ANAPHYLAXIS Urticaria may also be a feature of anaphylaxis, a severe and potentially fatal allergic reaction in which the blood pressure falls, resulting in light-headedness or even loss of consciousness.

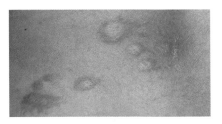

Urticaria is a rash of red and white lumps surrounded by inflamed skin. It is very itchy and can occur anywhere on the body.

IMPORTANT

Call an ambulance immediately if you or someone you are with develop the symptoms of angioedema or anaphylaxis. Epinephrine must be administered immediately.

IMMEDIATE RELIEF

- Try not to scratch the rash.
- Apply a cooling lotion, such as calamine lotion, to the rash as soon as you can.

TREATMENTS IN DETAIL

Conventional Medicine

If symptoms persist or recur, see your doctor, who may arrange a skin prick test (*see p.35*) to discover which substances might be the underlying cause. You can keep a diary to record the foods you have eaten and to list other potential triggers. Changes in diet may help in some cases (*see opposite*).

PRIMARY TREATMENT **ORAL ANTIHISTAMINES**, such as diphenhydramine, loratadine, desloratadine, and fexofenadine, may bring the fastest relief. Most of these are available without a prescription.

EPINEPHRINE Anyone with a severe allergy to bee stings, insect bites, or certain foods

One in five people will develop urticaria at some time in their life

should carry a self-injecting epinephrine device. Available by prescription, these devices can be lifesaving.

Nutritional Therapy

PRIMARY TREATMENT — **FOOD-EXCLUSION DIET** Evidence suggests that some cases of urticaria are caused by food sensitivity or by reactions to additives, such as monosodium glutamate (MSG), colorings, flavorings, preservatives, and aspartame. Try to identify and eliminate suspect foods from your diet (see p.39).

In infants, use of an extensively hydrolyzed casein formula instead of cows' milk reduced allergic symptoms, including urticaria. However, breast milk is better than any formula for babies.

Homeopathy

Case studies suggest that urticaria responds quite well to homeopathic treatment.

URTICA URENS is one of the primary homeopathic medicines for urticaria. Made from stinging nettles, it is appropriate when the skin is swollen, with raised areas that may be very itchy or sore. *Urtica urens* is specifically helpful when symptoms are made worse by contact with water and cold objects.

APIS MELLIFERA is made from irritated bees and is especially useful when urticaria is associated with angioedema.

ANARCARDIUM ORIENTALE is particularly appropriate for people who are extremely bad tempered, even violent, when their skin is bad. They may also get indigestion. Eating improves their indigestion and skin.

CALCAREA CARBONICA Many people with a tendency to urticaria have skin that reacts to a blunt point drawn across it so they can "write on their skin," a phenomenon known as dermatographism. *Calcarea carbonica* is the main medicine used to treat these individuals. Typically, those who respond to *Calcarea carbonica* are rather stout, solid both physically and mentally; they are calm, hardworking, conscientious, and stubborn. Beneath this solid exterior, they may have many fears and anxieties, particularly if they work themselves to the point of exhaustion. They sweat freely on the head and neck, especially at night.

Western Herbal Medicine

TREATMENT AIMS The affected area, the frequency of occurrence, and the severity of the symptoms, such as heat, swelling, and itchiness, are key clues for the herbalist. Especially in cases with no identifiable external triggers, an herbalist will take note of the following: the presence of other allergic symptoms that result from food sensitivity and allergic rhinitis; signs of toxicity, poor diet, and constipation; chronic infection, signs of impaired digestive function, including a deficiency in the secretion of gastric acid; and the emotional and psychological state of the affected person — in particular, if they suffer from nervous irritability and chronic anxiety.

The symptoms are best treated internally, although lotions and creams can help. In almost all cases, a herbalist prescribes remedies to aid digestion, liver metabolism, and detoxification.

NETTLES Remedies known to have antihistamine and antiallergy actions include nettle (*Urtica dioica* or *U. urens*). Nettle leaf has proven anti-inflammatory activity, and some clinical evidence suggests that it has an antiallergenic action as well. For urticaria, nettle leaf is best used as a tea. However, the nettle tea can also be applied as a lotion to relieve irritated skin. The ability of nettle leaf to relieve urticaria (nettle rash) is an

example of an herbal medicine curing "like with like." Although the hairs contain histamine, serotonin, and acetylcholine and provoke a painful inflammatory rash, they are deactivated when cooked.

OTHER HERBS Licorice (*Glycyrrhiza glabra*) and rehmannia (*Rehmannia glutinosa*) are antiallergenic and help relieve inflammatory skin rashes. Licorice also has a restorative action on the liver and adrenal glands.

German chamomile (*Matricaria recutita*), yellow dock (*Rumex crispus*), calendula (*Calendula officinalis*), and echinacea (*Echinacea* spp.) are also often used. However, caution is advised in using echinacea because an allergy to related plants is a common cause of urticaria.

Acupuncture

Traditionally, acupuncture has been used to alleviate both acute and chronic persistent urticaria. There have been no controlled trials, but case studies suggest that acupuncture may be of real value.

After a traditional Chinese diagnosis is made, treatment for urticaria may be repeated regularly, depending on the severity and persistence of the rash. Usually, treatment should be provided weekly, in the first instance, for 6–8 weeks to correct imbalances in the flow of energy through the meridians. Afterward, treatment is recommended every month or every three months to help maintain a good constitutional balance.

PREVENTION PLAN

The following may help prevent urticaria:

- Avoid identifiable substances to which you are sensitive
- Food exclusion diet
- Oral antihistamines

RINGWORM AND ATHLETE'S FOOT

Ringworm is a fungal infection of the skin that causes itchy, red, ring-shaped patches. It is not caused by worms, despite its name. Fungal infections may occur in many parts of the body and common forms affect the scalp and groin. When it affects the feet, the infection is known as athlete's foot. Ringworm may also affect the nails. Topical antifungal creams are the treatment of choice, although if your ringworm is persistent or widespread then you will need to take oral antifungal drugs. An alternative treatment for athlete's foot is tea tree oil.

WHAT ARE THE SYMPTOMS?

For ringworm:

- Red, scaly rash that appears in a small circle
- Itchiness of the affected area
- After 1–2 weeks, further circles may appear
- The circles grow larger and form a red, scaly ring, usually surrounding a central area of normal skin
- Ringworm of the scalp may cause scaling like dandruff. Alternatively, there may be round, scaly patches often with associated hair loss

For athlete's foot:

- Cracked, sore and itchy areas of skin on the bottom of the foot, often between the toes
- Flaking, white, soggy skin in the same areas
- Flaking on the sides of the foot
- Onychomycosis, a fungal infection of the nails, may cause whitening and thickening of the nails, often accompanied by crumbly white material under the nails

WHY MIGHT I HAVE THIS?

PREDISPOSING FACTORS

- Diabetes mellitis
- Genetic predisposition

TRIGGERS

- Contact with the fungus

WHY DOES IT OCCUR?

RINGWORM is caused by several species of fungus, such as *Microsporium*, *Trichophyton*, and *Epidermophyton*, that live on the skin of people and animals. These fungi thrive in warm, humid conditions, which is why ringworm is often seen in the groin area (the genitals, buttocks, and inner thighs) and on the feet.

Ringworm can affect people of all ages. Scalp ringworm is more common in children, while ringworm affecting the groin area (sometimes called jock itch) is much more common in men. People with conditions such as diabetes mellitus (*see p.314*) and AIDS (*see p.470*) that reduce their immunity to infection are particularly prone to ringworm.

Ringworm is spread by direct, skin-to-skin contact with an infected person or by sharing infected towels and hair brushes. The infection can also be caught from a

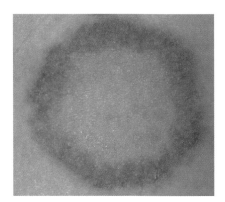

This red circle on the skin of the neck clearly shows the characteristic mark of ringworm. The circle is, in fact, skin that is recovering as the infection spreads outward.

dog or cat, although a pet may have ringworm without transfering it to its owner.

ATHLETE'S FOOT tends to be more common in adolescents and young adults. The fungus is usually caught through direct contact or from walking barefoot in warm, humid, communal areas, such as swimming pools and changing rooms.

TREATMENT PLAN

PRIMARY TREATMENTS

- Antifungal creams and drugs
- Anti-*Candida* diet

BACKUP TREATMENTS

- Homeopathic marigold therapy
- Western herbal medicine

For an explanation of how treatments are rated, see p.111.

SELF-HELP

IF YOU HAVE RINGWORM:

- Always keep your skin clean and dry.
- Apply a topical cream (*see p.179*) and/or powder to the rash every day.

IF YOU HAVE ATHLETE'S FOOT:

- Use only your own towel and thoroughly dry yourself, especially between your toes, after swimming or bathing.

- Dust your socks and shoes with athlete's foot powder each morning.
- Wear socks and shoes made from natural rather than synthetic materials to allow air to circulate around your feet.
- Change your socks every day.
- Sprinkle an antifungal powder and/or apply a topical cream (*see below*) between your toes twice a day.

TREATMENTS IN DETAIL

Conventional Medicine

Your doctor will probably diagnose ringworm by looking at the affected patches of skin. If confirmation is needed, laboratory tests on samples of skin, hair, or nail will identify the fungus responsible.

PRIMARY TREATMENT **TOPICAL ANTIFUNGAL CREAMS** If the infection is localized and affects just one area, then topical antifungal creams may be the best treatment. You can buy some of them over the counter but stronger creams are available only by prescription. Patches of ringworm and athlete's foot may be treated with prescribed topical creams containing antifungal drugs, such as miconazole or terbinafine. However, these drugs may cause some local irritation. Since ringworm and athlete's foot are chronic, they may need to be treated continuously.

ORAL ANTIFUNGAL DRUGS, such as griseofulvin, may be needed if your ringworm is more widespread, especially on the scalp. They are also sometimes taken for athlete's foot and nail infections. Your doctor can prescribe the drugs, which you will probably need to take for up to two months.

> **CAUTION**
>
> Oral antifungal drugs have a range of possible side effects; ask your doctor to explain these to you.

Nutritional Therapy

While research has yet to prove this, some people report relief from the symptoms of ringworm after following an anti-*Candida* diet (*For more details on* Candida, *see p.40.*)

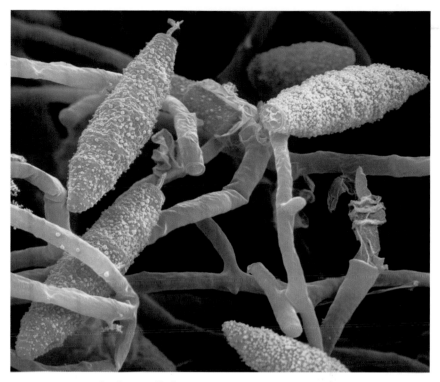

The fungus *Microsporum gypseum* is found in the soil and causes ringworm on the scalp and on the body. The yellow cylindrical structures produce the spores that spread the infection.

Western Herbal Medicine

TEA TREE OIL Applied topically, tea tree (*Melaleuca alternifolia*) essential oil is a popular complementary treatment for many kinds of fungal infections. One study found that tea tree cream was equivalent to 1% clotrimazole for treating toenail fungus. Another study found that a 10% tea tree oil cream was better than placebo for treating the symptoms of athlete's foot (tolnaftate was better at killing the fungi). Some people experience skin dryness or irritation with the use of tea tree oil.

EXTERNAL TREATMENTS An herbal practitioner may recommend other herbs for external use, but these have not been tested in clinical trials. If you have athlete's foot, try soaking your feet in an infusion of goldenseal (*Hydrastis canadensis*). Afterward, dry your feet and then dust them with powdered goldenseal. A cream prepared from marigold (*Calendula officinalis*) may relieve the itching. Another remedy you can apply each day to athlete's foot is a mixture prepared from marigold ointment and the essential oil of tea tree (*Melaleuca alternifolia*), clove (*Syzygium aromaticum*), or thyme (*Thymus vulgaris*).

For treating ringworm, try making a poultice from the green rind of the fruit of black walnut (*Juglans nigra*) or from lobelia (*Lobelia inflata*). Alternatively, you can try using a decoction of plantain (*Plantago major*).

AJOENE, a substance in garlic, has been found to be more effective than placebo for treating fungal infections of the skin. However, ajoene preparations are not currently available in the US and fresh garlic can burn the skin.

> **CAUTION**
>
> See p.69 before taking or using an herbal remedy. Do not use thyme oil if you are pregnant.

PREVENTION PLAN

- Keep your skin and feet dry, especially after bathing
- Avoid walking barefoot in changing rooms

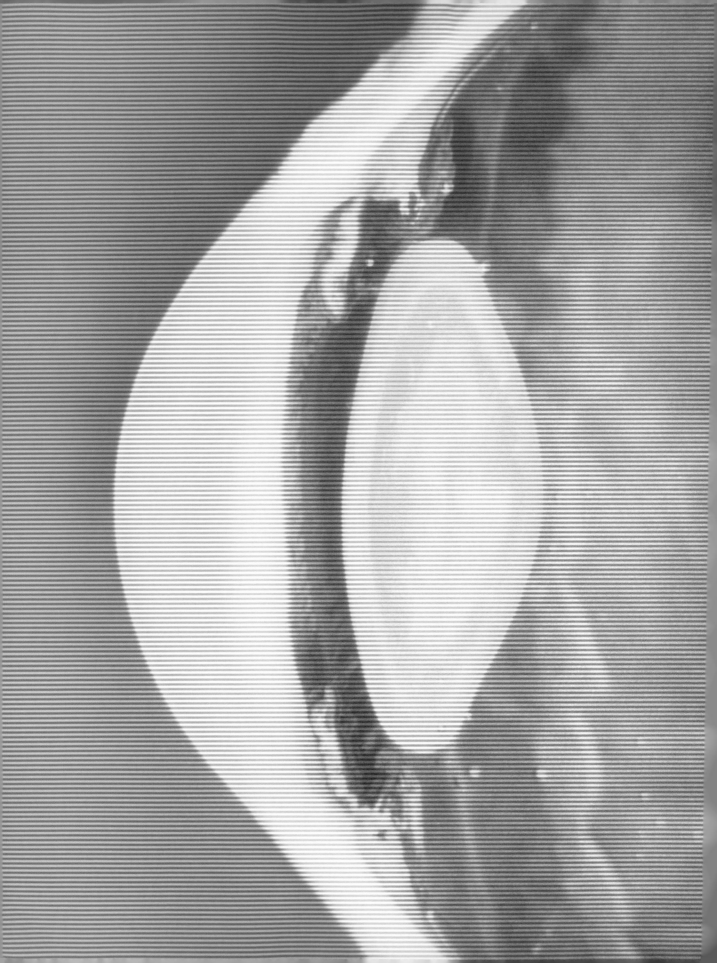

Eyes & Ears

When our sight and hearing are reduced we can become disoriented, unnerved, and isolated. Eating nourishing food, preventing excess strain, and refraining from smoking can keep the senses intact. If an ailment does develop, treatments ranging from visual and hearing aids to medication, surgery, and nutritional supplements are available.

WHAT ARE THE SYMPTOMS?

- Blurred vision
- Colors appear faded
- Increase in nearsightedness
- Halos and stars around bright light which may be worse at night

WHY MIGHT I HAVE THIS?

PREDISPOSING FACTORS

- Low levels of antioxidants in blood
- A diet lacking in antioxidants
- Increasing age
- Smoking
- Genetic factor
- Excessive sunlight
- Other sources of radiation

TRIGGER

- Free-radical damage

TREATMENT PLAN

PRIMARY TREATMENT

- Surgery

BACK-UP TREATMENTS

- Various nutritional supplements
- Environmental health measures

WORTH CONSIDERING

- Homeopathy

For an explanation of how treatments are rated, see p.111.

CATARACTS

A cataract is a cloudy area in the normally clear lens of the eye. It stops light rays from passing through the lens, leading to a reduced clarity of vision and, in some cases, blindness. One eye is often more severely affected, but cataracts may develop in both eyes. Since cataracts tend to develop over a long period of time, loss of vision is gradual and may not be noticed at first. Surgery is usually required although you can help slow their development with nutritional, homeopathic, and environmental means.

WHY DOES IT OCCUR?

Cataracts result from structural changes to protein fibers in the lens of the eye. The most common type is an age-related cataract, the exact cause of which is not known. However, various factors, including sunlight exposure, general health, and genes, are likely to play a role.

Other causes include eye injury, certain medications (such as long-term corticosteroids), diabetes mellitus (*see p.314*), and inflammatory diseases of the eye. People with Down syndrome are also at increased risk. For some people, the tendency to develop cataracts is hereditary and in rare cases, cataracts may be present from birth.

SELF-HELP

The following measures may help while waiting for cataract surgery or if you choose to manage without an operation:

- Have your eyes tested regularly to make sure glasses are correctly prescribed.
- Read with proper lighting.
- Use visual aids, available from an optician or eye clinic, including magnifying glasses (with an optional attached light source) and mini-telescopes that attach to glasses for looking across a room. A closed-circuit TV may help you read — a camera aimed at a page produces a magnified image on a TV screen.

IMPORTANT

If the symptoms of a cataract develop quickly, or you are experiencing pains in your eye, see a doctor immediately.

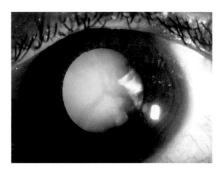

In a cataract, the lens of the eye becomes cloudy and opaque behind the pupil. The normally transparent lens loses its ability to transmit and focus rays of light, causing blurred or distorted vision.

TREATMENTS IN DETAIL

Conventional Medicine

PRIMARY TREATMENT **SURGERY** is the only treatment that can cure cataracts. However, your doctor will only recommend surgery if problems with your vision interfere with everyday activities such as driving and reading.

The operation is usually short, lasting around 15–30 minutes, and performed under local anesthetic. The surgeon makes a tiny cut — about 1/8in (3mm) long — in the eye and inserts a probe to remove the lens while leaving behind the lens capsule (the layer that encloses the lens). The surgeon places a plastic lens implant inside the lens capsule, which holds the new lens in the correct position.

After surgery, you may experience some blurring of vision and mild discomfort, both of which should last only a few days. Most people still need glasses after surgery, either for reading, distance vision, or both.

The operation is relatively risk-free. However, infection is a possible complication of the surgery, affecting about 1 in 1,000 people. It may lead to permanent loss of vision in the affected eye. Very rarely, bleeding inside the eye during surgery causes permanent loss of vision. For 1 in 300 people, the operation is more complicated than expected and further surgery is needed to complete the treatment.

After routine surgery, some people develop scar tissue in the lens capsule. This causes the same symptoms as the original cataract, but is easily treated with a painless five-minute laser procedure at an eye clinic.

Nutritional Therapy

ANTIOXIDANTS The development of a cataract is believed to be related to damage caused by destructive molecules called free radicals. Antioxidants, such as carotenoids (found in carrots, mangoes, and apricots) and vitamins C and E, neutralize the free

> **Cataracts are more common after the age of 75 but may be present from birth**

radicals. People with few antioxidants in their blood or diet may be at high risk of developing cataracts.

Some research claims that certain antioxidants, such as vitamin A, C, and E, may protect against UV damage to the lens of the eye. Other evidence suggests that taking 3000mg of N-acetylcysteine boosts levels of glutathione, which in turn neutralizes free radicals formed by UV light in the human lens. You should consider these supplements if you are exposed to sunlight on a regular basis.

CAROTENOID-RICH DIET Research shows that eating foods rich in nutrients known as carotenoids (especially lutein and zeaxanthin) is associated with a reduced cataract risk. In large epidemiological studies, lutein and zeaxanthin levels have been correlated with the risk of cataracts. In a small clinical trial, supplementation with lutein (15mg 3 times weekly for two years) appeared to improve vision in people who already have cataracts.

Good sources of lutein include spinach, kale, collard greens, romaine lettuce, leeks, peas, egg yolks, kiwi fruit, squash, black grapes, brussels sprouts, and green peppers. Zeaxanthin is found in mangoes, oranges, red peppers, nectarines, papayas, squashes, corn, honeydew, and egg yolks. Eating plenty of these foods may help prevent and slow down cataract formation.

NUTRITIONAL SUPPLEMENTS may slow the progression of age-related cataracts, but only if you take them for many years. A 2002 study found that, by taking a daily regimen of 18mg of beta-carotene, 750mg of vitamin C, and 600mg of vitamin E for three years, an age-related cataract will progress more slowly.

MULTIVITAMIN/MINERAL SUPPLEMENT A 2000 study revealed that people who took a multivitamin/mineral supplement that contained vitamin C and/or vitamin E for ten years experienced a 60 percent reduction in the risk of developing cataracts. Another study found that taking vitamin C supplements for ten years or more reduced the risk of cataract development by 70 percent. The evidence also suggests taking a daily dose of 500mg of vitamin C and 400 IU of vitamin E with a multivitamin/mineral supplement reduces the risk of cataract formation in the long term.

> **CAUTION**
>
> Consult your doctor before taking vitamin C with antibiotics or warfarin, or vitamin E with warfarin or aspirin (*see p.46*).

Homeopathy

There is no evidence that homeopathy can help treat cataracts. Homeopaths recommend *Cineraria* eye drops. A number of other medicines may be given orally, including *Calcarea carbonica*, *Calcarea iodatum*, *Causticum*, and *Silicea*.

CALCAREA FLUORICA pills may also be used, particularly for people who generally have lax connective tissues. They may presently be (or have been when younger) hyperextensible (double-jointed), with sway-back knees (knees that go beyond straight) and a tendency to hernias. They may also be arthritic with bony lumps on their fingers.

Environmental Health

UV-B RADIATION Exposure to UV-B (even in small amounts), primarily from the sun but also from welding or ironwork, causes a reaction in the lens that, over many years, contributes to the formation of certain types of cataracts. The risk may be increased because of holes in, or thinning of, the ozone layer. However, there is still some uncertainty about how serious the problem might be. The plastic or glass lenses in sunglasses block as much as 80–90 percent of offending rays and wearing a hat decreases exposure by 30–50 percent.

INFRA-RED RADIATION may also cause cataracts. Exposure to damaging levels, such as the extreme heat in steel making and glass blowing, has been reduced through shorter workdays and the use of furnace shields and protective eyewear.

IONIZING RADIATION, such as X-rays and nuclear fallout, causes cataracts that can take up to 20 years to develop. The risk from X-ray therapy for cancer can be reduced by using proper eye shields. Radiologists, radiation technicians, and dentists should also use adequate protection.

SMOKING is directly toxic to the lens and decreases the availability of antioxidants, such as vitamins C and E to the eye. Avoid smoke-filled places and don't smoke.

> **PREVENTION PLAN**
>
> The following measures should reduce your risk of developing a cataract:
>
> - Eat plenty of fruits and green-leaved vegetables
> - Minimize exposure of your eyes to sunlight, especially UV-B radiation
> - If you are a smoker, quit

MACULAR DEGENERATION

When the macula of the retina degenerates, central and detailed vision are progressively lost. People with macular degeneration have increasing difficulty reading and recognizing faces and often both eyes are affected. Of the two types, the dry form is the most common but the wet form is more likely to severely affect vision. Both types affect women more than men, are more common in people over 70, and may run in families. The dry form can be treated by low-power visual aids. A number of treatments are available for the wet form.

WHAT ARE THE SYMPTOMS?

In both the wet and dry forms of macular degeneration, the main symptoms are:

- A progressive deterioration in central vision
- Increasing difficulty reading, watching television, and recognizing faces
- Distortions of vision; for example, straight lines may appear wavy when looking at a crossword puzzle

In the dry form:

- Symptoms develop slowly

In the wet form:

- Symptoms develop more rapidly and vision distortion is more severe

WHY MIGHT I HAVE THIS?

PREDISPOSING FACTORS

- Increasing age
- Smoking
- High blood levels of cholesterol
- Excessive exposure to sunlight
- Low levels of zinc or vitamin E in the body
- Genetic factors
- Reduced carotenoid intake and subsequent reduction of macula pigment density

TRIGGERS

- Free-radical damage

WHY DOES IT OCCUR?

The macula is the central and most sensitive area of the retina. Located at the back of the eye, the densely packed cells of the macula are responsible for focusing the images that are reflected there from the front of the eye. It is a yellowish oval spot about ⅛in (3mm) to the side of the optic nerve. Light-sensitive cells in the macula depend upon underlying supporting cells for their survival and damage to these cells is the first stage of macular degeneration.

DRY MACULAR DEGENERATION Eighty-five percent of people who experience macular degeneration have the dry form. In this form, light-sensitive cells die in groups, leading to patchy loss of central vision. The dry form develops slowly over a period of 5 to 10 years.

WET MACULAR DEGENERATION The wet form of macular degeneration is far less common than the dry form but is responsible for almost all severe vision loss. In the wet form, blood vessels break through the damaged supporting cells and grow underneath the macula, where they may bleed or leak fluid. This eventually results in scarring in the macular cells, and returns even after it is surgically removed. The wet form develops much more quickly than the dry form, over a period of weeks or months.

UNDERLYING CAUSES The cause of macular degeneration has yet to be discovered. However, increasing age, high levels of cholesterol in the blood, and smoking all increase the risk, as may excessive exposure of the retina to sunlight.

One of the underlying causes of macular degeneration appears to be a reduction in the density of the macula pigment, which is related to dietary intake of carotenoids (specifically lutein and zeaxanthin).

TREATMENT PLAN

PRIMARY TREATMENTS

- Low-powered visual aids (*see Self-Help, p.185*)
- AREDS formula supplements
- Laser therapy
- Macular relocation surgery
- Radiotherapy

BACKUP TREATMENTS

- Nutritional therapy
- Western herbal medicine

For an explanation of how treatments are rated, see p.111.

IMPORTANT

If you experience a sudden decrease in your vision or a sudden onset or worsening of visual distortion, you should see an eye specialist immediately because these symptoms may indicate the wet form of macular degeneration.

HOW THE EYE WORKS

The cornea and lens of the eye focus light from an object and create an upside-down image on the retina. This image stimulates a multitude of light-sensitive cells (rods and cones), which generate a pattern of electrical impulses that are relayed by the optic nerve to the visual cortex at the back of the brain. Here, the pattern is decoded and the object is seen as being upright.

Rod and cone cells

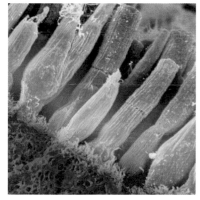

On the retina (pink) are rod cells (blue) which detect light intensity and cone cells (green-blue), which respond to color.

Anatomy of the eye

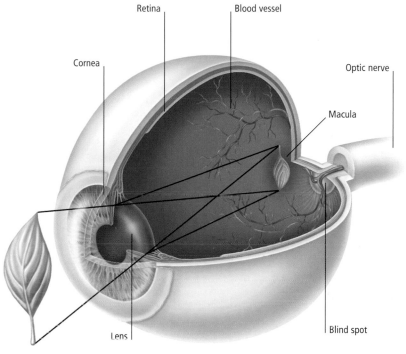

Changes in the shape of the lens enable the eye to focus the light rays on the macula, the most sensitive part of the retina.

LEGAL ISSUES Macular degeneration never causes total blindness because an affected person's peripheral vision is preserved. However, if you have macular degeneration, you may be able to register as legally blind and therefore be eligible for financial and social support.

SELF-HELP

`PRIMARY TREATMENT` If your sight is affected, the following may help:

- Read with good lighting.
- Use low-powered visual aids for reading or watching television. These are available from an optician or a visual aid clinic and include magnifying glasses and mini-telescopes (see p.182).
- Contact an organization established to address your needs, such as the National Association for Visually Handicapped.
- Order large-print editions of your favorite books. Many of these are available online.

TREATMENTS IN DETAIL

Conventional Medicine

Your doctor can make a diagnosis of both forms of macular degeneration by testing your vision and looking at your retina with an ophthalmoscope. Fluorescein angiography may be recommended to check for abnormal blood vessels in the retina and to detect the wet form. The test involves dilating the pupils with drops and injecting dye into an arm vein. Photos are taken with a special camera as the dye passes through blood vessels in the eye.

`PRIMARY TREATMENT` **LASER THERAPY** may be recommended if you have wet macular degeneration. There are two kinds of laser therapy — conventional laser therapy and photodynamic therapy.

Conventional laser therapy employs a high-energy beam to destroy new blood vessels. However, the laser also damages retinal tissue in the targeted area, so the treatment is only used when the new vessels are a distance away from the center of the macula. One result of the therapy will be a small blind spot close to the center of your vision.

Photodynamic laser therapy does not destroy retinal tissue and can be used to destroy new blood vessels at the very center of the macula, preventing them from doing further damage. This treatment is successful only in a select group of patients. It takes about 30 minutes to complete and can be carried out in an outpatient clinic.

If an eye specialist deems it appropriate, you will be injected with a special light-sensitive dye ten minutes before treatment begins. The dye will stick to the abnormal blood vessels in your eye, thereby helping the laser to single them out. You must avoid exposure to bright light for two days following treatment while your body eliminates the dye.

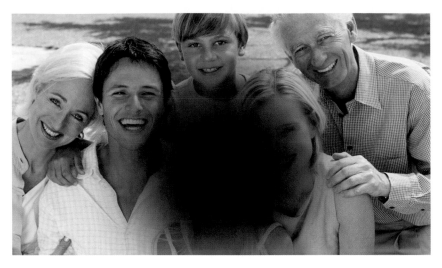

People with macular degeneration experience a blurred central vision, as this image represents, yet they can see details around the center because their peripheral vision remains unaffected.

After both types of laser therapy, the blood vessels may grow back over a period of years and treatment may need to be repeated. It is also important to understand that laser treatment aims to limit further visual loss and usually cannot improve currently impaired vision.

PRIMARY TREATMENT **MACULAR RELOCATION SURGERY** for the wet form of macular degeneration is the subject of ongoing research. It is the only treatment that can significantly improve your vision. Using keyhole surgery to get inside the eye, the retina is detached, rotated, and reconfigured so that the macula is relocated in an area of healthy supporting cells. The muscles that move the eye are also adjusted to allow for the change in the position of the retina.

Submacular surgery is similar to keyhole surgery and involves removing new blood vessels from underneath the retina with fine forceps and replacing the retina in the same position.

PRIMARY TREATMENT **RADIATION THERAPY** Some people with the wet form of macular degeneration can benefit from a focused beam of radiation therapy.

Nutritional Therapy

ANTIOXIDANTS, such as beta-carotene, can neutralize destructive molecules called free radicals that may be responsible for most cases of macular degeneration. Eating carotenoid-rich foods, such as red and orange peppers, apricot, cantalope, kale, and spinach, helps reduce the risk of developing macular degeneration.

LUTEIN AND ZEAXANTHIN Various research studies show that the antioxidant carotenoids lutein and zeaxanthin may provide protection against macular degeneration. A 2001 study found that individuals with the highest level of lutein and zeaxanthin in their retinas had an 82 percent lower risk of macular degeneration compared to those with the lowest levels of these nutrients.

High-dose lutein supplementation of 10mg every day for a year has been shown to reverse symptoms of age-related macular degeneration (AMD).

In addition to having potent antioxidant properties, lutein and zeaxanthin preferentially absorb blue light and therefore protect cells from this most damaging part of the visible spectrum (and hence they appear to be red, yellow, and orange). Zeaxanthin is specifically concentrated in the macula.

Lutein and zeaxanthin are important fat-soluble antioxidants that are absorbed along with fats in the diet. Therefore, supplements containing them should be taken alongside a meal that contains moderate levels of fat.

Foods that are good sources of lutein include spinach, kale, collard greens, romaine lettuce, leeks, peas, egg yolks, kiwi fruit, yellow squash, brussels sprouts, and green peppers. Foods rich in zeaxanthin include mangoes, oranges, sweetcorn, red peppers, nectarines, papayas, squash, and honeydew melons.

You can also supplement your diet with lutein and zeaxanthin — the recommended dose is 6mg of each per day.

SPINACH Eating spinach seems to be particularly beneficial for people who have macular degeneration. A 1999 case series conducted in men between the ages of 61 and 79 with early indications of macular degeneration, found that eating 4–7 servings of spinach a week caused some improvement in visual function tests.

OMEGA-3 FATTY ACIDS Eating fish may prevent the development of macular degeneration, probably due to the presence of omega-3 fatty acids. A 2001 study found that eating four portions of fish per week was associated with a 35 percent lower risk of macular degeneration compared to eating three or fewer portions each week. Try eating a portion of oily fish, especially salmon, trout, mackerel, herring, or sardines, at least 3 times a week to help prevent the condition. Alternatively, you can try taking 1000–2000mg of fish-oil supplements every day.

VITAMIN E AND ZINC also appear to have a protective role in macular degeneration. Studies show that low levels of both zinc and vitamin E are possible risk factors for having the condition. Vitamin E is found in vegetable oils, nuts, seeds, egg yolks, and green leafy vegetables, while zinc is found most readily in fish, seafood, meat, eggs, and tofu.

You may also be advised to take 400 IU of vitamin E along with 15–30mg of zinc each day. Taking zinc supplements over a long period can deplete the body of copper, so take 1–2mg of copper while taking 15mg of supplemental zinc.

CAUTION

Consult your doctor before taking AREDS formula or zinc with antibiotics, or omega-3 fatty acids, fish oils, vitamin E or vitamin C supplements with warfarin. (*see p.46*).

RED WINE Red wine contains appreciable levels of anthocyanins and a recent study found that consuming moderate amounts of wine may decrease occurrences of macular degeneration.

PRIMARY TREATMENT **AREDS FORMULA** The Age-Related Eye Disease Study (AREDS) was a government-funded, randomized controlled trial that looked at a combined nutritional treatment for preventing macular degeneration. Over 3,500 participants aged between 55 and 80, each with some degree of retinal changes ranging from mild to severe, were followed up over a six-year period. They received one of the following each day: (1) antioxidants, including 500mg of vitamin C, 400 IU of vitamin E, and 15mg (25,000 IU) of beta-carotene; (2) 80mg of zinc and 2mg of copper; (3) antioxidants plus zinc (with copper); (4) placebo.

Use of antioxidants reduced the risk of developing advanced age-related macular degeneration by 20 percent, while zinc lowered the risk by 25 percent. An even greater decline in risk was found when antioxidants and zinc were taken together, reducing the risk by 28 percent.

In addition, the combination of antioxidants and zinc led to a 27 percent decrease in the risk of eyesight worsening. Those with more severe retinal problems showed the greatest decrease in risk of developing age-related macular degeneration.

This clinical trial shows that nutrient supplementation in the AREDS formula has the potential to prevent and slow macular degeneration. However, whether a person will benefit from the AREDS supplement depends on the severity of his or her macular degeneration as assessed by an eye specialist. None of these supplements can improve vision that has deteriorated, but they may be able to prevent failing vision from becoming worse.

Western Herbal Medicine

Herbal medicine can help maintain eye health and sight if taken consistently for a long period of time. Specific studies indicate that anthocyanin antioxidants have a marked ability to slow or prevent the development of macular degeneration. Several herbal medicines, notably bilberry (*Vaccinium myrtillus*), contain high levels

of anthocyanins and may strengthen and stabilize the microcirculation within the eye. *Eyebright* (*Euphrasia officinalis*) is another effective herbal treatment.

BILBERRY The high level of anthocyanosides in bilberry may improve night vision. A review of placebo-controlled trials, however, revealed that no studies have tested people with eye diseases and more research is needed. Anthocyanosides strengthen capillaries, making them less liable to leak and cause damage to surrounding tissue.

The high level of anthocyanosides in bilberry increases the rate of regeneration of light-sensitive pigments in the retina and improves night vision.

Forty percent of Americans over the age of 75 are affected by macular degeneration

OTHER HERBS WITH ANTHOCYANOSIDES Other herbs that contain significant amounts of anthocyanoside include blackcurrant (*Ribes nigrum*) fruit, grape (*Vitis vinifera*) seed extract, and pine (*Pinus* spp.) bark extract.

OTHER HERBAL REMEDIES may also be useful in the treatment of macular degeneration. For example, hawthorn (*Crataegus* spp.), another herb with major anthocyanoside content, supports arterial and capillary health. Cornflower (*Centaurea cyanus*), the traditional French herb for eye problems, also has appreciable levels of anthocyanosides in its sky-blue petals.

Research is beginning to support the traditional use of eyebright (*Euphrasia officinalis*) for eye problems ranging from cataracts to conjunctivitis.

CAUTION

See p.69 before taking a herbal remedy and, if you are taking a prescribed medication, consult an herbal medicine expert first.

Environmental Health

SMOKING Since the 1960s, the list of uncurable ailments caused by long-term smoking has grown steadily. Macular

degeneration is the most recent addition to this list, according to medical studies of the last ten years. In fact, research has shown that smoking is the strongest environmental risk associated with the development of macular degeneration.

One US study traced the health patterns of smoking and nonsmoking women who were 50 to 59 years old. Their smoking habits were updated every 2 years for 12 years, and their retinas were also checked for degeneration. Results showed that women who smoked 25 or more cigarettes a day were 2.4 times as likely as nonsmokers to develop macular degeneration.

In addition to the obvious health benefits of giving up smoking, those who quit may experience improved long-term effects when treated with laser therapy.

SUNLIGHT Although the exact causes of macular degeneration are unknown, exposure to direct sunlight is believed to play a role in its development. You may try sunglasses that have UVA and UVB protection together with a visor to shade your face to prevent further vision deterioration.

Acupuncture

Two studies looked at about 100 patients with age-related macular degeneration whose condition improved following acupuncture treatment.

PREVENTION PLAN

The following may reduce your risk of developing macular degeneration:

- Eat plenty of fruit and green-leafed vegetables such as spinach
- Limit your exposure to UV light
- If you smoke, quit
- Control high cholesterol (*see p.32*)
- Take antioxidant and carotene supplements

WHAT ARE THE SYMPTOMS?

- Noises originating within the ear that resemble roaring, ringing, buzzing, whistling, or hissing

WHY MIGHT I HAVE THIS?

PREDISPOSING FACTORS

- Exposure to loud noises
- Temporomandibular joint dysfunction (*see p.280*)
- Ménierè's disease
- Osteoarthritis in the neck
- Exposure to environmental hazards

TREATMENT PLAN

PRIMARY TREATMENTS

- Masking devices or hearing aids
- Cognitive behavioral therapy

BACKUP TREATMENTS

- Antidepressants (if depression is factor)
- Ginkgo biloba
- Chiropractic and/or cranial manipulation
- Hypnotherapy

WORTH CONSIDERING

- Dietary changes
- Zinc and vitamin B (if deficiency is a factor)
- Homeopathy
- Environmental changes
- Acupuncture
- Relaxation training

For an explanation of how treatments are rated, see p.111.

TINNITUS

People with tinnitus hear sounds that originate in the ear itself. These noises may sound like roaring, ringing, buzzing, whistling, or hissing. They are usually continuous, although the intensity may vary and in some people episodes are brief. Tinnitus may be associated with hearing disorders but is usually a benign condition. It is helped by various measures including drugs, ginkgo herbal supplements, dietary changes, acupuncture, chiropractic, and other manipulation therapies. There are also psychological techniques to help you cope.

WHY DOES IT OCCUR?

There are currently over 50 million Americans who hear noises in the ear that do not exist in the outside world. However, researchers have yet to decode what causes tinnitus. It sometimes occurs for no apparent reason but is commonly associated with certain ear disorders, such as age-induced hearing loss (presbycusis), or Ménière's disease (a disorder of the inner ear that causes episodes of dizziness, nausea, and hearing loss, as well as tinnitus). In a study involving 1,002 chronic tinnitus patients, researchers concluded that temporomandibular joint disorder (*see p.280*) is probably a causal factor in cases if no other cause can be determined. Misaligned jaw boints or muscles may also cause tinnitus.

Up to 90 percent of tinnitus sufferers experience some degree of noise-induced hearing loss. Repeated exposure to loud sounds increases the likelihood of damage to the tiny hairs lining the inner ear. However, even a single exposure to music louder than 100 decibels can cause lifelong hearing damage.

Tinnitus may be associated with anemia and hyperthyroidism (*see Thyroid Problems, p.319*) and nutritionists believe that it is sometimes a symptom of blood-sugar fluctuation. Head injuries and treatment with certain drugs can also cause tinnitus. Other possible factors that may lead to tinnitus include wax buildup in the ear canal,

IMPORTANT

See your doctor if you develop tinnitus, especially if it affects one ear only.

certain medications, and ear or sinus infections. Tinnitus is also correlated with cardiovascular disease as well as head and neck trauma.

Tinnitus may affect both ears or one ear only, and range in volume from very subtle to excruciatingly loud. Tinnitus in one ear may be caused by a tumor affecting the nerve that carries information from the ear to the brain.

People with tinnitus may find that the constant sound in their ears distracts them and that they have difficulty concentrating. Some people with tinnitus have difficulty falling asleep at night (*see Sleeping Disorders, p.448.*) If tinnitus causes problems with day-to-day living, it may lead to depression (*see p.436*) and anxiety (*see p.414*).

TREATMENTS IN DETAIL

Conventional Medicine

Your doctor may arrange for hearing tests or other investigations to find an underlying cause for your tinnitus. Tinnitus is an individualized condition and treatments vary from person to person, so take time to discuss all possible options. Many therapies that may provide relief, and are worth trying, have yet to be clinically tested.

PRIMARY TREATMENT **MASKING DEVICES** Sometimes external noises, such as music, may help distract you from the noise in your ears. In addition, masking devices are available that you can wear in or behind the ears. These emit sounds that may help distract from the tinnitus. Masking devices can be conveniently inserted or removed according to the needs of the individual. For example, some environments may have enough external noise that the listener is more comfortable without the device. Hearing aids may be beneficial if you also have hearing loss.

ANTIDEPRESSANTS Tricyclic antidepressants may help relieve tinnitus when symptoms of depression are also present. Examples include amitriptyline, clomipramine, and imipramine.

> **CAUTION**
>
> Antidepressants can cause a range of possible side effects; ask your doctor to explain these to you.

OTHER DRUGS Many drugs are associated with causing tinnitus, especially some antibiotics and chemotherapeutic agents for cancer, quinine for leg cramps or malaria, and, most widely known, salicylate drugs (such as aspirin). A careful review of your prescription and nonprescription medicines can help pinpoint potential tinnitus-causing factors — for example, several combination nonprescription and prescription pharmaceuticals contain acetylsalicylic acid (aspirin). If you or your doctor are unsure whether you have had significant exposure to one of these compounds, laboratory tests that include bloodwork may help

Nutritional Therapy

DIETARY CHANGES Food sensitivity may be an occasional underlying cause of tinnitus. People with Ménière's disease may find that their tinnitus improves when they receive treatment for a specific allergy. (*For more information on identifying food sensitivities, see p.456.*)

Tinnitus may also be related to general dietary factors. If you have tinnitus, it can help to limit your intake of salt, red meat, dairy products, and tea and coffee, and consume plenty of fresh fruits and vegetables, nuts, seeds, extra-virgin olive oil, and water. An uncontrolled study showed improved symptoms of Ménière's disease in people who had followed this regime for a year. However, symptoms may abate by themselves over time. Since tinnitus can be a symptom of blood-sugar fluctuation,

---

TINNITUS MASKER DEVICE

A tinnitus masker is a small electronic device that fits in the ear and delivers continous "white" noise to block out the unwanted ringing and whistling sounds. To decide whether a masker may be useful, some specialists conduct a "tap test" in which the person with tinnitus stands close to a running faucet. If the sound of the water is enough to block out the tinnitus, a masker may be appropriate. The device is particularly useful during quiet periods in the day when the tinnitus noises are most noticeable.

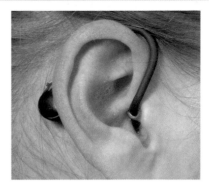

Looking like a hearing aid, a tinnitus masker fits discreetly in the ear.

---

controlling blood-sugar levels may also help. (*For details how to do this, see p.42.*)

> **CAUTION**
>
> Zinc and vitamin B_{12} can interact with certain drugs and other supplements; see p.46 for more information.

NUTRITIONAL SUPPLEMENTS Some people who have tinnitus have an underlying zinc deficiency. Taking zinc (at a dose of about 50mg per day) seems to be effective in some cases.

Vitamin B_{12} deficiency may play a role in the development of tinnitus. In one study, 47 percent of tinnitus patients were found to be deficient in vitamin B_{12}. This vitamin may be effective in treating tinnitus because it can enhance the conduction of nerve impulses used in hearing. If you have tinnitus, you should try taking 1mg of vitamin B_{12} every day.

Homeopathy

Although there are few studies that prove the effectiveness of homeopathic treatments for the symptoms of tinnitus, the results of some homeopathic treatments were comparable to those with conventional medications.

CHININUM SULPHURICUM AND CHENOPODIUM *Chininum sulphuricum* (quinine sulfate) is suitable when tinnitus is due to Ménière's disease with dizziness, ringing in the ears, and deafness. The rarely used homeopathic medicine *Chenopodium* may be useful when the person experiences unusual symptoms of deafness, particularly to the human voice, combined with sensitivity to loud sounds that hurt the inner ear.

GRAPHITES AND CAUSTICUM Constitutional features (*see p.73*) are important in prescribing *Graphites* and *Causticum*. People who respond to *Graphites* have ringing that is combined with deafness, which improves when there is background noise. They may also have skin trouble affecting the outer ear. People who respond to *Causticum* have tinnitus with a peculiar sensation of echoing, particularly of their own voice.

Western Herbal Medicine

There have been reviews of clinical trials of ginkgo biloba for tinnitus and it seems that ginkgo does not work for tinnitus as a primary complaint. Given the lack of many other efective treatments for tinnitus, you could consider trying ginkgo biloba for two months at a dosage of 120–200mg per day, keeping in mind that ginkgo does have side effects and could interact with medications you are taking.

Environmental Health

There are a variety of toxins in the environment that can contribute to tinnitus. Taking steps to decrease your daily contact with them may lessen the severity of the sounds in your ear.

HEAVY METALS There is evidence that exposure to heavy metals can lead to nerve damage, which is believed to be a cause of tinnitus. In order to prevent worsening of nerve damage, you should investigate your surroundings for lead or other heavy metals such as mercury. Send a sample of your tap water to a public health authority to have them check the water quality, and explore the possibility of toxic exposure at your workplace. Many foods contain mercury and other heavy metals, especially fish (particularly oily ocean fish, such as tuna, shark, and sword-fish) and products made from animal bones (such as some gelatins). Mercury levels are generally higher in larger, preda-tory fish. Therefore, canned tuna (made from the smallest of the fish) is likely to have lower levels of harmful mercury than fresh tuna steaks.

LOUD NOISES Injury to the cochlea in the inner ear is a frequent cause of tinnitus. One of the most obvious causes of cochlear damage is loud noise. If you know

are also an option, but reports say that these may actually worsen some cases.

OXYGEN THERAPY If you have had tinni-tus for less than three months, treatment with hyperbaric oxygen (oxygen at high pressure) can help relieve it. In one study, over 80 percent of people who started hyperbaric oxygen therapy between two and six weeks after the onset of tinnitus experienced improvement in the degree of tinnitus, while 35 percent of those who started therapy between six weeks and three months gained relief to some degree.

Bodywork Therapies

CHIROPRACTIC AND CRANIAL MANIPU-LATION Temporomandibular joint (TMJ) problems (*see p.280*), which may cause tin-nitus, can be treated by cranial osteopaths, sacro-occipital practitioners, craniosacral therapists, and dentists, depending on the cause of the jaw dysfunction.

A case report found chiropractic treat-ment effective for a 41-year-old woman

Mind–Body Therapies

PSYCHOTHERAPY AND RELAXATION EXERCISES Psychotherapy may be helpful for treating chronic tinnitus. Relaxation exercises may also be recommended (*for information, see p.99*). A 1999 article pre-sented an overview of tinnitus, its psychological effects, and application of psychological therapies for its treatment. This study concluded that psychological treatment for tinnitus, particulary cogni-tive behavioral therapy, is effective. Future studies hope to examine the effects of psychological treatments in relieving depression and sleep problems associated with tinnitus.

An uncontrolled study found that relax-ation training helped people manage stress better, which in turn reduced the extent to which tinnitus bothered them.

COGNITIVE BEHAVIORAL THERAPY Sev-eral studies have confirmed a correlation between psychological factors, such as anx-iety and depression, and severe tinnitus. Cognitive behavioral therapy can help tin-nitus by enabling you to cope better with stress and by alleviating depression.

Controlled studies have compared the effectiveness of cognitive behavioral train-ing for tinnitus with other therapies such as yoga. While yoga also helped tinnitus, cognitive behavioral therapy was shown to be of the greatest benefit and was the ther-apy that patients preferred. If you have tinnitus, you should consider having a course of cognitive behavioral therapy.

HYPNOTHERAPY One study showed that hypnotherapy may be as effective as either masking devices or counseling in the treat-ment of tinnitus.

> Close to one third of the US population experiences tinnitus to some degree

you will be exposed to loud noises, you should wear earplugs (look for kinds approved by a scientific laboratory). Even children exposed to sounds from toy guns and fireworks can suffer auditory damage and resulting tinnitus. Remember to wear ear protection when mowing the lawn. You may also try moving out of the closed air-space of a bathroom, or wearing earplugs, when using a hairdryer.

OTHER CAUSES There are many other causes of tinnitus. Carbon monoxide poi-soning is one, and a simple blood test to check for short- or long-term exposure to this deadly gas can determine whether it is responsible for your tinnitus.

HELPFUL STRATEGIES Some therapies for tinnitus make use of sound or electrical stimulation. Some people find that simply distracting themselves using a ticking clock or radio static can provide relief. Cochlear implants providing electrical stimulation

with ear pain, tinnitus, vertigo, some hear-ing loss, and headaches, whose symptoms were attributed to TMJ syndrome.

Chiropractic manipulation of the neck and cranium is claimed to improve tinnitus in cases not related to temporo-mandibular joint problems, especially when the condition is associated with an imbal-ance between the sympathetic and parasympathetic nerve supply to the region.

Acupuncture

There have been some positive case reports of acupuncture as an effective approach for tinnitus, but the few clinical trials evaluating this have been largely negative. A traditional Chinese diagnosis is necessary if acupuncture is used to treat tinnitus. Trying four to six treatments is always worthwhile to see if acupuncture can provide some relief. If acupuncture is to be effective, prolonged maintenance treatment may be required.

PREVENTION PLAN

To prevent tinnitus from occurring:

- Avoid loud noises

- Wear ear plugs during noisy activities

- Avoid exposure to hazardous materials such as heavy metals and carbon monoxide

- Review any long-term prescription drugs with your doctor

EARACHE

Earache usually results from disease of the ear, most commonly an infection in the middle or outer ear. Mild earache may be a symptom of the common cold. Sometimes, conditions affecting nearby structures may cause earache. Examples of this include temporomandibular joint disorder (*see p.280*) and shingles (*see p.165*) affecting the face. Depending on the cause, treatment for earache may involve traditional drugs, dietary changes, herbal medicine, and homeopathy. Cranial manipulation may also be helpful in some cases.

WHAT ARE THE SYMPTOMS?

Symptoms of middle ear infection include:
- Pain in the ear, which may be severe
- Fever
- Some hearing impairment
- Discharge from the ear if the eardrum ruptures

Symptoms of outer ear infection include:
- Itching and/or pain
- Discharge from the ear

There may be other symptoms associated with disorders affecting nearby tissues.

WHY MIGHT I HAVE THIS?

PREDISPOSING FACTORS

For inner ear infection:
- Upper respiratory tract infection, such as the common cold
- Food sensitivities

For outer ear infection:
- Swimming
- Eczema

TREATMENT PLAN

PRIMARY TREATMENTS
- Drugs for pain relief and to treat infection, if bacteria are present

BACKUP TREATMENTS
- Dietary changes

WORTH CONSIDERING
- Herbal medicine
- Cranial manipulation

For an explanation of how treatments are rated, see p.111.

WHY DOES IT OCCUR?

Earache is often due to germs that spread through the nasal passages and eustachian tubes to cause inflammation, swelling, and pain within the middle ear. Occasionally, earache results from a tumor located in the ear or in a nearby area, such as the throat.

Inflammation of the outer part of the ear (otitis externa) may be caused by a bacterial, viral, or fungal infection. Eczema is also a factor in outer ear infections.

Outer ear infections are often associated with increased moisture in the ear caused by swimming ("swimmer's ear") or working in a hot and humid environment. If you are a regular swimmer, be sure to thoroughly dry your ears after leaving the water to prevent infections from occurring. You may also try using a solution made of equal parts alcohol and water. Insert a few drops into the ear canal to help withdraw any remaining moisture.

CHILDREN Every year, about 1 in 5 children under the age of 4 experience a middle ear infection, known as otitis media. This often occurs when the eustachian tubes (which connect the middle ear to the nose, allowing fluid to drain) become clogged due to a common cold or allergies. The eustachian tubes in children are smaller than in adults, which can keep fluid from draining effectively. Otitis media may also be caused by a viral infection or by secondhand smoke.

IMPORTANT

If earache is severe or persistent, see your doctor immediately.

When children are very young, they may not associate their discomfort with a problem in their ear. Instead, they may vomit or have a fever, show signs of irritability, disturbed sleep, or pain when swallowing or chewing. More obvious symptoms of an ear infection are tugging at the ears, fussing when the ear is touched, or complaining of buzzing and ringing sounds. Recurrent middle ear infections may make a child more likely to develop chronic otitis media with effusion (glue ear, *see p.388*).

IMMEDIATE RELIEF

To reduce the pain of earache:
- Hold something warm against the ear, such as a hot water bottle wrapped in a soft towel.
- Analgesics, such as acetaminophen, ibuprofen, aspirin, or naproxen can also help. Never give aspirin to children under age 12.
- Chewing gum may help relieve the pressure of an infection in the middle ear.
- Eardrops are available over the counter.

TREATMENTS IN DETAIL

Conventional Medicine

The doctor will use an otoscope to examine your ears and may also look at your throat. If there is discharge from the ear, a sample may be sent to a laboratory so the infection can be identified. Additional tests may look for diseases in nearby areas.

PRIMARY TREATMENT **DRUGS** Analgesics, prescription or over the counter, may relieve the pain, which usually subsides

ANATOMY OF THE EAR

The ears are organs of both hearing and balance. There are three distinct parts to the structure: the outer, middle, and inner ear. The part of the ear that is visible is called the pinna — the outer part of the ear canal viewed without an instrument. The ear canal, which is lined with hairs and secretes protective wax, channels sound. It leads to the eardrum, which vibrates in response to soundwaves. The middle ear lies beyond the eardrum and is filled with air. It contains three tiny bones — the malleus, incus, and stapes — that transmit vibrations from the eardrum to the membrane of the oval window. This membrane separates the middle ear from the inner ear. To better show these features, diagrams are not to scale.

The outer, middle, and inner ear

Semicircular canals · Vestibular nerve · Incus · Oval window · Cochlea (cutaway) · Malleus · Ear canal · Pinna · Skull bone · Skull bone · Eardrum · Stapes · Vestibule · Eustachian tube

The ear canal runs from the pinna to the inner ear, which is situated inside the skull. The inner ear is filled with fluid and contains the cochlea, a shell-like structure **that is the sensory receptor for hearing. The inner ear also contains the vestibule and the semicircular canals, the organs reponsible for balance.**

---

after a week. Oral antibiotics may be prescribed for middle ear infections but most ear infections disappear on their own. Analgesic eardrops may also be prescribed.

To treat an outer ear infection, your doctor may carefully clean the ear and prescribe corticosteroid drops to relieve inflammation. If an infection is present, oral antibiotics or eardrops with an antibiotic or antifungal drug may be prescribed. Eardrops may cause some local irritation.

Other causes of infection are treated when possible. For example, antiviral drugs are prescribed for shingles that affects the face.

> **CAUTION**
>
> Drugs for ear infection can cause a range of possible side effects; ask your doctor to explain these to you.

Nutritional Therapy

PRIMARY TREATMENT **DIETARY CHANGES** Food sensitivity appears to be common in children who have recurrent otitis media (*see p.388*) and ear infections. In one study, the most common foods associated with otitis media were milk, eggs, beans, citrus fruits, and tomatoes. The elimination of suspect foods led to a significant reduction of otitis media symptoms in the majority of patients. Moreover, the reintroduction of suspect foods back into the diet tended to provoke a recurrence of otitis media. Some practitioners recommend restriction of dairy products and sugary food because they believe that these foods may impact immune function. (*For more about food sensitivities, see p.39.*)

Certain nutrients can help maintain healthy immune function which may prevent future ear infections. Probiotic supplements can also help counteract the digestive side effects that may occur while using antibiotics prescribed for ear infections. (*For more about these and other nutritional approaches to ear infection, see Otitis Media with Effusion, p.388.*)

Continuing to breast-feed infants beyond the age of four months may also offer some protection against future ear infection in children.

Homeopathy

Clinical trials and outcome studies suggest that homeopathy medicines are an effective treatment for acute otitis media. A double-blind placebo-controlled study on the effectiveness of homeopathic treatment for ear infections looked at children between the ages of 18 months and 6 years who had infections of the middle ear. The children were divided into two groups, with 36 children receiving real homeopathic treatment and 39 children receiving a placebo.

The study used eight different homeopathic remedies, which were prescribed for the children on an individual basis. The most frequently used treatments were *Pulsatilla, Chamomilla, Sulfphur,* and *Calcarea carbonica*. It was found that children who received one of the homeopathic treatments for their ear infections experienced less pain and fever after 24 hours than those who received the placebo.

For treatment at home, the remedies listed below may bring relief. If these do not work or seem inappropriate, consult a qualified homeopath. If conditions do not improve within 24 hours, then see your doctor.

KALIUM SULPHURICUM AND PULSATILLA The most commonly used homeopathic medicine for middle ear infection is *Kalium sulphuricum*. This treatment is appropriate when there is deafness as well as clicking in the ears while swallowing. The affected child often has thick discharge down the back of his or her nose. *Pulsatilla* is an appropriate medicine when there are similar symptoms but other features are present as well: the affected child tends to be weepy, whiny, and clingy, but quickly cheers up with attention. These children are often timid and indecisive.

CALCAREA CARBONICA Perhaps the next most common medicine for middle ear infection is *Calcarea carbonica*. Children who respond well to this homeopathic medicine get recurrent colds and tend to be large and chubby. They can be stubborn and have many fears (such as being afraid of the dark). They may wake up from frightening dreams and sweat freely, especially on the head.

Western Herbal Medicine

Middle ear infection can be a painful condition threatening to impair hearing in the affected ear. In serious acute cases, when the onset is likely to be sudden and pain severe, conventional treatment with antibiotics is preferred over herbal medicine. Herbal treatment for earache and ear infection is appropriate when symptoms are relatively mild or if earache is a recurrent problem that has not fully responded to antibiotic therapy.

The herbal approach seeks to determine factors that have enabled the condition to develop. For example, an herbalist will look for signs of chronic nasal infection or allergy or of chronic cold symptoms and congestion. All of these conditions weaken the immune system's resistance in the mucus-secreting tissue within the upper respiratory passageways. An herbalist may also look for signs of an acute upper respiratory tract infection, either viral or bacterial.

HERBS TO FIGHT INFECTION For self-help measures when infection is present, echinacea (*Echinacea purpurea* has better evidence than *angustifolia*) and elderberry (*Sambucus* spp.) taken orally are appropriate. For acute infection and in cases of chronic recurrence, visit a practitioner who will prescribe a combination of herbs. The mix is likely to include natural antibiotics to counter infection, such as antiviral garlic or immune tonics (e.g. thyme) to strengthen nonspecific immune activity (increase white blood cell activity). Both groups of herbs are important to counter infection but anti-inflammatory remedies such as licorice (*Glycyrrhiza glabra*) are often included to reduce swelling and ease pain. Plantain (*Plantago major*) or other astringents tone mucous membranes and reduce the secretion of mucus.

HERBS FOR PAIN RELIEF Other herbs may be used specifically for pain relief; Lavender (*Lavandula*) or German chamomile (*Larrea divaricata*) essential oils can be gently massaged into the area behind and in front of the ear, or 1–2 drops of oil (preferably warmed) can be applied to cotton balls and gently inserted into the ear. Another common treatment is mullein (*Verbascum* spp.) and garlic (*Allium saativa*) in olive oil; drops of this oil decoction can be used to relieve ear pain and perhaps fight infection due to the anti-inflammatory effects of mullein and antibacterial and antiviral effects of garlic. Drops should not be used if the ear drum is perforated.

> **CAUTION**
>
> See p.69 before taking an herbal remedy. If you are taking a prescribed medication, consult an herbal medicine expert first.

Bodywork Therapies

CRANIAL MANIPULATION Recurrent earache and glue ear in children are often treated by cranial osteopaths, chiropractors, and others who work on the craniosacral connection. Practitioners use very light pressure to evaluate the ease of motion and rhythm within the craniosacral system and to alter any imbalances. This may release stress and tension throughout the body and assist the body's own healing ability. Although there is little research so far to back up the effectiveness of cranial manipulation for middle ear problems, it may help if you or your child has a chronic condition affecting the middle ear. Cranial manipulation is just beginning to receive research attention designed to assess its effectiveness for treating ear problems.

> **PREVENTION PLAN**
>
> **The following may help:**
> - Breast-feed babies beyond four months
> - If problem foods could be a factor, try eliminating the most common ones (*see p.35 and p.39*)
> - Thoroughly dry your ears after a swim. Instill a few drops of a solution with equal parts water and alcohol

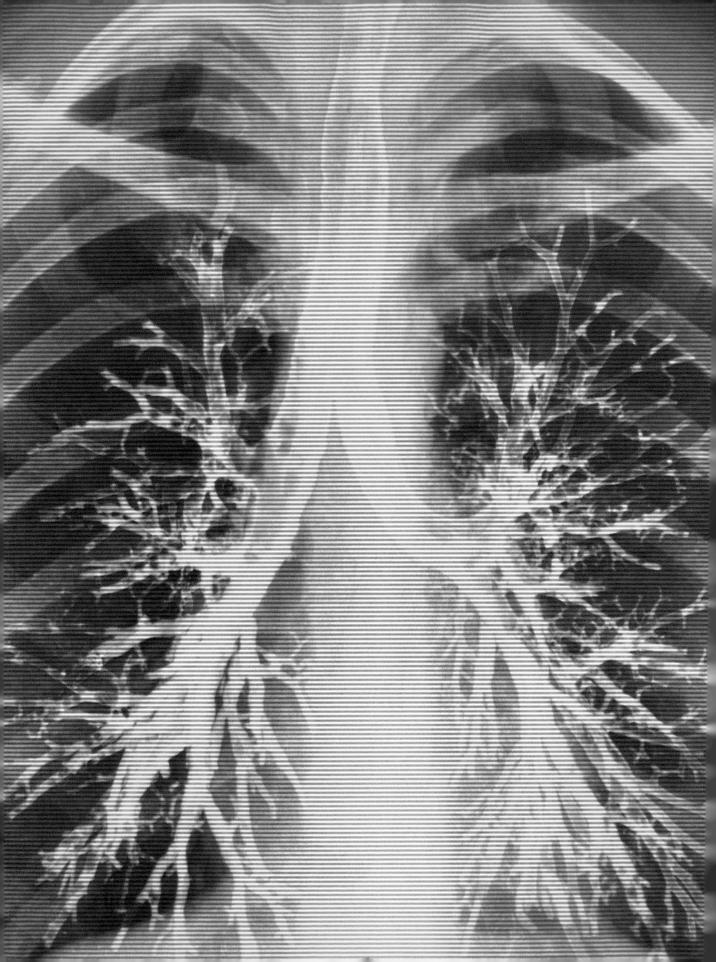

Respiratory System

We literally take in the outside world when we breathe. Protection from possible external toxins can be provided by environmental medicine, while herbal and nutritional therapies support the immune defenses. Although drugs can change how the lungs work at a cellular level, breathing is essentially physical. Bodywork therapies and exercises can optimize this mechanical process.

SINUSITIS

The sinuses are air-filled cavities in the head situated behind the nose and eyes and in the cheeks and forehead. They are lined with a mucus-secreting membrane and are connected to the nasal cavity by narrow channels. If the membrane in the sinuses and nose secretes too much mucus in response to infection or allergy, the condition may be called catarrh. If the membrane in the sinuses becomes inflamed, the condition is known as sinusitis. Drugs, lifestyle changes, homeopathy and manipulation therapy can all help to resolve these conditions.

WHAT ARE THE SYMPTOMS?

Symptoms of catarrh include:

- Persistently runny nose
- Cough and irritation caused by mucus running down the back of the throat

Symptoms of sinusitis include:

- Pain and tenderness in the face that may be worse when bending forwards
- Nasal discharge
- Nasal congestion or blockage
- Headache and possibly toothache, if the sinuses behind the cheeks are affected

WHY MIGHT I HAVE THIS?

PREDISPOSING FACTORS

- Infection
- Allergy
- Polyps in the nose
- Deviated septum
- Food sensitivity
- Yeast infection
- High levels of histamine in the body
- Trigger points in jaw muscles
- Upper chest breathing

WHY DOES IT OCCUR?

Excessive mucus production is frequently caused by an allergy, commonly occuring in allergic rhinitis (*see p.459*). In this case, symptoms usually stop once exposure to the allergen stops. The most common cause of sinusitis is a viral infection, such as a cold or flu (*see p.200*). If the channels connecting the sinuses to the nose become blocked, mucus may collect in the sinuses. In some cases, the mucus is infected with bacteria, worsening the condition. Blockage of the channels is more likely in people with an abnormality such as a deviated nasal septum or nasal polyps. Rarely, channels may be blocked by a tumor. People with reduced immunity, such as those with HIV infection (*see HIV and AIDS, p.470*) or taking immunosuppressants are at increased risk of sinusitis because they are more susceptible to infection.

Nutritionists' clinical experience suggests that food sensitivity is a common factor in sinusitis. Some foods, particularly dairy products but certain others as well, seem to induce mucus formation in the sinuses, causing congestion. Sensitive areas known as trigger points in the face and jaw can also increase mucus secretions in the nose and sinuses, causing or worsening sinusitis.

IMMEDIATE RELIEF

The following measures may help relieve your discomfort:

- Add a few drops of pine or eucalyptus essential oil to a bowl of steaming hot water. Lean over the bowl with a towel over your head and inhale for 5–10 minutes. Supervise carefully if using this method on children.
- Take a hot shower or bath, or run hot water in the bathroom and inhale the steam.
- Use a humidifier in your house.
- Take over-the-counter analgesics and nasal decongestants.

TREATMENT PLAN

PRIMARY TREATMENTS

- Drugs such as decongestants
- Drugs such as analgesics and possibly antibiotics
- Identification and elimination of problem foods

BACK-UP TREATMENTS

- Acupuncture
- Breathing retraining
- Surgery (if sinusitis is recurrent)

WORTH CONSIDERING

- Vitamin C and bromelain
- Homeopathy
- Western herbal medicine
- Environmental health measures
- Deactivation of trigger points and cranial manipulation
- Nasal specific technique

For an explanation of how treatments are rated, see p.111.

Conventional Medicine

Various treatments are available for sinusitis, some of which can be obtained over the counter.

PRIMARY TREATMENT **DRUGS** Nasal decongestants may help people in the short-term. However, their effect can gradually wear off after a week or so and symptoms may worsen when medication is stopped. Antihistamines may offer some improvement in runny nose and sneezing in colds. Analgesics may be taken to relieve the discomfort of sinusitis.

Antibiotics may be prescribed for sinusitis, but opinions vary over whether this is appropriate. Studies have shown that taking them may be helpful in some cases, but the potential benefits need to be weighed against possible side effects as well as the possibility of developing resistance to antibiotics. Sinusitis often clears up without treatment.

> **CAUTION**
>
> Drugs for rhinitis and sinusitis can cause a range of possible side effects; ask your doctor or pharmacist to explain these to you.

SURGERY Surgical treatment may be recommended to remove nasal polyps if sinusitis is recurrent, does not clear, or becomes chronic. Doctors will first recommend further exams, including sinus X-rays, CT scans, or ultrasound.

PREVENTIVE MEASURES Preventing dehydration by drinking plenty of water and by humidifying centrally heated air are also essential measures to help prevent rhinitis and sinusitis from developing.

Nutritional Therapy

PRIMARY TREATMENT **VITAMIN C** Histamine is associated with increased nasal and sinus congestion. There is some evidence that taking a high dose of vitamin C (3,000mg per day) can reduce histamine levels in people whose levels of this chemical are naturally high and in those whose blood levels of vitamin C are low. Taken at a lower dose of 2,000mg per day, vitamin C

ANATOMY OF THE SINUSES

The air-filled cavities in the skull known as the sinuses are located around the nose and eyes and in the cheeks and forehead. The sinuses are lined with glands that secrete mucus, which passes continuously through narrow channels leading from the sinuses to the back of the nose. This mucus traps small particles and moistens inhaled air. A further set of sinuses, known the sphenoid sinuses, is located deep within the skull behind the ethmoid sinuses.

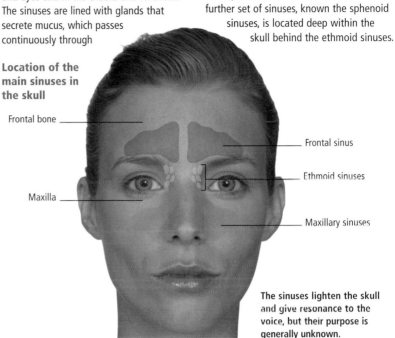

Location of the main sinuses in the skull

Frontal bone

Maxilla

Frontal sinus

Ethmoid sinuses

Maxillary sinuses

The sinuses lighten the skull and give resonance to the voice, but their purpose is generally unknown.

has been shown to help protect people who have allergic rhinitis (a significant predisposing factor for sinusitis) and are exposed to histamine. Research has also demonstrated that people who have chronic sinusitis have diminished antioxidant defenses against free radicals and therefore taking extra vitamin C corrects this imbalance.

BROMELAIN The enzyme bromelain, which is derived from pineapple, can be helpful in relieving the symptoms of sinusitis. Bromelain has the ability to break down protein in the body and may help loosen and clear sinus congestion. Bromelain is a form of natural decongestant and 500mg should be taken three times a day between meals in order to help prevent rhinitis and sinusitis.

> **CAUTION**
>
> Consult your doctor before taking bromelain and vitamin C with antibiotics, or vitamin C with the blood-thinning drug warfarin. (*For more information, see p.46.*)

PRIMARY TREATMENT **FOOD SENSITIVITIES** Dairy products (particularly milk and cheese) may cause certain people to produce excess mucus. Other common problem foods include white flour and bananas. Food sensitivity varies among individuals and, for this reason, is best assessed by a dietician on an individual basis (*see p.39 for details*).

In addition to particular food sensitivities, chronic sinus congestion is also often associated with poor diet, digestive function, and metabolism. In most traditional medicine systems, congestion is thought to result from inadequate processing of food. This gives rise to a buildup of waste products, which are eliminated via the mucous membranes. Dairy products and sugar are among the foods linked to chronic sinusitus and reducing or cutting them out of the diet is a good starting point.

Homeopathy

Homeopaths believe that individualized homeopathic treatment can go further in treating sinusitis than isopathy (treatment with homeopathic dilutions of allergens). As always with homeopathy, individualized treatment is important and many different homeopathic medicines may be appropriate, depending on the symptoms and the person who experiences them (*see p.73 and also Allergic Rhinitis, p.459*).

ALLIUM CEPA AND EUPHRASIA OFFICINALIS For acute rhinitis due to an

> ## The sinuses are not present at birth, but develop gradually throughout childhood

allergy or a cold, the medicine *Allium* (onion) provides a good illustration of the principles of homeopathy. The symptoms it treats are identical to those that you experience when cutting onions: sore, watery eyes, and a runny nose, often with sneezing. *Euphrasia* (made from the herb eyebright) may also be used. In practice, these medicines are often used together in a homeopathic complex.

HEPAR CALCAREUM SULPHURIS This medicine is appropriate for people who usually have a sudden onset of sharp pain above the eyes, usually without a nasal discharge. It may be accompanied by a sore throat — a feeling as if something sharp were stuck in the throat — or coughing and feeling chilly.

KALIUM BICHROMICUM Perhaps the most frequently used medicine to treat chronic or recurring sinusitis is *Kalium*. People who respond to this may have a headache either above the eyes or in the cheeks and a thick nasal discharge. Chronic sinusitis often responds well to homeopathy.

PULSATILLA may also be used to treat chronic sinusitis. People who respond to this remedy experience a nasal discharge that flows freely and feel better in fresh air. In addition, the nose becomes blocked and uncomfortable in a stuffy or overheated room The person who responds to *Pulsatilla* is usually mild-tempered, indecisive, or dithery and is easily moved to tears.

SILICEA is also recommended to treat sinusitis. People who respond to this

remedy seem to get every cold virus that is going around and are unusually sensitive to the cold temperatures. They often have cold, clammy hands and feet, weak, ridged nails, and fine or falling hair.

LYCOPODIUM is another remedy for sinusitis. Typically, people who respond to *Lycopodium* experience symptoms on the right side more than the left, or the problem starts on the right and moves to the left. Again, "whole person" characteristics are important. People who respond to *Lycopodium* are often rather reserved, intellectual types. They may get into a state of anxiety before doing anything important because they set themselves high standards and may be quite depressed. They often have digestive problems, particularly gas and bloating.

> **CAUTION**
>
> Many homeopathic medicines are neutralized by strong smells such as camphor, menthol, and eucalyptus. If you are using homeopathic medicine, do not use products containing these substances at the same time.

Western Herbal Medicine

Acute sinus problems respond well to herbal treatment.

HERBS TO RELIEVE SYMPTOMS Plantain (*Plantago lanceolata*) and elderflower (*Sambucus nigra*) are suitable herbs for self-treatment. Both herbs reduce sinus secretion and inflammation in the upper respiratory passageways. Elderflower has antiviral properties and can be used to treat allergy-related sinusitis. Teas made with chamomile (*Matricaria recrutita*) or linden flowers (*Tilea cordata*) are also helpful, easing sore and irritated nasal passageways. Linden flowers are considered especially helpful in treating sinus headaches. Either warm chamomile tea or

warm salt water may also be carefully used as a nasal wash (*see Nasal Cleanse, box, p.86*).

HERBS FOR DETOXIFICATION Practitioners are likely to prescribe herbs to promote detoxification and elimination, such as barberry (*Berberis vulgaris*) and goldenrod (*Solidago virgaurea*) and will seek to correct any underlying causes of toxicity, such as constipation. In acute rather than chronic states, herbs with established antimicrobial activity, such as echinacea (*Echinacea* spp.) and goldenseal (*Hydrastis canadensis*) are suggested, often in combination with cayenne pepper (*Capsiucm anuum*) and licorice (*Glycyrrhiza glabra*). Myrtol (*Myrrtus communis*) has also been effective when used as an aromatherapy.

> **CAUTION**
>
> See p.69 before taking a herbal remedy and, if you are taking prescribed medication, consult an herbal medicine expert first.

Environmental Health

ALLERGIES Inflammation of the nasal and sinus tissue typically precedes the actual infection of the sinuses and some existing conditions, such as allergic rhinitis (*see p.459*), are frequently associated with sinusitis. A study in New England linked the worsening of asthma and sinusitis with high pollen and mold counts caused by the El Niño winds in 1998.

AVOID DUST MITES AND MOLD If you are allergic to indoor allergens such as dust-mites or indoor molds, remove upholstered furniture and carpeting and wash bed linens at a high temperature. You should also eliminate dampness and mildew from your house.

AIR POLLUTION Numerous studies in Germany demonstrated the association between air pollution and the prevalence of chronic sinusitis (2). Ozone levels can fluctuate in the air and ozone can irritate the mucous membranes and may be central to the development of sinusitis (7). If you experience sinusitis regularly, limit your time outdoors on days when the pollution levels are high.

SMOKING Smoking is a strong risk factor for the development and prolongation of chronic sinusitis and catarrh. Many studies have supported this association and the effects of tobacco smoke on the lining of the upper respiratory tract, which includes the nasal passages and the sinuses, is immense. If you have sinusitis or other respiratory disease and you smoke, quitting should be a top priority.

WORKPLACE CHEMICALS Ammonia vapors have been linked to the development of chronic sinus disease, and people exposed to chlorine at work (or even in swimming pools) may be at risk of developing nasal congestion. In general, if you are prone to sinusitis, avoid swimming pools treated with chlorine, which irritates nose and sinus linings.

POLLUTANTS IN THE NOSE Nasal irrigation, preferably with a Neti pot or similar device, washes away many pollutants that are trapped in the nasal lining (*see box*).

AIR TRAVEL Traveling by air may worsen symptoms of sinusitis. With increasing altitude, the air pressure in a plane may be reduced, causing pressure to build up in your head and blocking your sinuses or the eustachian tubes in your ears. Chewing gum or drinking water during takeoff and landing may help the pressure in your sinuses and lessen pain. Some doctors recommend that you use either decongestant nose drops or inhalers before your flight. Be sure to stay well hydrated by drinking plenty of noncaffeinated beverages while on board. Avoid drinking alcohol because it causes nasal and sinus membranes to swell. A saline nasal spray also helps maintain moist nasal passages during a long flight.

Acupuncture

Acupuncture is widely used for the treatment of sinusitis and allergic rhinitis. Treating specific points on the lung and large intestine channel which runs over the affected area can be useful, but a traditional Chinese diagnosis is required first. Four studies that looked at the use of acupuncture as a treatment for in allergic rhinitis suggest that it may be of value, however, the studies are of poor quality. A number of Chinese studies, again largely uncontrolled and of poor quality, also claim great benefit for acupuncture in rhinitis. There is one relatively poor study of acupuncture on sinus pain, which indicates significant benefit. As always with acupuncture, treatment should be tried for at least six weeks to determine whether it is effective in that particular person, especially with a chronic sinus infection.

Bodywork Therapies

NASAL SPECIFIC (NS) TECHNIQUE Many chiropractors, naturopaths, and cranial osteopaths treat chronic sinusitis and sinus headaches with a combination of spinal manipulation, massage, and the "nasal specific" technique. This treatment involves inflating very small balloons within the nasal passages, thereby creating a change of pressure and, theoretically, a realignment of the nasal bones, which is believed to relieve congestion. In a case study, a 41-year-old woman's sinus headaches disappeared immediately following treatment involving NS. At the end of two months of treatment, her sinus headaches were significantly reduced both in intensity and in frequency.

TRIGGER-POINT DEACTIVATION Trigger points (particularly sensitive areas; *see p. 55*) in the face may influence mucus production in the nose and sinuses. These can be deactivated by acupuncture, as well as by manual pressure.

CRANIAL MANIPULATION This practice involves applying extremely gentle pressure to the bones of the head and face, sometimes working inside the mouth. There are a number of safe cranial techniques to help drain the sinuses.

Breathing Retraining

If a person's breathing is shallow, the blood can become too alkaline. This causes histamine levels to rise and may consequently result in allergic responses, which can contribute to rhinitis and sinusitis. Breathing retraining involves doing yoga-type diaphragmatic breathing exercises, which have been shown to be very effective in improving both the mechanics and efficiency of breathing. (*For a breathing sequence, see p.62.*)

NASAL CLEANSE

Put a pinch of salt in about 7oz (200m) of warm water in a neti pot. Stand over a sink, tilt your head back, and pour the water into one nostril, allowing it to flow freely out the other nostril. Repeat two to three times daily, increasing to four times daily during bouts of sinusitis. There is some evidence that a hypertonic (more concentrated) salt solution may be more effective, but the risk of damage to the mucosal tissue is increased, so do not increase the amount of salt.

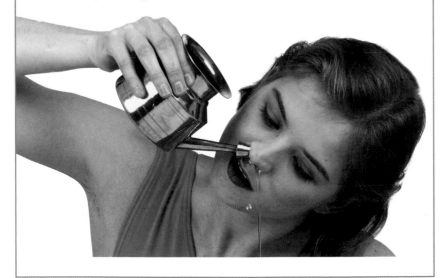

COLDS AND FLU

The common infections known as colds and flu are caused by viruses. There are at least 200 different viruses that cause the common cold, while true flu (or influenza) is caused by just two principal types of virus. Colds tend to have minor symptoms compared with flu, which usually causes a high fever and muscle aches. Treatment is directed at relieving symptoms and might include analgesics for muscle aches and decongestants for a blocked nose. Vitamin supplements, homeopathic and herbal medicines, and steam inhalations may also help.

WHAT ARE THE SYMPTOMS?

Symptoms of the common cold include:
- Sneezing
- Runny nose with discharge that is initially clear but sometimes becomes thick and green
- Mild fever and headache
- Sore throat and a cough

Symptoms of flu include:
- High fever, with sweating and shivering
- Aching muscles, especially in the back
- Severe exhaustion
- Frequent sneezing, runny nose, sore throat, and cough

WHY MIGHT I HAVE THIS?

PREDISPOSING FACTORS
- Exposure to others who have a cold or the flu
- Overwork and being "run down"
- Low immune function

IMPORTANT

If cold or flu symptoms persist for more than a week, or if symptoms of a secondary infection (such as earache or coughing up green or yellow sputum) develop, see your doctor. Babies, young children, the elderly and those with reduced immunity who develop flu symptoms should see a doctor immediately.

WHY DOES IT OCCUR?

Cold and flu viruses affect the upper respiratory tract and cause symptoms such as sneezing, runny nose, sore throat, and cough. Secondary bacterial infections that affect areas such as the ears, throat, or sinuses rarely develop as complications of either colds or flu.

The viruses responsible for colds and flu are all highly infectious and are spread in tiny airborne droplets from coughs and sneezes of infected people. They can also be spread by direct contact, often from hand to hand, and may live for hours on inanimate objects such as door handles, towels, or telephones.

Some people mistake a bad cold for the flu. Although many cases of influenza are mild, the flu tends to cause a high fever along with muscle aches and pains, symptoms that are not usually present in a cold.

Most people can expect to have between two and four colds a year. Children are more susceptible to colds compared to adults because they have not yet developed immunity to the viruses that cause colds.

There is no cure for the common cold or for flu. Both conditions tend to run their course in one to two weeks.

TREATMENT PLAN

PRIMARY TREATMENTS
- Rest and fluids
- Analgesics, NSAIDs, and decongestants
- Vitamin C and zinc
- Oscillococcinum and other homeopathic medicines
- Echinacea

BACKUP TREATMENTS
- Herbal medicines
- Regular exercise
- Environmental health measures

OTHER OPTIONS
- Chiropractic, osteopathy, massage
- Acupuncture
- Self-hypnosis

For an explanation of how treatments are rated, see p.111.

SELF-HELP

PRIMARY TREATMENT The following simple measures will help:
- Get plenty of rest.
- Drink lots of fluids, especially water.
- Take over-the-counter analgesics and decongestants to relieve symptoms.

TREATMENTS IN DETAIL

Conventional Medicine

It will probably not be necessary to see your doctor if you develop a cold or flu unless a secondary bacterial infection develops. Colds and flu are caused by viruses that cannot be treated with antibiotics. Elderly people and people with chronic conditions such as chronic lung conditions and diabetes mellitus may be offered immunization against flu. This needs to be repeated each year.

OVER-THE-COUNTER DRUGS
Cold and flu symptoms may
be relieved by analgesics and non-steroidal
anti-inflammatory drugs (NSAIDs), such
as acetaminophen or ibuprofen. Decongestants and cough remedies can be used to
soothe a scratchy throat. With both colds
and flu, it is important to drink plenty of
fluids, especially water.

PRESCRIPTION DRUGS If you only have a
cold, antibiotics do not help. They can
cause side effects such as diarrhea and
there is concern that over-prescription of
antibiotics is leading to increasing bacterial
resistance to them. Antibiotics are only
appropriate if a secondary bacterial infection develops. However, this does not
usually happen.

Antiviral drugs, such as neuraminidase
inhibitors, may be prescribed in some
cases. These drugs are recommended for
people with suspected flu ailments who are
over the age of 65 as well as those considered at risk because they have certain
chronic illnesses such as chronic lung
disease or diabetes mellitus. These may
also be prescribed for people who are
immunocompromised (their ability to
fight infection is impaired).

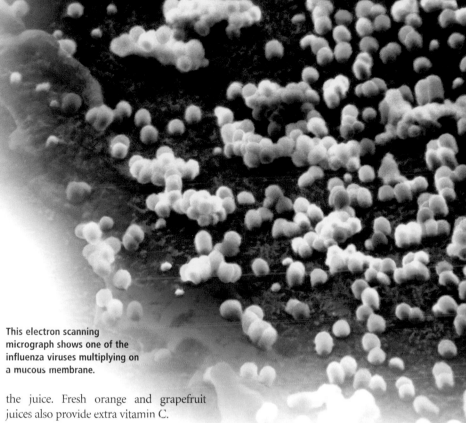

This electron scanning
micrograph shows one of the
influenza viruses multiplying on
a mucous membrane.

> **CAUTION**
>
> Over-the-counter and prescription drugs for
> colds and flu can cause side effects; ask your
> doctor or pharmacist to explain these to you.

Nutritional Therapy

VITAMIN C SUPPLEMENTS can
help prevent the common
cold, reducing the severity and duration of
symptoms in individuals who become
infected with the viruses that cause it. One
systematic review of 30 placebo-controlled
trials found evidence for high doses of vitamin C as a prophylaxis to limit the
duration and severity of colds, but it is
effective if not started until the symptoms
appear. Taking large doses of vitamin C can
sometimes cause diarrhea, but this clears
up once the dose is reduced. Try taking
500mg vitamin C per day to treat a cold.

You can eat foods rich in vitamin C as
well as taking supplements. Eat watercress
soup, fresh watercress, or juice it and drink

the juice. Fresh orange and grapefruit
juices also provide extra vitamin C.

ZINC Taking zinc lozenges
may shorten a common cold
but research results are mixed. Two systematic reviews came to slightly different
conclusions. One found that zinc lozenges
reduced symptoms after seven days, but
there were no differences after three or five
days. The second review (covering most of
the same trials) showed no improvement
in any cold symptoms after one week. A
subsequent study of people using an over-
the-counter zinc nasal gel within 24 hours
of a cold beginning showed they had a
shorter period of symptoms than did those
using a placebo. Start taking zinc gluconate
lozenges within 24 hours of the onset of
cold symptoms. Take one lozenge every
two hours throughout the day until symptoms disappear. Zinc may cause side
effects that include nausea and vomiting,
especially in children.

Although zinc gluconate is the most
commonly used form of zinc for treating
the common cold, zinc acetate may be an
even better form of zinc for this purpose.
Forms of zinc other than gluconate and
acetate should be avoided because they
may not release sufficient quantities of zinc
to be significantly effective. Also, the

lozenge should not contain citric acid, tar-
taric acid, mannitol, or sorbitol, since these
components can inactivate the zinc.

> **CAUTION**
>
> Consult your doctor before taking vitamin C
> with antibiotics or warfarin, or zinc with
> antibiotics. (*For more information, see p.46.*)

Homeopathy

A comparison of homeopathic and antibiotic treatments in children found that
those prescribed homeopathic treatment
had more positive results, fewer complications, and a higher quality of life compared
with those who were prescribed antibiotics.

OSCILLOCOCCINUM, a homeopathic speciality made by
Boiron, shows promise as a remedy for
reducing the duration of illness due to the
flu. This medicine is available as a treatment in the US as well as in France and
several other European countries.

ACONITE AND BELLADONNA are the most
commonly used single homeopathic

medicines for the early stages of colds and flu. Both should be started within a few hours of the onset of symptoms. People who respond to *Aconite* feel chilly, even though they may have quite a high fever, and may feel anxious. The skin is typically hot, red, and dry. They may be very thirsty for cold drinks and have a sensation of tingling on the tip of the tongue or lips.

People who respond to *Belladonna* often have a fever, the face is flushed and sweaty, and they may be confused — children may even hallucinate. The pupils are dilated, bright light and loud noises hurt, and sudden movement is painful. (Be aware that these symptoms can also be a sign of meningitis which needs immediate evaluation and treatment, *see p.391*).

GELSEMIUM may be useful after the initial stage of a cold or flu when the patient feels tired, weak, and tremulous and has profuse sweat but usually no thirst. *Gelsemium Sempervirens* is available in liquid or pill form in the US from manufacturers such as Boiron and WHP.

MERCURIUS SOLUBILIS AND EUPATO-RIUM PERFOLIATUM *Mercurius solubilis* is one of the most useful homeopathic medicines for colds that persist for three or four days. Symptoms often include a sore throat with swollen glands or thick green nasal discharge. People who respond to this medicine are always either too hot or too cold. They may have a great deal of perspiration and excessive saliva in the mouth. Their tongue feels sore and swollen, imprints of the teeth may visible around the edge of the tongue, and there may also be bad breath.

Eupatorium perfoliatum is a useful medicine for flu when there are a lot of muscular aches, as well as backache and pain in the eyes.

> **CAUTION**
>
> Many homeopathic medicines are neutralized by very strong smells (*see p.198*).

Western Herbal Medicine

Colds respond well to herbal self-help. Flu, caused by the influenza virus, is more serious than a cold, but taking herbs as soon as

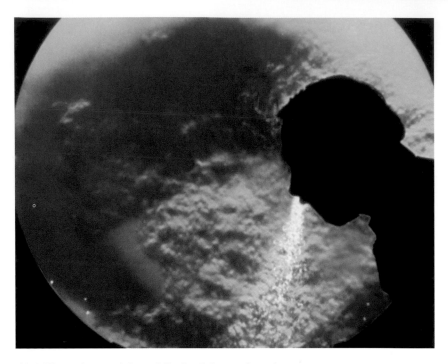

This Schlieren photograph (a specialized technique to show air turbulence) reveals what happens during a sneeze. Irritation of the nasal lining triggers a jet of droplets to erupt from the mouth and nose. An unprotected sneeze can travel 9ft (3m).

you start to feel ill can ease symptoms and decrease the duration of the symptoms.

SPICES At the first sign of a cold, infuse three slices of fresh ginger in a cup of boiling water for 10 minutes. Drink a cup every three or four hours. Ginger has a warming, stimulating effect that brings on a therapeutic sweat. A recent study has shown it has a significant action against four different strains of bacteria that may cause secondary infection following colds or flu. Cinnamon, cloves, and black pepper are also warming herbs.

PRIMARY TREATMENT **ECHINACEA** There are three types of echinacea: *Echinacea pallida, E. pallida* var. *angustifolia,* and *E. purpurea*. It is important to know the species and specific use of each so that you get the best effect. For example, none of the studies that tested echinacea for colds found that it could prevent their occurrence. Some studies that examined echinacea as a treatment for a cold once the symptoms were apparent have had mixed results, while one review of 16 trials suggested that, overall, echinacea does work. It appears that some forms of *Echinacea*

purpurea can decrease the duration of cold symptoms in adults, but it doesn't seem to work for children, or in college students when combined with *angustifolia*. Recent research casts doubt on the effectiveness of some preparations of *Echinacea angustifolia* root against some cold viruses.

ANDROGRAPHIS A promising new cold herb from India is *Andrographis paniculata*, used in Ayervedic and Chinese medicine. In one double-blind study, 208 people with upper respiratory tract infections were given either andrographis or a placebo. By the second day, the cold symptoms (runny nose and sore throat) in the andrographis group had improved compared to those given just the placebo. By the fourth day there was a significant improvement in cough, headaches, earache, and fatigue.

STEAM INHALATION Try a few drops of Olbas oil, eucalyptus oil (*Eucalyptus globulus*), or chamomile (*Matricaria recutita*) in a bowl, pour in boiling water and inhale the steam, while covering your head with a towel. One research study of chamomile steam inhalation using this method showed that it improved cold symptoms.

OTHER TRADITIONAL MEASURES Tea made by infusing elderflower (*Sambucus nigra*) and peppermint (*Mentha piperita*) and adding 3–4 slices of ginger is used for colds. Add yarrow (*Achillea millefolium*) if you have flu. Drink a full teacup of this every four hours. Alternatively, fresh hyssop (*Hyssopus officinalis*) tea is good for colds and flu. Add a teaspoonful of honey, especially manuka honey, to hot drinks. It has antibacterial properties and helps soothe sore throats.

Garlic (*Allium sativum*), mustard (*Brassica alba*), and horseradish (*Cochlearia armoracia*) have important properties that help combat colds and flu. As well as using them in cooking, you can try the old-fashioned remedy of soaking your feet in a mustard bath. Use a plastic bowl big enough to fit both your feet and pour 1gal (3 l) of hot water in, mixing three tablespoons of English mustard powder. Put your feet in the bowl for 10 minutes and cover your head with a towel while you do so in order to increase the heat in your head and sinuses. Do this morning and evening for the duration of your cold or flu symptoms.

Finally, tiger balm and Olbas oil may help ease congestion when applied externally. Rub tiger balm onto your chest and back, being careful not to get any in your eyes. Wash your hands carefully after application. Alternatively, apply Olbas oil to your temples and the back of your neck. Keep away from your eyes.

> **CAUTION**
>
> See p.69 before taking a herbal remedy and, if you are taking prescribed medication, consult an herbal medicine expert first.

Chinese Herbal Medicine

Traditional Chinese Medicine (TCM) practitioners believe adverse climatic factors can breach the body's defense system (called *Wei Qi*), causing colds and flu. In particular, wind is said to be "the initiator of 100 diseases." Wind combines with other disease-causing factors, such as cold, heat, and damp. Treatments aim to improve lung function, increasing the protection afforded by *Wei Qi*. Many treatments are said to "open the exterior" and produce a therapeutic sweat, which

drives out adverse climatic factors of wind, cold, heat, or damp.

One simple general remedy is soybean soup (*Cong Chi Tang*). This comprises stalks of green onion combined with prepared soybeans to which have been added perilla leaf (*Zi Su Ye* or *Perilla frutescens*), Quiang Huo (*Notopterygium incisum*), siler (*Fang Feng* or *Ledebouriella seseloides*), and schizonepeta (*Jing Jie* or *Schizonepeta tenuifolia*). In more severe wind-cold patterns, TCM doctors use stronger prescriptions, such as Schizonepeta-Ledebouriella Defeat Poison Powder (*Jing Fang Bai Du San*).

WIND-DAMP INVASION If the pattern is wind-cold damp invasion, you will have a heavy feeling in the head and feel tired, possibly with nausea, loss of appetite, bloating, and loose stools. In such cases a TCM doctor might prescribe Notopterygium Conquering Dampness Decoction (*Qiang Huo Sheng Shi Tang*).

WIND-HEAT INVASION Wind-heat colds and flu are marked by feelings of cold and heat in which heat predominates. The person may have a stuffy nose, a cough, and a sore throat. The classical remedy is the famous Honeysuckle and Forsythia Powder (*Yin Qiao San*) available in pill form. The timing of taking Yin Qiao San is important — it is recommended to take it as soon as one realizes the symptoms of Wind invasion. Another popular formula is Gan Mao Ling, which is used after the initial Wind-Heat invasion turns to Wind-Cold symptoms.

INVASION OF DRYNESS Another common pattern is invasion of dryness (said to be a feature of autumn colds and flus). The usual prescription for this syndrome is a variation of the Mulberry Almond Decoction (*Sang Xin Tang*).

INTERNAL DEFICIENCIES such as *Qi*, Blood, *Yin*, or *Yang* deficiency are treated with specific formulas. Two remedies from

the woad family that have antiviral properties, *Ban Lan Gen* and *Da Qing Ye,* are often added to cold formulas.

> **CAUTION**
>
> Do not use Chinese herbal remedies without first consulting an herbal medicine expert.

Environmental Health

AVOIDING CROWDS AND CONFINED SPACES The most obvious way to avoid getting colds or flu is to avoid crowds and confined areas during the peak cold season, which is early autumn, and the peak flu season, which is in the winter. You are at greatest risk of getting infected in highly populated areas such as in crowded living conditions, in schools, or on public transportation. A problem with preventing exposure to colds and flu is that people are most contagious from a day or so before they develop symptoms, making it difficult to identify contagious individuals.

KEEP YOUR HANDS AWAY FROM YOUR FACE Keep in mind that flu and colds can also be spread by inanimate objects such as towels, toys, and door handles that carry disease-causing germs. Germs commonly live on these objects for minutes or hours, sometimes even longer. If you touch a contaminated surface, germs can easily pass from your hand to your nose or mouth and lead to infection. Keep your fingers away from your nose, mouth, and eyes to avoid infecting yourself with viral particles that you may have picked up.

HAND WASHING Wash your hands regularly and thoroughly. One recent study done with hospital personnel showed the effectiveness of an alcohol-based hand rub, which was distributed widely in patient care areas. The result was a remarkable increase in those cleaning their hands effectively and consistently and a corresponding huge drop in infection rates. The

Antibiotics have no effect against viruses, which are the cause of colds and flu

convenience of handwashing with this hand rub was largely responsible for the results. Alcohol-based handrubs may be preferred because they are faster than hand washing, less drying to the skin, and easier to use. The effectiveness of these alcohol-based instant soaps against cold and flu viruses has been demonstrated.

HUMIDITY When mucus membranes become dry, it is easier for them to become infected with cold or flu viruses. Use a humidifier or put bowls of water near radiators or heat vents at home. One study emphasized the importance of maintaining an adequate humidity level at

> ## Colds are more frequent in children, due to their lower resistance to infection

home to prevent the mucous membranes in the nose from drying out. Drinking plenty of water helps protect mucous membranes as well.

BREATHING THROUGH THE NOSE This warms and humidifies the air before it reaches the lungs. Breathing through the mouth dries the throat.

OTHER MEASURES You can help prevent the spread of colds and flu by putting a second towel in the bathroom for healthy people to use. Remember to cover your nose and mouth with a tissue when you cough or sneeze, then throw the tissue away and wash your hands. Be sure to use tissues rather than a handkerchief. If you need to travel by air during the cold and flu season, drink plenty of water to combat dehydration. Wash your hands frequently while on board — you can also use alcohol handwipes. A nasal saline spray (preferably free of preservatives) can help keep your nasal passages moist and prevent dryness and cracking.

Acupuncture

Acupuncture is frequently used in China to treat acute (sudden and short-lived) conditions that usually resolve on their own, such as colds and flu. People in China

might be treated two or three times a day for colds and flu, often on the lung and large intestine meridian.

There are no clinical trials in this area, but many patients seek acupuncture for these conditions.

Practitioners believe that acupuncture can quickly stimulate an immune response that would be appropriate in acute viral infections such as colds and flu and would be likely to speed recovery.

Bodywork Therapies

LYMPHATIC DRAINAGE There is substantial evidence that using specific osteopathic methods, which are known collectively as lymphatic pump techniques, can increase the immune system's response to infection. These techniques work by markedly increasing levels of natural killer cells and B and T lymphocytes in the bloodstream (important components of the immune system) for up to 24 hours after the techniques have been applied. The increased levels of these cells appear to offer real advantages to the individual fighting infection of any sort.

MASSAGE, CHIROPRACTIC, AND OSTEOPATHY Immune enhancement in which levels of natural killer cells and B and T lymphocyte are significantly increased has also been observed in people after they have received general, nonspecific, massage. Similary, immune enhancement has been observed following specific chiropractic spinal manipulation. It is not clear how long this effect lasts or whether or not it would help colds.

The ways in which these methods improve immune function are not fully understood. However, it is thought that the osteopathic method stimulates production, or release from storage sites, of helpful immune substances. Massage is thought to reduce the presence of "stress hormones," thus improving the efficiency of the immune system. Chiropractic treatment is

thought to achieve its effect through the nervous system, in a similar way to osteopathic treatment. In order to benefit from these aspects of bodywork, consult a suitably qualified and licensed osteopath, chiropractor, or massage therapist.

Exercise

Lifestyle factors, including exercise, can strengthen (and also reduce) immune responses. A study of 50 women showed that a group taking regular exercise (walking briskly for 45 minutes, five days each week) had half as many colds as a group that did no exercise. People who exercise had more natural killer cells — one of the body's first lines of defense against viruses. However, most research suggests that while moderate exercise boosts immunity, too much leaves you prone to infection.

Mind–Body Therapies

Mental disharmony is known to undermine immunity. Major life events, such as moving to a new house or losing a loved one, also undermine immunity, as do high levels of anxiety. The accumulation of daily stresses may also adversely affect the immune system, which is why adequate rest and self-care can help boost immunity.

SELF-HYPNOSIS Studies have shown that stress reduces the immune responsiveness of the mucous membranes. Self-hypnosis might help people who are prone to colds when they are under stress. A study of medical students at exam time found that self-hypnosis incorporating imagery of the immune system can reduce the effects of stress on immune function. Results in the imagery group showed heightened immune function, improvements in mood, and fewer winter viral infections.

PREVENTION PLAN

The following may help to protect you against colds and flu:

- Eat a healthy diet rich in fresh fruit and vegetables.
- Wash your hands regularly and avoid crowds during cold and flu season.
- Get plenty of rest

ASTHMA

Asthma causes attacks of wheezing and shortness of breath. When someone with asthma inhales irritant particles, the immune system overreacts and produces histamine. This causes the muscle walls of the bronchi to contract, constricting the airways. Unless your asthma is mild, drugs are crucial for dilating airways and reducing inflammation. In integrated medicine, these are backed up with therapies to stretch the chest muscles and encourage easier breathing. Diet can play a part in susceptibility, so dietary change may be a key part of your plan.

WHAT ARE THE SYMPTOMS?

- Main symptom may be a persistent, dry cough
- Wheezing
- Feeling tight in the chest
- Shortness of breath
- Difficulty exhaling

Symptoms may be accompanied by:

- Sweating
- Feelings of panic
- Inability to complete a sentence due to shortness of breath

If an attack is very severe, symptoms may include:

- Wheezing that is inaudible because so little air is entering the airways
- Inability to speak properly
- Blue lips, tongue, and fingers due to lack of oxygen
- Exhaustion, confusion, and coma

WHY MIGHT I HAVE THIS?

PREDISPOSING FACTORS

- Allergies
- Smoking
- Genetic tendency
- Diet low in fatty acids

TRIGGERS (FOR EXISTING ASTHMA)

- Irritants, such as pollen
- Contact with birds or some animals
- Stress
- Beta-blockers and other drugs
- Cold air
- Exercise
- Respiratory infection

IMPORTANT

If you have symptoms, see your doctor for a diagnosis. Severe asthma attacks can be life-threatening without immediate medical treatment. If you have an attack, see Immediate Relief (*p.206*) and if necessary call a doctor or 911 or your local EMS. Never stop taking conventional medication for asthma without consulting your doctor.

WHY DOES IT OCCUR?

In an asthma attack, the immune system reacts to an inhaled substance and produces immunoglobulin E (IgE) antibodies. These substances stimulate the release of histamine in the lining of the airways which consequently become inflamed and swollen. The excess mucus that is produced can block the smaller airways. The resulting wheezing and shortness of breath can last for hours or days and be exhausting and, in some cases, life threatening. The airways of many people with asthma can become persistently inflamed over time. There is a wide range of factors that either trigger attacks or can make you more susceptible to them (*see left*). For some people, asthma is triggered by exposure to an allergen, such as pollen, dust mites, animal dander, or, less commonly, certain foods or food additives. This type of asthma tends to develop in childhood and can be genetic. It may appear along with hay fever and eczema.

In some cases, the first asthma attack is triggered by a respiratory infection. Some people develop occupational asthma as a result of exposure to workplace substances such as glues, resins, latex, and spray paints. Air pollution does not seem to cause asthma, but it may make existing asthma worse or act as a trigger. Stress can also bring on asthma attacks. In some people, exercise triggers attacks.

ASTHMA RATES WORLDWIDE The numbers of people with asthma have soared in recent decades in the US, Australia, New Zealand, and the UK. Australia has one of the world's highest asthma rates with 14–16 percent of children and 10–12 percent of adults affected. In Melbourne, over 25 percent of children have asthma.

Except in big cities, asthma rates in Asian countries are half those of developed countries. Asthma rates are increasing the fastest among the poor and the young. In the US, for example, the disease is particularly prevelant among young inner-city ethnic minorties. It would seem, therefore, that poverty, stress, pollution, race, and urbanization are key factors in the increase of the disease. But that does not explain why the world's highest rate of asthma is in Tristan da Cunha — a remote, unpolluted island in the South Atlantic.

TREATMENT PLAN

PRIMARY TREATMENTS

- Reliever and prevention drugs
- Avoiding environmental triggers

BACKUP TREATMENTS

- Food elimination diet
- Western and Chinese herbal medicine
- Breathing retraining

WORTH CONSIDERING

- Low-salt diet and other dietary changes
- Homeopathy
- Acupuncture
- Bodywork therapies and exercise
- Mind-body therapies

For an explanation of how treatments are rated, see p.111.

- Take your usual dose of inhaled medication on a regular basis, preferably using a spacer device.
- Stay calm and relax (but don't lie down).
- Try to breathe slowly for 5–10 minutes. If symptoms disappear, you can resume normal activities.
- If severe symptoms persist, call 911 or your local EMS. Use your inhaler every few minutes until help arrives.

TREATMENTS IN DETAIL

Conventional Medicine

Your doctor will consider possible triggers. He or she may assess your breathing by asking you to blow into a peak flow meter, a device that records the maximum flow of air you can produce when you exhale. This can be reduced if you have asthma and there may be a marked difference in morning and evening readings if your asthma is not adequately controlled. Your doctor may also arrange for you to have lung function tests to test your breathing, and you may also be gi ven allergy tests.

You will be asked to keep a record of your peak flow readings to monitor your condition and adjust your treatment or see the doctor as appropriate. He or she will assess your progress and alter your treatment if your symptoms are not being adequately controlled.

Asthma drugs are mainly taken with an inhaler, sometimes used with a "spacer" — a plastic device placed between the mouth and the inhaler, making it easier to inhale the drug and preventing it from sticking to the inside of the mouth and throat, which can increase the incidence of side effects. Spacers are especially useful for young children and elderly people, but everyone with asthma should use one. A nebulizer delivers drugs as a fine mist that is inhaled through a face mask or mouthpiece.

PRIMARY TREATMENT **RELIEVER AND PREVENTER DRUGS** Your doctor is likely to prescribe a reliever drug, such as salbutamol, to take when you have symptoms. These are short-acting bronchodilators that relax the muscles of the airways, allowing air to pass in and out more easily. Reliever drugs usually start working within

INHALING ASTHMA DRUGS

Inhaling is an efficient way of taking drugs for asthma because the chemicals reach the airways quickly. Very little of the medication enters the bloodstream so there are few side effects. In an asthma attack, the walls of the airways of the lungs constrict and excess mucus collects, so less air can pass through, which consequently makes breathing difficult. A few minutes after taking a reliever drug, the airway walls dilate and breathing becomes easier.

Effects of asthma drugs on the airways

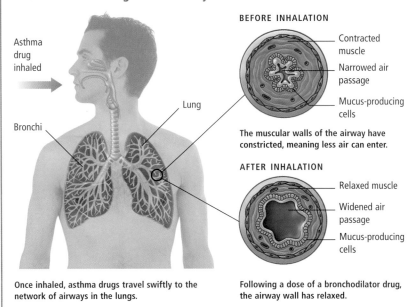

Asthma drug inhaled

Lung

Bronchi

BEFORE INHALATION

Contracted muscle

Narrowed air passage

Mucus-producing cells

The muscular walls of the airway have constricted, meaning less air can enter.

AFTER INHALATION

Relaxed muscle

Widened air passage

Mucus-producing cells

Once inhaled, asthma drugs travel swiftly to the network of airways in the lungs.

Following a dose of a bronchodilator drug, the airway wall has relaxed.

5–10 minutes of being inhaled, but their effects last for only a few hours. The doctor may tell you to take a reliever drug before you exercise.

You may have to take preventer drugs daily. These are mainly inhaled corticosteroids such as beclometasone, taken to reduce inflammation in the airway linings and make them less likely to narrow in response to triggers.

LONGER-ACTING BRONCHODILATORS, such as salmeterol may be prescribed. They also relax the muscles of the airways but unlike shorter-acting bronchodilators, their effects last up to 12 hours.

LEUKOTRIENE ANTAGONISTS may also be prescribed if symptoms persist. These work by dampening the allergic response and preventing narrowing of the airways.

ORAL CORTICOSTEROID DRUGS Courses of these drugs may also be prescribed for very severe asthma.

CAUTION

Asthma drugs can have a range of possible side effects; ask your doctor to explain these. People with asthma should avoid taking beta-blockers, aspirin, and nonsteroidal anti-inflammatory drugs (NSAIDs).

Nutritional Medicine

A FOOD EXCLUSION DIET is recommended (*see* p.39) since food sensitivities can be an underlying factor, especially in childhood asthma. In one study, 91 percent of children with respiratory allergies improved if they were put on a six-week diet that excluded common problem foods such as grains and dairy products.

FISH OILS may help since asthma may be related to an imbalance in fatty acids in the diet. Excessive amounts of omega-6 fatty acids (found in vegetable oils) and a relative lack of omega-3 fats (found in oily fish and some nuts and seeds) may promote inflammation of the airways which can aggravate asthma. Try cutting back on margarine and vegetable oils and eating at least two portions of oily fish a week (such as salmon, trout, herring, or mackerel). Children may also take 300mg of fish oil a day. A Cochrane review of randomized controlled trials of fish oils for asthma found the treatment harmless but its beneficial effects inconsistent.

> **CAUTION**
>
> Fish-oil supplements may affect the action of certain drugs, such as the blood-thinning drug warfarin; ask your doctor for advice.

A LOW-SALT DIET may help reduce asthma symptoms. Salt seems to increase the response of the airways to histamine, causing increased airway constriction. You should avoid adding salt to dishes and limit the amount of processed foods you eat. One study found that an additional 6.1g of salt per day made the symptoms worse for patients with asthma and increased their use of inhaled corticosteroid drugs. A low-salt diet (5–6g of salt per day) appears to have a favorable effect and reduces the need for antiasthma drugs. In another study of people with exercise-induced asthma, a low-salt diet improved and a high-salt diet worsened postexercise lung function.

VITAMIN C A low intake of vitamin C is thought to affect asthma. You can try taking 500mg–1g of vitamin C a day and 100mcg of selenium (adult doses), both of which are potent antioxidants. Children who weigh less than 100 lbs (40kg) should take half this dose and even less should be administered to smaller children.

MAGNESIUM may be helpful for people with asthma. Magnesium is found in nuts, seeds, and whole-grain foods. A study of children found that low intakes of magnesium were associated with poorer lung function. In children, eating fresh fruit has been related to fewer asthma symptoms and improved lung function. This protective effect was evident even in children who only ate fruit once or twice a week.

BREAST-FEEDING YOUR BABY may help reduce the risk of childhood asthma. One study found an increased risk of asthma if exclusive breast-feeding was stopped before the baby was four months old. Also, taking probiotics during pregnancy and then giving them to your baby may help prevent asthma. The gut microflora of infants who develop asthma appears to be different from those who do not develop it according to studies. In one study, the probiotic Lactobacillus GG was given to pregnant women who had at least one first-degree relative (or partner) with an allergic condition such as atopic eczema, allergic rhinitis, or asthma. After birth, the probiotic was also given to the child for six months. Probiotic supplements were found to significantly reduce the risk of early allergic disease in children who were at a high risk of developing it.

Homeopathy

There are three ways homeopathy can treat asthma: isopathy, acute treatment, and constitutional treatment (see p.73).

Isopathy involves taking homeopathic dilutions of allergens (such as dust mites or pollen). You should not take isopathic remedies when you have symptoms, since they work best during the "plateau" phase. The evidence for the effectiveness of isopathy is controversial, some is positive, some not. However, isopathy is only a small part of homeopathy and deeper effects can be achieved by whole person, individualized treatment.

Homeopathy can also be used for acute attacks of asthma when prescribed on the basis of a small number of typical "keynote" symptoms. There is little scientific research on individualized homepathy for asthma. The research that does exist is generally positive, although not conclusive. Notably, surveys that determine patient satisfaction with the results of homeopathic treatment are consistently positive.

ISOPATHY is helpful if you are sensitive to a known single substance, however if you do not have allergic asthma or have multiple sensitivities, it is unlikely to help. For dust sensitivity, take *House dust mite* 30C, two pills weekly. Do not take it during a flare-up because it works best during the quiescent phase. If asthma is triggered by pollen, start isopathy several months before the pollen season starts and stop a few weeks before the season ends.

ARSENICUM ALBUM is a remedy that is commonly used to treat asthma and is appropriate when the person affected feels chilly and very frightened during an asthma attack. People who respond to it frequently have dry skin problems including eczema and psoriasis.

> The Centers for Disease Control estimate that 15 million Americans suffer from asthma

KALIUM CARBONICUM, IPECACHUANA, AND ANTIMONIUM TARTARICUM *Kali carb* is another frequently used medicine, particularly for asthma that persists after a chest infection. Typically, asthma that responds to *Kali carb* is worse from 3–4 am. *Ipecachuana* is mostly given to children with asthma, particularly if they cough up a lot of mucus and feel sick. *Antimonium tart* may be appropriate if the child is coughing but when little mucus is brought up. The recommended dose is two pills of the 6C dilution every half hour when the child is having an attack. For long-term asthma, give two 6C pills three times a day.

Western Herbal Medicine

Herbal medicine can be helpful for people with asthma but the guidance of an herbal medicine expert is vitally important. An herbal medicine practitioner will assess the symptoms and prescribe a mixture of herbs to support easier breathing and reduce underlying allergies. The use of conventional medicines such as inhalers can be gradually reduced when symptoms and peak flow meter readings improve.

EPHEDRA used to be commonly prescribed herb for asthma, but with the recent ban by the Food and Drug Administration, ephedra products are no longer available. Ephedra (*Ephedra sinica*) contains ephedrine, a bronchodilator that eases spasm of the airways, but also causes serious side effects on the heart and vessels of the body. Instead, a mix that includes expectorants such as thyme (*Thymus serpillum*), elecampane (*Inula1 helenium*), and hyssop (*Hyssopus officinalis*) may be prescribed.

OTHER HERBS Antiallergic herbs, such as nettle (*Urtica* spp.) and ginkgo (*Ginkgo biloba*) leaf, are usually prescribed, and butterbur (*Petasites hybridus*) root may also be effective. Herbs such as marshmallow (*Althea officinalis*) soothe irritated mucous membranes lining the respiratory tract. Coltsfoot (*Tussilago farfara*) and wild cherry bark (*Prunus serotina*) may be recommended to ease coughing. Calming herbs such as chamomile (*Matricaria recutita*) and cramp bark (*Viburnum opulus*) are useful for relieving anxiety.

> **CAUTION**
>
> See p.69 before taking a herbal remedy. Do not self-treat with herbs for asthma; many are strong-acting with a range of side effects and can be dangerous if misused. Do not combine herbal and conventional asthma treatments without expert advice.

Chinese Herbal Medicine

In Ttraditional Chinese Medicine (TCM), asthma is equivalent to *Xiao Chuan* (wheezing and shortness of breath). TCM perceives asthma as primarily caused by phlegm that blocks the airways. TCM doctors distinguish between "cold" asthma (characterized by wheezing, shortness of breath, and a cough producing frothy white or clear sputum) and "hot" asthma (with hoarse breathing, a hacking cough, and yellow sticky sputum that may be difficult to cough up).

"COLD" ASTHMA *Xiao Qing Long Tang* (Lesser Blue Dragon Decoction) is the classic treatment for "cold" asthma. It warms the lungs, dispels cold and wind, relieves cold phlegm, and eases breathlessness.

"HOT" ASTHMA In "hot" asthma, the patient's tongue is red with a sticky, yellow coat and the pulse is rapid. Typically *Ding Chuan Tang* (Stop Asthma Decoction) is prescribed and clears lung heat, relieves phlegm, and "descends lung *Qi*."

SAIBOKU-TO This traditional Chinese herbal formulation has been shown to have a positive effect in treating asthma. The use of Saiboku-To can result in lowering the amounts of steroid medications needed to control chronic asthma. This formulation has also been found to have anti-inflammatory properties.

> **CAUTION**
>
> Do not self-treat with Chinese herbs.

Environmental Health

PRIMARY TREATMENT Environmental substances can trigger asthma attcks. The small airways of the lungs are susceptible to allergens, toxins, and irritants, and these should be avoided as much as possible.

PETS Indoor pets are a main cause of asthma attacks. If you have tested positive for allergies to pets (usually cats), the best option would be to avoid living with them. If this is not possible, the bedroom at least should become a "pet-free" zone. Regular pet bathing seems important. A vacuum cleaner with a high efficiency particle air (HEPA) filter may be useful. There is a lot of evidence, however, that early exposure to pets or farm animals reduces the incidence of asthma.

DUST MITES Another important perennial indoor allergen is the dust mite. These microscopic organisms live in bedding, upholstered furniture, and carpeting and leave behind highly allergenic droppings. A recent study suggests that using a mite-impermeable mattress cover as a single intervention is not effective. However, as part of a systematic approach that includes a weekly washing of bed linens in hot water, removal of as much carpeting from the house as is practical, elimination of stuffed toys on beds, and maintenance of home humidity levels below 40 or 50 percent, this measure may be very valuable. It is likely that reducing exposure to mites in the home will help people with allergies.

Installing a highly filtered closed vacuum system or using a vacuum cleaner with a HEPA filter are better alternatives than simple vacuuming.

MOLD AND COCKROACHES Numerous species of mold live around leaky pipes and in bathrooms that are not adequately ventilated. Removing obvious mold on surfaces and increasing ventilation in rooms where mold is found are useful steps. Also, cockroaches have been shown to be a significant asthma trigger. Appropriate removal, preferably without harmful pesticides, is an important step.

POLLEN Outdoor allergens are less controllable than indoor allergens and present more of a problem. Tree pollen, for example, can be blown for hundreds of miles, making life miserable for allergic individuals who do not even live near trees. Keep windows closed on days when the pollen count is high and use an air conditioner with an electrostatic micron-range furnace filter if possible. People with asthma should also avoid grass as much as possible and should not mow lawns or be present when grass is being cut. In the autumn, susceptible people should not rake leaves, since allergenic molds live in decomposing leaves and are a leading cause in cases of life-threatening asthma.

COLD AIR In cold weather, wearing a mask or scarf that allows air to be humidified and warmed is useful because cold, dry winter air can cause airway constriction in nearly all types of asthma. It is also important to breathe through the nose to provide humidification and warming of the air before it gets to the lungs.

ODORS Many people with asthma find that strong odors can trigger wheezing or chest tightness. These include strong cleaning solutions, perfumes, and car exhaust. When possible, avoid exposure to strong-smelling substances, especially in confined areas with inadequate ventilation. If exposure is inevitable, wear a respirator mask.

Acupuncture

Acupuncture is popular in China for asthma treatment. Although studies of acupuncture and asthma have been performed, a Cochrane review found most trials to be poor. Real acupuncture was no more effective than sham acupuncture in several clinical trials; however the "sham" points stimulated may have been active points for asthma. A review of acupuncture in asthma concludes that the trials are generally positive though very limited.

An acupuncturist will first make the traditional Chinese diagnosis (see p.82). The "pathogen cold" is frequently part of the diagnosis. He or she will then insert

showed no benefit of chiropractic for asthma. Randomized controlled trials and a Cochrane review concluded that there is insufficient evidence to support the use of manual therapies for asthma.

MASSAGE given regularly may help reduce stress and asthma symptoms. In a recent study (Field, 1998), children with asthma were given either 20 minutes of massage or regular relaxation instruction from their parents. Anxiety and lung function in the

method led to both reduced use of corticosteroid medications and improved breathing function.

Yoga

Yoga has been shown to be helpful in treating asthma.

Mind–Body Therapies

Although the exact mechanisms are not fully understood, stress may increase the demand for oxygen throughout the body, especially in the brain. If lung capacity is reduced due to asthma, this increased demand for oxygen may intensify stress.

Research shows a link between emotional distress and poor compliance with taking prescription medications. Taking asthma medication incorrectly is a common problem and can increase the severity of asthma symptoms. Studies have also shown that when stress increases, asthma symptoms may become exaggerated, although people under stress may be less able to judge their symptoms accurately and more likely to underestimate their severity. This could result in a severe attack not being treated in time. A review of relaxation therapies that have been used in the treatment of asthma concluded that muscular relaxation was the only relaxation technique that may improve lung function.

STRESS-MANAGEMENT PROGRAM A recent trial showed that a four-week self-administered program was very effective for people with asthma.

AUTOGENIC TRAINING AND MEDITATION Autogenic training, in which you learn mental exercises that help you teach your body to relax, can be useful in managing asthma. Alternatively, you could try meditation (see p.98). A study of transcendental meditation (TM) suggested that people who meditate had less severe asthma.

> Swimming is good exercise for asthma. The moist pool environment may be a helpful factor

acupuncture needles into various meridian points and will probably also use cupping and moxibustion to provide heat on the relevant acupuncture points. Some acupuncturists in China use embedded or permanent needles to treat asthma, but this is uncommon in other countries. You will probably need weekly treatment for 10–12 weeks to evaluate whether acupuncture is going to help you.

Bodywork Therapies

SOFT-TISSUE MANIPULATION (deep massage-type manipulation) can significantly relax the breathing muscles and mobilize the spine and ribs, making breathing easier. A recent study demonstrated that these methods can improve movement of the chest, increase air flow, and ease chronic asthma symptoms. Osteopaths, chiropractors, and physical therapists can provide soft-tissue manipulation.

If the nervous system is in "alarm" phase — when you are anxious — breathing becomes rapid and shallow and asthma symptoms increase. The vagal nerve, which runs from the neck, has branches that influence breathing function. Stimulation of the vagal nerve has been shown to help normalize the excessive degree of activity of the nerves, which can accompany asthma. A practitioner can manipulate the thoracic spine (the first four or five vertebrae below the neck) and the first joint of the neck to influence the activity of the vagal nerve, relax the diaphragm, and help ease asthma symptoms. The two best studies

children aged six to eight who were massaged improved more in the short term than those in the group that practiced relaxation. Children aged nine to 11 improved whether the treatment they received was massage or relaxation.

Exercise

Research shows that exercise helps people with asthma by improving fitness and breathing rate and increasing the amount of air movement through the lungs, which in turn improves oxygen supplies.

Breathing Retraining

Breathing retraining appears to be a promising treatment for asthma as many people suffering from asthma have evidence of dysfunctional breathing. Pursed lip breathing exercises improve the mechanics and efficiency of breathing. Inhale slowly through your nose and then, pursing your lips as if blowing up a balloon, exhale slowly for 4–6 seconds through your mouth. Practice for several minutes each day. In one study, patients who were taught basic yoga breathing, similar to the pursed-lip breathing described above, used less medication and had improved breathing function, which was still apparent four years after the study finished.

THE BUTEYKO METHOD is a similar form of breathing rehabilitation (with specific variations, including controlled breath-holding). Several studies of this Russian

PREVENTION PLAN

The following may help:
- Avoid known allergens
- Do not smoke
- Relax regularly

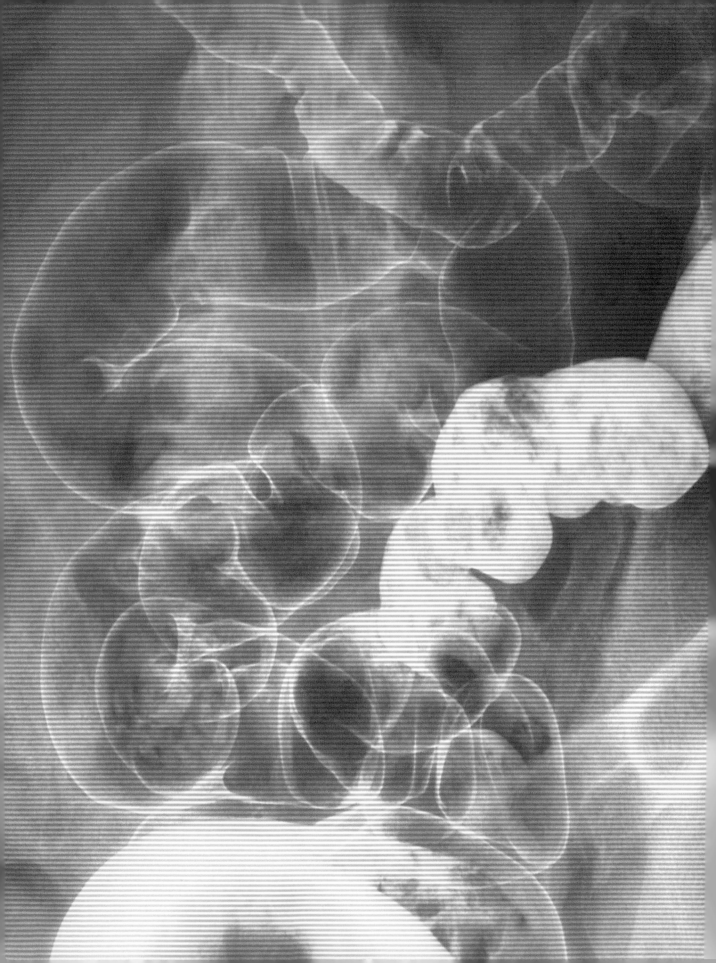

Digestive & Urinary Systems

The digestive and urinary systems convert food into fuel and nutrients, then excrete anything unwanted. Our nutrition, immune defenses, state of mind, and habitual posture can all affect these core systems. The holistic approach of integrated medicine works to counter stress and to support the digestive system's natural healing processes.

PEPTIC ULCER AND GASTRITIS

A peptic ulcer is an eroded area in the lining of the stomach or the duodenum, the first part of the small intestine. Gastritis is inflammation of the stomach lining, which may begin suddenly and be short-lived (acute) or may develop gradually and persist (chronic). Although once considered a stress-related disorder, doctors now realize that most people with ulcers or chronic gastritis have the bacterium *Helicobacter pylori* in their stomachs. Eradicating *H. pylori* is key to treating ulcers and chronic gastritis. Natural medicines may also help.

WHAT ARE THE SYMPTOMS?

Symptoms of peptic ulcers include:
- Pain or discomfort in the middle of the upper abdomen
- Loss of appetite and weight loss
- Nausea and occasional vomiting

Symptoms of gastritis include:
- Discomfort or pain in the middle of the upper abdomen

WHY MIGHT I HAVE THIS?

PREDISPOSING FACTORS
- Infection with *H. pylori*
- Smoking
- Drinking excessive amounts of alcohol
- Nonsteroidal anti-inflammatory drugs
- Foods that increase stomach acid secretion
- Trigger point activity

IMPORTANT

If you develop symptoms of peptic ulcer or chronic gastritis, see your doctor. Gastritis that is accompanied by gastroesophageal reflux disease (GERD), in which stomach contents are regularly regurgitated back up into the esophagus, should be treated by a doctor. GERD can contribute to esophageal cancer if left untreated.

WHY DOES IT OCCUR?

The bacterium *Helicobacter pylori* has been found to be associated with chronic inflammation and ulceration of the stomach and duodenal lining. The discovery of *H. pylori* in the early 1980s revolutionized the treatment of peptic ulcers. *H. pylori* may be found in the stomach lining of approximately half the population, but it is not known why it causes digestive problems in some people and not in others. It is thought that the bacteria may be transmitted orally.

How *H. pylori* contributes to peptic ulcers and gastritis is not known, but it may be that the body's immune response to the bacteria causes inflammation of the stomach lining. Gastritis and ulcers can also occur without an *H. pylori* infection.

Other factors that may play a role in the development of peptic ulcer and chronic gastritis include drinking large amounts of alcohol, smoking, and taking aspirin or nonsteroidal anti-inflammatory drugs (NSAIDs). Acute gastritis may follow an alcohol binge or severe illness. Stress does not cause ulcers, but it can reduce or increase acid production in the stomach and may have an effect on ulcers and gastritis.

Chronic gastritis and stomach ulcers tend to be more common in people over the age of 50, while duodenal ulcers tend to be more common in men between the ages of 20 and 45. Possible complications of peptic ulcers include bleeding and perforation, the latter in which the ulcer penetrates the thick walls of the stomach or duodenum, allowing contents to leak into the abdomen. If this happens, the affected person may vomit blood or pass blood in the stools, which may have a tarry appearance. Long-term infection with *H. pylori* may be associated with an increased risk of stomach cancer.

TREATMENT PLAN

PRIMARY TREATMENTS
- Drugs
- Lifestyle and dietary changes
- Surgery

BACK-UP TREATMENTS
- Nutritional therapy
- Acupuncture
- Western herbal medicine

WORTH CONSIDERING
- Homeopathy
- Bodywork therapies
- Exercise and yoga

For an explanation of how treatments are rated, see p.111.

SELF-HELP

PRIMARY TREATMENT If you have mild, infrequent gastritis, try these measures:
- Eat small, regular meals.
- Avoid spicy foods, caffeine, and alcohol.
- Sit down when you eat and eat slowly.

- Do not lie down right after eating; allow your body time to digest.
- Use antacids at the first sign of discomfort in the upper abdomen.

TREATMENTS IN DETAIL

Conventional Medicine

Your doctor may suspect that you have a peptic ulcer or chronic gastritis from a description of your symptoms, but tests are needed to confirm the diagnosis. If a peptic ulcer is suspected, a test for the presence of H. pylori may be done because studies have shown that eradicating H. pylori is beneficial both in healing a peptic ulcer and in preventing its return. Other tests might include endoscopy, in which a flexible viewing instrument is passed down the throat to examine the stomach and duodenum, and contrast X-rays of these areas. Endoscopy also allows the doctor to exclude the presence of stomach cancer, which may produce symptoms similar to those of a peptic ulcer. For acute gastritis, the doctor may suggest that you stop drinking alcohol and taking NSAIDs. Short-term treatment with antacid therapy, which also includes the H₂-receptor antagonists and proton pump inhibitors, may be needed.

PRIMARY TREATMENT **TESTS FOR H. PYLORI** There are two main tests that look for the presence of H. pylori.

In the breath test, the patient drinks a radioactive substance that is broken down into radiolabeled carbon dioxide by H. pylori if it is present in the stomach. A breath analyzer can then be used to detect the labeled CO_2 and, therefore, determine whether or not these bacteria are present.

Alternatively, a biopsy (a sample of the stomach lining) is taken during endoscopy. This can then be examined for the presence of H. pylori. A blood test that looks for antibodies to the bacteria is also available. However, a positive result in this test can indicate either a current or a previous infection.

Treating H. pylori infection (if present) as well as making lifestyle changes such as quitting smoking, reducing alcohol intake, and avoiding foods that exacerbate your symptoms are likely to help heal ulcers and relieve the symptoms of gastritis.

COMMON SITES OF PEPTIC ULCERS

The upper part of the digestive tract includes the esophagus, the stomach, and the duodenum. (The duodenum is the first part of the small intestine and is located just below the stomach.) Peptic ulcers affect the stomach and duodenum and are among the most common digestive disorders. Most peptic ulcers occur in the area known as the duodenal bulb. In the stomach itself, the most common site for ulcers is the lesser curvature.

The esophagus, stomach, and duodenum

PRIMARY TREATMENT **DRUG THERAPY** Your doctor may prescribe combination therapy, which may include a proton pump inhibitor (PPI) or some other antacid therapy to reduce stomach acid, with two different antibiotics. These are all taken for one to two weeks. You may have to continue to take the PPI for several weeks afterward.

In some cases, either the drug bismuth or an H₂-receptor antagonist may be prescribed instead of a PPI as part of combination therapy. Bismuth plays a role not only in healing the ulcer but also in treating H. pylori. Like PPIs, H₂-receptor antagonists reduce the amount of acid that is produced.

Overall, these regimes for eradicating H. pylori are successful in about 90 percent of patients, although the infection may recur. More than one antibiotic is given as part of the treatment because some strains of the bacteria are resistant to certain antibiotics. Smoking may slow the healing process, so quitting is often recommended.

PRIMARY TREATMENT **SURGERY** is reserved for repairing severe complications of ulcers, such as perforation.

CAUTION

Drugs for peptic ulcer and gastritis can cause a range of possible side effects; ask your doctor to explain these to you.

Nutritional Therapy

DIETARY CHANGES Certain foods may interfere with the healing of an ulcer. Sugar, alcohol, coffee, and decaffeinated coffee and tea have all been reported to increase stomach acidity, which may worsen or prolong an ulcer. There is also evidence to suggest that salt consumption is a risk factor for gastric ulcers. Research also suggests that eating salty food increases the risk of developing H. pylori infection and so increases the risk of gastritis and peptic ulcers. Avoiding these foods may help people who have a peptic ulcer.

VITAMIN A This vitamin is needed in the healing of mucosal tissue, including the linings of the stomach and intestines. One study found that vitamin A helped healing in people with stomach ulcers. A very high dose of vitamin A (50,000 IU, three times daily) was used in this trial, although clinical experience suggests that vitamin A at a much lower dose of 10,000 IU per day for women and 25,000 IU for men is safer and might be helpful for people with peptic ulcers. If you have a peptic ulcer, you could try taking vitamin A supplements at these lower doses.

ZINC This mineral is another nutrient that may help people with peptic ulcers. Like vitamin A, zinc enhances tissue healing. Animal studies suggest that zinc can protect rats from stomach ulceration. In one study, when people with gastric ulcers took zinc (at a dose of 88mg, three times daily), their ulcers healed three times faster than those taking a placebo. Clinical experience suggests that supplementing with 30mg of zinc per day (balanced with 2mg of copper per day) may help people with peptic ulcers. If you have a peptic ulcer, try taking zinc and copper at these dosages for three months to see if it helps.

> **CAUTION**
>
> Consult your doctor before taking vitamin A and zinc supplements with prescribed medications. Pregnant women and women trying to conceive should not take vitamin A supplements. (*See also p.46.*)

Homeopathy

The three most commonly used homeopathic medicines for gastritis and peptic ulcer are *Kalium bichromicum*, *Nitric acid,* and *Phosphorus*.

KALIUM BICHROMICUM People who respond to *Kalium bichromicum* have burning stomach pain, with a sensation of heaviness, nausea and vomiting; the vomit often contains stringy mucus. They may crave beer, although it makes their symptoms worse. These patients often also suffer from sinusitis or chronic catarrh.

NITRIC ACID The pains of people who respond to *Nitric acid* are typically described as sharp or piercing. They may crave rich or spicy food, although this makes the symptoms worse. Other symptoms include cracking at the edges of the mouth and also anal fissures, causing

severe pain after passing stool. These people may also have warts and hard, unforgiving personalities.

PHOSPHORUS is often appropriate, especially if the ulcers bleed easily. People who respond to this medicine vomit easily. They are thirsty, especially for iced drinks,

> Only about half of people with duodenal ulcers have the typical symptoms of pain and soreness

yet vomit even water a few minutes after drinking it. The pain is of burning character, and the symptoms are usually better in the morning and after a short nap. Those who respond to this medicine often have irrational fears and phobias, particularly of being alone in the dark and of storms. They may be may be oversensitive, "picking up vibes" too readily.

Western Herbal Medicine

Although self-treatment with herbal remedies can be helpful in treating ulcers and gastritis, professional treatment is recommended. Practitioners will combine key herbs to promote repair of mucous membranes, stimulate mucus secretion, counter inflammation and infection, and relieve associated symptoms such as acidity, indigestion, and pain. In the process, digestive health as a whole — including that of the stomach and duodenum — will normally be improved. Treatment will vary depending on the site of ulceration and severity of symptoms, although suppression of acid production within the stomach is not usually a central aim. The herbal approach typically focuses on strengthening and nurturing the digestive system.

DEMULCENT AND ASTRINGENT HERBS Licorice (*Glycyrrhiza glabra*), marshmallow root (*Althea officinalis*), and slippery elm (*Ulmus fulva*) are demulcent herbs, which have the ability to soothe and coat the stomach lining. They reduce inflammation and stimulate the rate of healing in the stomach lining.

In addition to being a demulcent, licorice is a powerful anti-inflammatory.

Clinical research indicates that licorice extracts are as effective as conventional treatments for treating peptic ulceration, with fewer relapses occurring after the treatment is stopped. However, side effects were frequent, mostly due to glycyrrhizin. Therefore, deglycyrrhizinated extracts of licorice should be used.

Astringent remedies, such as agrimony (*Agrimonia eupatoria*) and cranesbill (*Geranium maculatum*), may be used to tone mucous membranes, increasing resistance to inflammation and infection.

ANTIBACTERIAL AND OTHER HERBS Where infection, such as with *H. pylori*, is suspected or confirmed, antibacterial and immune-stimulant herbs may also be selected, such as echinacea (*Echinacea* spp.) and garlic (*Allium sativum*). Anti-inflammatory and carminative remedies, such as chamomile (*Matricaria recutita*) and marigold (*Calendula officinalis*), can also be important elements in balanced treatment. However, there is as yet little research to confirm the effectiveness of such herbs against *H. pylori*.

St. John's wort (*Hypericum perforatum*) macerated oil, which is a safe and effective anti-inflammatory and wound healer, is a common treatment for stomach ulceration and inflammation in Germany.

> **CAUTION**
>
> See p.69 before taking a herbal remedy and, if you are taking prescribed medication, consult an herbal medicine expert first.

Acupuncture

Acupuncture is used frequently in China for peptic ulcers, and a number of non-randomized studies have been done, all indicating a "good response." In one, over 90 percent of people treated felt significant improvement with acupuncture alone. Experiments have also suggested acupuncture may prevent duodenal ulcers in rats.

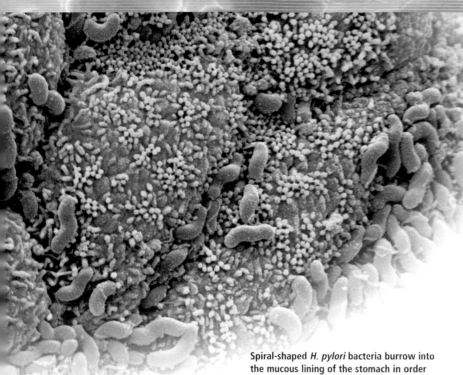

Spiral-shaped *H. pylori* bacteria burrow into the mucous lining of the stomach in order to survive the strongly acidic environment. They also produce urease, an enzyme that neutralizes gastric acids.

It is unlikely that acupuncture can help eradicate *H. pylori* where this is the cause of ulcers. However, it may help quite substantially with the symptoms of peptic ulcers and gastritis. A traditional Chinese diagnosis is required to prescribe and treat appropriate acupuncture points. Acupuncture modulates stomach acidity, thereby working as PPI or H₂ blockers.

Acupuncture treatment for peptic ulcer and gastritis is given weekly for a minimum of six to eight sessions. If the condition is acute, treatment may be given every day or every other day. When the symptoms subside, long-term constitutional acupuncture may be required to prevent recurrence, perhaps on a monthly basis.

Bodywork Therapies

MASSAGE THERAPY There is some surprising research evidence from China that massage is valuable in treating peptic ulcers. The question for researchers is whether it relieves stress, thereby influencing acid production in the stomach, or works on the autonomic nervous system in some way to reduce acid production directly. Until this is determined, the research must be treated cautiously. More recently, Russian researchers compared conventional medical treatment with a combination of deep reflex muscular massage and exercise. The massage and exercise may prolong remission of the condition and result in a lower frequency of recurrences of ulcers as well as associated gastrointestinal diseases.

The Russian team, in further studies, has reported that massage and exercise are at least as effective in treating peptic ulcer patients as medication.

OSTEOPATHY AND CHIROPRACTIC For about a century, osteopaths and chiropractors have manipulated the region of the spine from which the nerves to the stomach and duodenum emerge to treat uncomplicated peptic ulcers, as an adjunct to normal medical treatment.

Researchers in one study on the use of osteopathy concluded that routine use of conventional medication together with osteopathic manipulative treatment is generally sufficient to obtain relief from the symptoms of a peptic ulcer unless the condition has been caused by or is complicated by other factors.

TRIGGER POINT DEACTIVATION Trigger points (sensitive areas, *see p.55*) in the abdominal muscles can cause referred pain in the digestive organs. Abdominal pain may originate in either the muscles or the internal organs themselves. It is very easy for trigger-point activity to produce symptoms, especially pain, that can be confused with actual organ disease.

Since the joints of the spine and pelvis can be the cause of the muscular stresses that lead to trigger points developing in the first place, a comprehensive evaluation of pelvic and spinal mechanics, as well as of the muscles of the region, would clarify whether or not bodywork would be worth trying in a case of peptic ulcer.

Treatment to restore normal function to dysfunctional joints and muscles, including deactivation of trigger points, might include osteopathic, chiropractic, physical therapy, or massage and neuromuscular therapy.

Exercise

A number of research studies have shown that exercising regularly can help heal peptic ulcers and, in men, exercise may even be effective as a preventive measure. Russian research, for example, suggests that regular bicycling may be especially helpful by accelerating the ulcer healing process.

Yoga

Doing yoga exercises on a regular basis, particularly relaxing poses such as the corpse pose (*see p.226*), may be helpful if you have a peptic ulcer. Although stress is no longer thought to be the primary cause of peptic ulcers, persistent stress may make the pain of peptic ulcers worse and may be a factor in bringing on attacks. Learning to relax through regular yoga practice each day may make it easier to cope. Wear loose clothing and avoid doing any exercises within an hour after a meal.

PREVENTION PLAN

The following may help you avoid peptic ulcers:

- Avoid using aspirin and NSAIDs
- Do not smoke
- Moderate your alcohol intake
- Eat small, regular meals and avoid overeating and caffeine

CROHN'S DISEASE

The condition known as Crohn's disease is one of the inflammatory bowel diseases, in which the lining of the bowel becomes inflamed (*see also Ulcerative Colitis, p.227*). Crohn's disease can affect any part of the digestive tract from the mouth to the anus. However, it most commonly affects the last part of the small intestine (the ileum). There is no cure for Crohn's disease, but a variety of approaches, including drugs, dietary changes, and relaxation training, may help control symptoms and reduce the frequency of recurrences.

WHAT ARE THE SYMPTOMS?

- Weight loss
- Loss of appetite
- Diarrhea
- Abdominal pain
- Fever
- Depression

WHY MIGHT I HAVE THIS?

PREDISPOSING FACTORS

- Genetic tendency
- Cigarette smoking

TRIGGERS FOR CROHN'S DISEASE RELAPSES

- Bowel infections
- Stress
- Food sensitivities

WHY DOES IT OCCUR?

It is not known why Crohn's disease develops, but many theories have been proposed and there may be several causes. The disease sometimes runs in families and a number of genes have been identified that increase the risk of developing the disease. Past exposure to certain infections may also play a role. Most people who develop the disease do so before the age of 30, with the majority being between 15 and 30 when symptoms first appear.

Crohn's disease is a lifelong condition that is characterized by periods of remission (being well) and relapse (being ill). It is not known what triggers relapses. However, in some circumstances acute bowel infections may be a trigger. Stress may also have an effect, as may certain foods. Smokers are three times more likely to develop Crohn's disease and their symptoms may also be more difficult to control.

People with Crohn's disease may have other disorders, including joint disease, uveitis (inflammation of the eye), and erythema nodosum (a skin condition in which tender swellings appear, usually on the shins). Complications of Crohn's disease include the development of anal abscesses and fistulae (abnormal connecting channels between the bowel and surrounding areas). Intestinal narrowing or obstruction may also occur. Inflammation of the colon over a long period of time may also be associated with an increased risk of colorectal cancer.

TREATMENT PLAN

PRIMARY TREATMENTS

- Drugs for relapse and remission, including corticosteroids, aminosalicylates, and azathioprine
- Liquid diets

BACK-UP TREATMENTS

- Surgery (in severe cases)
- Eliminating sugar and problematic foods
- Probiotics
- Vitamin supplements

WORTH CONSIDERING

- Fish oils
- Homeopathy
- Bodywork and movement therapies
- Acupuncture

For an explanation of how treatments are rated, see p.111.

TREATMENTS IN DETAIL

Conventional Medicine

If your symptoms suggest Crohn's disease, the doctor will conduct several tests and investigations in order to make the diagnosis. These include endoscopy, in which flexible viewing instruments are passed both into the upper part of the bowel through the mouth and into the lower bowel through the anus. Doctors view the bowel lining to look for the characteristic changes that are caused by Crohn's disease. Biopsies (small samples of tissue) are taken from the lining of the intestines for microscopic examination.

IMPORTANT

If you experience unexplained weight loss and/or abdominal pain, see your doctor immediately.

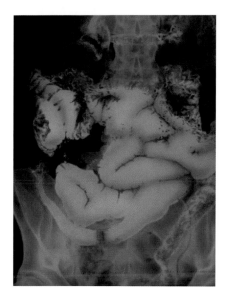

In this colour-enhanced contrast X-ray showing an intestinal tract affected by Crohn's disease, affected areas appear ragged and narrowed (top and right). In the centre is healthy tissue.

A barium X-ray will also be performed. A radioopaque fluid, either swallowed or passed down the digestive tract via a tube, outlines the lining of the bowel on a series of X-rays. This allows imaging of areas that cannot be viewed by standard endoscopy.

Treatment for Crohn's disease can be divided into treatment of relapse and maintenance of remission. More recent drugs may have a role to play in both these aspects of treatment. All treatments aim to reduce bowel inflammation and so reduce symptoms. Occasionally, simple antidiarrheal drugs such as loperamide may be prescribed to help control diarrhea. They work by slowing the passage of feces through the bowel.

PRIMARY TREATMENT | **DRUGS AND LIQUID DIETS FOR RELAPSE** Corticosteroids and special liquid diets are mainly used to treat relapses and will gradually be discontinued over time. Corticosteroids reduce inflammation in the bowels. Liquid diets contain precisely measured amounts of dietary components such as fats, carbohydrates, and proteins. In some cases, long-term steroids or frequent courses of steroids may be needed. For children, there is a risk of these drugs affecting growth, which is therefore carefully monitored. Corticosteroid therapy should never be suddenly discontinued.

PRIMARY TREATMENT | **DRUGS AND LIQUID DIETS FOR REMISSION** Remission of Crohn's disease is maintained by long-term use of certain drugs that may be combined with cortico-steroids and liquid diets. This treatment is used in some cases, depending on the severity of the disease, the part of bowel that is involved, and the presence of any other associated problems, such as abscesses or fistulae. These additional drugs range from those with mild anti-inflammatory properties, such as the aminosalicylate mesalamine, to immuno-suppressant drugs such as azathioprine. New drugs are being developed that target specific chemicals in the body that are known to play a part in inflammation, but the question of when these medicines should be used in the progression of the disease is still poorly understood. Antibiotics also play a role in treating inflammation, especially for disease occurring near the anus.

SURGERY Although every effort is made to avoid surgery, it may be necessary in some cases. If the symptoms persist despite the use of every suitable medication, a portion of bowel where the disease is uncontrolled may be removed. Surgery is used to

The American gastroenterologist Burrill B. Crohn first identified the disease in 1932

remove areas of the bowel that have become narrow if they are causing problems. A repair operation may also be carried in some situations where fistulae or abscesses have formed.

In some cases of Crohn's disease, an operation known as an ileostomy (in which the ileum, which is the last part of the small bowel, is connected to an artificial opening in the abdomen) may be necessary. Less commonly, a surgeon may have to carry out a colostomy (in which a similar procedure is followed with the colon — the large bowel).

CAUTION

Drugs for Crohn's disease can cause a range of possible side effects: ask your doctor to explain these to you.

Nutritional Therapy

ELIMINATING SUGAR People who have Crohn's disease may find it useful to eliminate refined carbohydrates from their diet, particularly sucrose. Experiments suggest that a low-carbohydrate diet can be effective in controlling the condition. In one study, people with Crohn's disease who followed a low-sugar, high-fiber diet had a 79 percent reduction in relapses requiring hospitalization compared with people who did not change their diet. In another study, people with Crohn's disease were fed either a high- or a low-sugar diet. Patients who had more active Crohn's disease fared better on a low-sugar diet compared with those eating larger amounts of sugar. Several people on the high-sugar diet had to stop eating sugar entirely because their condition worsened while on this regimen.

AVOIDING PROBLEM FOODS Identification and treatment of food sensitivities is often used in clinical practice to treat Crohn's disease. In one study, 77 patients were put on a diet excluding foods to which they were thought to be sensitive. Fifty-one of them (66 percent) remained healthy on the diet alone for up to 51 months and had an annual relapse rate of less than 10 percent. The most frequent symptom-provoking foods were wheat, dairy products, brassicas (cabbage, broccoli, and others), corn, yeast, tomatoes, citrus fruits, and eggs. (*For more information on food sensitivity, see p.456.*)

VITAMIN SUPPLEMENTS People who have Crohn's disease may have multiple nutritional deficiencies because they tend not to be able to absorb nutrients very effectively. Nutrients of particular importance are zinc, vitamin B_{12}, and folic acid, both because these nutrients can help repair the cells that line the intestinal tract and because people with Crohn's disease have been shown to be deficient in them. Try taking 30–45mg of zinc (balanced with 2–3mg of copper), 800mcg of vitamin B_{12}, and 800mcg of folic acid each day.

FISH OILS Crohn's disease is an inflammatory condition and excessive amounts of omega-6 fatty acids (found in vegetable oils and most processed and fast foods) combined with the relative lack of omega-3 fatty acids (found in oily fish, walnuts, and flaxseeds) seems to promote inflammation. Maintaining a balance between omega-6 and omega-3 fatty acids in the diet by avoiding excessive amounts of margarine, processed foods, and vegetable oils and including oily fish (such as salmon, sardines, trout, and mackerel), walnuts, and flaxseeds in the diet may be helpful in controlling the symptoms of Crohn's disease. One two-year study found

NITRIC ACID People who respond to *Nitric acid* are more likely to have painful splits in the skin (fissures) around the anus, which may cause pain for some time after passing a stool. There is also often a tendency to develop small, painful mouth ulcers (known as aphthae). The pain of the fissures and aphthae is described as being similar to the sensation caused by splinters. People who respond to *Nitric acid* are said to be rather bad-tempered, to bear grudges, and to be anxious about their health.

SULPHUR People who respond to *Sulphur* often experience diarrhea that feels hot and is often worse in the morning, forcing

Bodywork and Movement Therapies

General relaxation and massage as well as antianxiety breathing exercises and hypnotherapy are useful in easing the stress associated with inflammatory bowel disease (IBS) and other such diseases.

Exercise

Osteoporosis (*see p.308*) is a common complication of inflammatory bowel disease due to steroid treatment given for acute symptoms and because the absorption of nutrients by the intestine is reduced. People with Crohn's disease are at particular risk of developing osteoporosis.

Research indicates that taking regular weight-bearing exercise is beneficial. In a study on the effects of exercise on bone loss in people with the condition, participants following a low-impact exercise program for 12 months showed significant increase in bone density. This was enough to reduce the risk of osteoporotic fracture.

> Crohn's disease has become more common throughout the world in the past few decades

that diets high in oily fish (3.5–7oz/ 85–200g per day) substantially reduced the relapse rate in people with the condition. In addition, fish-oil supplements with the omega-3 fatty acids EPA and DHA might help control Crohn's disease due to their anti-inflammatory effect. If you have Crohn's disease, try taking 1g of concentrated fish oil one to three times a day.

PROBIOTICS Probiotic organisms (healthy bacteria) are believed to be important for maintaining a healthy lining in the gut. Probiotic supplements may help people with Crohn's disease. One study showed that probiotic treatment may allow for a reduction in steroid dosage.

the patient out of bed, and the odor of the diarrhea may be very offensive. These people also often have skin problems, especially itchy skin. In terms of personality, they are usually untidy and they may be outgoing, "larger than life" characters. They frequently feel the heat excessively.

PHOSPHORUS is useful when diarrhea is often bloody. People who respond to *Phosphorus* generally experience easy bleeding, including nosebleeds and easy bruising of the skin. There are sometimes accompanying liver problems, such as hepatitis.

Patients often feel run-down and tired, but are briefly better when rested and, therefore, usually feel better first thing in the morning. Mentally, these people tend to be sensitive and sympathetic to other humans and to the physical environment. They may be afraid of storms or of being alone in the dark.

Acupuncture

In order to treat Crohn's disease with acupuncture, a traditional Chinese diagnosis needs to be made, and patients may require quite lengthy treatment courses. While there have been a number of case studies indicating that acupuncture may be beneficial, there are no reliable clinical trials available in this field. However, in conjunction with other approaches, acupuncture may be especially valuable in symptom control.

Acupuncture has been reported to be effective in managing acute symptoms, and treatment may be required daily or every other day. Generally, however, people seek acupuncture for chronic and more persistent complaints, and for Crohn's disease weekly treatment for eight to ten weeks to assess whether there is some benefit would be appropriate. Further maintenance treatments may be required to avoid relapse.

> **CAUTION**
>
> Consult your doctor before taking fish oil, zinc, or folic acid supplements with existing medications. (*See also p.46.*)

Homeopathy

The treatment of Crohn's disease using homeopathy is likely to require individualized treatment from a qualified practitioner. Many different medicines may be appropriate in the treatment of this disease, including *Nitric acid*, *Sulphur* and *Phosphorus*.

Western Herbal Medicine

Certain phytochemicals (substances that occur naturally in plants) in herbs and spices have been found to interrupt one of the pathways causing the inflammatory response. Some of the most effective are peppermint oil (*Mentha piperita*), chamomile (*Matricaria recutita*), and turmeric (*Curcuma longa*).

> **PREVENTION PLAN**
>
> ● Do not smoke

COMMON DIGESTIVE DISORDERS

Indigestion is a term often used to describe common digestive disorders usually used to describe pain or discomfort in the upper abdomen. It may be caused by acid reflux, lactose intolerance, and some medications. When no underlying cause is found, a patient is often assumed to have nonulcer dyspepsia (NUD) Simple lifestyle and dietary changes do a great deal to help indigestion. Other approaches, including drugs, homeopathy, breathing exercises, bodywork and relaxation, and hypnosis can all help relieve indigestion and prevent future episodes.

WHY DOES IT OCCUR?

Indigestion occurs when the digestive tract becomes irritated. Food, especially rich, fried, or spicy food, alcohol, coffee, and certain drugs, such as aspirin and nonsteroidal anti-inflammatory drugs (NSAIDs) including ibuprofen, can irritate the digestive tract and cause indigestion. Smoking and being overweight increase a person's risk of developing indigestion. Stress can also cause the condition.

Indigestion may be accompanied by gastroesophageal reflux disease (GERD), also known as acid reflux or heartburn). In this condition, partially digested food is regurgitated from the stomach back into the esphagus. If GERD is persistent, digestive acids from the stomach can erode the esophageal lining, which unlike the stomach, is not protected by a layer of mucus.

The body can digest only so much food at once, so eating three large meals increases the risk of indigestion. Eating smaller meals throughout the day may help prevent indigestion.

Osteopaths and chiropractors believe that mechanical stress resulting from spinal restrictions or from trigger points in the back or abdomen can affect digestive function and may cause indigestion.

TREATMENT PLAN

PRIMARY TREATMENTS

- Drugs such as antacids
- Chewing properly
- Breathing retraining

BACKUP TREATMENTS

- Food combining
- Nutritional supplements and probiotics
- Homeopathy
- Bodywork therapies

WORTH CONSIDERING

- Psychological therapies

For an explanation of how treatments are rated, see p.111.

IMMEDIATE RELIEF

- Press the "belch button" to induce belching. This is located in the lower back just below the lowest rib (see p.221).
- Take homeopathic medicines *Nux vomica* or *Carbo vegetalis*.
- Take over-the-counter antacids.
- Drink a cup of peppermint, fennel, or ginger tea or eat a peppermint candy.

TREATMENTS IN DETAIL

Conventional Medicine

Indigestion may be relieved by lifestyle changes, including reducing intake of fatty and spicy foods, limiting or eliminating coffee and alcohol, reducing stress, quitting smoking, and eating smaller, more frequent meals. Avoid taking aspirin or NSAIDs, such as ibuprofen. You could also

INDIGESTION AND GASTROESOPHAGEAL REFLUX DISEASE (GERD)

Indigestion is often accompanied by gastroesophageal reflux disease (also known as acid reflux or heartburn), in which partially digested stomach contents are regurgitated up into the esophagus. GERD occurs when the lower esophageal sphincter does not work properly and allows acidic stomach contents back up into the esophagus. Too much food in the stomach or increased pressure in the stomach can cause the sphincter to relax. Long-standing GERD can result in pain and bleeding.

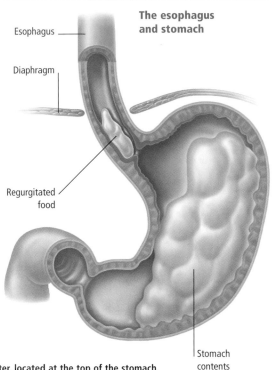

The esophagus and stomach

Esophagus

Diaphragm

Regurgitated food

Stomach contents

The lower esophageal sphincter, located at the top of the stomach, is a muscular one-way valve that normally keeps acidic stomach contents from being regurgitated back up into the esophagus. If the sphincter fails to work correctly, stomach contents can flow back up into the esophagus, causing discomfort and eventual damage to the esophageal lining.

try raising the head of your bed 2–4 inches to tilt your body slightly so that your head is higher than your feet. Propping yourself up with pillows does not work because it bends rather than tilts the body. These lifestyle changes may be combined with antacid drugs if needed.

For persistent symptoms, your doctor may recommend various exams to exclude certain underlying causes. These may include endoscopy, in which a flexible viewing instrument is used to examine the esophagus and stomach, and contrast X-rays of these areas. One of the various treatments described below.

PRIMARY TREATMENT **DRUGS** Several drugs are available to help reduce stomach acid secretion. These include proton pump inhibitors (PPIs) and H₂-receptor antagonists. Prokinetic agents, which reduce the time food spends in the stomach, may also be prescribed because they may be helpful for some patients with indigestion.

ELIMINATING HELICOBACTER PYLORI Often found in the stomach, this bacterium is associated with certain disorders of the stomach and duodenum (the first part of the small intestine), including chronic gastritis (inflammation of the stomach lining) and peptic ulcer (*see p.212*). Its role in indigestion is less clear; the impact of treating the infection with a course of antibiotics, usually with a proton pump inhibitor, is probably small.

> **CAUTION**
>
> Drugs for indigestion can cause a range of side effects; ask your doctor or pharmacist to explain these to you.

Nutritional Therapy

PRIMARY TREATMENT **CHEWING THOROUGHLY** can improve symptoms of indigestion. Each mouthful should be chewed to a creamy consistency before it is swallowed.

FOOD COMBINING may improve digestion. This involves eating protein-based foods (such as meat, fish, and eggs) at different times from carbohydrates (such as bread, potatoes, rice, and pasta). The body digests proteins and carbohydrates in distinct ways, so keeping them separated may make less work for the digestive tract. Food combining seems most useful in the evening, when the digestive capacity tends to be lower. (*For more information, see p.39.*)

NUTRITIONAL SUPPLEMENTS Sometimes indigestion may be the result of hypochlorhydria (low levels of acid in the stomach and/or low levels of digestive enzymes in the small intestine). A nutritionist may be able to suggest nutritional suplements to help remedy this.

PROBIOTICS Supplements containing healthy gut bacteria can promote good digestion. In one study, 30 patients with indigestion were given *Lactobacillus acidophilus* (two billion live bacteria per capsule) after breakfast. Symptoms of indigestion, such as pain, pressure, bloating, and flatulence, improved within two weeks. In patients with lactose intolerance (which may cause indigestion), tolerance of dairy products improved after taking probiotics.

Homeopathy

A range of homeopathic medicines may be used for indigestion. If the following fail to bring relief, consult a practitioner.

NUX VOMICA is the most frequently used homeopathic medicine for indigestion. It has been shown to be effective in clinical trials in Germany. *Nux vomica* is useful for indigestion triggered by too much food, especially when it is rich or fatty, or by alcohol. People who respond to *Nux vomica* often have nausea (sometimes with vomiting) and a bitter taste in the mouth. They are irritable and annoyed by inefficiency; their sleep may be poor, they often wake early and feel terrible in the morning.

> **CAUTION**
>
> Coffee can nullify the effect of *Nux vomica*; do not drink it if you are using this homeopathic medication.

CARBO VEGETABILIS is another possible treatment for indigestion. In people who respond to it, digestion seems slow and the stomach is bloated with a lot of burping.

LYCOPODIUM may be used for symptoms that include excess gas, craving sweets, feeling full quickly, and anxiety or depression.

Herbal Medicine

CHAMOMILE (*Chamaemelum nobile*) As a tea, it has a relaxing effect with digestive disorders and irritable bowel syndrome (IBS). Recent research has confirmed that a combination of relaxation, guided imagery, and chamomile tea is effective for children with recurrent functional abdominal pain.

GINGER (*Zanziber officinale*) Indigestion may be eased by candied root or ginger candy or by capsules of powdered root, 1g one to three times a day.

FENNEL (*Foeniculum vulgare*) A study comparing a combination product of caraway, fennel, peppermint, and wormwood to metoclopramide found that the herbal mixture was significantly more effective in treating heartburn and stomach cramps.

Bodywork Therapies

Spinal nerves can speed up or slow down digestion. The sympathetic and parasympathetic nerves control the body's unconscious actions, including heartbeat. The sympathetic nerves, which emerge from the upper spine, slow digestive function, while the parasympathetic nerves emerging from the top and bottom of the spine speed it up. Bodywork treatments on the back can thus affect digestive function.

CHIROPRACTIC AND OSTEOPATHY A chiropractic survey of almost 1,500 people showed that 70 percent of those with mechanical restrictions of the upper back had symptoms of indigestion. Of these, 22 percent felt relief after spinal manipulation.

DEACTIVATION OF TRIGGER POINTS Trigger points (sensitive areas in the abdominal muscles), can produce indigestion symptoms affecting the upper abdomen. Heartburn and a feeling of fullness are common effects of trigger points that lie

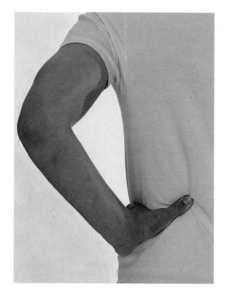

Pressing the "belch button" can ease indigestion by releasing trapped wind. Find the lowest rib on your back and feel for a tender point just below it. Press firmly for 5 seconds.

close to the center of the chest, on or just below the breastbone. Trigger points can be deactivated by manual pressure and stretching techniques used by osteopaths, massage therapists, and some physical therapists and chiropractors. One trigger point located in the lower back on either side and just below the lowest rib is known as the "belch button," since this is the common effect of pressing it (*see illustration, above*).

Breathing Retraining

PRIMARY TREATMENT **BREATHING CORRECTLY** Bloating and heartburn are caused by excessive swallowing of air (aerophagia). A common side-effect of rapid upper-chest breathing, it is also caused by eating too fast or talking and eating simultaneously. It can usually be improved slow, diaphragmatic (yoga-type) breathing methods, and correction of restrictions that develope in overused and stressed muscles and joints. See p.62 for a breathing sequence. If indigestion regularly bothers you, consider osteopathic treatment to relieve restrictions in overstretched joints.

Acupuncture

Several case series have demonstrated that releasing trigger points by acupuncture may be effective for treating indigestion.

Psychological Therapies

PSYCHOTHERAPY A 1990 study was used to determine whether brief psychodynamic-interpersonal (PI) psychotherapy was more effective than a psychological control treatment for patients with chronic, intractable nonulcer dyspepsia, and whether patients with abnormal gastric function responded differently from those with normal gastric function. At the end of treatment, there were significant advantages for the people who had received PI psychotherapy compared with the people in the control group. One year after treatment, the advantages remained.

A review of all available research into psychological treatments for indigestion concluded that psychodynamic psychotherapy and cognitive behavioral therapy may be used for nonulcer dyspepsia.

MOOD-IMPROVING TECHNIQUES If you have indigestion regularly, you may want to try psychological techniques such as guided imagery (*see p.100*) to improve your mood. A 2001 Cochrane review found that people who regularly had indigestion were more likely to be anxious, depressed, and pessimistic than the rest of the population. The review determined that psychological treatments, including psychotherapy, psychodrama, cognitive behavioral therapy, relaxation therapy, guided imagery, or hypnosis, improved patients' digestion. However, more studies to assess the role of psychological intervention in treating indigestion are needed in order to give a clearer picture.

PREVENTION PLAN

If you are prone to indigestion, try the following measures:

- Eat small meals at regular intervals
- Eat while sitting at a table rather than on a sofa
- Eat slowly and thoroughly chew food to a creamy consistency
- Maintain a normal, healthy weight
- Avoid alcohol, coffee, carbonated drinks, and spicy foods

IRRITABLE BOWEL SYNDROME

WHAT ARE THE SYMPTOMS?

IBS involves abdominal pain that may include:

- Pain relieved by defecation
- A change in the frequency of stool
- A change in the appearance of the stool

There may also be:

- Fewer than three bowel movements a week or more than three a day
- Hard or lumpy stools
- Loose (watery) stools
- Straining during a bowel movement
- Urgency (having to rush to have a bowel movement)
- A feeling that the bowel has not emptied completely
- Passage of mucus during defecation
- A feeling of fullness and bloating

Many people with IBS also have other symptoms that are not related to the digestive tract, such as headaches.

WHY MIGHT I HAVE THIS?

PREDISPOSING FACTORS

- Anxiety
- Depression
- Psychological stress
- Smoking

Irritable bowel syndrome (IBS) describes a combination of intermittent abdominal pain with constipation or diarrhea. The condition usually develops between the ages of 20 and 30 and is twice as common in women as in men. The symptoms typically persist for many years. Although it can be distressing, IBS does not lead to serious complications. There is no single treatment for IBS, but a combination of therapies including drugs, dietary changes, relaxation, and herbal preparations may bring relief.

WHY DOES IT OCCUR?

The cause of irritable bowel syndrome is unknown. It is classified as a functional disorder in which, although the intestines appear normal, they do not function normally. One theory is that the condition may result from abnormal contractions of the intestinal walls. Another factor in IBS may be food sensitivity, which may also cause symptoms similar to those of IBS.

In some cases, IBS first occurs following a gastrointestinal infection. There appears to be a genetic component because IBS seems to run in families. Stress, anxiety, or depression may be associated and can often make the symptoms worse.

In diagnosing IBS, the doctor may ask you whether the pain is relieved by defecation, whether you experience a change in the frequency of passing stools, and whether there has been a change in the appearance of the stools. An increased sensitivity to certain foods, such as lactose, fruit, or the artificial sweetener sorbitol, may cause symptoms that are similar to those caused by IBS.

IBS is not typically associated with pain that interferes with sleep, blood in the stool, weight loss, fever, or any physical abnormality. If you are experiencing any of these symptoms, you should see your doctor immediately.

IBS rarely begins after the age of 40. Therefore, any change in bowel habits that occur in middle age should be investigated by a doctor at once.

TREATMENT PLAN

PRIMARY TREATMENTS

- Antidiarrheal drugs and bulking agents
- Food elimination diet

BACKUP TREATMENTS

- Anti-muscarinics and anti-spasmodics
- Probiotics
- Western and Chinese herbal medicine
- Acupuncture
- Mind-body therapies

WORTH CONSIDERING

- Individualized homeopathy
- Breathing retraining
- Bodywork and movement therapies

For an explanation of how treatments are rated, see p.111.

IMPORTANT

- Consult your doctor if your IBS symptoms are severe, persistent, or recurrent or if you have rectal bleeding, blood in the stool, pain that interferes with sleep, or have unexpectedly lost weight.

- Consult your doctor if you are over 40 when symptoms first appear, since some gastrointestinal disorders may have similar symptoms.

- Keep a food diary to help you identify foods that bring on attacks so that you can avoid them.
- Make sure that you exercise on a regular basis.
- If stress is a factor in your IBS, practice relaxation or meditation daily.
- Try peppermint oil capsules.
- If constipation is a problem, take a gentle bulk-forming laxative regularly, but avoid stimulant and bran-based laxatives, which can make IBS worse.
- Do not smoke because smoking irritates the gastrointestinal tract.

Conventional Medicine

A diagnosis of IBS will usually be made if you have gastrointestinal pain but no abnormalities by radiologic tests and endoscopy. The doctor will review your symptoms and may refer you for investigations to exclude underlying disorders. Often, no medication is needed and the symptoms can be controlled with lifestyle and dietary changes and relaxation techniques. If specific treatment is needed, there are various options.

PRIMARY TREATMENT **ANTIDIARRHEAL DRUGS AND BULKING AGENTS** Antidiarrheal drugs, such as loperamide, may be helpful for people with diarrhea. There is some evidence to support the use of bulking agents, such as flaxseed husk, in the treatment of constipation associated with IBS. These drugs act by increasing the bulk of the stool and stimulating normal contractions in the wall of the gut.

ANTIMUSCARINICS AND ANTISPASMODICS Studies have shown that some antimuscarinics, such as atropine sulfate, and antispasmodics, such as dicyclomine, can help relieve the pain of IBS. These drugs are thought to reduce abnormal contractions in the gut by relaxing the muscles in the wall.

ANTIDEPRESSANTS Tricyclic or selective serotonin reuptake inhibitor (SSRI) antidepressants may relieve some of the symptoms of IBS.

> **CAUTION**
>
> Drugs for IBS can cause a range of possible side effects; ask your doctor to explain these to you.

Nutritional Therapy

PRIMARY TREATMENT **ELIMINATING SENSITIVE FOODS** Studies have shown that many people with IBS have food sensitivities. Gas and other IBS symptoms diminish when these sensitivities are discovered and the offending foods are eliminated from the diet.

Some people with IBS may not be able to digest the sugars lactose (found in milk) and fructose, found in high concentrations in fruit juice and dried fruit. The artificial sweetener sorbitol (found in diabetic and sugar-free products) can cause diarrhea. IBS patients may have lactose intolerance, in which case a lactose-restricted diet can markedly improve symptoms both in the short term and the long term. Fructose- and sorbitol-reduced diets in people with fructose malabsorption reduce gastrointestinal symptoms such as bloating, cramps, diarrhea, and other IBS symptoms. Milk, fruit juice, dried fruit, and products containing sorbitol might make their symptoms worse. (*For more information about food sensitvities, see p.456.*)

PROBIOTICS Imbalance in the organisms in the gut (gut dysbiosis) is common for people with IBS. One study found reduced numbers of "friendly" bacteria such as lactobacilli and bifidobacteria and higher numbers of harmful bacteria in those with symptoms of IBS. Two studies have shown symptom improvement with *Lactobacilli plantarum*; one study showed no effect of *Lactobacilli casei*.

Probiotics may be helpful to people with IBS. Some studies have shown improvements in pain and flatulence when people with IBS took probiotic supplements.

FIBER Fiber may help relieve the symptoms of IBS, but most studies find that people with IBS will generally not benefit by adding wheat bran to their diets. In fact, some people feel even worse after taking wheat-bran supplements. However, fiber from other sources, such as psyllium (20–30g per day of psyllium seed husk fiber), may alleviate symptoms.

Homeopathy

Two controlled studies in Germany published in the 1970s showed positive results for homeopathic treatment of IBS. However, these studies looked only at a single homeopathic medicine and, as with homeopathic treatments for many conditions, several medicines may be more appropriate. For dosing, two pills of all of the medicines discussed below should be taken twice daily in the 6C strength.

ARGENTUM NITRICUM may be indicated when anxiety is associated with IBS. The affected person has a lot of bloating and may have a craving for sweet foods.

PHOSPHORIC ACID may be indicated, particularly if a person's symptoms have been triggered by emotional stresses such as relationship difficulties or bereavement, and are associated with weakness of memory and difficulty concentrating. Diarrhea is usually a prominent symptom.

NUX VOMICA may be given for a frequent urge to pass stool, often with no result, and associated irritability and poor sleep.

> **CAUTION**
>
> Coffee can nullify the effect of *Nux vomica*; do not drink it if you are using this homeopathic medication.

Western Herbal Medicine

Even though insufficient research has been carried out, many people with IBS turn to herbal remedies to ease their symptoms. There are many traditional herbal remedies that can help a great deal in IBS. Since patients tend to react to remedies even at low doses, it is always a good idea to start any remedy at small doses, gradually increasing the strength as necessary.

PEPPERMINT OIL capsules appear to be an effective treatment for symptoms of IBS. A meta-analysis of five randomized controlled trials of peppermint oil for IBS suggests that it can be effective in relieving symptoms. In general, essential oils should not be taken internally, although peppermint is an exception. For IBS, the appropriate dosage of peppermint oil is 0.2–0.4 ml three times a day, taken in enteric-coated capsules.

CARMINATIVE HERBS Most important in easing spasms of the gut associated with IBS are so-called carminative (flatulence-relieving) herbs. In order to relieve pain, bloating, and flatulence, teas that are made from mixtures of the following carminative remedies may be effective: chamomile (*Matricaria recutita*), caraway (*Carvum*

ARTICHOKE LEAF EXTRACT shows promise in treating IBS as well as dyspepsia (indigestion). It is an ingredient in many over-the-counter remedies for IBS and relieves IBS symptoms in some patients. One analysis looked at the results of a study on dyspepsia and found benefits on bowel function and a decreased incidence of IBS by using artichoke leaf extract.

CONSTIPATION REMEDIES Aloe vera (*Aloe vera*) juice has a gentle, soothing effect on the bowel and is especially appropriate for people with IBS who have chronic constipation. Take a tablespoon of the

The use of anthraquinone-containing stimulant laxatives, such as aloe leaf, Chinese rhubarb root (*Rheum officinale*), senna (*Cassia angustifolia*), and cascara (*Rhamnus purshiana*), is generally avoided in the treatment of constipation associated with IBS. The intestines can become dependent on these strong laxatives.

SOOTHING HERBS There are several herbs that soothe the bowel. Slippery elm (*Ulmus fulva*) powder contains an abundance of mucilage (a sticky substance). When mixed with powdered ginger (*Zingiber officinale*), cinnamon (*Cinnamomum cassia*), and caraway, it helps reduce abdominal bloating. Slippery elm powder also combines well with cooked oatmeal. Other herbs that soothe an irritated bowel include marshmallow root (*Althea officinalis*) and fenugreek (*Trigonella foenum-graecum*). They work best if combined with pungent warming spices, such as ginger and cinnamon, and can be used to treat both diarrhea and constipation by helping restore normal bowel function.

> ## Irritable bowel syndrome is thought to affect 10–20 per cent of the general population

carni), fennel (*Foeniculum vulgare*), aniseed (*Pimpinella anisum*), cardamom (*Elletaria cardamomum*), garden mint (*Mentha arvensis*), spearmint (*Mentha viridis*), peppermint (*Mentha piperita*), dill (*Anethum graveolens*), lemon balm (*Melissa officinalis*), rosemary (*Rosemarinus officinalis*), and lovage (*Levisticum officinalis*).

These remedies combine well with bitter aromatics such as angelica root (*Angelica archangelica*), tangerine peel (*Citrus reticulata*), and bitter orange (*Citrus aurantium*). The bitter, aromatic combination is especially calming for an irritated gut. The carminative herb chamomile combines well with other relaxing herbs and help relieve IBS aggravated by anxiety.

HERBS TO AID BILE OUTPUT Painful bloating after eating fatty foods may be a result of poor bile output. In stimulating bile production and flow, these remedies enable the body to digest fats. Some herbs have an especially bitter action, which aids digestion. Wormwood (*Artemisia absinthium*), gentian (*Gentiana lutea*), and hops (*Humulus lupulus*) are extremely bitter and are prescribed in small doses. Hops act as a sedative and relaxes the bowel in low doses. Other bitter herbs that are effective for treating IBS include milk thistle (*Silibum marianum*), dandelion root (*Taraxacum officinale*), and globe artichoke (*Cynara scolimus*) leaves.

commercially extracted juice twice daily, but do not continue for more than 12 weeks because it will cause diarrhea. Do not confuse aloe vera juice with aloes, a violent cathartic.

Other remedies for the constipation caused by IBS include psyllium seeds. Psyllium is a soluble fiber, like oat bran, and has a gentle, bulk-forming effect on stool. Psyllium preparations have been researched for more than 20 years in the treatment of IBS and many people with constipation find them effective. However, the results of trials have been inconsistent and better research is needed. One trial showed that both psyllium and wheat bran were effective in normalizing stool consistency and frequency in IBS, but psyllium was better for improving stool frequency and reducing abdominal distension. Psyllium was considered preferable to wheat bran. These remedies work better for IBS that has more constipation than diarrhea; if there is more diarrhea, the remedies may actually make the condition worse.

Psyllium seeds (*Psyllium* spp.) often work best when they are stirred into a little warm water as a bulk laxative. Flaxseed (*Linum* spp.) is another alternative. A tablespoon a day taken with either oatmeal or yogurt is likely to ease constipation without any serious side effects. For these bulk laxatives to work effectively, drink a glass or two of water with them.

ANTI-INFLAMMATORY HERBS A partially blinded pilot study showed some effect on IBS symptoms by using a standardized extract of turmeric (*Curcuma longa*) for 8 weeks. Some experts recommend a dose of 300-400 mg up to three times daily.

HERBAL COMBINATION PRODUCTS Over-the-counter herbal products for IBS are popular in many countries. A recent randomized controlled trial compared two herbal combination products, both containing a mixture of several plant extracts, including bitter candytuft (*Iberis amara*), chamomile, and other extracts, with a bitter candytuft extract and a placebo (inactive substance). The patients taking the combination medicines had significantly fewer IBS symptoms than those taking either the bitter candytuft extract alone or the placebo.

OTHER REMEDIES A useful remedy for loose stools is arrowroot, which can be taken up to three times a day, flavored with a little ground cinnamon or nutmeg. Create a paste with two teaspoons of arrowroot compound and water or chamomile tea or combine it with yogurt. Taking commercially formulated charcoal tablets can also be effective for reducing the swing between loose bowel movements and constipation, in addition to helping reduce flatulence.

Chinese Herbal Medicine

There is no disease equivalent to IBS in Chinese medicine. Strategies for treating IBS are found in discussions of treating three diseases well known in China: diarrhea, constipation, and abdominal pain. The traditional treatment of these diseases allows modern TCM practitioners to discern a number of effective lines of treatment for IBS. TCM doctors will give appropriate dietary advice and, like Western doctors, will recommend that eating patterns must be regular. Meals should not be missed or eaten in a hurry.

RESEARCH There is important research that supports the use of Chinese medicine for IBS including a randomized controlled trial followed 116 patients with the condition. One-third were given capsules of a herbal formulation that was prescribed individually for them, another third were given a standard Chinese herbal mixture, and the final group were given a placebo (inactive substance). Treatment was continued for 16 weeks and those who received Chinese herbal medicines showed significant improvement. The people receiving individualized herbs did not benefit more than those taking the standard Chinese herbal preparations. However, during a follow-up 14 weeks after completing treatment, only those who received individualized treatment had maintained their improvement.

TREATMENTS Chinese practitioners diagnose and then prescribe herbs for a variety of conditions. The first is liver *Qi* (energy) stagnation. The most usual cause of this is emotional disturbance. Long-term resentment, anxiety, worry, or depression blocks

the flow of liver *Qi* that in turn disrupts the smooth flow of stomach, spleen, and large intestine *Qi* (digestive *Qi*), causing bloating, pain, flatulence, and diarrhea or constipation. In women, there may be accompanying PMS marked by mood swings as well as worsening IBS symptoms.

A second common pattern of symptoms is the deficiency of spleen and stomach with stagnation of *Qi*. In this case the patient is tired, especially after eating, and may experience bloating and dull pain after meals. A third pattern is deficiency of spleen with accumulation of "damp." People with this syndrome may have loose stools and feel fatigued. A fourth common pattern is "damp heat" in the large intestine. People with this syndrome may have bloating and abdominal pain and may experience rather explosive, foul-smelling bowel movements that may burn while passing. Lastly, if there is spleen and stomach *Yin* deficiency, the patient may complain of feeling hungry but not being able to eat much, as well as having abdominal bloating, dry lips, a dry mouth, and irregular bowel movements with difficulty passing stools.

Bodywork and Movement Therapies

The spinal nerves that govern digestive function can either speed up or slow down the organs of digestion. The sympathetic nerves emerge from the spine roughly between the shoulder blades and extend down to the lower back, and slow down digestive functions. The parasympathetic nerves, which emerge from the very top and very bottom of the spine, can restore digestive function to a normal state or speed it up. Another branch of the nervous

system exists in the abdomen itself, and this contains almost as many nerve cells as are found in the spine. Mechanical stress resulting from spinal restrictions or from trigger points in back or abdominal muscles can influence these "slowing down" or "speeding up" processes. Since IBS may involve a speeding up of bowel activities (diarrhea) and sometimes a slowing down (constipation), either branch of the nervous system may be involved.

CHIROPRACTIC AND OSTEOPATHY There have been no reliable clinical trials of chiropractic and osteopathic treatments for IBS. Clinical experience, however, suggests they can be useful. A case report illustrates the possible benefit of spinal treatment. The patient was a 25-year-old woman with a history of five years of diarrhea, abdominal pain, and cramping. On examination her spine was found to have a number of areas of marked restriction in the neck, middle, and lower back. She reported sustained improvement after chiropractic treatment that mobilized the restrictions in the spine. If you have IBS, a chiropractor or osteopath should be able to tell you whether spinal restrictions are contributing to your condition.

DEACTIVATION OF TRIGGER POINTS Trigger points are sensitive areas in muscles that usually cause pain or discomfort, not only where they are located but often in a generalized area. Those in the spinal or the abdominal muscles can cause symptoms in the intestinal tract itself. Research conducted nearly 50 years ago and confirmed by recent evidence shows that trigger points in the lower abdomen can cause or encourage diarrhea, one of the common symptoms of IBS. Trigger points can be deactivated by acupuncture as well as by manual pressure and stretching techniques as used by osteopaths, massage therapists (particularly those with neuromuscular therapy training), and some physical therapists and chiropractors.

> Although irritable bowel syndrome may recur throughout life, it does not usually get worse

RELAXATION FOR IBS

Visualisation and relaxation have both been shown to help relieve IBS symptoms. Each day, lie on the floor with a slim paperback under your head and a rolled towel under your knees. Close your eyes and relax fully for 20 minutes, visualising a soothing image such as a beach on a sunny day. Breathe deeply, exhaling slowly.

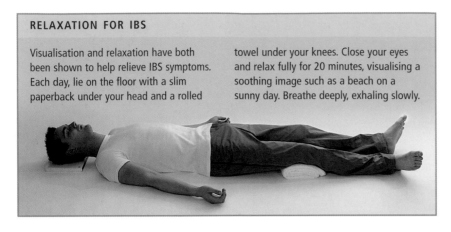

Breathing Retraining

IBS and fibromyalgia (*see p.298*) coexist in many patients. Studies have shown that patients who have IBS may also have significantly more tender points in muscles thannormal. Some experts suspect that the link between IBS and fibromyalgia might be a breathing rate disorder, such as hyperventilation. A common side-effect of rapid upper-chest breathing is elimination of too much carbon dioxide from the body. This can cause your bloodstream to become too alkaline (a condition known as respiratory alkalosis), making the smooth muscle layer around the digestive tract contract. This results in sluggish or interrupted digestion, leading to constipation. Breathing pattern disorders, such as a tendency to breathe using only the upper chest, can usually be improved or corrected by breathing rehabilitation, involving slow, diaphragmatic (yoga-type) breathing methods. Osteopathic correction of restrictions that may have developed in overused and stressed muscles and joints can also help.

Acupuncture

There are very few studies of acupuncture as a treatment for irritable bowel syndrome. One is a series of case reports that does suggest benefit, and the other is a randomized controlled trial that showed benefits for acupuncture in the short term. This study looked at the effects of acupuncture in seven IBS patients. The study found significant improvement in general well-being and in the patients' experience of bloating following acupuncture. However, this study did not include a placebo group, making it difficult to determine the degree to which acupuncture really helped.

Acupuncture is certainly a reasonable treatment option for IBS, with some evidence to sustain claims of benefit. However, a larger, double-blind, randomized controlled trial found no benefit of real acupuncture over sham acupuncture (both groups improved equally), so it is difficult to tell whether it is really useful.

Around 50 percent of people with IBS had their first attack during a major life event

Mind–Body Therapies

Depression is prevalent in IBS patients, as is diminished quality of life. IBS can affect sleep, sexual functioning, business and personal obligations, and social life. The condition may be further complicated by occurring with other conditions, such as fibromyalgia, chronic fatigue syndrome (*see p.474*), and thyroid problems (*see p.319*).

Since there are no definitive diagnostic tests, IBS is a diagnosis of exclusion. Drug treatment is geared toward symptom management, not a permanent cure. If you have IBS, you might want to consider mind–body therapies, such as relaxation or hypnosis (*see p.99*), since there is positive research supporting their use.

PSYCHOTHERAPY AND ANTIDEPRESSANTS are effective in patients with severe IBS. A study randomly allocated 257 patients with severe IBS to receive eight sessions of individual psychotherapy, 20mg daily of the antidepressant paroxetine, or routine care. Patients having psychotherapy or paroxetine felt better physically, but not psychologically, than those getting routine medical care. During the follow-up year, the patients who had psychotherapy maintained improvement in that they were less likely to need other medication or to see doctors. The improvement was not maintained in the paroxetine group.

RELAXATION, BIOFEEDBACK, AND HYPNOSIS Relaxation and biofeedback have shown success in improving symptoms of IBS and preventing the condition from recurring. One approach using relaxation therapy and medication was effective in two-thirds of patients who had not found relief using medication alone. Another approach using progressive muscle relaxation, thermal biofeedback, cognitive therapy, and education had a 50 percent success rate, and four years later those patients still showed improvement. Hypnosis has been shown to improve IBS symptoms, even in severe cases and in cases where psychotherapy had failed.

OTHER THERAPIES Mind–body techniques are effective in alleviating the symptoms of IBS and improving quality of life. A self-help program that includes Relaxation Response meditation or visualization can improve the ability of people with IBS to cope with abdominal pain and reduce or eliminate other symptoms. The need for medication may be reduced correspondingly. (*For details of these therapies, see pp.98–100.*)

PREVENTION PLAN

The following may help prevent IBS:

- Reduce stress
- Take regular exercise
- Avoid known problem foods

ULCERATIVE COLITIS

Ulcerative colitis is an inflammatory bowel disease (*see also Crohn's disease, p.216*), in which the colon (the large bowel) and/or the rectum (to which the large bowel leads) becomes inflamed and ulcerated. The disease may affect the rectum alone or may extend from the rectum up into the colon. Treatment involves a range of drugs and sometimes surgery. Dietary changes and supplements, homeopathic medicines and acupuncture may also play a useful role in controlling the symptoms and progress of ulcerative colitis.

WHY DOES IT OCCUR?

The exact cause of ulcerative colitis is not known. Since about one in ten people with ulcerative colitis has a relative with the condition or another inflammatory bowel disease, such as Crohn's disease, it is possible that genetic factors are involved. Overactive immune responses have also been proposed as a causative factor.

Ulcerative colitis usually starts between the ages of 15 and 35 and is a life-long condition that is characterised by periods of relapse (being ill) followed by periods of remission (being well). The symptoms vary from being mild to severe and generally become apparent over several days.

People who have ulcerative colitis often have other associated disorders, including liver disease, joint disease, uveitis (inflammation of the eye) and erythema nodosum

IMPORTANT

If you experience unexplained weight loss and/or abdominal pain, see your doctor without delay.

(a skin condition in which tender swellings appear, usually on the shins).

Unlike Crohn's disease, ulcerative colitis affects only the large intestine and/or the rectum and never affects the small intestine. People with ulcerative colitis whose disease is confined to the rectum alone tend to experience the fewest complications and have the best prognosis.

People who have ulcerative colitis are also at increased risk of developing colorectal cancer. The risk becomes significant about 10 years after the onset of the illness and is greatest when the whole colon is involved and there is also associated liver disease.

TREATMENT PLAN

PRIMARY TREATMENTS

- Drugs, such as aminosalicylates
- Fish oils

BACK-UP TREATMENTS

- Nutritional therapy
- Surgery

WORTH CONSIDERING

- Acupuncture
- Individualised homeopathy

For an explanation of how treatments are rated, see p.111.

TREATMENTS IN DETAIL

Conventional Medicine

The doctor will arrange investigations. Ulcerative colitis is diagnosed using colonoscopy, in which a flexible viewing instrument is passed up the bowel to examine its lining. Tissue samples (biopsies) are also taken for examination.

If ulcerative colitis is diagnosed, the aim is to control the disease with medical treatment. Several drugs are used to treat ulcerative colitis. The choice of drug depends on how much of the large bowel is involved, how severe the disease is and whether the aim is to treat a relapse or to maintain a remission.

PRIMARY TREATMENT **DRUGS FOR LIMITED DISEASE** If disease is limited to the last 25–30cm of the colon or less, it can be treated by liquid or foam enemas or suppositories which are given directly into the rectum. These may contain mild anti-inflammatory agents, such as amino-salicylates or corticosteroids.

PRIMARY TREATMENT **DRUGS FOR EXTENSIVE DISEASE** If the disease affects a large portion of the colon, oral drugs are required. Aminosalicylates can be used if the disease is mild. However, their main role is in the long-term maintenance of remission and possibly to protect against the development of cancer.

Generally, for more extensive disease or for symptoms that fail to respond to aminosalicylates, a course of corticosteroids will be recommended. These drugs reduce inflammation. The starting dose will be continued for a few weeks and then the dose will be gradually reduced; corticosteroids should not be stopped suddenly. For some people with ulcerative colitis, long-term steroids or frequent courses of steroids may be necessary, too. In children, there is a risk that steroids may affect growth and, for that reason, their use is carefully monitored.

DRUGS TO MAINTAIN REMISSION Azathioprine is an immunosuppressant drug, which helps maintain remission and which may be prescribed for persistent disease as it is thought that ulcerative colitis may be due in part to autoimmune factors. Azathioprine is also known as a steroid-sparing agent and may allow reduction of the steroid dose in people who require high doses or prolonged use of steroids.

PROBIOTICS Some early research has suggested that probiotics ("friendly" microorganisms that are present naturally in the large bowel) may help maintain remission in ulcerative colitis (see Nutritional Therapy, opposite).

SURGERY Surgery may be considered for severe disease that persists despite medical treatment or when high doses of steroids are needed on a regular basis to control the symptoms. There are various options. For example, the colon may be removed but the rectum left in place. The ileum (lower

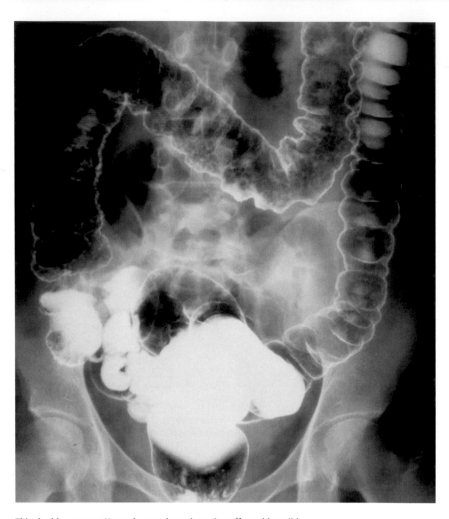

This double contrast X-ray shows a large intestine affected by mild ulcerative colitis. An abnormal mucosal pattern appears as mottling in the ascending colon, which can be seen on the left side of the X-ray. The white areas show barium, the contrast medium.

end of the small bowel) is then connected to an opening on the abdominal wall to form an ileostomy and the stools are collected in bags placed over the opening. It may be possible to reconnect the small bowel and the rectum at a later date or to remove the rectum and connect the small bowel to the anus. In some cases, the ileostomy is permanent. If part of the colon is left in place, the disease may recur in the remaining section.

Toxic megacolon is a serious condition that occurs in very severe cases of ulcerative colitis. In toxic megacolon, the motion of the intestinal wall stops and the colon rapidly becomes distended. Immediate admission to hospital is necessary and the patient is monitored very closely. If the condition does not improve after a few

days of treatment with intravenous steroids and antibiotics, surgery to remove most or all of the colon (known as colectomy) will be required. An ileostomy will be necessary if the entire colon is removed.

COLONOSCOPY Regular surveillance with colonoscopy is recommended for individuals with ulcerative colitis from about 10 years after the onset of the illness. This is done to check for the development of colorectal cancer.

Regular colonoscopy is especially important if the disease affects the entire colon and is accompanied by liver disease. Even if most of the colon has been surgically removed, surveillance is still needed because cancer may develop in the small amount of colon left in place.

Nutritional Therapy

ELIMINATING PROBLEM FOODS People affected by ulcerative colitis may benefit from identifying and eliminating problem foods from their diet (*For more information, see p.39.*)

PRIMARY TREATMENT **FISH OIL SUPPLEMENTS** Ulcerative colitis is an inflammatory condition. Excessive amounts of omega-6 fatty acids (found in vegetable oils) and a relative lack of omega-3 fatty acids (found in oily fish, walnuts and linseeds) seems to promote inflammation.

Maintaining a balance between omega-6 and omega 3-fatty acids in the body may be helpful. This can be achieved by avoiding excessive amounts of margarine and vegetable oils and including oily fish (such as salmon and mackerel), walnuts and flaxseeds in the diet. Studies suggest that taking fish oil (which has anti-inflammatory properties) might be useful in treating ulcerative colitis. In one study, ulcerative colitis patients taking fish oils were able to reduce their dosage of steroid medication by 50 per cent. However, the relapse rate after one year was the same as in another group taking olive oil capsules.

It was found that fish oil supplementation also resulted in weight gain and reduced intestinal inflammation in those taking it. If you have ulcerative colitis, you could try taking fish oil providing 3g EPA and 2g DHA per day.

PROBIOTICS Supplements of beneficial gut bacteria, such as *lactobacillus* and *bifidobacteria*, may be useful in treating ulcerative colitis. One study found that a probiotic supplement was effective in preventing flare-ups of chronic pouchitis (a major long-term complication in ulcerative colitis) in ulcerative colitis patients.

In another study, a group of 15 patients were treated with a mix of beneficial bacteria for one year. Eighty per cent of these patients were still in remission from the condition at the end of the year-long study.

FOLIC ACID Ulcerative colitis is linked to an increased risk of colon cancer, especially when the disease is long-standing. Studies show that people with ulcerative colitis who have been taking folic acid supplements or who have high blood levels of folic acid have a reduced risk of colon cancer compared to people with the condition who do not. People with ulcerative colitis who are taking the drug sulphasalazine, which inhibits the absorption of folic acid, appear to be at particular risk of developing folic acid deficiency. Folic acid supplementation may therefore be important for people with ulcerative colitis, especially for those taking sulphsalazine. If you are taking this drug, try taking 1mg of folic acid per day.

Homeopathy

Records of patients treated at the Tunbridge Wells Homeopathic Hospital suggest that most patients treated with individualised homeopathy (*see p.73*) for ulcerative colitis were helped considerably.

Among the most important homeopathic treatments for this condition are *Mercurius corrosivus*, *Arsenicum album* and *Phosphorus*.

MERCURIUS CORROSIVUS This homeopathic medicine is indicated when the condition is acute and the "keynote" symptom is tremendous tenesmus, which is a constant but ineffective urge to pass a stool, often at its worst just after having passed a stool. Only a little faeces may actually be passed, but they often contain a lot of blood. People affected may also have bladder tenesmus accompanied by a very sore mouth or throat.

ARSENICUM ALBUM can be very helpful in the acute situation when the patient feels very ill, cold and anxious, and may even fear he or she is about to die. Although the patient may indeed be quite ill, they generally feel worse than they are. The stool is typically thin, watery and foul-smelling and there is burning pain in the rectum. It can also be useful in a less acute situation for tense, anxious, chilly patients who may also have skin trouble or at least very dry, flaky skin.

> Doctors suspect ulcerative colitis may be an autoimmune disease, but there is no proof as yet

PHOSPHORUS In patients who respond to *Phosphorus* there is a lot of bleeding; the stools may be copious but often there is not much pain. The patient is tired and weak, although a bit better for rest, and hence feels better in the morning. The patient is often thirsty, especially for cold, refreshing drinks. In terms of personality, *Phosphorus* types are very sensitive, both to the physical and human environment. They are emotionally "up and down", but can be sympathetic and vivacious.

Acupuncture

There are a number of Chinese trials that have looked at the use of acupuncture for inflammation of the colon, but often the diagnosis is unclear and the quality of the trial is poor. There are no good controlled trials analysing the use of acupuncture in proven ulcerative colitis, although acupuncture is widely used for this condition. A traditional Chinese approach is needed for both diagnosis and treatment. It is essential to visit a qualified practitioner and to tell them of any prescribed drugs taken.

Circumstantial evidence and case reports suggest that acupuncture may be of real value in treating acute colitis, but treatment may need to be quite prolonged. Initially, treatment should be given on a weekly basis, or more frequently if the condition is very acute. If there is no obvious improvement after six to eight sessions, it is questionable whether continuing acupuncture treatment will be of value.

GALLSTONES

Hard masses that form from substances in the gallbladder are known as gallstones. They are made from the digestive bile which is stored in the gallbladder and contain cholesterol, pigments, and salts. Most gallstones consist of a mixture of cholesterol and pigments. Gallstones are more common in women and in people of Scandinavian and Native American origin. Surgery may be necessary if gallstones are troublesome or cause the gallbladder to become infected. Other treatment options include lithotripsy, dietary changes, and acupuncture.

WHAT ARE THE SYMPTOMS?

- Upper abdominal pain that may range from mild to severe
- Nausea and vomiting

WHY MIGHT I HAVE THIS?

PREDISPOSING FACTORS

- Being overweight
- Diabetes
- Pregnancy
- Diet high in fat
- Genetic factors
- Sickle-cell anemia and other blood cell disorders
- Lack of physical activity

TRIGGERS

- Changes in spinal joints
- Trigger points in abdominal muscles

IMPORTANT

If you develop any of the the symptoms of gallstones, see your doctor immediately.

WHY DOES IT OCCUR?

In many cases there is no obvious reason for gallstone formation. However, stones made up mainly of cholesterol are more likely in people who are very overweight, and a diet high in animal fats may increase the risk of developing this type of gallstone. A tendency to develop gallstones may run in families, suggesting that a genetic component may be involved. Stones made up mainly of pigment may form if there is excessive destruction of red blood cells which occurs in some hereditary blood disorders. Symptoms arise if a gallstone blocks the ducts that carry bile from the gallbladder to the gut. Symptoms tend to occur after a fatty meal, which causes the gallbladder to contract. In some cases gallstones cause no symptoms.

TREATMENT PLAN

PRIMARY TREATMENTS

- Weight-loss diet (if overweight)
- Surgical removal of the gallbladder
- Shockwave lithotripsy

BACKUP TREATMENTS

- Endoscopic retrograde cholangiopancreatography (ERCP)
- Dietary changes
- Western herbal treatments
- Acupuncture

WORTH CONSIDERING

- Vitamin C and phosphatidyl choline
- Homeopathy
- Bodywork therapies

For an explanation of how treatments are rated, see p.111.

TREATMENTS IN DETAIL

Conventional Medicine

If your doctor suspects that you have gallstones, he or she will conduct tests that include an ultrasound scan of the upper abdomen. Gallstones that are not causing any symptoms (those that are picked up incidentally during other tests) do not require treatment.

If you have gallstones, your doctor will probably advise you to reduce your intake of animal fats. If you are overweight, you may be advised to lose weight.

PRIMARY TREATMENT **SURGERY** If gallstones are causing symptoms, cholecystectomy (removal of the gallbladder) may be recommended. This may be performed traditionally or, more often, by laparoscopic ("keyhole") surgery. Occasionally, stones develop in the remaining bile duct.

PRIMARY TREATMENT **SHOCKWAVE LITHOTRIPSY** Other treatment options are used less and tend to be reserved for people for whom surgery may be dangerous. In shockwave lithotripsy, ultrasound waves generated by a machine are directed to shatter the stones and let the fragments pass through the bile ducts and into the gut.

OTHER TREATMENTS Occasionally, drugs such as ursodeoxycholic acid are given to dissolve cholesterol stones, but this a slow process that takes several months to complete and is only used in certain patients.

Gallstones in the bile duct may be treated using a procedure known as endoscopic retrograde cholangiopancreatography (ERCP), in which a flexible viewing tube with surgical attachments is passed down the esophagus to view and treat the stones.

> CAUTION
>
> Surgery and other procedures for gallstones carry some risks; ask your doctor to explain them to you.

Nutritional Therapy

PRIMARY TREATMENT **WEIGHT LOSS** Obesity is often a factor in gallstone formation, and obese women have been found to have seven times the risk of developing gallstones compared to women of normal weight. Losing weight may help reduce the risk of gallstone problems. However, extreme, rapid weight loss has been shown to actually increase the risk of gallstone formation, so if you need to lose weight, do so slowly and sensibly.

Other risk factors for gallstone formation during weight loss include a very low-calorie diet with no fat and a high level of certain blood fats called triglycerides. People who want to lose weight should follow a sensible eating plan and avoid extreme, "crash" diets. Slow, steady weight loss will probably help reduce the risk of gallstones in the long term. (*See p.444 for more information on obesity and weight loss.*)

DIETARY CHANGES In general, your diet should be rich in fiber. This may reduce the risk of developing gallstones. A diet high in refined carbohydrates (such as sugar, white bread, and white rice) appears to increase risk of gallstones. Refined carbohydrates may increase the production of cholesterol in the liver, which in turn may increase the risk of gallstone formation by raising the level of cholesterol in the gallbladder. The best protection includes a diet that is based on foods including whole-grain bread, brown rice, beans, fruits, and vegetables.

FORMATION AND LOCATION OF GALLSTONES

Gallstones usually result from an imbalance in the chemical composition of bile, a substance produced by the liver that is stored in the gallbladder. Gallstones form in the gallbladder but may travel from there into the cystic duct. They may also pass into the common bile duct and from there into the duodenum. If stones become impacted in a duct, they cause severe upper abdominal pain and nausea.

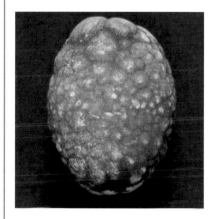

Cholesterol precipitates out of the bile to form crystals, which coalesce together to create a gallstone.

The gallbladder and bile ducts

Cystic duct

Gallbladder

Gallstone in cystic duct

Gallstones

Gallstone in common bile duct

Gallstones form in the gallbladder but may then travel to the bile ducts, where they sometimes become impacted.

Many people with gallstones, particularly those who are overweight, are advised to avoid fat in their diet. However, some studies show that a diet containing moderate amounts of fat may slow or prevent gallstone formation, possibly because dietary fat stimulates the gallbladder to empty, which may help the flow of bile and, thereby, preventing gallstone production.

In one study, obese individuals on a weight loss program had no gallstone formation. The authors of the study attributed this to the fact that their diet contained significant amounts of fat (26g of fat per day). In another study, two groups of obese people were put on very low-calorie diets (a known risk factor for gallstone formation). One group was given only 3g of fat per day, while the other was allowed 12.2g of fat per day. Weight loss was achieved in both groups of patients, but while gallstones developed in more than 50 percent of people following the lower fat diet, no one on the higher fat regimen developed gallstones.

The type of fat eaten also seems to be important. There is some evidence that a diet that is high in vegetable fat is a risk factor for gallstone formation, while fat from fish (omega-3 fatty acids) seem to be protective.

Include oily fish (such as salmon, mackerel, and sardines) as part of your weightloss program to help prevent the development of gallstones.

VITAMIN C helps convert cholesterol into bile acids that are involved in the digestion of fat in the body. In animals, vitamin C supplementation can reduce the formation of gallstones. A study on humans demonstrated that vitamin C (2000mg per day for four weeks) altered bile acid formation in a way that would be expected to reduce cholesterol gallstones formation. Vitamin C supplement use has also been associated with a decreased prevalence of gallstones. If you are concerned about preventing gallstones, try taking 500–1000mg of vitamin C a day.

PHOSPHATIDYLCHOLINE (a purified extract of lecithin) is one of the components of bile that may help protect against gallstone formation. If there is too little phosphatidylcholine or too much cholesterol in the bile, the risk of gallstones increases. Some studies have shown that 300–2000mg of phosphatidylcholine per day may be helpful in preventing and treating gallstones.

If you have gallstones or are concerned about developing them, try taking a daily supplement of phosphatidylcholine within this dosage range.

> **CAUTION**
>
> Vitamin C supplements can interact with certain drugs, including the blood-thinning drug warfarin; ask your doctor for advice. (*See also p.46.*)

Homeopathy

Homeopaths recommend the following medicines for the people who have a tendency to form stones in the gallbladder. *Berberis vulgaris* and *Chelidonium majus* are prescribed based on symptoms, while *Calcarea carbonica*, *Lycopodium*, and *Natrum sulfuricum* are prescribed on a "constitutional" basis (*see p.73*) *Colocynthis* may also be given in certain cases.

BERBERIS is indicated for those who are often nauseous and drowsy after eating, and have a tendency to develop kidney stones and gout.

CHELIDONIUM Where *Chelidonium* is indicated, there may be intermittent jaundice and pain radiating to the tip of the right shoulder blade. This may be accompanied by headache, which is usually on the right side.

CALCAREA CARBONICA The person who responds to *Calcarea carbonica* is typically stocky and solidly built, with a tendency to being overweight. He or she tends to be a phlegmatic type, solid, stubborn, and hard-working, but this calm exterior may conceal anxieties and fears about things such as serious illness. These people may also have bad dreams. They tend to be chilly and yet sweat a lot, especially on

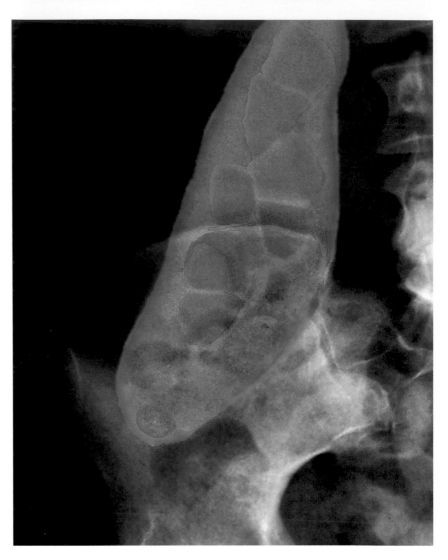

This color-enhanced X-ray shows a gallbladder containing gallstones which appear as red masses in the center of the picture. Gallstones cause problems when they become stuck in the cystic or common bile duct. The pain is from continued contraction of the duct against the stone, not from bile in the duct.

the head and neck. They often crave eggs, especially soft-boiled.

LYCOPODIUM The type of person who responds to *Lycopodium* is typically rather quiet and reserved, disliking large social gatherings. They are often thoughtful, conscientious people who worry in advance of important occasions and may be quite depressed. They take their responsibilities very seriously. They often crave sweets and may feel hungry when they start eating, but quickly feel full. These people often suffer from bloating and gas. They tend to be at their worst in the afternoon, typically between 4 and 8pm.

NATRUM SULPHURICUM People who respond to this remedy feel worse when they are exposed to dampness in any form (examples include such things as wet weather and damp housing). Apart from gallstones, these people may also have a cough that produces sputum, along with stiff joints and a stiff back, all of which are made worse by moisture. They may also have warts.

COLOCYNTHIS Finally, *Colocynthis* may be indicated in gallstone colic — when the gallstone gets stuck in the bile duct, causing severe, colicky pain that comes in waves and is relieved by doubling over.

Western Herbal Medicine

Many herbs can increase bile flow but where gallbladder health is poor and gallstones are large or long-standing. Conventional treatments (including surgical removal of the gallbladder) may prove to be the best option.

Herbal treatment is most effective when it is started when scans show relatively few, small stones. At this time, the primary problem may be gallbladder congestion and remedies can be selected to help flush our debris from the gallbladder and bile ducts. Self-help treatment can be safely undertaken in the early stages of gallstone formation, but professional treatment is best to help choose the best option the many herbs available.

HERBS TO CLEAR THE GALLBLADDER There have been no clinical trials of herbal medicines for gallstones. However, many herbal remedies, known as choleretics, directly stimulate bile production by the liver. As a result, an increased quantity of more dilute bile flows through the bile ducts into the small intestine.

Over time, the increased bile flow encourages cleansing of the gallbladder, reducing the size of stones so that they can be passed without discomfort. Choleretic herbs form the basis of treatment where multiple small gallstones are present.

Clinical research since the 1930s confirms that globe artichoke (*Cynara scolymus*) has a marked ability to increase bile production, lower cholesterol levels (which is important in cholesterol-based gallstones), and relieve dyspepsia (indigestion-like pain) and other symptoms.

Greater celandine (*Chelidonium majus*) is also beginning to be used in this way, although it has traditionally been viewed as a treatment for spasmodic pain arising from the gallbladder.

Milk thistle (*Silibum marianum*) may also be used to treat gallstones. It is best known for its ability to protect the liver but it is also an antioxidant and choleretic herb. Peppermint (*Mentha piperita*), which has long been used to relieve both nausea and dyspepsia, also appears to relax the bile ducts and gallbladder and thereby increase the scope for clearance of gallstones. Finally, turmeric (*Curcuma longa*) is a valuable remedy for gallbladder inflammation and is a powerful anti-inflammatory and choleretic.

OTHER MEASURES Other approaches may also be appropriate, especially those improving diet and digestive function.

> **CAUTION**
>
> See p.69 before taking an herbal remedy and, if you are taking prescribed medication, consult an herbal medicine expert first.

Chinese Herbal Medicine

Li Dan Pai Shi Tang, a Chinese herbal formula composed of *Lysinachiae, Autemisiae Scopaniae, Curcumae, Aromaticae Citrus Aurantitum Saussurea Lappa,* and *Rheum Palmatinum,* promotes the secretion and discharge of bile and eliminating gallstones. These effects have been confirmed by clinical practice.

> **CAUTION**
>
> Do not self-treat with Chinese herbal remedies; consult a specialist.

Acupuncture

TRADITIONAL CHINESE TREATMENT While acupuncture treatment for gallstones is common in China, it is far less common in the US, Canada, and Europe. The Chinese usually give daily treatment to help expel the gallstones under close medical supervision. Several large, nonrandomized clinical studies have shown that clearly demonstrate the discharge of gallstones after treatment with acupuncture.

It is thought that acupuncture works by dilating the common bile duct and causing the gallbladder to contract simultaneously. Ultrasound has shown that 7 to 10 percent of people have had complete clearance of stones and a further 15 percent had a significant reduction in the number of stones.

A dramatic increase in gallstones eliminated in the stool is also found after acupuncture treatment. Stones pass through the common bile duct and into the duodenum, from where they pass through the remainder of the digestive system until they are eliminated.

Treatment needs to be intensive over a relatively short period of time, with two or three hours of treatment given on a daily basis for three or four days.

Bodywork Therapies

Osteopaths believe that improvement in gallbladder function, including reduction of associated discomfort and pain (both before and after surgery), can be achieved by appropriate osteopathic manipulation of the spine.

GALLBLADDER DYSFUNCTION AND THE SPINE This theory holds that there is an important connection between the way the gallbladder functions and the condition of the middle of the thoracic spine (the part of the spine that runs through the chest), from which the gallbladder derives its nerve supply. Osteopaths believe that dysfunction of the gallbladder is linked to changes in the spinal joints, due to a feedback from the distressed organ to the tissues in and around the nerve root emerging from the spine.

DEACTIVATION OF TRIGGER POINTS Pain relating to active trigger points (sensitive areas) in the abdominal muscles can produce symptoms that are almost identical to the pain experienced in the gallbladder region when gallstones are present.

Relief from this pain is often possible when these trigger points in the abdominal muscles are deactivated. Trigger-point activity can have far-reaching effects that spread beyond the muscle housing the trigger point itself.

Symptoms that may be caused by trigger points, such as pain in the gallbladder region, can often be relieved by acupuncture (*see above*) as well as by manual pressure and the stretching techniques that are used by osteopaths, massage therapists (particularly those with a neuromuscular therapy training), and some physical therapists and chiropractors.

> **PREVENTION PLAN**
>
> **To reduce your risk of gallstones:**
> - Keep your weight within a normal range

HEPATITIS

Inflammation of the liver, whatever the cause, is known as hepatitis. The liver has a variety of vital functions including processing nutrients, regulating blood-sugar levels, breaking down toxic chemicals (such as alcohol), making proteins needed for blood clotting, and producing digestive bile. Hepatitis may be acute (short-term), lasting less than six months, or chronic (long-term), lasting for more than six months. Hepatitis requires medical attention but there are also things you can do to help yourself, including a change in diet and taking supplements.

WHAT ARE THE SYMPTOMS?

Initial symptoms of acute hepatitis may include:

- Fatigue and a feeling ill
- Poor appetite
- Nausea and vomiting
- Fever
- Pain or discomfort in the upper right side of the abdomen

Several days later, the following symptoms may appear:

- Yellowing of the whites of the eyes and the skin (jaundice)
- Pale stools and dark urine

Symptoms of chronic hepatitis may include:

- Loss of appetite and weight loss
- Fatigue
- Yellowing of the whites of the eyes and the skin (jaundice)
- Widespread itchiness
- Abdominal discomfort and possible swelling

WHY MIGHT I HAVE THIS?

PREDISPOSING FACTORS

- Ingestion of water or raw shellfish from water that contains sewage (hepatitis A)
- Eating contaminated food in high-risk areas (hepatitis A)
- Contact with blood (hepatitis B, C)
- Needle sharing (hepatitis B, C)
- Unprotected sexual intercourse (hepatitis B)
- Acetaminophen use, especially with excessive alcohol consumption
- Drug use
- Herb use
- Exposure to chemicals that are toxic to the liver (e.g. toluene)
- Exposure to drugs toxic to the liver (e.g. phenytoin)

WHY DOES IT OCCUR?

Many conditions can cause hepatitis, but the most common is infection with a hepatitis virus. There are several viruses, of which the most common are hepatitis A, hepatitis B, and hepatitis C. Other lesser known types of the virus include hepatitis D and hepatitis E. In addition, other hepatitis viruses are likely to be discovered in the future. Non-infectious causes of hepatitis include excessive alcohol consumption and side effects of medication.

The hepatitis A virus is transmitted through contaminated food or water and can be found in the urine and feces of infected people. Infection with the hepatitis A virus is always acute and does not become chronic.

The hepatitis B virus is spread by contact with infected bodily fluids, such as blood. It can be transmitted by drug users sharing needles and by sexual intercourse. Infection with the hepatitis B virus can cause both acute and chronic hepatitis.

The hepatitis C virus is transmitted mainly by needle sharing and blood transfusions (although all blood is now tested for hepatitis C) and, less commonly, by sexual intercourse. The hepatitis C virus can cause either acute or chronic hepatitis, although it is the most common cause of chronic hepatitis.

Acute hepatitis may either cause no symptoms, or symptoms may be so mild that they go unnoticed. If hepatitis is caused by a virus, the time from infection to appearance of symptoms varies from 2–3 weeks for hepatitis A to 1–5 months for hepatitis B.

Acute hepatitis may become severe and in some cases may progress to liver failure, a life-threatening condition in which the liver is unable to carry out its functions. Severe acute hepatitis is relatively common following an acetamenaphen overdose but occurs only rarely with hepatitis A and B infections.

Roughly one-third of acute hepatitis infections with type B or C viruses become

TREATMENT PLAN

PRIMARY TREATMENTS

- Drugs including antivirals and corticosteroids

BACKUP TREATMENTS

- Liver-supporting diet
- Liver transplant (for liver failure)
- Vitamin C
- Milk thistle, glycyrrhizin, and other liver-protective herbs

WORTH CONSIDERING

- Environmental health measures
- Homeopathy
- Acupuncture

For an explanation of how treatments are rated, see p.111.

IMPORTANT

If you develop symptoms that suggest hepatitis, see your doctor without delay. If left untreated, some types of hepatitis can lead to irreversible liver damage.

THE LIVER AND ITS FUNCTIONS

The liver converts molecules from the bloodsteam into either simpler or more complex forms, depending on the body's requirements. The liver consists of thousands of lobules, tiny units about 1/25in (1 mm) wide that process blood. Each lobule is surrounded by branches of the portal vein, hepatic artery, and bile duct. Processed blood is returned to the heart through the inferior vena cava. The liver also produces digestive bile, which is then stored in the gallbladder.

The liver, gallbladder, and pancreas

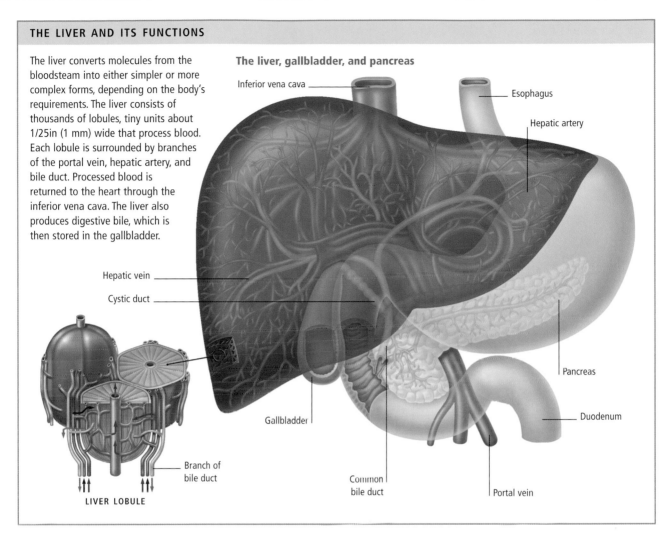

Inferior vena cava

Esophagus

Hepatic artery

Hepatic vein

Cystic duct

Pancreas

Duodenum

Gallbladder

Branch of bile duct

Common bile duct

Portal vein

LIVER LOBULE

---

chronic. In the other two-thirds of cases of chronic hepatitis, the condition develops gradually with no apparent previous illness. Some people may be unaware of having a previous episode of acute viral hepatitis until the symptoms of chronic hepatitis appear or until routine blood tests assessing liver function are found to be abnormal. Other causes of chronic hepatitis include autoimmune diseases (where the body's immune system produces antibodies against its own tissues).

Chronic hepatitis can progress to cirrhosis — irreversible liver damage that may cause liver failure. Both of these conditions are associated with an increased risk of developing liver cancer.

Some people with hepatitis caused by hepatitis B, D, and possibly C continue to carry the virus in their blood. They can pass the virus although they do not develop symptoms themselves.

TREATMENTS IN DETAIL

Conventional Medicine

The treatment of both acute and chronic hepatitis depends on the underlying cause. In many cases of acute hepatitis, no specific treatment is necessary.

Hepatitis A requires no specific treatment. It usually lasts 3–6 weeks and, in most cases, the prognosis is good. Similarly, acute hepatitis B requires no treatment; most people make a complete recovery.

PRIMARY TREATMENT **ANTIVIRAL DRUGS** People who develop chronic hepatitis may be treated with antiviral agents, such as interferon, which is given by injection, usually for about four months. Interferons are proteins produced by the body in response to viral infections; synthetic versions are used to treat certain diseases.

Interferon produces a response in up to half of those treated, but relapses may occur. The antiviral drug lamivudine is also used. It is taken orally for about a year and is generally well-tolerated. Other antiviral treatments and immunomodulatory agents are being studied and appear promising for hepatitis B. Treatment with a combination of antiviral drugs (often including interferon), usually for about six months, may be appropriate and is effective for some cases of chronic hepatitis C.

PRIMARY TREATMENT **OTHER MEASURES** In other types of chronic hepatitis the underlying conditions are treated. Hepatitis that results from autoimmune disease is treated with long-term corticosteroids and sometimes azathioprine, which reduces the activity of the immune system. If liver failure occurs in acute or chronic hepatitis, a liver transplant may be necessary.

> **CAUTION**
>
> Drugs for hepatitis can cause a range of possible side effects. Ask your doctor to explain these to you.

Nutritional Therapy

PRIMARY TREATMENT **LIVER-SUPPORTING DIET** People with hepatitis should avoid anything that puts stress on the liver, including acetaminophen, alcohol, and high-dose vitamin A. *(For more information on a diet to support the liver, see p.42.)*

VITAMIN C Vitamin C may help people with hepatitis. In addition to its immune system-stimulating and antiviral properties, this nutrient is also known to promote tissue healing, and may therefore help reduce the risk of long-term liver damage.

Vitamin C may also be useful for combating free radical damage that is a common a factor in people with hepatitis. Clinical experience suggests that 2g of vitamin C taken three times a day while symptoms persist may be helpful. In the longer term, individuals with hepatitis might benefit from taking 1g of vitamin C, twice a day. If you have hepatitis, try taking vitamin C at these dosages.

VITAMIN E Vitamin E is another antioxidant vitamin that may help people with hepatitis, who often have low levels of this nutrient. A study demonstrated the ability of vitamin E (1200 IU per day of the d-alpha-tocopherol form for eight weeks) to prevent one aspect of liver damage (fibrogenesis cascade) in hepatitis C patients. Another study found that vitamin E supplementation might be effective in the treatment of chronic hepatitis B . People with hepatitis may benefit from taking 800–1200 IU vitamin E per day.

CATECHIN This bioflavonoid compound, found in green tea, has antioxidant action and may help neutralize free radicals generated by substances toxic to the liver. One study found that catechin supplementation was effective in treating hepatitis in some individuals. Try taking 500–750mg catechin, three times a day if you have hepatitis.

> **CAUTION**
>
> Consult your doctor before taking vitamin C with antibiotics or warfarin, or vitamin E with warfarin or aspirin. These vitamins can affect the action of these drugs. (*See also p.46.*)

Homeopathy

PHOSPHORUS is the usual homeopathic medicine for acute hepatitis, particularly for hepatitis A and acute alcoholic hepatitis. People for whom *Phosphorus* is indicated are tired and weak, although rest helps somewhat so they feel better in the morning. Those who respond to this medication often have pain under the right ribs and loss of appetite, although they are often thirsty, especially for cold, refreshing drinks, and they like ice cream.

ARSENICUM ALBUM is another medicine for acute hepatitis. In this case, the "picture" is similar to that of *Phosphorus*, but the people who respond to *Arsenicum album* are also very anxious and chilly and there may be edema (accumulation of fluid) and ascites (accumulation of fluid in the abdomen). *Arsenicum album* may also be appropriate for chronic hepatitis.

LACHESIS may also be indicated for patients whose face is a dark reddish blue hue or if they have bleeding gums and hemorrhoids. Patients are talkative and may be aggressive or paranoid. *Lachesis* may also be indicated for chronic hepatitis.

LYCOPODIUM AND NATRUM SULPHURICUM can both be indicated for hepatitis. People who respond to *Lycopodium* often experience bloating, indigestion, and right-sided migrainous headaches. Patients are typically rather reserved and their symptoms are worse between 4 and 8pm.

People who respond to *Natrum sulphuricum* often have pale, bulky stools with diarrhea, especially in the morning. They always feel worse when the weather is wet and may be very depressed.

Western Herbal Medicine

Herbs should never be used in place of conventional medicine but they can be used as a complementary treatment. when they may provide the most effective treatment for acute and chronic hepatitis. Self-treatment is not appropriate; you should always seek treatment from an herbal medicine expert

In determining treatment for hepatitis of all types, the herbal practitioner will assess and prioritize specific areas requiring treatment. These include support and protection of liver function, stimulating the elimination of toxins other than via the liver (e.g. by the kidneys or through sweating), managing fever, stimulating immune function, and countering viral infection.

HERBS TO FIGHT INFECTION If treating an acute condition, the main priorities will be to stimulate immune resistance and support normal liver function.

Herbs such as echinacea (*Echinacea* spp.), garlic (*Allium sativum*), phyllanthus (*Phyllanthus amarus*), and St. John's wort (*Hypericum perforatum*) figure prominently in prescriptions. All four have broad antiviral activity, while St. John's wort and its active constituents hypericin and pseudohypericin have specific activity against the hepatitis A, B, and C viruses, as well as against the Epstein-Barr virus.

Schisandra (*Schisandra chinensis*) is a plant used in traditional Chinese and Japanese medicine, usually in herbal mixtures. One small study of a Japanese herbal mixture (called TJ-108) containing schisandra found that it may be an antiviral effective in treating hepatitis C.

While hepatitis A offers a chance for full recovery, hepatitis B and C herbal treatments primarily aim at preventing the development of chronic hepatitis.

LIVER-PROTECTIVE HERBS For herbal treatment of sub-acute or chronic hepatitis, the herbal medicine expert will

> ## Liver specialists report an increase of acute alcoholic hepatitis

primarily use hepatoprotective (liver-protective) herbs, which have specific antioxidant action on liver tissue, protecting it against damage and cirrhosis (scarring of the liver. Such herbs also help to normalize liver function.

Key hepatic herbs include dandelion root (*Taraxacum officinale*), bupleurum (*Bupleurum falcatum*), and globe artichoke (*Cynara scolymus*). Many other herbs and medicinal foods, such as wormwood (*Artemisia artabinthium*) and beets (*Beta vulgaris*), have antioxidant and protective activity for the liver.

Meta-analyses mention some effects of milk thistle (*Silybum marianum*) and its flavanolignans (known collectively as silymarin) on mortality and liver function tests in people with chronic hepatitis, but milk thistle does not seem to control the viral load or liver anatomy. More research is needed to determine how milk thistle might act with conventional therapies.

A review of several randomized trials suggested that glycyrrhizin (an extract of the licorice plant) may reduce the complications of chronic hepatitis C in patients who do not respond to interferon. Several trials showed that the liver functioned better after treatment with glycyrrhizin. Studies performed in 1997 and 2002 showed that long-term treatment with glycyrrhizin might prevent liver cancer in patients with chronic hepatitis C.

> **CAUTION**
>
> See also p.69 before taking an herbal remedy. Hepatitis is not suitable for self-treatment with herbs. Always consult an herbal medicine expert.

Chinese Herbal Medicine

Some Chinese medicinal herbs may work in chronic hepatitis B. It is important to choose a practitioner who has an expertise in treating hepatitis.

Environmental Health

The liver is the body's chemical factory. It is responsible for breaking down and metabolizing drugs and for processing environmental and other toxicants. These activities can bring it into contact with a variety of hepatotoxins (compounds that are toxic to the liver).

Many hepatotoxins have specific effects on just one area of the liver or on one type of cell in the liver. Others cause a certain type of damage to the liver, such as fatty changes or fibrosis, which are not technically classified as hepatitis but nevertheless put the organ under stress.

People with existing hepatitis should avoid hepatotoxins and anything else that could further injure, or cause stress to, liver cells. In practice, this entails eating organically grown foods, avoiding smoky atmospheres, drinking filtered water, and not taking drugs or supplements that may be metabolized through the liver, such as alcohol and common over-the-counter medicines that contain acetaminophen.

HEPATOTOXIC MEDICINES Many drugs are hepatotoxic. Acetaminophen is a common cause of hepatitis. The most common medications that cause acute or chronic cases of hepatitis are methyldopa, isoniazid, nitrofurantoin, phenytoin, and oxyphenisatin.

If you take any of these medications, your doctor should follow the recommended monitoring guidelines, ordering blood tests to check your liver enzymes; you may need to change drugs if the tests show any evidence of liver damage.

HEPATOTOXIC CHEMICALS AND METALS Certain chemicals and metals can damage the liver. If your job involves working with hepatotoxic chemicals (such as toluene, chloroform, solvent mixtures, or trichloroethylene) or heavy metals (such as lead, mercury, and manganese), it is important to follow safety instructions such as using protective gloves, suits, eyewear, or respirators.

If you are frequently exposed to these chemicals or metals you should have a blood test to check your liver function for possible damage. An environmental health practitioner can advise you on how to avoid the chemicals to which you are regularly exposed. Taking a daily supplement of the herb milk thistle (*see Western Herbal Medicine, above*) can help to protect your liver from damage caused as a result of exposure to toxins.

OTHER HEPATOTOXINS There are certain natural compounds from plants that may be hepatotoxic and should be avoided. Examples include alflatoxin, which comes from a fungus that infects peanuts, tree nuts, and certain bacteria. To protect yourself from naturally occuring hepatotoxins, be sure that you discard any nuts that appear old, shriveled, or moldy. Since alcohol is also considered a hepatotoxin, limit the amount of alcohol you drink and avoid it altogether if you have hepatitis.

Acupuncture

Acupuncture is of no proven value in acute infective hepatitis, although it has been used to improve symptoms in patients with hepatitis B and C. It may provide relief from symptoms, but there is little hard evidence to support these claims.

If acupuncture is used to help with chronic hepatitis, weekly treatments should be provided for at least eight to ten weeks. If after this period there appear to be clinical benefit, then regular constitutional acupuncture may be required on a monthly or trimonthly basis to help maintain the improvement.

Remember that you should always inform your doctor if you have an infective form of hepatitis. Particular care should be taken with respect to exposure to blood products and needle disposal, cases of hepatitis due to inadequately sterilized needles have been reported. Make sure your acupuncturist uses only disposable needles.

> **PREVENTION PLAN**
>
> **The following measures will help protect you from hepatitis:**
>
> - Drink alcohol in moderation
> - Practice safe sex
> - If you use intravenous drugs, never share needles
> - Get immunized against hepatitis A if you are traveling to a developing country where it may be prevalent
> - If you are a healthcare worker, make sure you are immunized against hepatitis B
> - Avoid eating raw shellfish
> - Minimize use of drugs and potent herbs

For an explanation of how treatments are rated, see p.111.

CYSTITIS

In cystitis, the lining of the bladder becomes inflamed, causing frequent, painful urination. About half of all women have at least one attack of cystitis in their lives, and some women have recurrent attacks. In men, cystitis is rare and is often associated with a disorder of the urinary tract. In some cases of cystitis, short courses of antibiotics may be given. Analgesics may help with any discomfort. There are also herbal, homeopathic, dietary, and other strategies to help prevent cystitis from recurring.

WHAT ARE THE SYMPTOMS?

- Burning pain when urinating
- Frequent and urgent need to urinate, with only a little urine each time
- A feeling that the bladder has not been emptied completely

If a bacterial infection is causing cystitis, symptoms may also include:

- Pain in the lower abdominal region and sometimes in the lower back
- Fever and chills
- Smelly or cloudy urine
- Blood in the urine

WHY MIGHT I HAVE THIS?

PREDISPOSING FACTORS

- Wiping incorrectly after a bowel movement
- Menopause
- Yeast overgrowth
- Diabetes mellitus

TRIGGERS

- Sexual intercourse
- Diaphragm use
- Trigger points in muscles in the pelvic area

IMPORTANT

If you suspect that your child may have cystitis, see a doctor immediately. In children, cystitis needs prompt treatment because it may otherwise progress to a kidney infection and eventually to kidney damage.

WHY DOES IT OCCUR?

Cystitis is often caused by a bacterial infection, most commonly by the bacteria *Escherichia coli*, which normally lives in the intestines. While a urinary tract infection (UTI) may occur anywhere along the urinary tract, cystitis is the term for a UTI that only affects the bladder and urethra. Women are more likely to be affected than men, probably because they have a shorter urethra (the tube that leads from the bladder to outside the body), which makes it easier for the bacteria to pass up into the bladder. Bacteria from the vagina or anus may enter the bladder during sex or when wiping after a bowel movement. The risk of bacterial cystitis is increased if the bladder is not emptied fully during urination, allowing bacteria to multiply in the urine that remains behind.

People with diabetes mellitus may be particularly susceptible to cystitis (among other reasons, their urine may contain glucose which the bacteria can feed on). Postmenopausal women may also be at increased risk, due to changes in the urinary tract that occur with age and as a result of lower levels of female sex hormones in the body.

Recurrent bouts of cystitis are often associated with yeast overgrowth in the body. Beneficial bacterial organisms are athought to exert a controlling effect on organisms around the female genitalia that may cause bladder infections, such as *E. coli*. In yeast overgrowth, lower levels of healthy organisms around the urethra make it more likely that unwanted organisms can infect the bladder.

Pelvic pain and frequent urination that do not respond to antibiotics may be due to interstitial cystitis, an uncommon condition in which the lining of the bladder becomes chronically inflamed.

There are a number of measures that you can take to relieve the discomfort of cystitis.

TREATMENT PLAN

PRIMARY TREATMENTS

- Antibiotics (for bacterial cystitis)
- Pure cranberry juice (unsweetened or extract)
- Increased water intake

BACKUP TREATMENTS

- Bearberry and other Western herbs
- Probiotics
- Dilating the urethra for interstitial cystitis

WORTH CONSIDERING

- Anti-Candida diet
- Individualized homeopathy
- Chinese herbal medicine
- Trigger point deactivation

SELF-HELP

- Drink plenty of fluids (about eight 8oz glasses per day and more in hot weather). This helps flush the bacteria out of the bladder. Drinking cranberry juice as an alternative to water, may be particularly helpful (*see p.240*).

- Urinate shortly after intercourse and before going to bed.
- Take analgesics and hold something warm, such as a heating pad or hot water bottle, against your abdomen.
- Avoid caffeinated beverages, which may further irritate the bladder.

TREATMENTS IN DETAIL

Conventional Medicine

PRIMARY TREATMENT **ANTIBIOTICS** The doctor may send a urine sample to be tested for evidence of infection. While waiting for the results he or she may prescribe an antibiotic, which studies show resolve the majority of cases of bacterial cystitis. Another antibiotic may be prescribed once the results are back.

Studies have shown that a long course of low-dose antibiotics, usually for 6–12 months, significantly reduces the rates of recurrent cystitis. Alternatively, if cystitis seems to be related to sexual intercourse, some women may be prescribed antibiotics to take as suppositories. Studies have shown that these can prevent cystitis.

OTHER TREATMENTS Further tests, such as ultrasound scanning, may be recommended to look for an underlying disorder of the urinary tract in women who have recurrent bacterial cystitis or for men who have a single episode. If your doctor suspects that you have interstitial cystitis, he or she may recommend that you see a urologist. Dilating the urethra during cystoscopy (viewing the inside of the bladder through an instrument inserted into the urethra) may be one treatment option. Postmenopausal women may find that estrogen creams applied around the urethra help relieve their symptoms.

Nutritional Therapy

PRIMARY TREATMENT **DRINKING WATER** throughout the day can help flush out organisms before they can cause infection. Aim to drink at least eight 8oz glasses of water each day.

ELIMINATING YEAST FROM THE BODY Clinical experience suggests that taking

---

THE URINARY TRACT

The kidneys filter waste products from the blood and pass them into the bladder with excess water, as urine. The urinary tract consists of the two kidneys, the ureters (which connect the kidneys and bladder), the bladder, and the urethra (which leads from the bladder to outside the body). The lower urinary tract differs in men and women. In men, the urethra is longer and passes through the prostate gland. In women, the shorter urethra passes directly to the opening in front of the vagina.

Sexual differences

The male bladder sits above the prostate gland and the male urethra passes through it. The male urethra is about 8in (20cm) long and carries either urine or semen out through the penis.

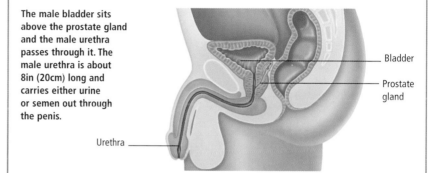

Urethra

Bladder

Prostate gland

MALE

The female bladder sits below the uterus and the female urethra carries urine directly to an opening located in front of the vagina. In women, the urethra is about 1½in (4cm) long.

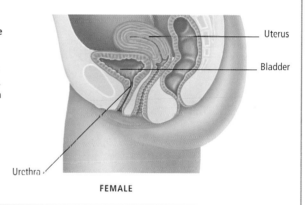

Uterus

Bladder

Urethra

FEMALE

---

steps to control yeast organisms, such as *Candida albicans*, in the body can help prevent recurrent urinary tract infections (*for information, see p.40*).

PROBIOTICS are supplements containing "healthy bacteria," which seem to be particularly useful in controlling unwanted organisms. Probiotic organisms are believed to compete with and crowd out the unhealthy organisms around the vagina, hence helping prevent infection. Probiotic microorganisms, such as *lactobacilli*, also make the bladder environment more acidic, and this helps prevent the growth of unwanted organisms. In one study, weekly probiotic pessaries containing *lactobacillus* reduced the recurrence rate of cystitis infections in women.

Herbal Medicine

TRADITIONAL HERBS for cystitis and urinary tract infections include agrimony (*Agrimonia eupatoria*), barleywater (made from barley, *Hordeum distychum*), bearberry (*Arctostaphylos uva-ursi*), bilberry (*Vaccinium myrtillus*) fruit and leaves, buchu (*Agathosma betulina*), couchgrass (*Agropyron repens*), cranberry (*Vaccinium macrocarpon*), garlic (*Allium sativum*), goldenrod (*Solidago virgaurea*), goldenseal (*Hydrastis canadensis*), heather flowers (ling, *Calluna vulgaris*), horsetail (*Equisetum arvense*), hydrangea (*Hydrangea arborescens*), juniper (*Juniperus communis*), ladies mantle (*Alchemilla xanthochlora*), marshmallow root (*Althea officinalis*), matico leaves (*Piper angustifolia*), nettle

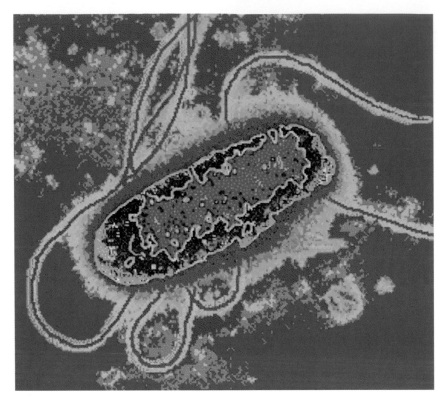

The bacterium *E. coli.* is one of the main causes of cystitis. It normally inhabits the intestines without causing problems, but may infect the bladder by traveling up the urinary tract.

(*Urtica dioica*), parsley (*Petroselinum crispum*), parsley piert (*Alchmilla arvensis*), pellitory of the wall (*Parietaria judaica*), pipsissewa (*Chimaphila umbellata*), plantain (*Plantago lanceolata*), shepherd's purse (*Capsella bursa-pastoris*), wild carrot (*Daucus carota*), and yarrow (*Achillea millefolium*). To date, few of these herbal remedies have been investigated for the treatment of UTI, but given the emergence of strains of bacteria resistant to antibiotic treatment, research should be carried out into this largely untapped and potentially invaluable resource.

PRIMARY TREATMENT **CRANBERRY JUICE** is perhaps the best-researched remedy for the treatment of UTI. It is a nutraceutical (functional food) that is bought as much for its reputation for allaying urinary tract infections as for its taste. It was once assumed that cranberry was effective because it acidified the urine, thereby inhibiting bacterial growth. However, it has been discovered recently that the action of cranberry juice is probably due to its condensed tannins (proanthocyanidins), which appear to prevent the adherence of harmful bacteria to urinary epithelial cells. If bacteria cannot stick to the walls of the urinary tract, they are washed out of the system.

However, a Cochrane systematic review of research on the use of cranberry juice for urinary infections has highlighted significant flaws in the accumulated data. The reviewers commented that both the small number and the poor quality of the trials gave no reliable evidence for the use of cranberry juice or any other cranberry products in the treatment of UTI. Nevertheless, data from laboratory studies and clinical trials (including one that was published after the Cochrane review) seem to support the use of cranberry as a useful treatment. More research, however, is needed to test its efficacy.

People subject to recurrent UTI who are prescribed long-term antibiotic therapy are ideal candidates for cranberry treatment. Two to three glasses of juice a day should be sufficient. It is important, however, to purchase pure juice products, avoiding those products that merely have cranberry flavor on top of a base of high-fructose corn syrup. Those with diabetes should use sugar-free preparations. A recent Canadian trial revealed that cranberry tablets provided the most cost-effective prevention for UTI.

OTHER REMEDIES Bearberry (*Artostaphylos uva-ursi*) is a close relative of cranberry with a similar longstanding reputation for curing UTI. It has exhibited an antibacterial action on a wide range of infecting organisms including *Staphylococcus aureus*, *Bacillus subtilis*, *Escherichia coli*, *Mycobacterium smegmatis*, *Shigella sonnei* and *Shigella flexneri*.

In one study, an herbal mix that included bearberry (*Artostaphylos uva-ursi*), hops (*Humulus lupulus*) and peppermint (*Mentha piperita*) was used to treat patients with enuresis and painful and difficult urination. Approximately 70 percent of the 915 patients who participated reported improvement after six weeks of treatment with this regimen.

Buchu (*Agathosma betulina*) is a traditional remedy of the indigenous people of South Africa and was taken for UTI by the early Dutch settlers there. In a laboratory study an alcoholic extract of buchu was found to be effective against infecting organisms causing UTI.

Nettle leaf has been approved in Germany for inflammatory disease of the lower urinary tract and prevention of kidney stones, and is useful for chronic cystitis. Couchgrass (*Elymus repens*) is also recommended in Germany for UTI.

Goldenseal has a reputation as a urinary antiseptic. This herb contains a substance known as berberine, which has a broad-spectrum action against many bacteria, including *E. coli*.

Almost half of all women will have an attack of cystitis at some point in their lives

Chinese Herbal Medicine

In Traditional Chinese Medicine (TCM), *Lin* disease (*Lin Zheng*) includes a variety of disorders characterized by pain associated with urination, some of which correspond to cystitis and other UTI.

There are several varieties of *Lin* disease, but heat is characteristic of most of them. TCM doctors distinguish between "full" (*Shi*) and "empty" (*Xu*) conditions. There are three varieties of heat *Lin*: damp heat, heart fire, and liver fire.

Some people repeatedly have persistent symptoms of cystitis despite several courses of antibiotics. Such cases may not be caused by harmful bacteria; in western medicine this is known as interstitial cystitis. This phenomenon may be due to other *Lin* patterns, one of which is liver *Qi* stagnation (*Qi Lin*). Once again, it has an emotional basis. The classic prescription is Aquilaria Powder (*Chang Xiang San*). Another pattern that may occur in chronic cystitis and may not respond to antibiotic treatment is fatigue *Lin*. After making a diagnosis, the TCM doctor treats the underlying cause, which may be kidney *Yin*, *Qi*, or *Yang* deficiency or spleen deficiency.

Homeopathy

Homeopathy can be particularly helpful in interstitial cystitis, in which no infective organism can be found but urination is frequent and painful nonetheless.

STAPHYSAGRIA (made from a type of wild delphinium) is the most frequently used homeopathic treatment. A clinical trial showed it to be effective, helping when symptoms include a constant desire to urinate. Symptoms are frequently triggered by trauma (including sexual intercourse), and there may be a background of apparent or suppressed anger or indignation, sometimes related to sexual assault or abuse.

OTHER REMEDIES *Equisetum* often helps in chronic or recurrent cystitis in children, which may be associated with bed wetting. Pain at the end of urination is typical of the cystitis that responds to this medicine.

An enlarged prostate gland can increase the likelihood of developing cystitis

Cantharis is the classical homeopathic medicine for acute cystitis with severe pain when urinating and tenesmus, which is the sensation of needing to urinate again as soon as you have finished.

Bodywork Therapies

TRIGGER POINTS are sensitive spots in the muscles that can refer pain to other parts of the body (see p.55). As far back as the early 1950s there were reports that symptoms similar to those of cystitis could be the result of trigger-point activity in the muscles of the abdomen.

According to leading researchers of trigger point therapy, urinary frequency, urinary urgency, and kidney pain may be referred from trigger points in the skin of the lower abdominal muscles. Injection of an old appendectomy scar has relieved frequency and urgency, and increased the bladder capacity from 240ml to 420ml.

More recent research confirms these findings and has shown how the effects of trigger-point activity can spread. In some cases it may have effects that reach well beyond obvious muscle and joint pain.

TRIGGER-POINT DEACTIVATION Symptoms resulting from trigger points, such as those of cystitis, may be relieved manually, as well as by injection. A recent study involved 42 people with "chronic cystitis" whose main symptoms were painful urgency and frequency of urination. Following manual treatment of trigger points in the pelvic muscles, 35 of these people (83 percent) reported moderate to marked improvement, with some being completely relieved, after up to 14 years of experiencing these symptoms.

Trigger points can be deactivated either by acupuncture treatment or by using various manual pressure and stretching techniques. These treatments may be provided by osteopaths, massage therapists (particularly those with neuromuscular therapy training), and some physical therapists and chiropractors.

CHIROPRACTIC AND OSTEOPATHY If you experience recurring attacks of cystitis, it may be that a back problem is either causing or contributing to it. The nerve supply to the bladder derives from the lower back, and some studies have suggested that irritation of these lower back nerves can also affect bladder function. A chiropractor, an osteopath, or a physical therapist trained to use manipulative techniques can evaluate your condition and provide the appropriate treatments.

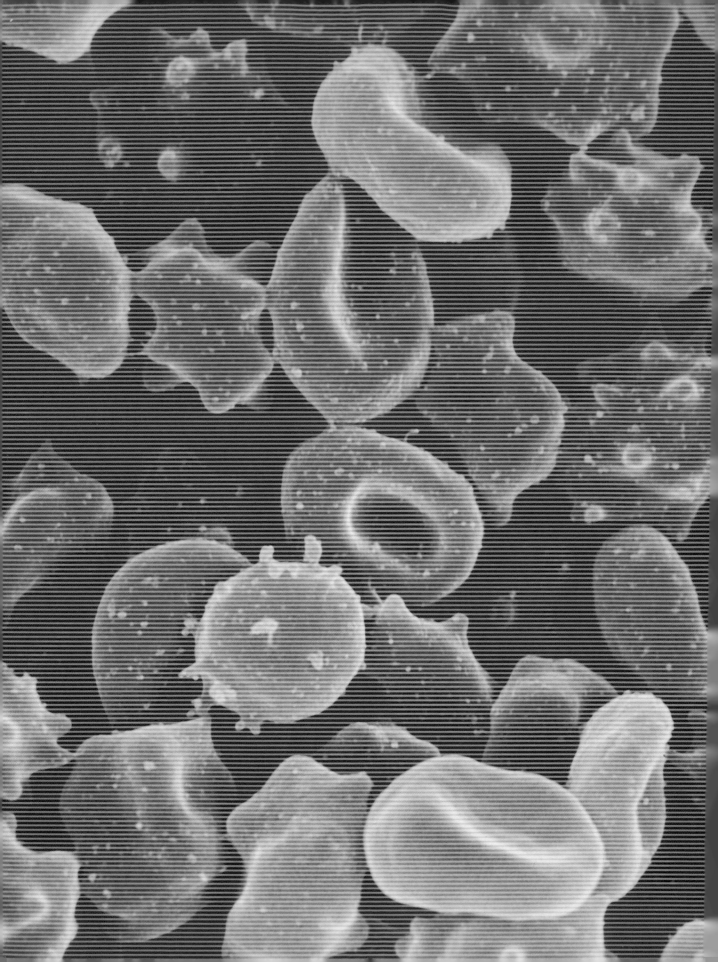

Circulatory System

Circulating blood carries food and oxygen to all parts of the body. Problems can develop if the heart loses its power or rhythm, or if flow through the vessels is disrupted. Surgery and drugs are available for certain circulatory illnesses while a healthy lifestyle and complementary therapies help restore health and well-being.

HYPERTENSION

Persistently high blood pressure, also known as hypertension, affects as many as 1 in 5 adults in the US. It puts strain on the heart and arteries, and can damage delicate tissues, such as the eyes and kidneys. The higher the pressure, the greater the risk that serious complications, such as a heart attack or stroke, will develop. Integrated treatments offer ways of lowering blood pressure, including drugs, supplements, regular exercise, osteopathy, chiropractic, massage, herbs, homeopathy, yoga, and other stress-reduction techniques, and lifestyle changes.

WHY DOES IT OCCUR?

Blood pressure varies naturally with activity, rising during exercise or times of stress and falling when we rest. It also varies among individuals and increases with increasing weight and age.

In most people with hypertension, there is no obvious cause for the condition. However, lifestyle and genetic factors may both contribute. High blood pressure increases with age and is more common in men than women. It tends to run in families and is more common in people of African–American descent. Risk factors for the condition include stress, a high alcohol intake, a diet high in salt, and excessive weight.

Older people are more prone to hypertension because their arteries become less flexible with age, a condition known as atherosclerosis. The condition may be aggravated by too much stress. In a few cases, kidney disease or a hormonal disorder may be the cause. Some drugs, including oral contraceptives and corticosteroids, may also cause hypertension.

BLOOD PRESSURE IN PREGNANCY Hypertension may occur in pregnancy for reasons that are largely unknown. The high blood pressure may be a symptom of preeclampsia, a condition that often develops in pregnancy. The condition may occasionally cause convulsions if the blood pressure becomes very high and therefore must be monitored closely by a doctor. However, not all pregnant women with hypertension have preeclampsia. Blood pressure usually returns to normal after birth but the condition may recur in subsequent pregnancies.

IMPORTANT

If you are experiencing symptoms that suggest that your blood pressure might be high, you should see your doctor as soon as possible to have it checked.

SELF-HELP

PRIMARY TREATMENT Try the following to reduce the risk of hypertension and coronary artery disease (*see p.252*):

- Maintain a healthy weight.
- Eat a diet low in salt and saturated fat and rich in vegetables, fruit, and oily fish.
- Drink alcohol in moderation (less than 21 units per week for men and 14 units per week for women).
- Exercise regularly (primarily aerobic exercise, such as brisk walking).
- Stop smoking.

TREATMENTS IN DETAIL

Conventional Medicine

When your blood pressure is raised, your doctor will make an assessment to exclude an underlying cause, look for risk factors, and assess whether vulnerable organs — in particular the heart, eyes, and kidneys — have been damaged.

Unless your blood pressure is very high, your doctor will monitor it and suggest self-help measures that may help lower your blood pressure before considering drug treatment. These include maintaining a healthy weight, moderate alcohol intake, and regular exercise.

PRIMARY TREATMENT **ORAL DRUGS** If the self-help measures (*see left*) fail to lower your blood pressure sufficiently or if your blood pressure is very high, your doctor may prescribe a variety of medications. When you start the drugs, and what drugs you take, depend on various factors, including the level of your blood pressure, your age, and the presence of other diseases. Various medications can control blood pressure and reduce the risk of organ and tissue damage.

Thiazide diuretics, such as hydrochlorothiazide, are often the first medications to be prescribed. They have been found to reduce the risk of stroke associated with hypertension. Thiazide diuretics cause the kidneys to excrete more water and salts than usual, thus reducing the volume of circulating blood.

Antihypertensives may be prescribed instead, or in addition, to diuretics. Antihypertensives work in various ways — most dilate (widen) the blood vessels throughout the body or reduce the force with which the heart pumps blood. Your doctor will weigh the side effects of antihypertensives against the potential benefits, such as reducing the risk of a stroke or coronary artery disease.

Groups of antihypertensives include:
- Beta-blockers, such as atenolol, which have been shown to reduce the risk of complications in people with hypertension. These block the effect of epinephrine and norepinephrine, two chemicals produced by the body that increase the heart rate and raise blood pressure.
- Angiotensin-converting enzyme (ACE) inhibitors, such as captopril, dilate the body's blood vessels so that the blood pressure falls.
- Calcium-channel blockers, such as nifedipine, block the entry of calcium ions into the muscle in arterial walls. The muscles relax, allowing the walls to dilate and causing the blood pressure to fall.
- Other antihypertensives include aspirin, alpha-blockers, such as doxazosin, and angiotensin II receptor blockers, such as losartan.

CAUTION

Drugs to combat high blood pressure have a range of side effects: ask your doctor to explain these to you.

HOW THE HEART PUMPS BLOOD

In every heart beat there are two main phases as the blood is pumped out of the ventricles (systole) and then as blood fills the atria (diastole). One-way valves between the chambers of the heart open and close in sequence, controlling the direction of blood flow. The timing of the systolic contractions and diastolic relaxation are synchronized by the heart's pacemaker (known as the sinoatrial node), which sends out electrical impulses to the muscles in the atria and ventricles.

The cycle of the beating heart

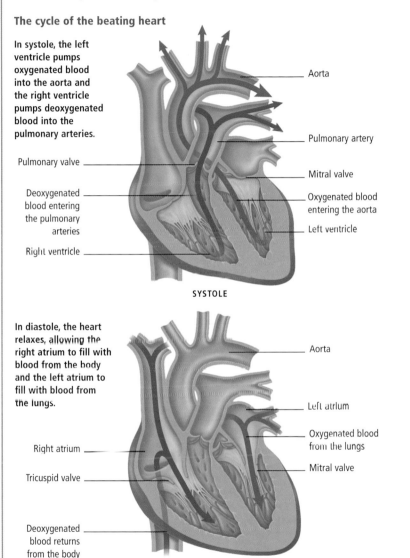

In systole, the left ventricle pumps oxygenated blood into the aorta and the right ventricle pumps deoxygenated blood into the pulmonary arteries.

Pulmonary valve

Deoxygenated blood entering the pulmonary arteries

Right ventricle

Aorta

Pulmonary artery

Mitral valve

Oxygenated blood entering the aorta

Left ventricle

SYSTOLE

In diastole, the heart relaxes, allowing the right atrium to fill with blood from the body and the left atrium to fill with blood from the lungs.

Right atrium

Tricuspid valve

Deoxygenated blood returns from the body

Aorta

Left atrium

Oxygenated blood from the lungs

Mitral valve

DIASTOLE

Nutritional Therapy

LOWER SALT LEVELS Some peple have salt-sensitive hypertension, which responds well to reducing dietary salt. One meta-analysis that pooled the results of several trials showed that reducing salt in the diet to approximately 5g per day had a significant effect on the blood pressure in individuals both with and without hypertension. It is worth trying a low-sodium diet while monitoring your blood pressure to see whether or not it has an effect. If possible, try to reduce your salt intake by not adding salt during cooking or at the table. You should also avoid processed and packaged foods because these tend to have a high salt content.

MEASUREMENT OF BLOOD PRESSURE

Blood pressure is expressed as two values measured in millimeters of mercury (mmHg). The upper figure, known as the systolic pressure, refers to the pressure of the blood when the heart contracts. The lower figure, known as the diastolic pressure, refers to the pressure of the blood when the heart muscle relaxes between contractions. The blood pressure of a young adult should not be more than about 120/80 mmHg. Definitions vary but, in general, high blood pressure is defined as being higher than 140/90 mmHg.

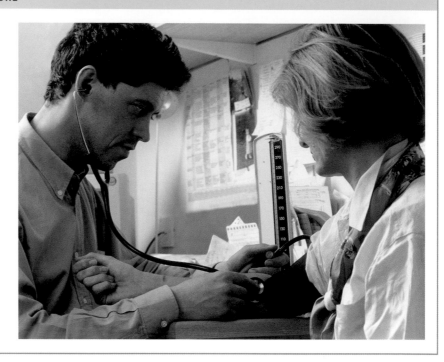

An inflatable cuff is wrapped around the upper arm. The doctor listens to the blood flow through a stethoscope. When he can hear the heart beat he records the systolic pressure, when the sound disappears he notes the diastolic pressure.

RAISE POTASSIUM LEVELS While the sodium in salt tends to raise blood pressure, potassium tends to lower it. One study demonstrated that eating a potassium-rich diet (one with plenty of fresh fruits and vegetables), together with a low sodium diet, can help lower blood pressure.

REDUCE CAFFEINE A review of many trials indicates that coffee consumption (average of 5 cups per day) increases blood pressure and could therefore contribute to hypertension. In trials with younger participants, the effect of coffee drinking on blood pressure was greater than normal. People with hypertension are recommended to reduce or eliminate coffee from their diet.

SUPPLEMENTS Calcium has been reported to help reduce blood pressure, although not by much. However, individuals sensitive to salt may get significant benefit. Try taking 1,000mg of calcium supplements per day for a 12-week period.

Magnesium supplements may also help reduce blood pressure. The recommended dose is 300–500mg of magnesium per day. Another nutritional agent that may help is Coenzyme Q_{10}. The recommended dose is 50mg of Coenzyme Q_{10}, twice a day.

One systematic review has found that fish-oil supplementation in doses of 3g daily modestly lowers blood pressure.

> **CAUTION**
>
> Consult your doctor before taking, calcium, magnesium, and CoQ_{10}, because they can interfere with other medications (*see p.46*).

Homeopathy

If you have hypertension, consult a practitioner for a suitable remedy.

BARYTA CARBONICA, according to one study, helps reduce high blood pressure in patients with arteriosclerosis (hardening of the arteries) and helps people who are mentally slow and timid, and those whose feet sweat offensively.

SULPHUR People who respond to *Sulphur* are sensitive to, and dislike, heat. These people tend to have congestive phenomena, such as congested hemorrhoids, red lips, congestive headaches, and burning feet. (*See also Constitution & constitutional prescribing, p.73.*)

AURUM MURIATICUM People who respond to *Aurum muriaticum* often have palpitations or extra systoles. They may be deeply depressed, lacking in self-confidence, and bad tempered — they can also get very angry over small things. They are worse in winter and may suffer from sinusitis.

LACHESIS is often appropriate for women with hypertension that starts during their perimenopausal period, although it can also be used successfully for men. People who respond to *Lachesis* are generally excitable and loquacious. (*See also Constitution & constitutional prescribing, p.73.*)

GLONOINUM is a symptomatic medicine that is usually given in fairly low dilution (6C), two or three times daily. The kind of symptoms that suggest *Glonoinum* may be appropriate include throbbing or pulsating in the head or neck, and attacks of glowing heat in the face.

Western Herbal Medicine

DIAGNOSIS Herbal practitioners use a wide range of medicinal plants to normalize blood pressure, whether it is raised or lowered. As in most cases where no identifiable cause can be found for raised blood pressure, the selection of specific remedies depends on assessment of immediate needs, such as relaxation and weight loss, and of underlying factors, such as constipation.

A naturopath or other herbal medicine expert assesses your pulse and blood pressure over several visits, as well as checking your cholesterol, LDL, HDL, and triglyceride levels (*see p.34*). These are linked to other signs that reflect your overall state of health. Important factors include signs of oxidative damage and atherosclerosis, capillary tone, venous congestion, constipation, and nerve and muscle tone. If kidney or endocrine factors cause high blood pressure, these require treatment in their own right.

PRIMARY TREATMENT **HAWTHORN** Regarded as a "food for the heart," hawthorn (*Crataegus* spp.) is a heart tonic that contains antioxidants that dilate the blood vessels (vasodilator). As a result, it is a key treatment for hypertension when it is associated with atherosclerosis. It is also a recommended treatment wherever there is a long-term increased load on the heart (*see Coronary Artery Disease and Heart Attack, p.252*). Although it was previously thought that hawthorn should not be used with digoxin, a recent human study found no evidence of an interaction.

> **CAUTION**
>
> Consult an expert in herbal medicine before taking hawthorn extracts because they may interact with other medicines.

OTHER REMEDIES Dandelion (*Taraxacum officinale*) leaf has traditionally been used as a diuretic that helps reduce blood pressure. Clinical studies since the 1950s have confirmed this activity. Rich in potassium, dandelion leaf is thought to minimize the risk of potassium loss that is commonly associated with diuretics.

Cramp bark (*Viburnum opulus*) is an antispasmodic herb that is used to relax the muscles in the walls of arteries. Linden flowers (*Tilia europea*) are both diaphoretic (they promote sweating) and relaxant, with the potential to lower elevated systolic blood pressure. Garlic may be somewhat effective because it increases the elasticity of the arterial wall.

Environmental Health

The causes of hypertension are difficult to ascertain, as conventional medicine acknowledges when using the generic term "essential hypertension" to describe the seemingly complex and undescribed causes of this common problem. However, compelling environmental associations with hypertension warrant a closer look.

LEAD As with so many other diseases, there is ample evidence that hypertension is linked to long-term lead exposure. Do the following to minimize exposure:

- Limit your exposure to lead-containing paints in older homes.
- Run water for at least a minute through household pipes that may contain lead-containing solder.
- Use cold, not hot, tap water (or filter your water with an approved portable filter, or reverse osmosis system).
- Do not use leaded crystal or improperly glazed ceramics for eating or drinking.
- Check that remedies, including calcium supplements, are free from lead before you use them.
- Take precautions if you use lead solder either for a hobby or professionally.

Exposure to significant amounts of lead can be detected by testing the blood or, in cases of long-term exposure, by measuring the amount of lead that as been incorporated into bone. Chelation (binding a metal and filtering it from the bloodstream by chemical means) is one way of dealing with lead in the body, but there is no guarantee that it will work, even in acute high-dose lead poisoning.

Supplementing your diet with calcium (*see Osteoporosis for RDA table, p.309*) may work, since it takes preference over lead when the metals are absorbed and incorporated in the body.

CADMIUM Several studies suggest that cadmium may also be involved in causing hypertension. To limit your level of cadmium, avoid zinc processing plants and eat organ meats and shellfish in moderation. If you are a smoker, quit immediately. If you are exposed to cadmium, take lead-free calcium supplements in recommended amounts (*see Osteoporosis for RDA table, p.309*). Do not exceed the recommended daily allowance for calcium because too much calcium can cause cardiac and other problems.

POLYCHLORINATED BIPHENYLS (PCBs) A strong incentive for everyone to convert to a vegetarian diet is the correlation between PCB levels and hypertension.

Every 2 pounds of weight you lose can lower your blood pressure by 2.5/1.5 mmHg

PCBs, which have caused thinning of eggshells in some birds, are most often found in animal fat and in certain fish.

AIR POLLUTION Some evidence suggests that exposure to air pollution directly relates to elevated blood pressure. People with heart disease are more susceptible to worsening cardiac problems and even death from dangerous levels of air pollution. There are several reports of large numbers of people succumbing to heart disease during periods of intense air pollution.

COLD WEATHER Exposure to cold temperatures may be linked with one of the dreaded complications of hypertension — ischemic stroke (*see p.148*). Blood pressure varies more than normal in colder temperatures, which may account for the increase in heart and stroke conditions during the winter. You should avoid strenuous exercise during especially cold weather.

Acupuncture

Established high blood pressure may produce a range of different symptoms, some of which can be relieved by acupuncture. These may include excessive fatigue and headaches. However, there is no evidence that the use of acupuncture alone, even in the long term, will produce a sustained and safe normal blood pressure.

Acupuncture may help if it is combined, in prolonged treatment, with appropriate dietary and conventional medicine. Occasionally, acupuncture may relieve adverse reactions from antihypertensive drugs.

Acupuncture needs to be used on a weekly basis, and probably for eight to ten weeks, to obtain a consistent initial response. If acupuncture treatment is effective then it will often need to be repeated on a monthly basis for a prolonged period.

Bodywork Therapies

Evidence suggests that osteopathic manipulation, focused on those spinal areas from where the nerve supply to the kidneys emerges, may help reduce high blood pressure. This manipulation encourages the kidneys' role in fluid elimination. Cranial

> Hypertension affects approximately 75 percent of people over the age of 75

manipulation can lower high blood pressure in some cases.

Any therapy that reduces stress will probably lower high blood pressure, if only temporarily. For example, massage has been shown to effectively reduce diastolic blood pressure (the lower of the two figures when blood pressure is measured; *see How the heart pumps blood, p.245*).

Yoga-type Breathing

A simple yoga-type breathing method may lower blood pressure after a stressful episode. Slowing the rate of breathing (*see Anxiety, p.414*) has been shown to be as effective in lowering blood pressure in people with mild hypertension as medication.

In addition to the breathing benefits, the movements and postures of traditional yoga can produce a significant lowering of blood pressure, often enough to allow a reduction in medication.

Aerobic Exercise

In one study, it was found that mildly hypertensive white women who did aerobic exercise for 30 minutes were able to reduce their blood pressure for up to seven hours following the exercise. However, a later study showed that this response is not the same in African–American women, whose blood pressure rose or stayed the same. In fact, aerobic exercise may adversely affect the blood pressure of black women.

Weight loss is helpful in reducing high blood pressure, and exercise is better than dieting. Aerobic exercise is more effective at helping reach a healthy weight than a low-calorie diet alone.

Finally, there is another benefit of exercise for people with hypertension. Between 20 percent and 45 percent of people experience "white coat hypertension" — their blood pressure rises when it is measured by a nurse or physician. Research has shown that this tendency disappears if they exercise regularly.

Mind–Body Therapies

STRESS The relationship between stress, emotions such as anger and hostility, and cardiovascular health is becoming increasingly clear. The link between anger or hostility and heart disease is well documented (*see Coronary Artery Disease and Heart Attack, p.252*). In addition, people who are very hostile are also more likely to engage in unhealthy lifestyle behaviors, such as smoking and eating a high-fat diet, which increase the risk of hypertension.

Studies have demonstrated that there is a link between increased feelings of hopelessness and cardiovascular disease. One Finnish study showed that men who did not have hypertension but reported high baseline levels of hopelessness were three times as likely to develop hypertension during the four years of follow-up.

In many respects, anger/hostility, depression/hopelessness, and anxiety can be viewed as the emotional and behavioral consequences of stress. In other words, they are what happens when people perceive that they do not have the internal or external resources to meet the demands or challenges of life.

Experiencing occasional feelings of anger, concern, and sadness is normal. However, when these mood states become more frequent or even chronic, it is a clue that the normal stresses and challenges of life are no longer being managed effectively. This chronic activation of the stress response can not only wear away the quality of mental and emotional health and well-being, but it can also have a significant effect on physical health and well-being, especially cardiovascular health in general and blood pressure in particular.

BIOFEEDBACK has been demonstrated to be effective in lowering blood pressure and, when combined with general relaxation strategies, maintaining lower blood pressure over extended periods of time. Using biofeedback to increase peripheral blood flow and temperature (as an indication of blood vessels dilating) has also been shown to lower blood pressure.

JOB STRAIN is a type of stress characterized by situations of high demand (excessive amounts of work) but low control (little input about the workload). One study focused on 40 men who had mild to moderate high blood pressure while they were at work. When these men were faced with tasks that they felt were dictated by external demands over which they had little control, their blood pressure increased. However, when they were faced with tasks that they felt they could meet with their own self-pacing (internal control), their blood pressure remained either normal or just borderline high.

SENSE OF CONTROL Practicing mind-body skills such as relaxation and yoga can help restore a sense of control and calm. These strategies provide a safe, effective means of maintaining normal blood pressure levels, even in demanding work situations.

PREVENTION PLAN

To prevent hypertension:

- Eat a diet low in salt and saturated fat, high in fruit, vegetables, and oily fish
- Exercise regularly
- Give up smoking if you are a smoker

ANGINA

Angina is a chest pain that is often brought on by physical activity and is relieved by rest. The pain is due to an inadequate supply of oxygen to the heart muscle that usually results from coronary artery disease (*see p.252*). The flow of oxygen-rich blood to the heart may be adequate when the body is at rest, but becomes inadequate during exertion. The integrated approach to treatment combines lifestyle measures and drugs such as aspirin, beta-blockers, and nitrates, with nutritional supplements and stress-relieving therapies, such as relaxation.

WHAT ARE THE SYMPTOMS?

- A heavy or tight pain in the middle of the chest that may spread to the neck and down one or both arms, usually the left
- The pain may be accompanied by breathlessness
- If severe, angina may also occur when resting

WHY MIGHT I HAVE THIS?

PREDISPOSING FACTORS

- Smoking
- A high-fat diet
- Lack of exercise
- Excess weight
- High blood pressure
- Diabetes mellitus

TRIGGERS

- Physical exertion
- Cold, windy weather
- Extreme emotions, such as excitement
- Blood-sugar imbalance

IMPORTANT

If you develop symptoms of angina, see your doctor immediately. If you have established angina and attacks become more frequent or occur at rest, or if you have a severe attack or pain that is not relieved by fast-acting nitrate spray or pills, seek medical help immediately. Do not take sildenafil (Viagra) or other drugs for erectile dysfunction.

WHY DOES IT OCCUR?

When deposits of fatty acids build up on the internal walls of the coronary arteries (atherosclerosis), they form plaque that restricts the flow of blood to the heart. Angina is likely to occur when the coronary arteries are too narrow to allow the heart muscle to receive the oxygen needed for exercise. Toxic substances accumulate in the muscle, causing cramplike pain.

Angina is less common in women than men until the age of 60, probably due to estrogen, the female hormone that protects against coronary artery disease (*see p.252*). After menopause, the protection wears off.

Smoking, a high-fat diet, lack of exercise, excess weight, high blood pressure (*see p.244*), and diabetes mellitus (*see p.314*) are all risk factors for coronary artery disease.

Angina is often brought on by exertion, but may also be triggered or worsened by exposure to cold, windy weather, and extreme emotions, such as excitement.

IMMEDIATE RELIEF

Angina is usually relieved by rest and using a fast-acting nitrate spray or pill. If pain persists despite these measures, seek medical attention immediately.

TREATMENTS IN DETAIL

Conventional Medicine

TESTS If your doctor suspects angina, you will undergo various medical exams. Blood tests look for conditions such as high cholesterol levels and diabetes mellitus. An ECG, or electrocardiogram (a recording of the electrical rhythm of the heart), is routinely taken, but results are likely to be normal between episodes of angina. However, an ECG taken while exercising on a treadmill may indicate both the presence and severity of coronary artery disease.

Echocardiography (ultrasound scanning of the heart) may be used to assess the

TREATMENT PLAN

PRIMARY TREATMENTS
- Lifestyle changes
- Oral drugs for symptom relief and prevention

BACKUP TREATMENTS
- Angioplasty
- Coronary artery bypass grafting
- Blood-sugar stabilizing diet
- Magnesium and coenzyme Q$_{10}$

- Breathing retraining
- Mind–body therapies

WORTH CONSIDERING
- L-arginine and L-carnitine
- Exercise
- Bodywork therapies
- Acupuncture

For an explanation of how treatments are rated, see p.111.

functioning of the heart muscle. It sometimes might be necessary to have coronary angiography, which involves the injection of a dye into a blood vessel in the arm or groin. The dye travels in the blood to the heart and its progress through the coronary arteries is monitored on a screen and recorded on X-rays. Coronary angiography may be used to confirm the diagnosis and will show where and to what extent the arteries have become narrow.

PRIMARY TREATMENT **LIFESTYLE CHANGES** You will need to take stock of your lifestyle and make significant changes: if you are smoker, quit; if you lead a sedentary life, exercise regularly (under medical advice); and, if you need to, lose weight. Your doctor may prescribe drugs to help lower your lipid levels as well as suggest a low-fat diet (*see Cardio-protective diets, p.255, and The Ornish approach, p.256*).

PRIMARY TREATMENT **ORAL DRUGS** Taking 75mg of aspirin every day can reduce the risk of a heart attack (myocardial infarction). Fast-acting nitrate drugs, in the form of a spray or pill, are used to relieve pain.

You may be prescribed one of a variety of drugs to prevent angina from occurring. There are three main drug groups.

Beta-blockers, such as atenolol, reduce the heart's rate and the force with which it contracts. This puts less stress on the heart muscle, reducing its demand for oxygen.

Long-acting nitrates, such as isosorbide mononitrate, relax the walls of the coronary arteries, improving blood supply to the heart muscle and widen the blood vessels around the body, making it easier for the heart to pump blood.

Calcium-channel blockers, such as amlodopine and diltiazem, also relax the walls of the coronary arteries and reduce the force of the heart's contraction. Some also make the heart beat more slowly.

> **CAUTION**
>
> Drugs for angina can cause side effects: ask your doctor to explain them to you.

ANGIOPLASTY aims to relieve angina by widening the affected arteries (*see p.253*). A catheter with a deflated balloon at its end

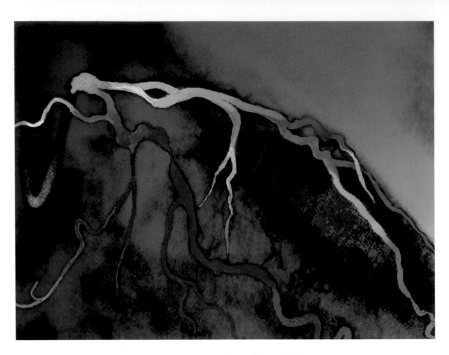

An angiogram is a contrast X-ray that is used to detect abnormalities, such as narrowing, in the coronary arteries of the heart. Dye is injected into the blood vessels to make them clearly visible on the X-ray.

is inserted through an artery in the groin and then passed through the veins to the affected coronary artery. It is inflated several times to widen the narrowed artery. The doctor is guided by images on a screen. There is a relatively small risk of myocardial infarction or of a split in the artery, which necessitates bypass grafting. Sometimes, a tube called a stent is placed in the artery to keep it open and reduce the risk of it becoming narrowed again.

CORONARY ARTERY BYPASS GRAFTING also aims to relieve angina. A blood vessel taken from the leg or chest is used to bypass the narrowed part of the artery. This treatment may be offered if symptoms are still present despite drug therapy and if angioplasty is inappropriate. Possible complications include a small risk of a stroke.

Nutritional Therapy

A BLOOD-SUGAR BALANCING DIET may be important in controlling angina. When blood-sugar levels fall, the body secretes epinephrine to stimulate the liver to release sugar. Epinephrine may trigger angina because it increases the oxygen demands of the heart muscle and can induce spasm in the coronary arteries (*See also p.42*).

MAGNESIUM SUPPLEMENTS are often useful in treating angina. Important for energy production, magnesium also enhances heart muscle function and reduces the risk of spasm and constriction in the coronary arteries. There is evidence that magnesium deficiency may be a factor in angina. A randomized double-blind study performed in the US, Israel, and Austria found that 365mg per day of magnesium citrate for 6 months lessened exercise-induced angina and increased exercise duration. The normal recommended dose is 500–1,000mg per day. Magnesium can cause diarrhea.

COENZYME Q_{10} (COQ$_{10}$) is a nutrient that is also essential for energy production in the body. One study showed that taking 150mg of CoQ$_{10}$ per day significantly lengthened the amount of time it took for angina to affect a person during exercise.

L-ARGININE, an amino acid, may be useful for people with angina. It appears to operate by helping blood vessels dilate, which might enable more blood to reach the heart muscle. L-arginine supplements have been shown to improve exercise tolerance in people with angina. The recommended dose is 2g of L-arginine per day.

L-CARNITINE supplements can help transport fat into parts of the body's cells called mitochondria, where energy is produced. Studies show that taking 1g of L-carnitine twice a day can improve heart function and reduce angina symptoms.

Breathing Retraining

There is evidence that spinal or soft-tissue problems can produce symptoms identical to those of "real" (i.e. cardiac) angina. Called pseudoangina, chest pains mimicking angina can also occur in people with and without coronary artery disease, when excessive upper-chest breathing causes spasm in otherwise normal blood vessels of the heart. Pseudoangina can be diagnosed when the usual indicators, following blood tests and ECGs, are absent.

One study suggests that up to 90 percent of noncardiac chest pain can be brought on by hyperventilation (HVS) and other breathing pattern disorders (BPD) (see p.57). It is therefore important that chest pain associated with HVS/BPD is investigated, so that heart disease can be excluded as a diagnosis and breathing retraining started (for exercises, see p.62).

A condition called Prinz-Metal angina refers to people whose chest pain can be provoked by an exercise test — pain comes on within six minutes or less — but who have normal cardiac arteries. More common in women than men, the condition is helped by breathing retraining (see p.62).

Exercise

Based on evidence of benefit in cardiovascular rehabilitation, people with angina should follow a graduated and prescribed exercise program. For moderate angina, this is at least as effective for symptom control as coronary angioplasty or stenting.

Bodywork Therapy

TREATING PSEUDOANGINA Spinal restrictions and disk degeneration can cause symptoms identical to angina, without any cardiac involvement. No controlled studies have been done. A series of 164 cases were reported in medical literature, with all patients experiencing angina symptoms, neck and arm pain, and headaches. About one quarter needed spinal surgery, but most were treated with nonsurgical methods such as intermittent traction, hard collars, stretching of neck muscles, and anti-inflammatory medication.

A 1976 report studied the lower neck region in seven pseudoangina cases. Surgically removing the damaged disks or using soft collars provided relief in five cases.

The thoracic spine can be a major source of pseudoangina. In a coronary unit at a Swedish hospital, pseudoangina resulting from thoracic spinal dysfunction (known as T4 Syndrome) was the third most common diagnosis after coronary thrombosis and true angina. Treating the spinal causes by manipulation has been shown to relieve "angina-like" symptoms, often in as little as one treatment, with no return of symptoms up to ten years later.

DEACTIVATE TRIGGER POINTS Many cases of pseudoangina result from trigger points (see p.55) in the pectoral muscles, as well as in various shoulder and neck muscles. In one report, angina-like pain, palpitations, and shortness of breath cleared up following treatment of the trigger points by lidocaine injections, as well as massage, hydrotherapy (hot packs, ice packs, and whirlpool), and muscle stretching.

Trigger points can also be deactivated by acupuncturists, osteopaths, massage therapists (those with neuromuscular therapy training in particular), and some physical therapists and chiropractors.

Acupuncture

Several small studies indicate that acupuncture can help angina over a two-year period. Treatment resulted in the avoidance of surgery in about 61 percent of patients and the possible halving of a myocardial infarction (heart attack) during the two-year period. However, the studies do not prove that acupuncture is an effective alternative to surgical intervention. While acupuncture does not alter the underlying coronary artery disease that triggers angina, it can apparently modify the outcome. The treatment is usually given weekly for two months. If the therapy is helpful, long-term maintainance treatments may be needed.

> According to recent US health statistics, more than six million Americans have angina

Mind-Body Therapies

STRESS MANAGEMENT combined with exercise yields tangible, positive benefits for the reduction of angina. According to research, those with angina should engage in mind–body techniques such as meditation, deep breathing, or guided imagery (see p.99). Results from a 1997 study suggest that mind–body techniques that induce relaxation can reduce the frightening and dangerous chest pain of angina.

Many people with angina report a poor quality of life, including higher levels of both anxiety and depression. In 1999 and 2000, newly diagnosed patients from York followed the "Angina Plan," a cognitive behavioral disease management program. Patients suffered less anxiety and depression and had fewer angina episodes, a reduced need of glyceryl trinitrate, and none of the physical limitations reported at the beginning of the study. Participants also changed their diet and increased their daily walking.

PREVENTION PLAN

The following should reduce your risk of developing angina:

- Eat a diet high in vegetables, fruit, and oily fish, but low in saturated fat

- Exercise regularly, such as brisk walking or cycling, for 30 minutes, five or more days per week

- If you smoke, quit

- If you are diabetic, control blood sugar

CORONARY ARTERY DISEASE

In coronary artery disease (CAD), sometimes called coronary heart disease, one or more of the coronary arteries becomes narrowed and blood flow to the heart is restricted. Exertion or stress, which increase the oxygen demands of the heart muscle, may bring on symptoms such as chest pain and even a myocardial infarction (heart attack). Frontline treatments include lifestyle changes, aspirin, and lipid-lowering drugs. In some cases, angioplasty or bypass surgery may be recommended. Various nutritional therapies will help, as will managing stress.

WHAT ARE THE SYMPTOMS?

- In the early stages of CAD there may be no symptoms
- Later, angina (see p.249) may develop

If a heart attack occurs, the individual may experience:

- Persistent, severe pain in the chest that may spread up into the neck and down the arm — the pain may occur while resting
- Sweating
- Shortness of breath
- Nausea and vomiting

WHY MIGHT I HAVE THIS?

PREDISPOSING FACTORS

- Smoking
- Genetic factors
- A diet high in certain fats
- Lack of exercise
- Excess weight
- Hypertension
- Diabetes mellitus
- High intake of trans-fatty acids
- Oxidized cholesterol
- Raised triglyceride levels
- Raised homocysteine levels
- Anger, hostility, anxiety, depression

TRIGGERS (FOR EXISTING CAD)

- Physical exertion, cold, windy weather, extreme emotions, and excitement
- Blood-sugar imbalance

WHY DOES IT OCCUR?

The coronary arteries branch from the aorta and supply the heart muscle with oxygenated blood. Coronary artery disease (CAD) is usually due to atherosclerosis, in which fatty deposits build up on the lining of the coronary artery walls. These deposits narrow the arteries and restrict the flow of blood through them, thus reducing the supply of blood to the muscles. If one of the arteries becomes blocked, a heart attack, which is also known as a myocardial infarction, occurs and the heart muscle is damaged.

CAD caused by atherosclerosis is more likely if you have a high blood cholesterol level and if you eat a diet high in fats. Smoking, a lack of exercise, excess weight, high blood pressure (see p.244), and diabetes mellitus (see p.314) are all risk factors.

CAD is more common with increasing age and may sometimes run in families. The risk of developing CAD is generally lower in women than in men — until they reach the age of 60, when the risk for both sexes becomes approximately the same. The lower risk of CAD for a woman is thought to be due to the protective effect of the female hormone estrogen during the fertile part of her life. This protection against CAD wears off gradually after menopause (see p.339).

CAD may be an underlying factor in arrhythmias (see *Palpitations, p.258*) and heart failure, in which the heart becomes too weak to pump blood around the body effectively. Chronic heart failure may occur in the elderly, causing excess fluid in the lungs and tissues, as well as shortness of breath and swollen ankles.

TREATMENT PLAN

PRIMARY TREATMENTS

- Lifestyle changes (see *Self-Help*)
- Thrombolytic, anti-angina, and other drugs
- Cardiac rehabilitation program (following a myocardial infarction)

BACKUP TREATMENTS

- Nutritional therapy
- Cardioprotective diet
- Moderate aerobic exercise
- Breathing retraining
- Ornish approach
- Stress management

WORTH CONSIDERING

- Acupuncture

For an explanation of how treatments are rated, see p.111.

IMPORTANT

If you experience any of the symptoms of CAD, consult your doctor immediately. (*See also Angina, p.249.*)

PRIMARY TREATMENT If you have or want to reduce the risk of CAD, take the following measures:

- Stop smoking.
- Eat a diet low in saturated fats.
- Lose weight if necessary.
- Exercise regularly according to medical advice.
- Take a lipid-lowering drug if prescribed by your doctor.
- Take a blood-pressure lowering drug if your blood pressure is high.
- Consider taking a low dose of aspirin (75mg) every day to reduce the risk of a heart attack. (Check with your doctor because taking aspirin is not appropriate for everyone, particularly those who have asthma.)

TREATMENTS IN DETAIL

Conventional Medicine

TESTS If you are experiencing chest pain, your doctor may suspect CAD and will probably conduct tests to confirm this. Tests may include an electrocardiogram (ECG) to record the electrical rhythm of the heart and an exercise test to determine how your heart performs under stress.

If the tests indicate that your heart is not receiving enough blood, you may need a coronary angiography. A dye injected intravenously highlights your coronary arteries under an X-ray and reveals where they are blocked or narrowed.

If your doctor suspects that you have had a myocardial infarction, your heart rhythm will be recorded on an ECG at regular intervals. The ECG recordings will allow your doctor to look for changes characteristic of a heart attack and monitor progress. A series of blood tests will measure the levels of certain enzymes that are produced by damaged heart muscle.

PRIMARY TREATMENT **THROMBOLYTIC DRUGS**, such as streptokinase, may be given if a heart attack is confirmed. These drugs aim to break down the clot (thrombus) blocking the coronary artery in order to minimize the damage to the heart muscle. Taking aspirin can also help the process. The drug treatment for angina (a related problem) is described on p.250.

ANGIOPLASTY

In an angioplasty, a less invasive alternative to open-heart surgery, a tiny balloon is inflated to open up a coronary artery that has become clogged with fatty deposits. The patient, who is usually awake throughout, has a mild sedative and a local anesthetic. Then a catheter (a hollow tube) carrying the balloon is inserted into a blood vessel in the groin and guided, with the help of X-rays, through the arteries to the blockage. The surgical procedure follows four stages.

The four stages of an angioplasty

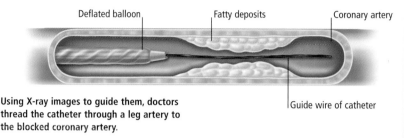

Using X-ray images to guide them, doctors thread the catheter through a leg artery to the blocked coronary artery.

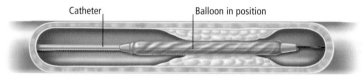

The balloon is now positioned correctly. Patients sometimes report feeling a slight tugging sensation when it is in place.

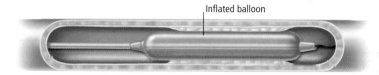

The balloon is inflated for up to two minutes, stretching the artery wall and increasing its diameter.

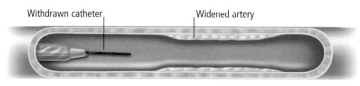

The balloon is deflated and withdrawn. Substantially more blood can now flow through the coronary artery.

PRIMARY TREATMENT **SURGERY**, such as an angioplasty or a coronary bypass (*see Angina, p.249*), may be needed to widen or bypass narrowed coronary arteries.

CORONARY CARE After a heart attack, you may need to be monitored in the coronary care unit for about two days where you may be given oxygen and a pain-relieving drug such as diamorphine. In the short term, you may need to receive intravenous drugs, such as beta-blockers, which aim to slow the heart rate.

PRIMARY TREATMENT **LONG-TERM TREATMENT** Ongoing treatment for CAD may include aspirin and beta-blockers, which can help reduce the risk of a myocardial infarction. Drugs that are called angiotensin-converting enzyme (ACE) inhibitors may also improve the prognosis in some cases. They dilate (widen) blood vessels around the body, thereby making it easier for the heart to pump blood.

Lowering cholesterol with drugs and diet (*see below*) can also reduce the risk of further myocardial infarctions and strokes.

Following a myocardial infarction, you can gradually increase your activity levels. Exercise appropriately and follow a cardiac rehabilitation program which will focus on various aspects of life after a heart attack such as diet and quitting smoking. Emotional support is also very important.

> **CAUTION**
>
> Heart drugs can cause side effects; ask your doctor to explain these to you.

Nutritional Therapy

PRIMARY TREATMENT What you eat partly determines whether or not your coronary arteries will gradually accumulate cholesterol and other fats on their internal walls. (*See also Angina, p.249.*)

HEALTHFUL AND UNHEALTHFUL FATS The type of fat we eat has an important bearing on the development of CAD (*see p.34*). While much emphasis has been placed on the need to avoid saturated fat in the diet — red meat, dairy products, and eggs — some evidence suggests that the role it plays in heart disease may not be so important after all.

There is mounting evidence to suggest that fats known as "partially hydrogenated" and trans-fatty acids (*see p.34*) are a more important risk factor for CAD. These hard fats found in many fast foods, baked goods, processed foods, and margarine are associated with an increased risk of heart disease. They should be avoided if possible.

The omega-3 fatty acids in oily fish such as salmon, trout, mackerel, sardines, and herring, have several effects in the body that would be expected to reduce the risk of CAD. For example, they can raise the levels of "healthy" high-density lipoprotein (HDL) cholesterol, reduce blood pressure, and thin the blood. According to experts,

eating one or two portions of fish each week or supplementing your diet with 1g of concentrated fish oils per day, is likely to reduce the risk of heart disease.

TRIGLYCERIDES Raised levels of blood fats known as triglycerides appear to be another risk factor for CAD. Raised triglycerides often occur with accumulation of body fat around the middle of the body ("apple-shaped" bodies), insulin resistance (which may lead to diabetes in time), and high blood pressure. Together, these conditions are the metabolic syndrome (known sometimes as Syndrome X), which is present in about 20 percent of the adult population in the US. Its importance as a risk factor for CAD development is well established. Fish-oil supplements can help reduce the triglyceride level, too.

HOMOCYSTEINE LEVELS Raised levels of a substance called homocysteine appear to be a major risk factor for CAD and heart disease. Homocysteine is a breakdown product of the amino acid methionine, and is normally converted in the body to a harmless substance called cystanthionine. However, this conversion is dependent on the presence of vitamins B_6, B_{12}, and folic acid. A deficiency of one or more of these nutrients might cause homocysteine levels to rise. Higher intakes of folic acid and vitamin B_6 in the diet are associated with a decreased risk of CAD.

Anyone who has a raised homocysteine level (as determined by a blood test) should take 10mg of vitamin B_6, 50mcg of vitamin B_{12}, and 400mcg of folic acid per day.

VITAMIN E Much attention in CAD prevention focuses on the need to control the level of cholesterol in the blood. However, it is when cholesterol becomes damaged through a process known as oxidation that it has the propensity to settle on the inside of the body's arteries. Vitamin E is an antioxidant nutrient that can protect cholesterol from oxidation.

Vitamin E may also help prevent heart disease through its ability to thin the blood. Two studies (one on men and one on women) found that taking vitamin E supplements (100 IU or more per day) for two or more years was associated with a 20–40 percent reduction in the risk of CAD. However, other studies do not back up these findings.

VITAMIN C Evidence is beginning to emerge that vitamin C may protect against CAD, especially if it is taken with vitamin E. But the protective factor probably applies only to people with poor dietary intake of the vitamins.

A 16-year follow-up study of over 80,000 nurses suggested that increased vitamin C intake reduced the risk of CAD. After factoring out other risks for CAD, such as age, smoking, and exercise, the women who took vitamin C still had a significantly lower risk of CAD. As a result, taking 1g vitamin C each day in conjunction with vitamin E supplements may help reduce the risk of CAD.

MULTIVITAMIN/MINERAL SUPPLEMENT taken daily may be a good way to protect against CAD. Studies have found that a

88 percent of men and 83 percent of women in the US consume too much saturated fat

daily intake of a multivitamin is associated with a lower risk of CAD. Many nutrients within the mineral supplement, such as vitamin E, vitamin C, copper, and selenium, may be beneficial in reducing the risk of CAD.

BIOFLAVONOIDS are phenolic compounds that are present in a wide range of foods and medicinal plants. Many studies indicate that flavonoids are anti-inflammatory, antiviral, and able to dilate blood vessels. Most importantly, they are antioxidants, able to neutralize free radicals and reduce their formation.

Bioflavonoids are found in nuts, cereals, olive oil, vegetables, fruits, berries, tea, red wine, dark chocolate, and many herbs (*see p.255*). Many of these foods are part of a so-called Mediterranean diet.

POLYPHENOLS Extracted from the purple grape skins in red wine, polyphenols have been shown to inhibit the formation of endothelin-1, a chemical that makes blood vessels constrict. It seems that the polyphenols reduce the stickiness of blood and protect the lining of the blood vessels of the heart by producing nitric oxide. In this way, not only red wine but also dark grape juice can reduce atherosclerosis and heart disease.

CHOLESTIN, a Chinese red-yeast rice supplement, contains lovastatin, a naturally occurring statin and other compounds that lower cholesterol. Cholestin has been shown to lower raised levels of cholesterol and triglycerides in blood serum.

> **CAUTION**
>
> Consult your doctor before taking omega-3 fatty acids or fish oils with warfarin, or zinc with antibiotics, or vitamin E with warfarin or aspirin, or vitamin C with antibiotics or warfarin (see also p.46).

Cardioprotective Diets

In parts of France and other Mediterranean countries, death from heart disease is significantly lower than in developed countries elsewhere despite a high consumption of fat and saturated fats. The reason advanced for this cardio-protective effect is the diet accompanied by regular consumption of red wine. A long-term

> An estimated 84 percent of people who die of coronary artery disease are age 65 or older

study of 89,299 male physicians found that drinking moderate amounts of red wine (one or two glasses a day) reduced overall mortality. However, there was no benefit from drinking more!

The people of Okinawa, a collection of islands between Japan and Taiwan, commonly live active, independent lives well into their 90s and 100s. Their rates of obesity, heart disease, osteoporosis, memory loss, and breast, colon, and prostate cancer rank far below those in other industrialized countries, and their age at menopause is higher. Researchers point to their mainly vegetable diet, which includes plenty of onions and soy, giving high levels of antioxidant bioflavonoids and carotenoids. In addition, a slower decline in sex hormones that appears to be linked to diet and lifestyle is believed to contribute to the impressive cardiovascular health of the Okinawans.

WHAT DIET? In 2002, a review looked at 147 studies of dietary factors and their relationship to CAD. The factors included fat, cholesterol, omega-3 and omega-6 (polyunsaturated) fatty acids, carbohydrates, glycemic index, fiber, folate, and dietary patterns.

The review concluded that there are three effective strategies for preventing CAD. First, replace saturated fats with unsaturated fats. Second, increase the amount of omega-3 fatty acids that you derive from fish, fish-oil supplements, or plant sources in the diet. Third, eat a diet that is high in fruits, vegetables, nuts, and whole grains, and low in refined grain products.

As yet, it is unclear just how much or in what proportion each of these is important. Nor is there certainty about the precise role played by essential plant substances such as antioxidant vitamins minerals, flavonoids, and lycopenes. However, the authors suggest that a diet containing these components, combined with regular exercise, no tobacco, and staying at your ideal body weight could prevent most cases of CAD.

GARLIC AND ONIONS contain organosulfur compounds that reduce the stickiness of human blood platelets and appear to confer cardiovascular benefits on those who eat them regularly. In addition, they reduce levels of unhealthy fats in the blood and can help lower blood pressure.

The protective effect of garlic (*Allium sativum*) is attributed to its ability to reduce arterial plaque and atherosclerosis and to protect the lining of the blood vessels in the heart. Garlic also appears to inhibit cholesterol manufacture in the liver and to increase the excretion of cholesterol. It may also relax the heart muscle and maintain the elasticity of the aorta.

TEA (*Camellia sinensis*) has cardioprotective properties because it is rich in catechins and polyphenols that are antioxidants. A study carried out on black tea consumption found that drinking tea appeared to improve the function of the coronary blood vessels in patients with CAD. In a Japanese study, people who drank at least ten cups of green tea a day had a decreased risk of death from cardiovascular disease.

TOMATOES contain lycopene, an antioxidant carotenoid which has the ability to inhibit cholesterol synthesis and prevent heart disease. Tomatoes are also a good source of beta-carotene, flavonoids, potassium, folic acid, vitamin C and E — all of which may work together to maintain a healthy heart.

OTHER CARDIOPROTECTIVE FOODS Several studies suggest that eating plenty of fruit and vegetables is associated with a reduced risk of CAD.

Substantial epidemiological evidence indicates that diets rich in fiber and whole grains are associated with decreased risk of CAD. Studies show that eating whole-grain foods can also help reduce the risk of CAD, by up to 30 percent if you eat more than three servings per day.

Legumes also seem to have a beneficial effect on the heart. Soy has been shown to reduce "bad," low-density cholesterol (LDL), while increasing the ratio of "good," high-density cholesterol (HDL).

> **CAUTION**
>
> Consult your doctor before taking medicinal doses of garlic at the same time as anticoagulant drugs (see p.69).

Western Herbal Medicine

From across the world, epidemiological evidence makes the case that common compounds found in traditional plant remedies help maintain a healthy heart. If you have coronary artery disease, an herbal medicine expert may prescribe a one or more of these plant remedies.

HAWTHORN (*Crataegus monogyna* or *Crataegus laevigata*) flowers are rich in bioflavonoids and the spring leaves are high in oligomeric proanthocyanidins (OPCs). These bioflavonoid antioxidants are about 20 times as potent as vitamin C and 50 times as potent as vitamin E.

OPCs protect the heart by binding to the surface of blood vessel (endothelial) cells where they neutralize harmful free radicals. OPCs can also be found in grape-seed (*Vitis vinfera*) extract.

Hawthorn extract strengthens the power of the heart muscle, increases blood flow through the coronary arteries, and appears to keep the rhythm of the heartbeat regular. This research demonstrated that patients with heart disease taking hawthorn found their breathlessness and fatigue improved significantly compared to patients on a placebo.

GINKGO (*Ginkgo biloba*) can improve circulation and is used to treat CAD, Standardized ginkgo biloba extract (GBE) helps normalize the circulation of the blood and exerts a beneficial effect on the lining and tone of the blood vessels. GBE reduces the stickiness of blood platelets that can lead to coronary artery blockage and heart disease.

MOTHERWORT (*Leonurus cardiaca*) is another herb with a long folk use for treating cardiac debility, rapid heartbeat, and anxiety affecting heart function.

OTHER HERBS AND SPICES Several kitchen herbs and spices have a beneficial effect on the heart. Rosemary (*Rosmarinus officinalis*) contains phenolic diterpenes that reduce "bad" low-density lipoprotein (LDL) cholesterol in the blood. The antioxidants present in cinnamon (*Cinnamon verum*) bark neutralize free radicals. Turmeric (*Curcuma longa*) has anti-inflammatory activity and can help lower cholesterol levels and reduce the symptoms of angina pectoris. Ginger (*Zingiber officinale*), a close relative of turmeric, prevents the aggregation of blood platelets and may therefore be helpful in patients with coronary artery disease.

TERMINALIA ARJUNA The bark of this Ayurvedic remedy is a source of OPCs and bioflavonoids that not only strengthen the power of heart muscle but the bark also relieves angina as well as the frequency of angina attacks.

> **CAUTION**
>
> See p.69 before taking a herbal remedy and, if you are taking prescribed medication, consult an herbal medicine expert first.

Aerobic Exercise

Doing aerobic exercise on a regular basis is commonly associated with protection against heart disease. However, exercise is usually beneficial for people with existing heart disease, too. Among the benefits of aerobic and general exercise are decreased risk of conditions such as thrombosis, myocardial ischemia (which involves symptoms such as angina), and stroke.

If there is a history of heart disease, a patient should follow a graduated exercise program based on research evidence in cardiovascular rehabilitation and prescribed by a physical therapist.

One remarkable study that was conducted over a period of 33 years revealed that aerobic exercise, when performed 3–4 times each week, slows down the aging process of the heart.

Another long-term (13-year) research study involving 10,000 men showed that regular exercise helps prevent strokes as well as helping people recover from them. In the study, walking, stair-climbing, dancing, cycling, and gardening all reduced the risk of stroke. The lowest risk was associated with walking 12mi (20km) or more a week.

Research strongly suggests that regular participation in moderate-intensity (non-aerobic) activities, such as walking and gardening, for at least 60 minutes per week, provide almost the same heart health benefits as regular and more intense aerobic activity.

Current exercise levels protect the heart, not an earlier history of physical exercise. Researchers have demonstrated that it is never too late to start exercising.

Breathing Retraining

Hyperventilation and altered breathing patterns can aggravate existing cardiovascular disease by reducing oxygen delivery to the tissues, including the heart itself, and by causing contractions of the smooth muscles surrounding the blood vessels. Breathing retraining (*see p.62*) may be helpful in easing these stresses to the heart, as well as lowering general levels of anxiety. Physical therapists and yoga instructors can help you learn better breathing habits.

Acupuncture

Acupuncture cannot treat the primary causes of CAD, but it may act to dilate the coronary arteries, sometimes providing effective long-term treatment. A study using coronary arteriograms has shown that acupuncture can dilate coronary arteries. The authors suggested that this might be the basis of a useful treatment for angina and CAD.

More than one million Americans have heart attacks each year

Mind–Body Therapy

STRESS can have a "double whammy" effect in cardiovascular health. First, it can impact the body directly—the chronic overproduction of stress hormones, such as epinephrine and cortisol, negatively affect the cardiovascular system.

Second, stress can indirectly contribute to poor cardiovascular health when people respond to it with unhealthy behavior such as poor diet, lack of exercise, smoking, and excessive alcohol.

PHYSIOLOGICAL EFFECTS Stress affects the cardiovascular system in a number of ways. It speeds up the heart rate, raises blood pressure, and increases the tendency for blood clots to form. Blood vessels throughout the body become narrow and the arteries that supply blood to the heart muscle constrict.

As blood flow becomes more turbulent it can injure the lining of the arteries and, over time, to blockage of the arteries as the body attempts to heal these injuries.

HOSTILITY AND ANGER Numerous studies have demonstrated a strong link between higher levels of hostility and anger and heart disease. In one of the most famous studies, physicians who scored high in a measure of hostility at the age of 25 were seven times more likely to have died from heart disease (as well as from other causes) 25 years later than physicians who were not hostile.

People who have higher levels of hostility are also more likely to engage in

Overall, the clinical and research literature suggests that symptoms of depression represent a significant risk factor for cardiovascular disease. For example, a study of 1,190 medical students discovered that the presence of clinical depression proved to be a risk factor for later coronary artery disease.

THE MANAGEMENT OF STRESS In many respects, hostility–anger, anxiety, and depression–hopelessness can be viewed as the emotional and behavioral consequences of stress, or what happens when people perceive that they do not have the internal or external resources to meet the demands or challenges of life.

Experiencing occasional feelings of anger, concern, and sadness is normal. However, when these mood states become more frequent or even chronic, it is a clue that normal life stresses and challenges are

various relaxation techniques (*see p.99*) and stress-coping strategies, were significantly less likely to have a recurrent coronary event, such as a heart attack, at the five-year follow-up.

If you have CAD, ask your doctor about participating in a stress-management program or taking up meditation or guided imagery (*see p.98*).

THE ORNISH APPROACH The Lifestyle Heart Trial was initially published in 1990 and updated in 1998. It follows the approach that was initially devised by Dean Ornish in the 1980s and entails a low-fat diet, combined with a program of quitting smoking, taking up aerobic exercise, participating in some form of stress-management training, and obtaining psychological support.

The Ornish approach is a good example of the benefits of integrating mind–body therapies with nutritional changes. Patients exercise for an hour three times a week, participate in group therapy sessions, and learn to manage their stress with techniques that are adapted from yoga and meditation. They also follow a rigorous high-fiber diet that provides the following calorie breakdown: 10 percent comes from fat, 15–20 percent from protein, and 70–75 percent from complex carbohydrates.

Research suggests that the Ornish approach can reverse and prevent CAD without drugs or surgery. These findings have been replicated at many different sites throughout the US since 1983. The longer the regimen is continued, the more the follow-up heart scans demonstrate continued improvement and reversal of the atherosclerosis.

Vegetarians have a lower mortality rate from coronary artery disease than meat-eaters

unhealthy lifestyle behaviors such as smoking and high-fat diets. In a 1983 study, Finnish men with the highest levels of expressed anger were at twice the risk of having a stroke during eight years of follow-up.

Research published in 1996 examined a sample of 1,305 men who did not have coronary artery disease at the beginning of the study. Among these men, those who reported the highest levels of anger were three times as likely to experience either a nonfatal heart attack or fatal heart disease at the follow-up, which was conducted seven years later.

ANXIETY AND DEPRESSION Studies have also demonstrated a link between both anxiety and depression (including hopelessness) and cardiovascular disease. For example, several large-scale, community-based studies have shown significant relationships between anxiety disorders and deaths from heart disease. Other studies have demonstrated the relationship between both anxiety disorders and worry and coronary artery disease.

no longer being managed effectively. Not everyone who is clinically "stressed" reacts this way; the tendency to do so may be genetically determined.

The chronic activation of the stress response can not only wear away at the quality of mental and emotional health and well-being but it can also have a significantly negative effect on a person's physical health, especially his or her cardiovascular health.

Given the clear link between stress and cardiovascular health, it is not surprising that clinical research shows that stress-management techniques (*see p.99*) can be effective in treating and preventing coronary artery disease.

One of the best examples of this comes from a study by James Blumenthal and his team of researchers at Duke University. They conducted a trial in which individuals with documented coronary artery disease followed an exercise program, a stress-management program, or the usual medical treatment for five years. Those individuals receiving stress-management training, which included instruction in

PREVENTION PLAN

The following measures should reduce your risk of developing coronary artery disease:

- Eat a diet that is high in vegetables, fruit and oily fish, but low in salt and saturated fat

- Exercise regularly, such as brisk walking or cycling for 30 minutes, five or more days of the week

- If you smoke, quit

PALPITATIONS

Palpitations are an awareness of the heartbeat, which may be felt either as normal in rate and rhythm or may be sensed as irregular and/or rapid. It is normal to sense the heartbeat when nervous, excited, or as a result of exertion, but sometimes there is a trigger that needs to be eliminated or an underlying arrhythmia that needs medical attention, so diagnosis is essential. Treatment includes drugs to control the rhythm of the heart, as well as supplements, manipulation therapy, breathing retraining, and mind–body therapies, such as relaxation.

WHAT ARE THE SYMPTOMS?

- Awareness of the heartbeat

Additional symptoms may be experienced, depending on the cause:

- Palpitations with panic attacks may be associated with nausea and excess sweat
- Palpitations associated with atrial fibrillation may be accompanied by light-headedness and shortness of breath
- Palpitations associated with other rapid arrhythmias may be accompanied by shortness of breath, fainting, and chest pain

WHY MIGHT I HAVE THIS?

PREDISPOSING FACTORS

- Underlying arrhythmia
- Overactive thyroid gland
- Anemia

TRIGGERS

- Caffeine
- Nicotine
- Alcohol
- Anxiety
- Panic attacks

IMPORTANT

Consult your doctor if you experience palpitations, especially if they are irregular or recurrent. Seek urgent medical attention if they are accompanied by other symptoms, such as chest pain.

WHY DOES IT OCCUR?

Rapid, regular palpitations may occur repeatedly in people who are prone to persistent anxiety and panic attacks (*see p.414*), as well as in people who have certain medical disorders, such as an overactive thyroid gland (*see Hyperthyroidism, p.319*) and anemia.

Palpitations may also occur as a side effect of certain medications, such as calcium-channel blockers, which are used to treat angina (*see p.249*) and hypertension (high blood pressure; *see p.244*), so you should ask your doctor if palpitations are a side effect of any prescribed medication. Palpitations may also be triggered by stimulants, such as caffeine and nicotine.

TREATMENT PLAN

PRIMARY TREATMENTS

- Drugs including beta-blockers

BACKUP TREATMENTS

- Nutritional therapy
- Homeopathy

WORTH CONSIDERING

- Bodywork therapies
- Breathing retraining
- Acupuncture
- Relaxation and other mind–body therapies

For an explanation of how treatments are rated, see p.111.

ARRHYTHMIAS There are two types of arrhythmias that commonly cause palpitations, slow arrhythmias (known as bradyarrhythmias) and fast arrhythmias (tachyarrhythmias). While most tachyarrhythmias originate in the sinus node, premature ectopic beats are arrhythmias of unknown origin.

Premature ectopic beats are early heartbeats that are next followed by a normally delayed heartbeat, which may be felt as a "thud" in the chest. Ectopic beats are usually no cause for concern and are often associated with stress (*see p.408*) or the use of nicotine, caffeine, and alcohol. However, occasional ectopic beats may cause discomfort or they may be a symptom of an underlying heart disorder, such as coronary artery disease (*see p.252*).

Atrial fibrillation is a type of tachyarrhythmia in which the atria (the upper heart chambers) contract irregularly and very rapidly. Some of the electrical impulses that cause these contractions trigger rapid and irregular contractions of the ventricles (the lower heart chambers). This arrhythmia is often present continuously and may be symptomless. However, it may cause palpitations when it occurs in episodes.

TREATMENTS IN DETAIL

Conventional Medicine

DIAGNOSIS Your doctor may arrange tests to exclude nonheart causes, such as hyperthyroidism. If the doctor suspects an underlying arrhythmia, your heart rate may be recorded over a 24-hour period by a portable monitor attached to a strap that can be worn around your body.

Whether palpitations are due to panic attacks, anxiety, an excess of a stimulant such as coffee, a disrupted heart rhythm (arrhythmia), or another medical disorder such as anemia, the underlying cause needs to be avoided or treated.

PRIMARY TREATMENT **DRUGS** Some arrhythmias require treatment with drugs. Ectopics are not usually treated unless they are bothersome, in which case the doctor may prescribe beta-blockers. Recurrent episodes of atrial fibrillation may also be treated with beta-blockers or certain anti-arrhythmic drugs, for example, flecainide or propafenone.

CAUTION

Beta-blockers and anti-arrhythmic drugs have a range of side effects; ask your doctor to explain these to you.

HEART RHYTHMS

An electrocardiograph (ECG) is a machine that is used to measure the electrical activity of a person's heart. Electrocardiography is a safe and painless diagnostic technique that can show whether a heart beat is normal or is affected by a disrupted rhythm (arrhythmia). Signals detected by electrodes that are attached to the skin on the chest, ankles, and wrist reveal the electrical activity in various parts of the heart, which shows up as a trace recorded on paper in the ECG machine.

Normal and disrupted heart rhythms

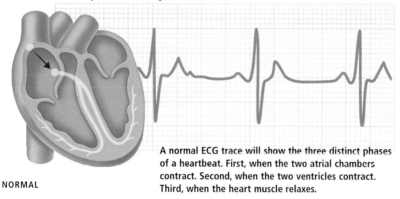

NORMAL

A normal ECG trace will show the three distinct phases of a heartbeat. First, when the two atrial chambers contract. Second, when the two ventricles contract. Third, when the heart muscle relaxes.

SINUS TACHYCARDIA

In sinus tachycardia ("tachy" means fast), the rhythm of the electrical pulse from the sinoatrial node (the heart's pacemaker) is over 100 beats per minute.

ATRIAL FIBRILLATION

In atrial fibrillation, the heart rate is rapid and irregular. The atrial chambers contract weakly between 300 and 500 beats every minute. The ventricles beat up to 160 times every minute.

Nutritional Therapy

CAFFEINE can increase the pulse rate and may even trigger abnormal heart rhythms. If you experience palpitations, try to reduce or eliminate caffeine (found in coffee, tea, and cola) from your diet. Some herbs, including mate and guarana, also contain caffeine, as do ephedra and other stimulant herbs.

OMEGA-3 FATTY ACIDS Some evidence suggests that eating fish and fish oils (omega-3 fatty acids) may help maintain a normal heart rhythm. If you suffer from palpitations, either eating oily fish (salmon, mackerel, sardines, herring, and trout) or taking fish-oil supplements may benefit you.

MAGNESIUM appears to be important for maintaining a normal heart rhythm, with several studies showing that intravenous magnesium may be useful in the treatment of various types of arrhythmia. One study of people who had abnormal heart rhythms (and heart failure) found that oral magnesium helped. Taking 300–600mg of magnesium supplements per day may be an effective dose for people who are experiencing palpitations and/or arrhythmia.

COENZYME Q₁₀ (COQ₁₀) seems to possess the ability to stabilize the heartbeat of individuals who have arrhythmias. In one study, 100mg per day of CoQ_{10} (in addition to the standard treatment) was effective in reducing palpitations in the majority of patients with congestive heart failure.

CAUTION

Consult your doctor before taking either CoQ_{10} or omega-3 fatty acids/fish oils with warfarin (see p.46).

Homeopathy

SPIGELIA ANTHELMIA is frequently used by homeopaths to treat palpitations, at times with other medicines chosen to suit the individual. It is most effective when the palpitations are accompanied by facial pain or migraine, usually left-sided and involving the eye. Sometimes, in those whom the medicine benefits, a hot drink seems to help control the palpitations.

LACHESIS The palpitations in people who respond to *Lachesis* are often accompanied by a sensation of constriction in the chest and/or hot flashes. In women, the problem often starts at menopause and tends to be at its worst just after waking in the morning. In general, the patient is hot and hates tight clothes, especially collars. They may be depressed, moody, or irritable, and are sometimes very talkative.

NATRUM MURIATICUM People who may find *Natrum muriaticum* useful have palpitations that seem to be triggered by mental exertion, or sometimes by lying down. Typically, the heart seems to "skip a beat" every few beats. But the key to this medicine is the "mental profile": people who respond to it often have masked depression — they may be very depressed, but hide it. This profile may have been triggered by a psychological trauma: a bereavement or relationship break-up, for instance, which they have never talked about. Although they put on a brave face, privately they feel desperately depressed.

NUX VOMICA Overindulgence in food or alcohol may trigger the palpitations in people who respond to *Nux vomica*. The problem is often worse early in the morning (between 5:00 AM and 6:00 AM). The person is often very bad-tempered; the palpitations may be triggered by a fit of bad temper or a frustrating incident.

Bodywork Therapies

Much of the heart's regular rhythmic contraction is triggered by an internal nerve supply, which is rather like a local generator that is independent of the overall power supply. The external nerve supply to the heart that helps it adapt to the demands of life come from different areas of the spine.

The sympathetic nerves that "speed up" the heart rate arise from the first five spinal segments below the neck (thoracic spine), while the parasympathetic nerves that slow down the heart rate come from the vagus nerve, which emerges from the spine in the neck region. Imbalances in nerve supply, sometimes associated with spinal dysfunction, can disturb the rhythm of the heart, and palpitations may be one result of this.

OSTEOPATHY AND CHIROPRACTIC Someone with a heart problem will almost always have identifiable and palpable changes in those areas of the spine that feed the nerves to it. Appropriate osteopathic or chiropractic manipulation of the spinal joints of the neck and upper back can influence and, at times, assist in returning irregular heart rhythms to normal.

DEACTIVATE TRIGGER POINTS Another reason for an uneven heart rhythm can be trigger-point activity (*see p.55*) between the fifth and sixth ribs, in the intercostal or pectoral muscle fibers a little to the right side of the breast bone. Pressure into, and stretching of, the local contractions surrounding the trigger point can deactivate it and ease the symptoms it may be causing.

Breathing Retraining

People who habitually breathe just from the upper chest automatically exhale excessive carbon dioxide and so increase the alkalinity of their blood. This breathing pattern can disrupt the normal oxygen supply to the heart, at times causing it to beat abnormally.

An upper-chest breathing pattern also creates a great deal of additional work for particular muscles, including the intercostals and pectorals, that may house trigger points involved in heart arrhythmia (*see above*). Breathing retraining (yogictype patterns) can help restore normal nerve and oxygen supply to the heart, easing disturbances such as palpitations.

Acupuncture

Case reports and studies published in China suggest that acupuncture may be able to treat some causes of palpitations. Certainly, acupuncture relieves anxiety; it appears to have a powerful effect on the parts of the nervous system, particularly the autonomic nerves, that may trigger palpitations.

Acupuncture can sometimes be used to relieve palpitations as they occur, but may also have an effect in more chronic and persistent symptoms. Try six to eight treatment sessions on a weekly basis to see if the palpitations improve. If they do, your acupuncturist can decide, depending on symptoms, on further treatment.

> One type of palpitation — atrial fibrillation — affects 3–5 percent of people over 70

Mind–Body Therapies

Palpitations can be a symptom of organic ischemic heart disease, such as coronary artery disease, or of anxiety, social phobia, and the tendency to manifest anxiety in physical symptoms. They are more prevalent in people who are highly sensitive to bodily sensations and who experience a greater number of minor daily irritants.

RELAXATION AND BIOFEEDBACK are two mind–body techniques that, with regular practice under medical supervision and/or used regularly at home, can help an individual prevent the onset of heart palpitations. Although the research is still not definitive, it seems very likely that practicing them regularly could help people with palpitations cope better and perhaps reduce the severity of palpitations when they occur.

PREVENTION PLAN

The following may help prevent palpitations:

- Practice relaxation regularly
- Avoid stimulants such as caffeine

VARICOSE VEINS

Varicose veins are swollen veins beneath the skin that occur mainly in the legs. They may cause discomfort and look unsightly, but they are not harmful. If left untreated, they often get worse. If self-help measures, such as losing weight and regular walks, do not prevent the veins from worsening, surgery may be needed. Eating foods rich in anthocyanidins, hydrotherapy, compression stockings, homeopathic medicines, and herbal remedies may also help relieve the symptoms and slow progression of the condition.

WHAT ARE THE SYMPTOMS?

- Easily visible blue, swollen, and distorted veins that bulge beneath the skin and are more prominent when standing
- Aching or pain in the affected leg, especially after prolonged standing
- In severe cases, the skin over a varicose vein may become thin, dry and itchy — eventually, an ulcer may form

WHY MIGHT I HAVE THIS?

PREDISPOSING FACTORS

- Excess weight or obesity
- Inherited tendency
- Pregnancy
- Prolonged standing
- Straining while constipated

TREATMENT PLAN

PPRIMARY TREATMENTS

- Self-help measures (*see right*)
- Surgery (sclerotherapy or stripping)

BACKUP TREATMENTS

- Horse chestnut and other Western herbal remedies
- Daily exercise
- Hydrotherapy
- Compression therapy

WORTH CONSIDERING

- Nutritional therapy
- Homeopathy

For an explanation of how treatments are rated, see p.111.

WHY DOES IT OCCUR?

Normally, blood in the legs collects in the superficial veins just below the skin and is transferred to deep-lying veins by small blood vessels called perforating veins. Valves in the veins prevent the blood from flowing away from the heart. If valves in the perforating veins do not close properly, the blood flows back into the superficial veins, causing them to swell and become distorted. These are the varicose veins. (*See illustration, p.262.*)

Weakness of the valves in the veins may be an inherited problem, but the general reason varicose veins develop is not known. The condition is more common in people who are overweight or obese. It is also more common in women, especially during pregnancy when the female hormone progesterone, which causes veins to dilate, is produced in greater quantities.

Standing in one position for a prolonged period of time may encourage the development of varicose veins, and some believe that straining while constipated may also be a predisposing factor.

SELF-HELP

PRIMARY TREATMENT The following measures may prevent varicose veins from appearing or worsening and may help relieve aching and discomfort:
- Lose weight, if necessary.
- Avoid standing for long periods of time.
- Take daily walks.
- Keep your legs elevated above your hips while sitting.
- Avoid sitting with your legs crossed.
- Avoid clothes that constrict circulation in your legs.

TREATMENTS IN DETAIL

Conventional Medicine

Your doctor will be able to diagnose varicose veins from the appearance of your legs. If they are not severe, the doctor will advise self-help measures that you can try on your own (*see Self-Help, left*).

PRIMARY TREATMENT **SURGERY** may be needed if varicose veins are unsightly or causing you discomfort, or if an ulcer develops. In sclerotherapy, a chemical is injected into the affected veins, causing the walls to stick together and preventing blood from entering.

Alternatively, the perforating arteries of the affected varicose vein may be tied off so that blood cannot enter. In some cases, the entire effected vein is removed (known as stripping).

CAUTION

Surgical procedures for varicose veins may lead to complications; ask your doctor to explain these to you.

Nutritional Therapy

PREVENT CONSTIPATION Some evidence suggests that constipation causes varicose veins. The theory that straining to pass feces during constipation raises the pressure in the abdomen, which is transmitted to the veins of the legs. If you are susceptible to varicose veins, you may benefit from a high-fiber diet containing fruit, vegetables, beans, legumes, oats, seeds, and nuts to prevent constipation.

PROANTHOCYANIDINS (or procyanidins) may help to alleviate varicose veins, possibly by strengthening the walls of the veins. Studies have shown them to be useful in treating varicose veins. If you have varicose veins, incorporate proanthocyanidins in your diet. Good sources include red wine, dark chocolate, cranberry juice, apples, blueberries, grapes (especially the skin), peanuts, and bilberries.

Homeopathy

If you have varicose veins, consult a practitioner who can recommend the most appropriate remedy for you.

POIKIVEN A clinical trial has shown that the homeopathic complex *Poikiven* is effective in treating varicose vein symptoms.

HAMAMELIS is among the most commonly used homeopathic medicines for varicose veins. It may be taken by mouth or can be applied topically to the affected areas. In individuals who respond to *Hamamelis*, there is a feeling of heaviness and distension, made worse by the heat, as well as easy bruising.

VIPERA is a useful medicine for treating inflamed varicose veins — a condition called thrombophlebitis in which a person feels a throbbing pain that can be relieved by elevating the legs.

CALCAREA FLUORICA People who respond to this deeper-acting constitutional medicine (*see p.73*) may have lax connective tissues. When younger, they may have been hyperextensible (double-jointed) or had swayback knees (knees that bend beyond straight). Alternatively, they may have a tendency to develop hernias.

PULSATILLA is a constitutional medicine (*see p.73*) in which the pain of varicose veins is relieved by elevating the legs. People who respond to *Pulsatilla* may also have a tendency to develop chilblains.

LACHESIS A marked feature in people who respond to *Lachesis* is their intolerance of wearing anything tight around their legs. In women, the symptoms are worse before a menstrual period and may also be triggered by menopause.

HOW VARICOSE VEINS DEVELOP

The veins that lie deep in the leg collect deoxygenated blood and return it to the heart. The contraction of leg muscles helps this process. Within every vein, there are one-way valves that prevent the blood from flowing backward. Blood at the surface of the legs is channelled into the deep veins by superficial veins. Sometimes the valves in the superfical veins fail, causing the vein to bulge.

Normal and varicose veins

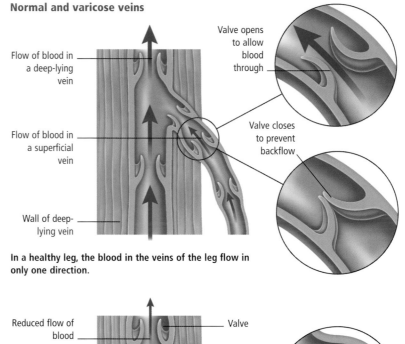

Flow of blood in a deep-lying vein

Flow of blood in a superficial vein

Wall of deep-lying vein

Valve opens to allow blood through

Valve closes to prevent backflow

In a healthy leg, the blood in the veins of the leg flow in only one direction.

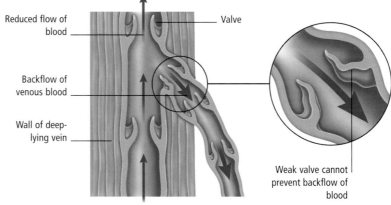

Reduced flow of blood

Backflow of venous blood

Wall of deep-lying vein

Valve

Weak valve cannot prevent backflow of blood

When the valves in a superficial vein weaken, they allow a backflow of blood.

Western Herbal Medicine

Herbal medicine can be used to strengthen vein walls, reduce fluid leakage resulting from varicose veins, and improve venous circulation to and through the liver. When prescribing herbal medicines, practitioners take into account the health of the affected veins and the cardiovascular system as a whole. They assess your weight, rate of healing, tissue repair, and liver function. Treatment generally needs to be continued for an extended period of time. You may need to take butcher's broom (*Ruscus aculeatus*) and apply a remedy, such as witch hazel (*Hamamelis virginiana*), to the affected leg for a minimum of six months.

HORSE CHESTNUT (*Aesculus hippocastanum*) is the herb of choice for chronic venous insufficiency, a different and more serious condition than varicose veins that is associated with swollen, discolored legs. Horse chestnut extract contains a complex mix of saponins and other active constituents. Many clinical trials confirm its ability to strengthen and tone the walls of veins, reduce swelling (edema) and fluid leakage from incompetent veins, and decrease capillary permeability. Theoretically, horse chestnut extract may help heal varicose veins as well. Horse chestnut extract also reduces the risk of deep vein thrombosis (DVT), in which blood clots form in the deep veins of the legs.

In one clinical trial, horse chestnut extract was as effective as using support stockings in relieving the symptoms of chronic venous insufficiency. Other clinical trials endorse the extract's use in the treatment of varicose veins during pregnancy, and in the treatment and relief of hemorrhoids, which have similar causes to varicose veins. Pynogenol has a synergistic effect with horse chestnut extract.

OTHER REMEDIES include butcher's broom, an anti-inflammatory with strong clinical evidence for use in chronic venous insufficiency and increased vascular permeability. Though poorly researched, yarrow (*Achillea millefolium*) is a traditional herb that can widen blood vessels, stimulate tissue healing, and provide a tonic for veins.

Varicose in Ancient Greek means "grapelike," referring to the appearance of veins

Bilberry (*Vaccinium myrtillus*) is a powerful antioxidant and capillary tonic.

> **CAUTION**
>
> See p.69 before taking a herbal remedy and, if you are taking a prescribed medication, consult an herbal medicine expert first.

EXTERNAL TREATMENTS include aloe vera (*Aloe vera*) juice to promote tissue repair, witch hazel for its astringent and anti-inflammatory properties when applied to the skin, and butcher's broom extract.

Gotu kola (*Centella asiatica*) is a well-researched Ayurvedic herb. Extracts have been found to improve the tone and function of varicose veins and recover the tone of connective tissue.

Exercise

German research showed that medically supervised exercise can relieve pain and reduce the tendency for the legs to swell. It can also heal leg ulcers, which may result if the dermatitis gets infected.

Hydrotherapy

Combining exercise and hydrotherapy appears to benefit varicose veins. According to a Swiss study, thermal hydrotherapy with sulfurous water, with elastic compression of the legs, reduces pain and swelling.

Italian hydrotherapy research examined the effect of spa treatment on 2,504 patients with primary or secondary varicose veins. For 15–20 days, the patients were treated with active and passive physical therapy using mineral waters. Nearly half the patients returned to the spa the next year for the same treatment. The researchers concluded that "the occurrence of acute venous episodes, working days missed, number and duration of hospital admissions, drug consumption, and physical therapies were all significantly reduced in the year following thermal therapy."

Compression Therapy

Minor forms of varicose veins affect about 40 percent of the population, 10 percent show major varicose veins, and 3 percent suffer from chronic venous insufficiency.

The mechanical support of regularly wearing compression stockings assists circulation and reduces symptoms of varicose veins. Elastic bandages may be more effective for applying pressure in a precise location and are used for compression therapy during the acute phase while support stockings, providing uniform pressure, are used to maintain the result. In more severe cases, joint mobilization, walking exercises, and draining the lymph from the affected areas may be used to reduce the swelling.

EXERCISES TO PREVENT VARICOSE VEINS

Whenever you have to sit for long periods of time, it is important to exercise your leg muscles every 30 minutes or so. If you sit still for hours at a time, the veins in the legs become compressed and it becomes harder to return blood to the heart. Blood begins to pool in the veins, putting pressure on the valves.

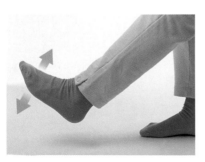

Slip your shoes off and raise your left foot slightly off the ground. Gently flex your foot up and down ten times. Repeat with the other foot.

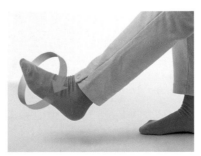

Rotate your left ankle ten times to the left, as if drawing a circle with your big toe, and then ten times to the right. Repeat with the other foot.

PREVENTION PLAN

The following may help prevent varicose veins from developing:

- Lose weight, if necessary
- Don't stand for long periods of time
- Exercise regularly

RAYNAUD'S DISEASE

In Raynaud's disease, spasm of arteries supplying the fingers or toes restricts their blood supply, causing them to become pale. In addition, there may be feelings of numbness or tingling in the affected fingers or toes. Exposure to cold and handling frozen items can trigger an attack. Treatment involves keeping hands and feet warm and taking nifedipine and other circulation-enhancing supplements, such as niacin or inositol hexaniacinate. Occasionally, surgery may be necessary.

WHAT ARE THE SYMPTOMS?

- Numbness or tingling in fingers or toes that may develop a painful burning sensation
- Change of color in the affected fingers or toes — they first become pale, then blue, and finally red as blood flow is restored to the tissues
- In severe cases, ulcers may form at the tips of fingers or toes

WHY MIGHT I HAVE THIS?

PREDISPOSING FACTORS

- Autoimmune disorder
- Beta-blockers and other drugs

TRIGGERS

- Exposure to cold

TREATMENT PLAN

PRIMARY TREATMENTS

- Keeping hands warm and stopping smoking (see Self-Help)
- Nifedipine (in some cases)

BACK-UP TREATMENTS

- Low back surgery (occasionally)
- Niacin or inositol hexaniacinate
- Ginkgo extracts
- Acupuncture

WORTH CONSIDERING

- Magnesium supplements
- Homeopathy
- Exercise
- Mind–body therapies

For an explanation of how treatments are rated, see p.111.

WHY DOES IT OCCUR?

The name of the condition can be confusing. If there seems to be no apparent cause, it is called Raynaud's disease. However, when the cause is known, it is called Raynaud's phenomenon.

Various disorders may underlie the condition, including autoimmune disorders (in which the body's immune system produces antibodies that attack its own tissues) such as rheumatoid arthritis (see p.293) and systemic sclerosis, a rare connective tissue disease that affects many organs and tissues of the body, including blood vessels. Buerger's disease, a rare condition in which the small arteries of the legs become inflamed due to smoking, can also cause Raynaud's phenomenon. Some drugs, such as beta-blockers, can produce symptoms of Raynaud's phenomenon as a side effect.

SELF-HELP

PRIMARY TREATMENT The following measures may help treat symptoms:

- Layer your clothing and keep your hands and feet warm with thermal gloves and socks.
- If you are a smoker, quit. Nicotine constricts arteries.
- Discontinue use of beta-blockers.

TREATMENTS IN DETAIL

Conventional Medicine

A diagnosis of Raynaud's disease is made from a description of the symptoms and a physical examination. The doctor may require additional tests to determine an underlying cause.

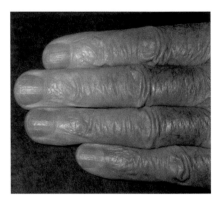

When Raynaud's disease affects the hands, blood supply to the tips of the fingers is restricted, causing them to turn white.

PRIMARY TREATMENT **NIFEDIPINE,** a calcium-channel blocker that helps relax blood vessel walls, may be prescribed. The drug is also used to prevent angina attacks and to treat high blood pressure.

> **CAUTION**
>
> Nifedipine may have side effects; ask your doctor to explain these to you.

PRIMARY TREATMENT **LOWER BACK SURGERY** may, in very severe cases, be necessary to cut nerves that control constriction of the arteries supplying the feet.

Nutritional Therapy

MAGNESIUM People with Raynaud's disease may have low levels of magnesium or suffer from abnormal magnesium metabolism. Magnesium deficiency can cause spasms in small blood vessels and worsen the symptoms. Taking 300–500mg of magnesium per day may reduce the frequency and severity of your condition.

NIACIN The ability of vitamin B$_3$ to enhance circulation is well known. One form of this vitamin, niacin, can induce a skin flush in doses as low as 50–100mg per day.

An alternative is inositol hexaniacinate, a compound of inositol (loosely classified as a B vitamin) and niacin. It appears to help enhance circulation without the side effects that commonly occur with niacin. Taking 500mg of inositol hexaniacinate 2–4 times a day may help control the symptoms of poor circulation, although it may take up to two months to see any improvement.

There is limited clinical evidence that L-arginine can also reverse digital necrosis by improving circulation.

> **CAUTION**
>
> Consult your doctor about the possible side effects of niacin and before taking magnesium with ciproflaxin, warfarin, or spironolactone (see p.46).

Homeopathy

Raynaud's disease can respond well to homeopathy. Among the more frequently indicated medicines are *Agaricus*, *Carbo vegetabilis*, *Secale*, and *Silica*.

AGARICUS is appropriate when the symptoms are very painful and feel like "splinters of ice." The individual may also have itchy chilblains or suffer from twitching or tics.

CARBO VEGETABILIS People who respond to *Carbo vegetabilis* have sluggish circulation and their fingers and toes often turn a blotchy reddish blue, often with burning pain. They may also have varicose veins (see p.261) or hemorrhoids. Their digestion is also sluggish, with bloating and gas, or they may be short of breath. They often look flushed and congested, and feel better if there is a breeze.

SECALE People who respond to *Secale* have blood vessel spasms and their fingers turn white and feel very cold to the touch. They experience a burning pain that gets worse, at least in the short term, from warming up.

SILICEA People who respond to *Silicea* are said to have a "frog handshake" — their hands are cold and damp. Although cold, their hands and feet are sweaty and their nails are weak with lengthwise ridges. People who respond to *Silicea* may have other "constitutional" features (see p.73).

Western Herbal Medicine

GINKGO A randomized, controlled trial of a standardized ginkgo extract showed that it was more effective than a placebo in reducing the number of attacks of Raynaud's disease per week.

> **CAUTION**
>
> See p.69 before taking an herbal remedy. Ginkgo may interact with other medicines; consult an herbal medicine expert first.

Bodywork Therapies

Crowding, compression, and irritation of the nerves and blood vessels in the narrow space between the collar bone, the shoulder blade, and the first rib are collectively known as thoracic outlet syndromes, or TOS. The symptoms may be virtually identical to Raynaud's disease — very cold hands that appear sweaty and blue, and feelings of numbness or tingling. This condition may sometimes follow injury, but it may also be the result of other causes, including excessive growth of the first rib or an extra rib in the neck.

Chiropractic manipulation, aimed at relieving the crowded space between the upper ribs, the shoulder blade, and the collar bone, can relieve TOS symptoms by improving circulation to the hands.

Acupuncture

Four clinical trials of varying quality all conclude that acupuncture is of value in treating Raynaud's disease. It particularly helps in the short term but also possibly has a preventative effect. The clinical improvement in "attacks" correlates well with an improved flow of blood flow through the hands.

At a time when you know you are likely to experience Raynaud's symptoms — for example, in the winter — you should start a course of treatment over a period of six to eight weeks.

Mind-Body Therapies

Stressful life events can influence the sympathetic nervous system responsible for spasms of the small blood vessels (vasospasms) that are associated with Raynaud's disease. As a result, the spasms, which can be quite painful, may be amenable to mind–body treatment.

Research has demonstrated that a number of mind–body therapies such as clinical biofeedback, autogenic training, and progressive relaxation, can help with treatment. However, there does not appear to be any distinct advantage of one technique over the other.

Mind–body techniques can be combined with conventional drugs such as sympathetic blocking agents, that reduce the impact of stress on the nervous system.

TEMPERATURE BIOFEEDBACK or regular relaxation may help improve symptoms of Raynaud's disease. A 1979 study examined the possible benefits of relaxation and finger temperature biofeedback in people with Raynaud's disease.

After six weeks, both the combined treatment group and the relaxation-only group showed consistent increases in the finger temperatures with a resulting decrease in Raynaud's symptoms and discomfort. However, there was no difference between the groups. At a two-year follow-up, many of the patients reported that improvements were sustained and they had less severe and less frequent episodes of Raynaud's discomfort.

A 1987 research summary of the use of mind–body interventions with Raynaud's disease revealed that temperature biofeedback reduces reported symptom frequency and enables patients to voluntarily increase finger temperature and capillary blood flow as long as one year after treatment. Moreover, the improvement in symptoms persisted for up to three years.

> **PREVENTION PLAN**
>
> **The following may help prevent Raynaud's disease:**
>
> - Avoid cold conditions
> - If you are a smoker, quit

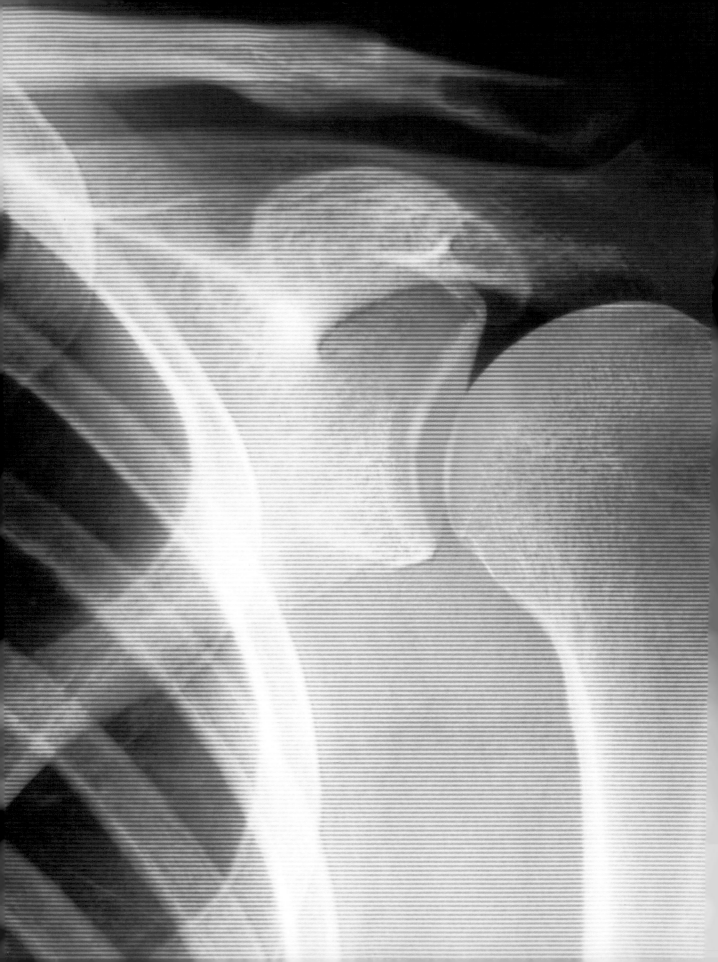

Musculoskeletal System

We rarely appreciate the amazing engineering of the muscoloskeletal system until something goes wrong. The aim of integrated medicine is to keep muscles, bones, and joints working well throughout life. Acupuncture can be as effective as analgesics for certain conditions, and surgery can sometimes be avoided with appropriate bodywork and movement therapies.

WHAT ARE THE SYMPTOMS?

- Pain in the back or the neck, which may be mild or severe
- The pain may come on suddenly or develop over a period of days or weeks
- Persistent numbness in a limb or persistent weakness of certain movements may reflect pressure on a nerve root

WHY MIGHT I HAVE THIS?

PREDISPOSING FACTORS

- Habitual poor posture
- Stress
- Certain occupations, such as working on computers
- Pregnancy
- Joint dysfunction or muscle spasm
- Prolapsed disk
- Muscle and ligament pain
- Degenerative disease

TRIGGERS

- Sports injury
- Whiplash
- Lifting a heavy object awkwardly

TREATMENT PLAN

PRIMARY TREATMENTS

- Rehabilitation program
- Chiropractic, osteopathy, and massage
- Acupuncture

BACKUP TREATMENTS

- Postural therapies and exercise
- Homeopathy
- Mind–body therapies

WORTH CONSIDERING

- Nutritional therapy

For an explanation of how treatments are rated, see p.111.

BACK AND NECK PAIN

Back and neck pain may have a variety of causes and descriptions. The pain is usually centered around the vertebrae of the spine, from the neck to the sacroiliac joints of the pelvis. Causes include muscle and ligament injuries, problems derived from habitually poor posture, and chronic joint disorders. Back pain commonly affects the lower back. Treatment focuses on resolving the underlying problem or, at the very least, bringing short-term relief to acute pain or long-term management of chronic pain.

WHY DOES IT OCCUR?

The spine is an intricate network of bones, nerves, muscles, ligaments, tendons, and cartilage. Back and neck pain can result from acute physical injury, such as a pinched nerve, strained muscle, torn ligament, or compressed cartilage. These can be caused by various means, such as whiplash — often from a car accident — (see right), lifting a heavy object, engaging in a strenuous, unaccustomed activity, or exercising without warming up. Back pain and the injury causing it may become worse with continued activity, so it is best to consult a doctor about the level of activity that is appropriate for you.

Lower back pain can accompany pregnancy due to changes in posture and the softening of ligaments in the pelvis. Adopting poor posture (a common occurrence in people who work on computers) for a prolonged period of time can cause neck or back pain. Stress can also result in neck pain, often in combination with tension headaches.

Persistent pain in the back or neck may also be caused by joint disorders such as osteoarthritis (see p.289) and ankylosing spondylitis (see p.305). Vertebral fractures

resulting from osteoporosis (see p.308) may also cause severe back pain. (See also Sciatica, p.272, and Prolapsed Disk, p.274.)

SELF-HELP

The following measures may help bring relief from an acute attack of back and neck pain:

- Apply an ice pack or bag of frozen peas to the area of maximum pain. Use for 5–10 minutes each hour.
- Hold a hot-water bottle wrapped in cloth over the painful area if the pain affects muscles or ligaments.
- Take analgesics, such as aspirin or ibuprofen.
- Practice therapeutic exercises for lower back pain, such as the pelvic tilt and the passive extension.

TREATMENTS IN DETAIL

Conventional Medicine

Your doctor will examine your spine and posture, testing your reflexes and looking for areas of tenderness and numbness. You may have tests, such as X-rays, to look for an underlying condition, which will be treated where possible.

PRIMARY TREATMENT **REHABILITATION PROGRAM** If your pain is due to an injury, you may require only analgesics, rest, and, in some cases, physical therapy. Fractures and other damage may need specific treatment.

If your pain is related to posture or stress, analgesics or nonsteroidal anti-inflammatory drugs (NSAIDs) may be prescribed for a short period. Physical

IMPORTANT

If back pain is associated with difficulty controlling your bowel or bladder, you may have a disorder putting pressure on the spinal cord and should see a doctor at once. If you have an area of persistent numbness, consult a doctor immediately.

WHIPLASH

A car accident, in which the collision comes unexpectedly from behind, is the most familiar cause of whiplash. Anyone who is in the car will feel their head thrown violently backward and forward. Their neck vertebrae curve one way and then the other and the ligaments take the strain because the muscles were not primed for the impact. The ligaments are overstretched and may be torn. Vertebral disks, muscles, and facet joints may all be damaged in the process.

Strain on the neck

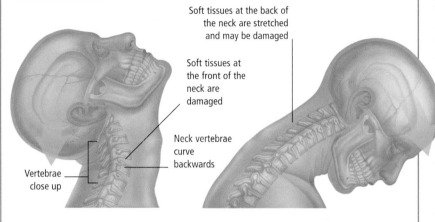

Soft tissues at the back of the neck are stretched and may be damaged

Soft tissues at the front of the neck are damaged

Neck vertebrae curve backwards

Vertebrae close up

When the force of the collision comes from behind, the head is suddenly thrown back. The strain is felt most by the soft tissues at the front of the neck's vertebrae.

When the force of the collision comes from in front, the head is suddenly thrown forward. The soft tissues at the back of the neck feel the strain most of all.

therapy may also be recommended to help relieve both muscle spasms and pain.

As part of your rehabilitation program, you may need expert advice on posture (*see p.62*), relaxation techniques, and, in some cases, counseling to help you cope with stress. Occupational therapists can help if the pain appears to be work-related.

> **CAUTION**
>
> NSAIDs may have side effects; ask your doctor to explain these to you.

Nutritional Therapy

VITAMIN C Collagen is largely responsible for the strength and resilience of the disks of cartilage between the vertebrae in the spine. One report found that a daily dose of 1,500–2,500mg of vitamin C, which plays an important part in the formation of collagen, can alleviate back pain and reduce the need for disk surgery. If you are experiencing back or neck pain, you may benefit from long-term supplementation with 1,000mg of vitamin C, taken twice a day.

GLUCOSAMINE SULFATE is a constituent of intervertebral disks. Clinical experience suggests that 500mg of glucosamine sulfate, two or three times a day, may help stimulate the healing and repair of damaged disks.

VITAMIN D may help in the treatment of chronic back pain. One study in 2003 examined individuals who had experienced low back pain with no obvious cause for more than six months. After treatment with 5,000 or 10,000 IU of vitamin D each day for three months, every individual with a previously low level of vitamin D showed clear signs of improvement. Vitamin D supplements may have special significance for those who have little exposure to sunlight, since most of our vitamin D supplies come from the action of sunlight on the skin.

> **CAUTION**
>
> Consult your doctor before taking vitamin C with antibiotics or warfarin, or vitamin D with verapamil (*see p.46*).

Homeopathy

In a clinical trial published in 2002, individualized homeopathy was shown to be at least as effective as physical therapy for lower back pain. Evidence from clinical trials also suggests that different forms of homeopathic medicines may help in the various conditions that underlie back pain, including osteoarthritis and fibromyalgia. These medicines include topically applied creams and gels, such as SRL gel (which contains *Symphytum*, *Rhus toxicodendron*, and *Ledum*).

RHUS TOXICONDENDRON AND BRYONIA *Rhus toxicodendron* is one of the most commonly used medicines for back pain, particularly if there is rapid stiffening up when the person wakes up during the night due to stiffness.

By contrast, if the pain is relieved by remaining very still, and hence by a support (for example, a collar or corset), then *Bryonia* may help.

OTHER HOMEOPATHIC MEDICINES may be helpful in the treatment of back or neck pain, but they need to be prescribed on constitutional grounds (*see p.73*). These include *Sepia*, which is often useful for inflammation that involves the sacroiliac joints, and *Natrum muriaticum*. Those for whom *Sepia* and *Natrum muriaticum* is indicated find that they can obtain relief from a firm cushion placed in the small of the back. These people may also be depressed but they hide their feelings.

Nux vomica may help patients who have back pains in which muscle spasm is an important factor.

Bodywork and Movement Therapy

Both short- and long-term treatment solutions need to be determined for back and neck problems that involve either joint dysfunction or complex imbalances between different muscle groups. Such conditions may be brought on by injuries, such as whiplash (*see above left*); years of misuse of the body — for example, by adopting poor sitting postures, or awkward and incorrect postures when working or playing sports); or by disuse of the body — for example, a lack of exercise).

PRIMARY TREATMENT | **CHIROPRACTIC, OSTEOPATHY, AND MASSAGE** At first, it is important to ease symptoms and return to normal activity as soon as possible. Once your doctor has ruled out a serious disorder, a number of bodywork approaches may help. These include chiropractic, osteopathy, and massage, as well as deactivation of local trigger points (which can be responsible for neck and back pain), yoga, stretching, ultrasound, hydrotherapy, and exercise.

AVOID BED REST Evidence suggests that there is no point in taking to your bed to rest (unless it is totally necessary — for example, if you have an acute disk prolapse).

A review of many studies concluded that bed rest has no positive effect for lower back pain and may even be slightly harmful. You should start to move around as soon as your pain will allow. Most people affected by backache recover in three to four weeks, with or without treatment.

POSTURAL THERAPIES AND EXERCISE If backache is a problem, you need to learn how to keep your spine and pelvis supple (and the supporting muscles strong and stable). You also need to avoid movements and positions that put the joints at risk of strain, which means being particularly careful when bending and lifting.

Experts cannot agree whether, in both the short and the long term, manipulation of the body is more effective than exercise, and/or reeducation, in helping relieve back pain. In the short term, there is evidence that osteopathic and chiropractic manipulation can help your period of recovery be more comfortable at least.

However, because acute back pain commonly recurs in the long term, reeducating your posture by learning new ways of standing, walking, sitting, and working is very important in preventing further episodes of back and neck problems.

TREATMENT TO RESTORE FUNCTION once the back has become painful may involve the stretching of tight muscles, the mobilization of restricted joints, and the learning of better habits of use, such as postural reeducation using the Alexander technique (*see p.62*).

ACHIEVING CORE STABILITY There is very good evidence that maintenance of strong abdominal muscles — the transversus abdominis (the transverse abdominal muscle) in particular — as well as spinal supporting muscles, such as the multifidi (the multifidus muscles), is the key to a back that remains pain-free. Most backcare professionals now teach basic exercises to achieve this so-called "core stability." The Pilates exercise system is one good example of a program that can help prevent back pain from recurring.

AVOID RISKY POSTURES Sometimes, simple changes can reduce the chance of the back pain recurring. For example, one of the most vulnerable times for the low back is early morning, soon after getting out of bed. Some movements, such as bending forward (for example, putting on socks), can strain the back.

Avoiding such "high-risk" activities early in the morning, or after sitting for any length of time, can help prevent both injury and reinjury. Research has shown that avoiding early morning bending helps recovery from acute low back pain.

MASSAGE A review of eight randomized, controlled trials for lower back pain concluded that massage may be beneficial, especially in combination with exercise and education.

TRIGGER POINTS

People who either adopt an unhealthy posture for prolonged periods or are feeling an acute attack of neck pain, may develop a trigger point (*see p.55*). As a result, a muscle in the neck or shoulders may develop a knot of tension, which is tender when pressed, sending out a wave of pain across the area of the body that is already affected. Some of the ways of relaxing these trigger points include massage, dry needling by an acupuncturist, passive stretching exercises, or physical therapy.

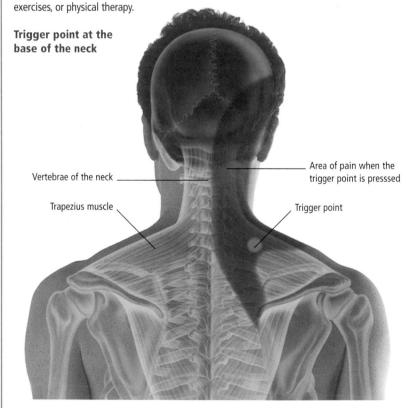

Trigger point at the base of the neck

Vertebrae of the neck

Trapezius muscle

Area of pain when the trigger point is presssed

Trigger point

When a person feels a pain in the muscles down one side of the neck or in the top of the trapezius muscle, a trigger point may develop at the point where the base of the neck meets the shoulder. When this sensitive knot of tension is touched or pressed, a wave of pain may spread through the same muscles that were hurting in the first place, from the base of the skull to the tip of the shoulderblade.

Acupuncture

PRIMARY TREATMENT There is strong evidence that acupuncture is an effective treatment for both back and neck pain. Studies with long-term follow-ups have suggested that it achieves 60–70 percent of pain relief even a year after treatment.

A limited number (usually between four and eight) of acupuncture treatments can have a prolonged beneficial effect on chronic back or neck pain. Moreover, the need for analgesics or anti-inflammatory drugs can be substantially reduced for prolonged periods.

However, scientists continue to debate how much of acupuncture's effect is due to activating the right acupoints and whether "sham" acupuncture — placing the needles at inappropriate spots or at locations not thought to contain acupuncture points — would have exactly the same effect.

Treatment for back or neck pain is usually given on a weekly basis. Anybody contemplating acupuncture for this condition should assume that six to eight treatment sessions will produce some initial benefit. Further treatment should be based solely on the need for symptom relief and continued improvement.

Mind–Body Therapies

In both the US and the UK, back pain is a leading cause of absenteeism from work and one of the most common reasons why people visit their doctors.

The psychosocial symptoms of chronic pain have been well documented and include anger, anxiety, depression, low perceived quality of life, low self-efficacy, and poor coping skills.

HELPFUL APPROACHES Daily relaxation, meditation, or guided imagery (*see pp.98-100*) may help. Studies demonstrate the effectiveness of cognitive behavioral measures, including relaxation, meditation, and guided imagery, in reducing pain perception, visits to the doctor, and analgesic use, and increasing feelings of well-being and self-efficacy in painful conditions.

A Swedish study of 253 people with neck and back pain found that cognitive behavioral intervention, including relaxation and imagery, reduced progression to chronic disability by 88 percent.

PAIN-FREE WAYS TO SIT DOWN AND GET DRESSED

Bending from the waist first thing in the morning is a "high-risk activity" (*see p.270*) that can exacerbate back pain. Here are some tips on how to get dressed and get up from a chair without stressing the back. In addition, choose clothes that are easy to put on and take off, such as slip-on shoes and loose trousers.

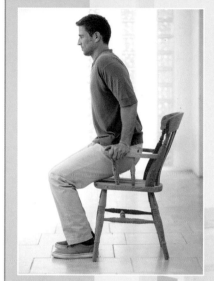

If you have back pain, choose chairs with arms. To sit down or get up, position your feet close to the chair legs. Place your hands on the arms and lever yourself up or down. Try to keep your back as straight as you can.

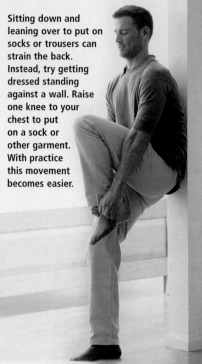

Sitting down and leaning over to put on socks or trousers can strain the back. Instead, try getting dressed standing against a wall. Raise one knee to your chest to put on a sock or other garment. With practice this movement becomes easier.

PAIN RELIEF Research shows that mind–body therapies (*see p.94*), as well as the use of home-based practices, such as meditation and guided imagery, can be effective treatments for relieving pain from back and neck conditions. For example, at the University of Massachusetts School of Medicine, meditation was found to be successful in a mixed group of chronic pain patients, including those with back pain. The actual location of the pain did not appear to make a difference.

In a study into the relief of tension headaches, a group practicing relaxation and imagery were three times as likely to report major pain reduction — a very striking magnitude of difference.

Relaxation and imagery has also significantly reduced pain in studies involving patients with cancer, arthritis, fibromyalgia, hemophilia, and migraine headaches. In all follow-up studies, improvements in pain, function, and mental outlook were sustained for as long as 18 months.

Overall, it is clear from this research that mind–body interventions, as well as the use of mind–body practices, such as meditation and guided imagery, by patients at home can be an effective complementary treatment for general chronic pain conditions, including back and neck pain.

PREVENTION PLAN

The following may help you to prevent back and neck pain:

- Always warm up before and cool down after sports or other physical activity
- Develop good postural habits — for example, when sitting for long periods of time or moving heavy objects
- Do back exercises to keep your body supple and flexible
- Practice relaxation skills and breathing exercises.

SCIATICA

Sciatica is pain that can occur anywhere along the course of the sciatic nerve, which runs from the buttock down the back of the leg (*see also Back and Neck Pain, p.268*). Most people have at least one episode of sciatica in their lives. Often, only one leg is affected. The pain usually disappears gradually over the course of a week or two, but it may recur. Treatment aims to treat the underlying cause where possible, to relieve the pain, and to encourage the patient to remain active through exercise training programs.

WHAT ARE THE SYMPTOMS?

Symptoms may be mild or severe, and include:

- Shooting pain down one or both legs, made worse by movement
- Tingling or numbness in the affected leg
- Muscle weakness in the affected leg
- Difficulty walking if the sciatica is severe

WHY MIGHT I HAVE THIS?

PREDISPOSING FACTORS

- Changes in the spinal column due to a prolapsed disk or osteoarthritis
- Changes in posture during pregnancy
- Anatomical abnormality in the path of the sciatic nerve

TRIGGERS

- Sudden heavy strain in the back

TREATMENT PLAN

PRIMARY TREATMENTS

- Treatment of underlying cause
- Pain-relieving and muscle-relaxant drugs
- Physical therapy or chiropractic

BACKUP TREATMENTS

- Homeopathy
- Dynamic back exercises
- Osteopathy
- Acupuncture

WORTH CONSIDERING

- Vitamin B_{12}

For an explanation of how treatments are rated, see p.111.

WHY DOES IT OCCUR?

The sciatic nerves are the largest nerves in the body and the main nerve in the legs. The roots of the sciatic nerve emerge from the lower spinal cord, merge together in the buttock, and run down the back of the thigh. They branch above the knee and then extend to the lower leg and the foot.

Sciatica is caused by compression of, or damage to, the sciatic nerve, usually at the point where the nerve roots emerge from the spinal cord. The most common cause of the compression, particularly among 20 to 40-year-olds, is a prolapsed disk (*see p.274*) in the spinal column that presses on a spinal nerve root. This kind of sciatica is usually sharp and well delineated, and may be accompanied by tingling or numbness in the affected leg. Sitting in an awkward position for long periods is a possible cause. In some cases, the cause is unknown.

When leg pain is less sharp, it may still be due to a prolapsed disk. However, some practitioners believe that this kind of leg pain can be produced by irritation or trigger points in the lower back or buttock muscles, or by strain or inflammation in the ligaments of the sacroiliac joint at the bottom of the back. Changes in posture that put extra pressure on the sacroiliac joint may cause pregnant women to develop sciatica during the last months of pregnancy. This usually disappears after childbirth.

IMPORTANT

The pain of sciatica normally starts to subside after a few days, but if it does not improve within two weeks consult your doctor.

SELF-HELP

The following measures may help bring relief from the pain of sciatica:

- An ice pack applied to the area of maximum pain for 5–10 minutes each hour.
- A hot-water bottle wrapped in cloth and held over the painful area. Don't do this if there is active inflammation.
- Analgesics, such as acetaminophen.
- Therapeutic exercises for the lower back, such as pelvic tilt and passive extension.

TREATMENTS IN DETAIL

Conventional Medicine

Your doctor will carry out a full examination to assess your spinal column and legs. This may be followed by X-rays of the lower back and other tests, such as magnetic resonance imaging (MRI), if a disk prolapse is suspected (*see p.274*).

PRIMARY TREATMENT **DRUGS** Your doctor will treat the underlying cause where possible. Analgesics and NSAIDs may both relieve the pain of sciatica. Keeping mobile (under medical advice) may help relieve the pain and increase the speed of recovery. You may need physical therapy.

Muscle relaxants, such as diazepam, are sometimes prescribed for acute sciatica to relax muscles in the back if there are spasms, but only on a short-term basis due to the risk of dependence.

CAUTION

NSAIDs and muscle relaxants have various side effects; ask your doctor to explain these to you.

SCIATIC NERVE

A sharp pain shoots down one leg when a sciatic nerve is pinched as it leaves the spinal cord between the second sacral vertebra and the fourth lumbar vertebra. The area of pain may stretch from the hip to the calf.

Back view showing sciatic nerve

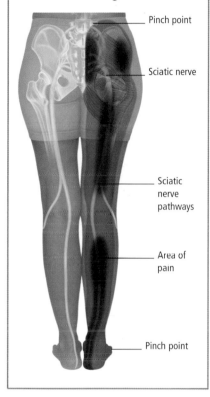

- Pinch point
- Sciatic nerve
- Sciatic nerve pathways
- Area of pain
- Pinch point

Nutritional Therapy

VITAMIN B₁₂ In 2000, a study found that an intramuscular injection of 1mg of vitamin B_{12} every day for two weeks effectively alleviated the lower back pain associated with lumbago or sciatic neuritis. In addition, participants did not need to take as much acetaminophen.

Homeopathy

The following homeopathic medicines may help with sciatica. Each should be taken in the 6C dilution. Take two pills 4 times daily.

BRYONIA ALBA is useful for people whose sciatica improves when their back is supported (for example, with a brace) and when they keep still. It is also appropriate if movement (for example, a sneeze or a cough) makes the sciatica worse. Thirst, dry mouth, and headache are other common symptoms.

COLOCYNTHIS may be for people whose sciatica improves if they lie on the affected side and are warm. Symptoms are accompanied by bad temper and irritability.

NUX VOMICA If warmth makes the sciatica feel better, but stress or overwork makes it worse, *Nux vomica* may help. It is also indicated when the pain is worse in the morning and/or accompanied by irritability.

RHUS TOXICODENDRON If gentle movement, stretching, or warmth relieves the pain, or if immobility and cold wet weather make it worse, then *Rhus tox.* is indicated. It is also appropriate for people who sleep restlessly or who have a skin rash with fine blistering.

OTHER REMEDIES *Hypericum* suits those who have a shooting pain down the course of the sciatic nerve or whose symptoms began after a back injury. *Magnesia phosphorica* is useful when sciatica improves with heat or pressure, gets worse with cold, or is accompanied by cramps.

CAUTION

Do not drink coffee if you are taking *Colocynthis* and *Nux vomica.*

Exercise

DYNAMIC BACK EXERCISES All the available evidence suggests that prolonged bed rest can be harmful, so people with sciatica are recommended to remain active. But the question is "How active?".

A 1991 study revealed that, irrespective of sex, age, duration, and degree of severity of the back trouble, or of preexisting sciatica or X-ray findings of damage, people with sciatica derived most benefit from a dynamic training program of back exercises. The study did not include people with clinical signs of current lumbar nerve root compression (disk herniation).

In 1999, research showed that people with lower back pain and sciatica had a significant reduction in symptoms after a program of Mensendieck exercises. Named after a Danish therapist, these exercises correct body postures and increase consciousness of posture to prevent injuries and sore muscles. Similar to but different from Pilates, they may be available from physical therapists or specialized instructors.

Bodywork Therapies

PRIMARY TREATMENT **PHYSICAL THERAPY AND CHIROPRACTIC MANIPULATION** are equally beneficial for individuals with lower back pain. However, in a 1998 study, even people who followed the advice of an educational booklet on the best ways to look after the spine (such as posture) experienced benefits that were almost as good.

OSTEOPATHY Sometimes the sciatic nerve runs through the small piriformis muscle that connects the sacrum to the top of the leg rather than under it. The nerve may be compressed here by muscle spasm, causing sciatica (*see Neuropathy, p.127*). Effective osteopathic soft-tissue manipulation can release the muscle in many cases. When this fails, surgery may be required.

Acupuncture

Acupuncture is promising for lower back pain but not proven. The cause of sciatica makes a difference. If it is generated by mechanical back pain, then acupuncture should be effective, often with relatively few treatments. If it is caused by nerve compression as a result of a prolapsed disk, then acupuncture is likely to be less effective with more treatments required. A Western acupuncture technique is usually used: the tender areas are needled and sometimes electrical stimulation is given following the pain from the lower back down to the foot. Treatment is given twice a week for very acute pain, or weekly if the pain is less acute. If there is no benefit after six to eight sessions, it is probably wise to stop.

PREVENTION PLAN

To reduce the risk of sciatica:

- Follow a back exercise program

PROLAPSED DISK

A prolapsed disk occurs when the soft core of the cartilage between two vertebrae pushes outward. The disk inflames the surrounding tissue, causing swelling. If the outer coat ruptures, it is called a herniated disk. In both conditions, the bulge produced presses on local nerves, causing pain, commonly in the leg (*see Sciatica, p.272*). Prolapsed (slipped) disks occur most commonly in the lower back, but disks in the neck and, rarely, in the upper back may also prolapse or herniate. Treatment aims to relieve the pain and restore the health of a damaged disk.

WHAT ARE THE SYMPTOMS?

Symptoms may appear gradually over a period of weeks or can appear suddenly. They may include:

- Pain in the affected area
- Muscle spasm and stiffness around the affected area that make movement difficult

If a spinal nerve is affected, the following symptoms may also be present:

- Severe pain, tingling, or numbness in a leg, or, if the neck is affected, an arm
- Weakness or restricted movement in the leg or arm

In a few cases, when a disk herniates, it puts pressure on the cauda equina (a bundle of nerves that emanate from the lower parts of the spinal cord). This requires emergency treatment. Symptoms of this may include:

- Inability to urinate
- Loss of bowel control
- Numbness around the anus
- Shooting pains down the legs

WHY MIGHT I HAVE THIS?

PREDISPOSING FACTORS

- Bad posture

TRIGGERS

- Lifting a heavy weight

IMPORTANT

If you develop impaired bladder or bowel function combined with other symptoms of a prolapsed or herniated disk you should get immediate medical attention.

WHY DOES IT OCCUR?

The vertebrae of the spine are separated and cushioned by shock-absorbing disks consisting of a strong, fibrous outer layer and a soft, gelatinous core. When a prolapse or herniation occurs, the shape of the disk is distorted. Pain results when the inflamed and swollen surrounding tissues and the disk itself press upon the spinal cord or a spinal nerve as it emerges from the spinal cord. The initial symptoms are often back pain and spasms. This gradually fades over several days but leg pain may become more severe.

Around the age of 25, the disks begin to dry out and become more vulnerable to prolapse or herniation due to the normal stresses of daily life and minor injury. A disk may sometimes be damaged by a sharp bending or twisting movement or by lifting a heavy object incorrectly. Around the age of 45, fibrous tissue forms around the disks, eventually stabilizing them and making them less prone to damage.

SELF-HELP

PRIMARY TREATMENT If you have the symptoms of a prolapsed or herniated disk, try the following:

- Take analgesics (aspirin, acetaminophen, or ibuprofen) to ease the pain.
- Relax and lie flat on your back to reduce the pressure on your spine. If this is still uncomfortable, then try bending your knees at right angles and supporting your calves with pillows.
- Soothe tight muscles with a hot water bottle held against the most painful part of your back. Or, wrap a pack of crushed ice cubes in a towel and apply to the area for 15 minutes every few hours.
- Get up and move around carefully as soon as the pain allows.
- Avoid lifting anything for three months or as advised by your doctor. Avoid heavy lifting in the long term and don't drive for long periods of time.
- Get plenty of rest.

TREATMENT PLAN

PRIMARY TREATMENTS

- Analgesics and relaxation (*see Self-Help, right*)
- Treatment for cervical disk prolapse
- Treatment for lumbar disk prolapse
- Anesthetic injections
- Surgery (in some cases)

BACKUP TREATMENTS

- Bodywork therapies

WORTH CONSIDERING

- Nutritional therapy
- Acupuncture

For an explanation of how treatments are rated, see p.111.

TREATMENTS IN DETAIL

Conventional Medicine

The doctor can usually make a diagnosis from a description of symptoms and an examination of the back. In some cases, an X-ray may be needed to exclude other

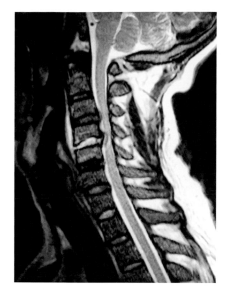

Nerves supplying the limbs, and those providing bowel and bladder control, run through the spinal cord in the neck. A prolapsed cervical disk in the MRI scan (above) may cause pain and weakness in the neck and arm or lower down the body.

causes of pain. Tests, such as magnetic resonance imaging (MRI), may be used to establish the site and severity of the prolapse. A prolapsed or herniated disk often spontaneously returns to normal.

PRIMARY TREATMENT **TREATMENT FOR CERVICAL DISK PROLAPSE** Symptoms caused by a cervical disk prolapse (in the neck) often settle with rest and analgesics. A neck brace may be needed for support. In more extreme cases, a period of traction in the hospital may help relieve pain and other symptoms.

Occasionally, for very severe and persistent pain, surgery may be performed to remove the affected disk. Vertebrae in the neck may be fused to avoid making them unstable and to relieve the original symptoms. However, this restricts the movements of the cervical spine.

PRIMARY TREATMENT **TREATMENT FOR LUMBAR DISK PROLAPSE** Symptoms of lumbar disk prolapse (in the lower back) tend to decrease with rest, analgesics, and muscle relaxers, such as diazepam (only for a short period due to the risk of dependence). Physical therapy is often recommended to help relieve muscle spasms and speed up recovery.

PRIMARY TREATMENT **ANESTHETIC INJECTIONS** To relieve the pain of a prolapsed disk, a local anesthetic may be injected into the epidural space (the space surrounding the membranes that envelop the spinal cord). Alternatively, a local anesthetic, sometimes in combination with a corticosteroid drug, may be injected near the affected disk to help relieve pain and swelling.

PRIMARY TREATMENT **SURGERY** may be considered if the symptoms still persist after several weeks, if they are becoming worse, or if the pain is severe. If there is pressure on the cauda equina (at the base of the spine), surgery must be performed immediately.

A disk may be removed either by traditional surgery or by microdiskectomy, a relatively new procedure in which the surgeon removes the disk through a small incision, while watching images of the procedure provided by a camera inserted through another small incision. The results from these two types of surgical approaches are similar in terms of the relief of symptoms, although the recovery period following traditional surgery is likely to be longer. Following removal of a disk, there may be some residual pain and stiffness due to new stresses placed on the back.

In some cases, instead of removing the disk to relieve the symptoms, the affected disk may be softened by an injection of a softening agent called chymopapain in a procedure known as chemonucleolysis.

> **CAUTION**
>
> Drugs and surgery for prolapsed disk may have side effects; ask your doctor to explain these to you.

Nutritional Therapy

GLUCOSAMINE SULFATE is a basic building block of disk tissue. Clinical experience suggests that 500mg of glucosamine sulfate, 2 or 3 times a day, may help stimulate healing and repair within damaged disks. (*See also Back and Neck Pain, p.268*)

Bodywork Therapy

RESOLVING DISK-RELATED LOWER BACK PAIN Studies show that various strategies can assist in the early resolution of disk-related lower back pain. These include supervised "McKenzie-concept" exercises (involving repetitive extension, or arching, of the back when lying face down and strengthening the "core stability" of abdominal and lower back muscles), traction, use of a cold pack on the affected area, and mobilization of the muscles and joints.

CHIROPRACTIC is a valuable treatment for herniated lower back and neck disks. Its ability to alleviate these conditions is supported by a great deal of evidence (including scan images). In one study, CT scans showed that the resolution of symptoms following manipulation was accompanied by a reduction in disk prolapse in 75 percent of larger herniations and 40 percent of smaller ones.

PENS UNITS Pain management of sciatica (*see p.272*) caused by disk prolapse has been effectively controlled by use of PENS units. This involves passing a mild electrical current through needles inserted into the painful areas. PENS is more effective than the more widely used TENS, which involves passing the current over the pain area instead of through the tissues. PENS is available at pain control clinics and some acupuncturists. However, it is not recommended for self use.

ALTERNATIVES TO SURGERY Intradiskal electrothermal therapy (IDET) is an alternative surgical intervention that heats the damaged tissues in order, many believe, to speed up the process of reabsorption of disk fragments. Results of a 2002 study revealed that, two years after IDET, a significant improvement in pain level and physical functioning (sitting, standing, and walking) was observed, and overall quality of life was much improved. More than 80 percent of the patients reported they were satisfied with the procedure.

A 2002 Swedish study found that when disk prolapse occurs in the neck (often causing major pain in the arms), supervised, intermittent, on-the-door, neck traction resulted in complete symptom resolution within three weeks. On-the-door traction is widely available for self-use and involves a person, either seated or standing, using a harness or other form of material attached to a piece of equipment that hooks onto the top of a door.

THERAPEUTIC BACK CARE EXERCISES

Regular strengthening exercises are a key part of a back care program to avoid further injury, but you should always first consult a physical therapist or doctor. The following exercises strengthen the extensors (the muscles used to straighten the back and limbs) and the deep stabilizing muscles of the abdomen so they can protect the spine. Do ten repetitions each day to start. For best results, you should combine them with exercises to stretch your hamstrings — tight leg muscles contribute to back problems.

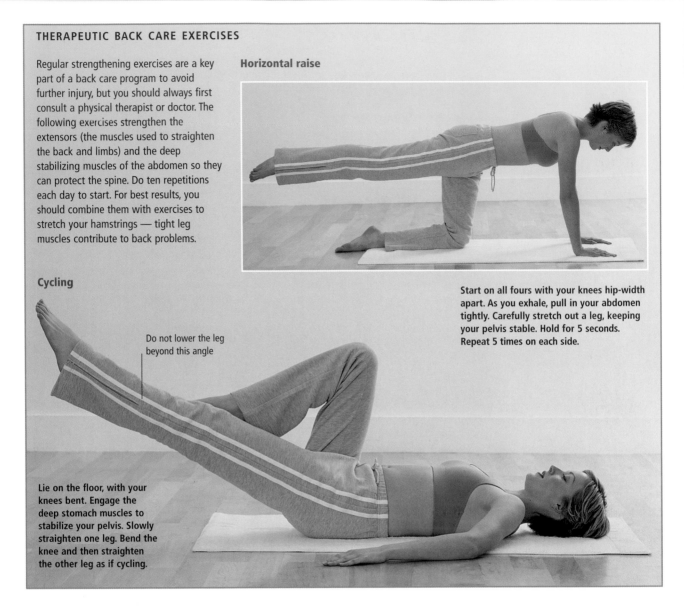

Horizontal raise

Start on all fours with your knees hip-width apart. As you exhale, pull in your abdomen tightly. Carefully stretch out a leg, keeping your pelvis stable. Hold for 5 seconds. Repeat 5 times on each side.

Cycling

Do not lower the leg beyond this angle

Lie on the floor, with your knees bent. Engage the deep stomach muscles to stabilize your pelvis. Slowly straighten one leg. Bend the knee and then straighten the other leg as if cycling.

RECOVERY AFTER SURGERY In a 2001 study, 294 patients with disk degeneration were treated by surgery or by different types of physical therapy. Two years after treatment, 63 percent of the surgical group reported they were "much better" or "better" after surgery and that their "back to work rate" was also significantly better than those who had not received surgery.

However, after surgery, exercise is an essential part of any rehabilitation plan. A systematic review of research made the following conclusions:

- Intensive exercise programs begun 4-6 weeks after surgery get faster results than mild exercise programs begun at the same time. In the long term, however, there is no difference between intensive

and mild exercise programs with regard to overall improvement.

- There is no strong evidence for the effectiveness of supervised training as compared to peforming home exercises.
- It is not known whether active rehabilitation programs should start immediately after surgery or later.
- There is no evidence that patients need to have their activities restricted after first-time lumbar disk surgery.

Acupuncture

Prolapsed disks are very difficult to treat with acupuncture, largely because of the pathology. However, if they impinge on a nerve root and causes symptoms of neuro-

logical stress, the pain is likely to be intense, persistent, and last for many weeks. In these cases acupuncture is one way to manage the pain, even though it cannot treat the underlying condition. In many cases, prolapsed disks clear up on their own.

PREVENTION PLAN

The following help you keep the spine healthy:

- Mackenzie exercises, Pilates, or other core strengthening exercises
- Advice on posture and lifting

SPORTS INJURIES

Athletes and others who exercise strenuously risk sports injuries, such as strains, sprains, bursitis (*see p.284*), ligament injuries, stress fractures, and joint dislocations. Such injuries often occur in people who are new to a sport, beginning exercise after a long period of inactivity, or who fail to warm up properly before exercising. Sports injuries may occur suddenly or develop gradually as a result of repeated stress. Treatment aims to relieve pain and restore function; options include using analgesics, physical therapy, manipulation, and homeopathy.

WHAT ARE THE SYMPTOMS?

Depends on the injury
- Pain
- Swelling
- Stiffness

WHY MIGHT I HAVE THIS?

PREDISPOSING FACTORS
- Lack of fitness
- Failure to warm up/cool down properly

TRIGGERS
- Violent contact
- Overuse of a joint or muscle
- Accidental injury

TREATMENT PLAN

PRIMARY TREATMENTS
- R I C E (Rest, Ice, Compression, Elevation) (see Immediate Relief, right)
- Analgesics and NSAIDs
- Treatment for dislocated joints, fractures, ruptured Achilles tendons, and other specific injuries
- Physical therapy
- Bodywork and movement therapies

BACKUP TREATMENTS
- Nutritional therapy
- Acupuncture
- Homeopathy

For an explanation of how treatments are rated, see p.111.

WHY DO THEY OCCUR?

Any part of the musculoskeletal system can be injured while playing a sport. Bone injuries commonly occur in contact sports, such as football. Repeated jarring of small bones in the feet can lead to stress fractures in runners. Joint injuries can happen in almost any sport and dislocation of a joint is always a risk in contact sports.

Injuries to ligaments and tendons, the fibrous bands of tissue that hold the musculoskeletal system together, are also common and often result from falling or jumping. Tendinitis occurs when tendons are inflamed.

Two common types of tendonitis are tennis elbow and golfer's elbow, which affect the outer and inner sides of the elbow respectively — they are named after the sports in which they classically occur, although they are not restricted to these. Plantar fasciitis, common in long-distance runners, affects the sole of the foot. Less commonly, tendons may rupture; the Achilles tendon at the back of the ankle is particularly susceptible to this.

Finally, muscle injuries, such as strains, can occur in any sport, especially if you fail to warm up properly before starting.

DIFFERENT SPORTS Each sport has its own hazards, no matter how much time is spent training. For example, golf produces the highest level of back problems of any professional sport. Many are spine-related because the spine absorbs a great deal of the strain caused by rotation of the hips, knees, and shoulders.

Lower back pain, as well as shoulder and neck pain, is commonly reported by runners. Gymnastics is the sport associated with most lumbar spinal injuries. In swimming, certain strokes such as the butterfly produce enormous stress on the bones and muscles of the lower back, especially in young swimmers. Thoracic pain and round back deformities are common in young women who do the breast stroke because of the repeated round shoulder-type stroke motion.

More young players experience injuries in soccer than in any other sport. Damage to certain bones, muscles, or tendons develops over a period of time due to too much repetitive activity. Gifted youngsters are asked to train and play competitively at ever-younger ages, which in many cases leads to tragic consequences.

IMMEDIATE RELIEF

PRIMARY TREATMENT R I C E Analgesics such as aspirin, or ibuprofen are likely to be needed. However, R I C E is the best immediate treatment for most injuries:
- Rest: sit or lie down with the injured part comfortably supported.
- Ice: apply ice or a bag of frozen peas to the injured part for 10–15 minutes.
- Compression: bandage a thick layer of fabric around the injured part.
- Elevation: raise and support the injured part to reduce blood flow and prevent further swelling.

IMPORTANT

If you think you have injured yourself while involved in a sport or physical activity, don't continue — stop, get immediate relief, and seek a medical opinion.

Conventional Medicine

Doctors can often make a diagnosis based on your symptoms and an examination, although X-rays may be needed to look for fractures. Sometimes, additional investigations, such as CT scanning, enable a doctor to look at the affected area in more detail.

PRIMARY TREATMENT **ANALGESICS AND NSAIDS** The treatment varies depending on the injury. In all cases, analgesics are likely to be needed. Tendinitis, ligament damage, and muscle strains are usually treated by rest and sometimes with NSAIDs.

PRIMARY TREATMENT **TREATMENT FOR FRACTURES** involves holding the fragments of bone in position, often with a cast, so that they heal strongly; surgery may first be needed to return displaced fragments to their original position.

PRIMARY TREATMENT **TREATMENT FOR DISLOCATED JOINTS** In a dislocation, the displaced joint may need to be manipulated into the correct position and then held immobile, so that the surrounding tissues can heal and return to keeping the bones of the joint in position.

PRIMARY TREATMENT **TREATMENT FOR RUPTURED ACHILLES TENDON** If an Achilles tendon ruptures, the two ends of the tendon are held together with a plaster cast; this is sometimes preceded by surgery. Following treatment, patients must avoid exercise for approximately four months.

PRIMARY TREATMENT **PHYSICAL THERAPY,** and sometimes ultrasound treatment (to cool or heat tissues), form a part of treatment for many injuries. When enough time has passed after your injury to begin exercising, always wear the correct clothing and use quality equipment. Warm up and cool down, and avoid overusing your muscles and joints.

BURSITIS Bursas are fluid-filled sacs separating tendons from bones and ligaments. They are easily inflamed and irritated by strong repetitive movements (*see also Bursitis, p.284*). For example, the psoas bursa over the hip joint is commonly injured by

hurdlers and in martial arts and step classes. Doctors who specialize in sports injuries can recommend training modifications to avoid recurrences.

> **CAUTION**
>
> NSAIDs have side effects; ask your doctor to explain these to you.

Nutritional Therapy

BROMELAIN For joint or ligament sprains, take 500mg of the pineapple extract bromelain, three times a day on an empty stomach. If you do this as soon as possible following a sprain, a study shows that the edema (fluid retention) and inflammation may be alleviated.

A 10-minute warm-up before exercise can prevent most sports injuries

CHONDROITIN AND GLUCOSAMINE are important components of cartilage and may help recovery from cartilage, ligament, or tendon damage. In a 1984 study, athletes with damaged knee cartilage who received 1,500mg of glucosamine sulfate per day for 40 days, followed by 750mg of glucosamine sulfate per day for a further 100 days, either experienced a complete cure or were at least able to resume training.

In a 2003 study, people with knee pain that may have been caused by prior injury experienced pain relief and improved function after taking 2,000mg of glucosamine each day for eight weeks. No studies have looked specifically at chondroitin sulfate in sports injury, though in practice, 1,200mg per day seems to be an effective dose.

DIMETHYL SULFOXIDE (DMSO) A double-blind trial of DMSO has demonstrated its therapeutic value in the treatment of bursitis, as well as for acute strains, sprains, and tendonitis.

Homeopathy

Many medicines may be indicated due to the wide range of sports injuries, strains, and overuse problems. Although they can-

not treat the underlying injury of a break or tear, many homeopathic cures can greatly relieve the pain of sports injuires.

ARNICA MONTANA is frequently the most appropriate homeopathic medicine for sports injuries. It is used for muscle over-strain and bruising and is particularly suitable for achiness or sensitivity to lying down. *Arnica* was previously thought to enhance performance, but recent studies have indicated otherwise.

OTHER REMEDIES The most common medicine for enthesitis is *Ruta graveolens*, but others including *Bryonia alba* and *Rhus toxicodendron* may also be used. In people who respond to *Bryonia*, the typical symptom is sharp pain from particular movements, such as lifting a heavy object.

The symptoms are relieved by firm support, such as an elastic brace. Similar symptoms elsewhere — for instance, in the knees (a common injury in soccer players) — may also respond to *Bryonia*, if they improve with support. *Rhus toxicodendron* can help a range of different injuries that show marked improvement from taking time to properly warm-up.

TISSUE AFFINITIES Some homeopathic medicines have specific tissue affinities. For example, *Symphytum* is used for bone fractures, such as the metatarsal stress fractures in the feet common in professional soccer players and long-distance runners. *Ledum* is used for black eyes.

Bodywork and Movement Therapies

PRIMARY TREATMENT **PHYSICAL THERAPY, OSTEOPATHY, AND CHIROPRACTIC** The object of manipulation treatments, such as physical therapy, osteopathy, chiropractic, sports massage, and neuromuscular therapy, is to achieve rapid resolution of sporting injuries and restore optimal function. A practitioner will assess the injury and take the most suitable

STRETCHING TO PREVENT INJURIES

Injuries can occur if stiff muscles are pushed beyond their natural range of motion during vigorous activity. Stretching elongates tight muscle fibers and increases flexibility and range of movement. Stretch before your activity for a few minutes to warm the muscles and afterward for at least 10 minutes to reduce soreness. The muscles in the legs and feet work hard during sports, so protect them with the following exercises.

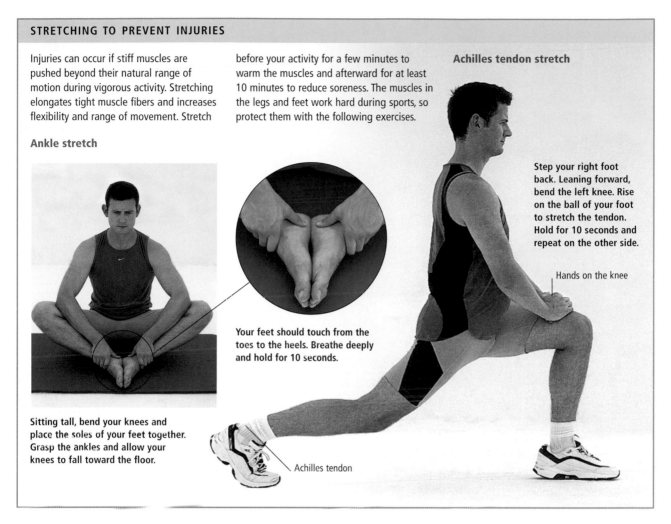

Ankle stretch

Sitting tall, bend your knees and place the soles of your feet together. Grasp the ankles and allow your knees to fall toward the floor.

Your feet should touch from the toes to the heels. Breathe deeply and hold for 10 seconds.

Achilles tendon

Achilles tendon stretch

Step your right foot back. Leaning forward, bend the left knee. Rise on the ball of your foot to stretch the tendon. Hold for 10 seconds and repeat on the other side.

Hands on the knee

---

action — for example, freeing and loosening whatever is tight or restricted, and toning and improving both the strength and function of whatever tissue is weak.

However, the most basic advice for dealing with a recent injury is summarized as R I C E — rest, ice, compression, and elevation (*see Immediate Relief, p.277*).

An osteopathic perspective on sporting-related injuries and dysfunction starts from the principle that the body has an built-in capacity to cope with and adapt to most of the normal (and many abnormal) demands placed upon it (*see Adaptation, p.53*).

One major mistake made in treating sports injuries is neglecting to respect the natural healing process. Practitioners advise against returning to activity too soon after an injury — time is needed to allow tissue inflammation to calm and tissue repair to be consolidated.

The body's response to soft-tissue injury follows a predictable sequence: there is an inflammatory phase, a repair phase, and a maturation (or rebuilding) phase. Manual therapy should not start until tissue repair is well established — usually about four weeks after the injury. The timing of the three phases is fairly predictable, but varies with the severity, extent, and type of tissue injured, as well as the age, general health, and nutrition of the injured person.

Within that framework, treatment must avoid retarding repair and recovery, but also too much rest and inactivity, which can cause loss of strength and muscle bulk.

Acupuncture

Acupuncture in sports injuries is directed both at relieving pain and accelerating healing. It is widely used by sports physical therapists and can be very effective in the treatment of injury to joints and the surrounding ligaments and tendons as well as muscle. It is vitally important that a clear diagnosis is made: acupuncture may take away the pain of a stress fracture but in the long term it may cause more damage.

Trigger points (*see p.55*) commonly occur in injured muscles. They cause pain that can be local or referred (experienced some distance away). Acupuncture or local anesthetic injection can successfully treat trigger-point pain; the more acupuncture that can be given immediately following the injury, the better. Initial daily treatment is ideal, followed by weekly, or twice weekly, treatment.

PREVENTION PLAN

The following should help you to prevent sports injuries:

- Warm up and cool down properly
- Exercise regularly

TEMPOROMANDIBULAR JOINT DISORDER

The temporomandibular joint connects the lower jawbone (mandible) to the temporal bone of the skull. In temporomandibular joint disorder (TMJ), the joint and its associated muscles and ligaments do not work together properly, causing pain. Treatment may involve orthodontic work, analgesics, chondroitin and glucosamine supplements, acupuncture, physical manipulation, and mind–body therapy.

WHAT ARE THE SYMPTOMS?

- Tenderness in the jaw
- Headaches
- Aching pain in the face and sometimes the ears — the pain may be caused by chewing or opening the mouth widely, as when yawning

There may also be other symptoms, including:

- Difficulty opening the mouth
- Locking of the jaw
- Clicking noises from the joint when the mouth is opened or closed

WHY MIGHT I HAVE THIS?

PREDISPOSING FACTORS

- Osteoarthritis
- Malocclusion

TRIGGERS

- Stress

TREATMENT PLAN

PRIMARY TREATMENTS

- Orthodontic treatment
- Acetaminophen or NSAIDs for pain and muscle spasms (*see Self-Help*)
- Chondroitin and glucosamine

BACKUP TREATMENTS

- Surgery
- Physical therapy (mouth-opening exercises)
- Chiropractic and other bodywork therapies
- Acupuncture
- Mind–body therapies

For an explanation of how treatments are rated, see p.111.

WHY DOES IT OCCUR?

The temporomandibular joint allows the jaw to move in all directions so that the teeth can bite and chew food efficiently. TMJ disorder is often due to spasm of the muscles responsible for chewing. The spasm is commonly a result of clenching the jaw or grinding the teeth. Stress may be a factor in both of these. If the teeth do not meet properly (malocclusion), there may be additional stress on the temporomandibular joint.

TMJ disorder may also be the result of an injury that displaces the joint. Rarely, the condition is due to arthritis. The condition is more common in women.

SELF-HELP

PRIMARY TREATMENT The following measures may help you reduce muscle spasm and relieve pain:

- Massage the muscles of the jaw.
- Apply heat to the painful area with a warm towel or a covered hot-water bottle containing warm water.
- Ease the pain with acetaminophen or NSAIDs.
- Eat soft foods until the pain settles. Avoid chewy foods, such as bagels, and do not chew gum.

TREATMENTS IN DETAIL

Conventional Medicine

Your doctor or dentist may arrange X-rays of your jaws and teeth. Other imaging tests, such as magnetic resonance imaging (MRI), may also be needed to diagnose TMJ disorder.

PRIMARY TREATMENT **ORTHODONTIC TREATMENT** The underlying causes are treated when possible. For example, orthodontic treatment appliances may be recommended to improve the bite (how the teeth come together) and a device is available that can be fitted over the upper or lower teeth at night to prevent grinding and clenching.

SYMPTOM RELIEF Treatment aims to reduce muscle spasms and relieve pain (*see Self-Help, left*). Relaxation techniques may help to relieve associated stress.

SURGERY Occasionally, in severe cases when symptoms persist and there is an underlying problem, surgery is recommended to restructure the joint.

> **CAUTION**
>
> NSAIDs may cause side-effects: ask your doctor to explain these to you.

Nutritional Therapy

PRIMARY TREATMENT **CHONDROITIN AND GLUCOSAMINE** supplements may help people with TMJ. Glucosamine is believed to help regenerate cartilage, while chondroitin is said to enable cartilage to remain hydrated and hence keep its resilience. Clinical experience and scientific studies suggest that a combination of both can help people with TMJ who might have osteoarthritis of this joint.

In one study, people with osteoarthritis of the temporomandibular joint took 1,500mg of glucosamine hydrochloride and 1,200mg of chondroitin sulfate daily

TEMPOROMANDIBULAR JOINT DISORDER 281

THE TEMPOROMANDIBULAR JOINT

The temporomandibular joint is located where the temporal bone meets the mandible (jaw) bone. Between the two bones lies a disk of cartilage called the meniscus that allows the joint to open and close like a hinge, but also to move backward, forward, and from side to side. The two temporomandibular joints are subjected to great deal of pressure during the process of chewing food.

Section through a temporomandibular joint

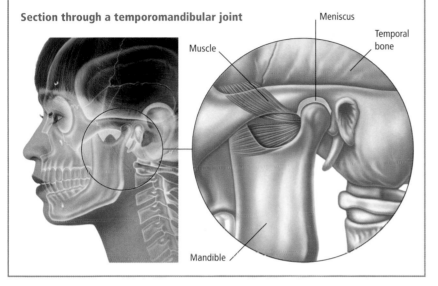

Labels: Muscle, Meniscus, Temporal bone, Mandible

---

for 12 weeks. Glucosamine and chondroitin supplements relieved pain and tenderness in the joint, and reduced the amount of analgesics needed.

In another study, 50 patients with osteoarthritis of the same joint took 3,200mg of glucosamine hydrochloride and 2,400mg of chondroitin sulfate each day, together with 2,000 mg of vitamin C for three months. At the end of the study, 80 percent of patients reported a decrease in both the noises coming from the joint, and the pain. If you have TMJ, take 1,500–3,000mg of glucosamine hydrochloride (or glucosamine sulfate) with 1,200–2,400mg of chondroitin sulfate.

Physical Therapy

Temporomandibular joint disk displacement is the cause of many people's TMJ problems. A research study evaluated non-surgical treatments, such as splints to correct malocclusion, mobilization of the jaw, and pain medication. The results suggested that TMJ caused by anterior displacement of the disk is likely to improve with only minimal (i.e., nonsurgical) treatment.

Another study showed that people with painful TMJ disk displacement made a greater improvement when they received physical therapy (for example, mouth-opening exercises) and analgesics than they did if they received no treatment at all. At the same time, approximately 75 percent of patients were successfully treated without analgesics and using only active and passive (i.e. assisted) jaw movement exercises, correction of body posture, and relaxation techniques.

Bodywork Therapies

Where exercise and/or splint therapy fails to correct anterior disk displacement, active manipulation may be called for, followed by a splint, according to a Chinese study. Chiropractic manipulation of the temporomandibular joint and associated muscles has been shown to be a useful approach in correcting imbalances related to TMJ pain and dysfunction.

DEACTIVATION OF TRIGGER POINTS Muscular imbalances associated with TMJ disorder may involve the active presence of trigger points (*see p.55*), particularly in the temporalis muscles. However, pain may be the result of three distinct problems: a TMJ disk or joint, trigger points in a muscle (e.g. the temporalis), or trigger points resulting from another joint, such as in the cervical spine. Each requires separate treatment. Trigger points can be treated by injection, acupuncture, self-stretching, or by a combination of neuromuscular techniques that manipulate soft tissues.

Acupuncture

Trials comparing acupuncture with placebo treatments have indicated that it is likely to be of substantial benefit in treating the pain of TMJ. Treatment is usually based on needling the tender points around the temporomandibular joint and pain can be relieved for months and sometimes years after relatively few treatments. As with all painful conditions, four or five weekly acupuncture sessions will be enough to know whether this approach is likely to prove effective.

Mind–Body Therapies

BIOFEEDBACK AND COGNITIVE BEHAVIORAL SKILLS TRAINING (CBST) may help counter any underlying stress that may be perpetuating symptoms, according to research. In 1977, a pioneer study showed that electromyographic (EMG) biofeedback could be effective in people who suffered from long-term pain that was related to the temporomandibular joint. The patients were trained to be aware of tension in the jaw. In 2000, a study assigned almost 100 patients with chronic TMJ to one of four groups for treatment: biofeedback, CBST, biofeedback and CBST, or a control. Results showed that the three treatment groups reported significantly decreased pain and improved mood. Patients who were in the biofeedback group were the most significantly improved of all when compared to the control group, which did not get any treatment.

PREVENTION PLAN

The following may help prevent the development of TMJ disorder:

- Seek dental advice about malocclusion
- Try to stop clenching your jaw or grinding your teeth

FROZEN SHOULDER

Frozen shoulder is pain and stiffness in and around the shoulder joint that severely restricts movement. Often caused by injury to the shoulder or following a bout of capsulitis (in which the joint is warm, tender, and swollen), it occurs most frequently in people over 40 and is more common in women and in those with diabetes. It can last for up to two years. The integrated healing plan centers on manipulation therapies, which aim to stretch and strengthen shortened, weakened muscles. It also includes drugs to relieve pain and therapies such as yoga and the Alexander technique to improve posture and mobility.

WHAT ARE THE SYMPTOMS?

Symptoms usually develop slowly over weeks or months and may include:

- Pain in the shoulder which is severe in the early stages and often worse at night
- Over time, decreasing pain but increasing stiffness and restricted movement of the joint
- Sometimes, pain extending down the arm to the elbow

WHY MIGHT I HAVE THIS?

PREDISPOSING FACTORS

- Diabetes mellitus
- Poor posture
- Prolonged immobility of the shoulder
- Trigger points below collarbone
- Repetitive tasks, such as digging or painting walls
- Diet rich in omega-6 and deficient in omega-3 fatty acids

TRIGGERS

- Injury to the shoulder

TREATMENT PLAN

PRIMARY TREATMENTS

- Physical therapy, osteopathy, or chiropractic

BACKUP TREATMENTS

- Analgesic drugs
- Homeopathy
- Nutritional therapy
- Alexander technique, Pilates, yoga, and massage
- Acupuncture

For an explanation of how treatments are rated, see p.111.

WHY DOES IT OCCUR?

Frozen shoulder may result from an injury to the shoulder region that causes inflammation, or it may occur if the shoulder is immobilized for a long period of time. Often, the cause is unknown.

In many cases, frozen shoulder develops over months or years. If your posture is slumped, with your head forward and shoulders rounded, it puts the joints under stress (*see feature box, right*). Over time, especially if the muscles have to perform heavy, difficult, or repetitive tasks (such as yardwork, painting walls, or playing tennis — particularly serving) the shoulder may become inflamed. The inflammation can be restricted to the shoulder joint capsule itself or may involve tissues just outside the capsule. If this happens, scar tissue may develop that severely restricts movement of the shoulder.

Sensitive areas known as trigger points (*see p.55*) can create a painful shortening of the muscles that control the shoulder joint (the rotator cuff group). This situation is more likely to occur when poor posture changes the relationship of the bones in the shoulder, thereby causing increased mechanical stress on the rotator cuff group of muscles.

There are other situations in which the muscles, ligaments, and tendons of the complex shoulder joint become irritated, inflamed, and restricted, resulting in frozen shoulder. These include nerve entrapment, muscle spasm, calcification of muscle attachments, activation of trigger points, and partial dislocation of the shoulder joint due to injury or repetitive strain.

IMMEDIATE RELIEF

To reduce the swelling and pain:

- Wrap a bag of frozen vegetables in a hand towel or use an ice pack applied on the painful area for 10 minutes once every hour.
- Alternatively, fill an empty soft-drink can with water, seal with tape, and freeze. Roll the can over the area for 3–5 minutes every hour.
- Take analgesics for the pain.

TREATMENTS IN DETAIL

Conventional Medicine

If your symptoms suggest frozen shoulder, see your doctor to arrange an X-ray to exclude an underlying disorder.

PAIN-RELIEVING DRUGS, such as nonsteroidal anti-inflammatory drugs (NSAIDs) may be prescribed to relieve the pain. For severe pain, a course of oral corticosteroids may be prescribed, or a corticosteroid drug may be injected into the shoulder joint to give relief from pain and stiffness.

> **CAUTION**
>
> NSAIDs may cause side effects; ask your doctor to explain these to you.

Nutritional Therapy

OMEGA-3 AND OMEGA-6 FATTY ACIDS Excessive amounts of omega-6 polyunsaturated fatty acids (found in vegetable oils)

HOW A FROZEN SHOULDER DEVELOPS

If you habitually hunch your shoulders and poke your head forward, the socket into which your upper arm slots (glenoid fossa) will be further forward than if your posture were upright (as in the X-ray below). The rotator cuff muscles that link the shoulder joint to the humerus will need to work under immense mechanical stress. Over time, this may lead to the shoulder becoming inflamed, restricted, and painful.

Inflammation of the shoulder

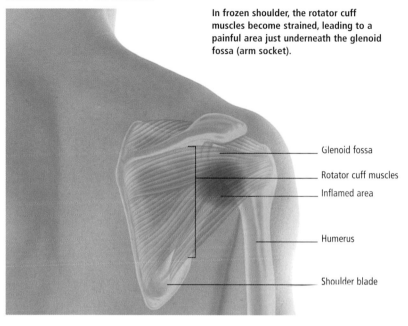

In frozen shoulder, the rotator cuff muscles become strained, leading to a painful area just underneath the glenoid fossa (arm socket).

Glenoid fossa

Rotator cuff muscles

Inflamed area

Humerus

Shoulder blade

and a relative lack of omega 3 fatty acids seem to promote inflammation. Eating foods that are rich in omega-3 fatty acids can help reduce the inflammatory component of frozen shoulder. For example, omega-3 fatty acids are found in some nuts and seeds, especially walnuts and flaxseeds, and in oily fish (including salmon, sardines, mackerel, and herring). If you have repeated bouts of frozen shoulder, you may benefit from eating these foods regularly.

Homeopathy

The homeopathic preparation *Formica rufa*, injected subcutaneously (under the skin, rather than into the joint as with steroid injections), often helps relieve the pain of frozen shoulder. The special injectable preparation must only be given by a qualified practitioner.

Several homeopathic medicines may be helpful, especially if given early in the inflammatory stage. The most commonly suitable homeopathic medicine for this condition is *Rhus toxicodendron*. In people who respond to this medicine, the pain of frozen shoulder is eased by gentle movement of the joint. Take two 6C pills, 3 times a day.

Bodywork and Movement Therapies

PRIMARY TREATMENT **PHYSICAL THERAPY, OSTEOPATHY, AND CHIROPRACTIC** are all highly recommended for frozen shoulder. Once a shoulder has become very painful and movement is significantly restricted, the healing process is often lengthy and requires careful and regular treatment by a qualified practitioner, as well as self-treatment, to rehabilitate the joint. In some very severe cases of frozen shoulder, surgery may be necessary.

Visit a practitioner or a doctor who practices manual medicine as soon as your condition is diagnosed. As with most chronic joint problems, the process of developing a frozen shoulder starts with minor discomfort and mild restriction of movement. Do not neglect the problem at this stage. It is likely to develop increased irritation and inflammation, and ultimately the formation of scar tissue and severe restriction of movement.

Treatment of the condition in the early stages is likely to include identifying muscular imbalances, stretching shortened muscles, toning and strengthening weakened muscles, and deactivating trigger points. Your therapist may also advise on the correct way to stand, sit, and move, since poor posture can be a major cause of stress in the muscles, tendons, and ligaments.

There are many cases recorded of spontaneous recovery of frozen shoulder, after approximately 30 months — evidence of the self-healing potential of the body.

ALEXANDER TECHNIQUE AND PILATES If poor posture contributes to the problem, try some lessons in the Alexander technique. This may be useful in improving posture over a period of 6–12 months. Pilates may also benefit your posture.

YOGA AND MASSAGE Yoga may help relax you, relieve stress, and stretch tight muscles. Massage also has this effect.

Acupuncture

Of five clinical studies, four support the use of acupuncture in treating the pain associated with frozen shoulder. The negative study was carried out in the 1980s but was poorly constructed.

Acupuncture should be used in the early stages of shoulder pain to prevent the development of frozen shoulder. If frozen shoulder is established, acupuncture often offers pain relief after a substantial number of treatments, but physical therapy is still required. Usually, frozen shoulder needs weekly treatment for 10–12 weeks before significant improvement occurs.

PREVENTION PLAN

The following may help prevent the development of frozen shoulder:

● Stretching and strengthening exercises to keep the shoulder strong and flexible

BURSITIS

In bursitis, the fluid-filled sac (bursa) that surrounds a joint and cushions it against friction becomes inflamed, leading to tenderness and swelling. Movement of the joint may also be restricted. The knee is the most common site for bursitis but the elbow (tennis elbow) and other joints, such as the hip, may also be affected. Treatment aims to reduce inflammation and relieve pain.

WHAT ARE THE SYMPTOMS?

- Pain and swelling in the affected joint
- Restricted movement in the affected joint

WHY MIGHT I HAVE THIS?

PREDISPOSING FACTORS

- Overuse of a joint

TRIGGERS

- Injury
- Unaccustomed exercise
- Bacterial infection

TREATMENT PLAN

PRIMARY TREATMENTS

- Rest
- NSAIDs
- Fluid drainage and corticosteroid injections

BACKUP TREATMENTS

- Antibiotics (for infective bursitis)
- Surgery (if the condition recurs)
- Acupuncture
- Bodywork therapies

WORTH CONSIDERING

- Homeopathy
- Nutritional therapy

For an explanation of how treatments are rated, see p.111.

WHY DOES IT OCCUR?

Bursitis may develop after an injury or unaccustomed exercise. Some joint diseases, such as rheumatoid arthritis (*see p.293*) and gout (*see p.302*), increase the risk of bursitis. Rarely, the condition may be due to a bacterial infection.

Overuse of the joint, or repeated or prolonged stress to the joint, may also be involved. This is reflected in the traditional names for bursitis: housemaid's knee may be due to excessive kneeling, weaver's bottom (which affects the bursa overlying the pelvic bones that you sit on) is named after weavers who shuffled up and down long benches as they worked their looms. Golfers may also suffer from bursitis affecting the elbow. This condition is popularly referred to as tennis elbow.

Bursitis usually improves on its own if you rest the affected joint, but this may take several weeks.

IMMEDIATE RELIEF

Try the following to help relieve the pain and discomfort of bursitis:

- Get plenty of rest. In particular, ischial bursitis (weaver's bottom) is often helped by sitting on either a foam rubber or an inflatable ring.
- A "warming" compress (which is sometimes paradoxically called a cold compress) can help ease discomfort and swelling. Wring out a double layer of fabric in very cold water and wrap it around the joint. Immediately cover this with a layer or two of an insulating washcloth or woolen material so that no damp edges protrude. The goal of this wrapping is to allow the cold cotton to become warm. Fix the compress in place with a safety pin and leave for 2–8 hours or even overnight.

TREATMENTS IN DETAIL

Conventional Medicine

PRIMARY TREATMENT **REST AND DRUGS** Your doctor will examine the affected joint and will probably recommend that you rest it to allow the inflammation to subside. You may be prescribed NSAIDs to help this process and if the condition is caused by a bacterial infection, antibiotics will be prescribed.

PRIMARY TREATMENT **INJECTIONS AND SURGERY** If symptoms persist or are very severe your doctor may drain fluid from the bursa and inject it with a corticosteroid to relieve the inflammation. In a few cases — if, for example, the condition recurs — the bursa may be removed.

> **CAUTION**
>
> Medication and surgery for bursitis may cause side effects; ask your doctor to explain these to you.

Nutritional Therapy

OMEGA-3 FATTY ACIDS Studies have shown that taking omega-3 fatty acids reduces the inflammation and pain associated with bursitis. The omega-3 fatty acids eicosapentaenoic acid (EPA) and docosahexaenoic acid (DHA), given at doses of 378mg and 259mg respectively per day for two months or longer, have been found to reduce inflammation, and may therefore help people with bursitis.

Omega-3 fatty acids can be found in some nuts and seeds, especially walnuts and flaxseeds, but the main dietary source is oily fish, such as mackerel, trout, herring, salmon, and sardines. Eating plenty of these

CORTICOSTEROIDS TO RELIEVE BURSITIS

An injection of corticosteroids, known as an infiltration, into the bursa of a joint is an effective way of relieving the pain and inflammation associated with bursitis. One of the advantages of such local injections is that compared to oral administration of corticosteroids, there are fewer side effects to the body as a whole. The knee and shoulder are two of the joints that benefit from corticosteroid injections.

Treating bursitis in the shoulder

The subacromial bursa is one of three regions of the shoulder that benefit from corticosteroid injections when it is inflamed.

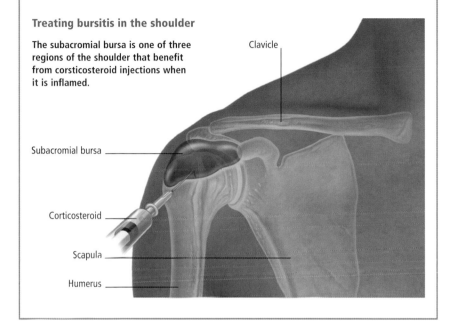

Clavicle

Subacromial bursa

Corticosteroid

Scapula

Humerus

---

foods may help reduce the symptoms of bursitis. Another option is to take 1,000mg of concentrated fish oil, once or twice a day.

DIMETHYL SULFOXIDE (DMSO) A double-blind trial of DMSO has demonstrated its therapeutic value in the treatment of bursitis, as well as for acute strains, sprains, and tendonitis.

> **CAUTION**
>
> Consult your doctor before taking either omega-3 fatty acids or fish oils with warfarin (see p.46).

Homeopathy

Several homeopathic medicines are available to help ease the sypmtoms of bursitis. *Apis mellifera*, *Ruta graveolens*, and *Sticta* should be taken in the 6C strength. Take two pills 2 or 3 times daily.

APIS MELLIFERA is among the most important remedies for bursitis. It is a good illustration of the principle of homeopathy. The symptoms of bursitis resemble those of a bee sting, and the remedy *Apis* is made from live bees. The medicine is likely to help when the onset of bursitis is acute with much pain and swelling. The bursa is very sensitive to pressure, but cold applications may relieve the pain.

RUTA GRAVEOLENS The most commonly suggested medicine for less acute situations is *Ruta graveolens*, made from the herb rue. It is appropriate when the affected region feels weak and bruised, and gentle movement provides some improvement. *Ruta graveolens* is available as a pill or a cream.

STICTA is more commonly used for sinusitis, but is sometimes useful for knee bursitis.

Acupuncture

Painful conditions, such as tennis elbow, appear to respond very well to acupuncture, but few clinical trials have looked specifically at bursitis. Some small studies or case reports indicate that acupuncture is immediately and rapidly effective — treatment is usually based on needling local tender areas and does not necessarily require a traditional Chinese diagnosis. Acupuncture can be safer and sometimes swifter than conventional treatments.

Acupuncture treatment should be given on a weekly or twice-weekly basis. If there is no benefit after five or six sessions, it may be best to stop the treatment.

Bodywork Therapies

DEACTIVATE TRIGGER POINTS At times, bursitis is accompanied by active trigger points (see p.55) in the area. For example, in subacromial bursitis in the shoulder joint, trigger points in the pectoralis, supraspinatus, or teres major muscles often create more pain than the bursitis itself.

Manual methods such as applying pressure to the tender area or stretching, as well as acupuncture or a local anesthetic injection can deactivate such trigger points and markedly reduce the pain. However, this may do little to change the actual bursitis.

PAIN RELIEF Treating the bursitis involves releasing shortness or tightness in the muscles attached to the joint. At the same time, hydrotherapy, ice packs, and/or hot and cold compresses can ease swelling and reduce discomfort. Lymphatic drainage massage (see p.62) will help reduce fluid pressure around the joint.

HEEL PADS of foam rubber or felt may be used to treat bursitis in the heel joint (calcaneum) to elevate the heel, pad the bursa, and minimize shoe pressure. An orthotic (shock-absorbing foot support) may also help prevent abnormal heel motion.

GRADUATED EXERCISES, in which you gradually increase your effort or number of repetitions, are an important part of careful rehabilitation as the bursitis eases. These stretch short or tight muscles and tone weakened muscles.

PREVENTION PLAN

The following may prevent bursitis:
- Avoid overuse of particular joints

REPETITIVE STRAIN INJURY

Prolonged, repeated movements of one part of the body can lead to repetitive strain injury (RSI). It most commonly affects muscles and tendons in the arms, and is sometimes known as upper limb disorder. RSI may be associated with stress in the workplace or at home. Treatment involves pain relief, reducing inflammation, manipulation, acupuncture, homeopathy, and making changes in the way you work.

WHAT ARE THE SYMPTOMS?

The symptoms of RSI develop gradually and may only be present during the repeated activity at first. They may include:

- Pain, aching, tingling, and restricted movement in the affected area
- In some cases, tissue swelling in the affected area

WHY MIGHT I HAVE THIS?

PREDISPOSING FACTORS

- Occupations that involve repetitive movements
- Poor posture
- Stress
- Low thyroid function
- Vitamin B₆ deficiency

TREATMENT PLAN

PRIMARY TREATMENTS

- Ergonomic changes in work practices (*see Self-Help and Ergonomics*)
- Symptom relief with analgesics, nonsteroidal anti-inflammatory drugs (NSAIDs), and physical therapy

BACKUP TREATMENTS

- Vitamin B₆
- Bodywork and movement therapies
- Acupuncture
- Stress-management program

WORTH CONSIDERING

- Homeopathy
- Nutritional therapy

For an explanation of how treatments are rated, see p.111.

WHY DOES IT OCCUR?

In repetitive strain injury, muscles or tendons become damaged over time due to movements that repeatedly subject them to strain and do not allow them sufficient time to recover. Tendinitis, tenosynovitis, and carpal tunnel syndrome (*see p.152*) may cause symptoms similar to RSI.

People who perform repeated movements on a daily basis, such as those who use a keyboard or work on a production line, are particularly at risk of developing RSI, as are musicians and athletes.

Skeletal muscles contain two types of fiber — Type 1 and Type 2 (*see p.51*). When the muscles, such as those in the arm, are overused repetitively, the Type 1 fibers shorten, while the Type 2 fibers weaken. Over time, an imbalance occurs in which muscles may not be able to perform their functions normally and other muscles are inappropriately brought into action. The end result is a painful, cramp-like tension in the area and an inability to perform normal movements and actions.

Inflammation at the point where a tendon attaches to a bone, a condition known as tendonitis, may be part of RSI. Tennis elbow and golfer's elbow are the two common types of tendonitis affecting the arms. They affect the outer and inner sides of the elbow respectively.

IMPORTANT

Consult your doctor if you develop the symptoms of RSI. Once it becomes long-term, the condition is much more difficult to treat.

SELF-HELP

PRIMARY TREATMENT If you have the symptoms of RSI or wish to prevent the condition, take the following steps:
- If your condition is work-related, inform your employer and request an ergonomic assessment of your work space (*see p.287*).
- Seek occupational health advice on how to relieve the strain placed on your muscles and tendons.
- Take regular breaks from repetitive activity.

TREATMENTS IN DETAIL

Conventional Medicine

Your doctor will examine you and ask whether you perform repetitive activities. Tests, such as X-rays, may be arranged to exclude an underlying condition.

PRIMARY TREATMENT **SYMPTOM RELIEF** Your doctor may recommend analgesics, NSAIDs, or physical therapy to help relieve the pain and inflammation.

CAUTION

NSAIDs may cause a range of side effects; ask your doctor to explain them to you.

Nutritional Therapy

REDUCED THYROID FUNCTION If you have symptoms such as sensitivity to cold, cold hands and feet, dry skin, and lethargy, your RSI may be related to a reduction in the function of your thyroid gland (*see Thyroid Problems, p.319*).

VITAMIN B₆ DEFICIENCY may, according to some doctors, be a major factor in the development of RSI. This vitamin, which is necessary for normal functioning of nerve cells, reduces inflammatory reactions in soft tissues. Foods rich in vitamin B₆ include lean meat, fish, poultry, eggs, dairy products, nuts, soybeans, brown rice, whole-grain cereals, and potatoes.

Studies show that many people with RSI derive significant relief from taking B₆ supplements. The recommended dosage is 100mg of B₆ three times a day for three months, followed by a good B-complex supplement containing at least 25mg of B₆, taken daily.

VITAMIN B₂ can also be effective, even more so if you take it with vitamin B₆, according to research. Take 100mg of vitamin B₂ each day for three months, followed by a B-complex supplement containing at least 25mg of vitamin B₂ each day.

BROMELAIN is an extract from pineapple that has natural anti-inflammatory proper-ties and can be useful in the treatment of RSI, especially when taken in conjunction with vitamin B₆. The recommended dose is 500mg of bromelain, taken three times a day on an empty stomach.

> **CAUTION**
>
> Consult your doctor before taking vitamin B₆ with levodopa or phenobarbital (*see p.46*).

Homeopathy

BRYONIA ALBA is the classic medicine for inflammation of tendons and the sheaths that surround them. People who respond to *Bryonia* typically have a sharp pain from particular movements, so much that they may suddenly drop heavy objects. Pain, tenderness, and sometimes visible swelling occurs along the course of the tendon.

People who respond to *Bryonia* find their symptoms are relieved by elasticized wrist support. They may have an associated stiff neck with a headache, which is worse after sudden movements and being jarred, but which is relieved by support, such as a soft collar. Thirst and a dry mouth may be accompanying symptoms.

RUTA GRAVEOLENS is another homeopathic medicine that may help people who have RSI affecting the ligaments and tendons. They have a feeling of weakness, especially in the wrists. *Ruta graveolens* is one of the most frequently indicated medicines for enthesitis. Eyestrain from long periods in front of a VDU or computer screen may also respond to this medicine.

CONSTITUTIONAL MEDICINES tailored to the constitution of particular individuals may be required for more complex and longstanding cases of RSI. The most common medicine is *Calcarea carbonica*. Typically, those who respond to this medicine constantly strain their arms from slight overexertion. They easily get cramps in their hands and elsewhere. Often, their hands and feet are sweaty and they have lower back pain.

Psychologically, people who respond to *Calcarea carbonica* are often fed up and jaded from long periods of overwork and may become very anxious about their ability to cope with their workload. As workers, they are usually reliable and conscientious, if rather plodding. Bad dreams and sweating on the head at night are among their other associated symptoms.

Ergonomics

PRIMARY TREATMENT If you are experiencing RSI, it is most important that you review the ergonomics of the way you work. Examine your posture and activities, and look again at the implements you use regularly, such as desks, chairs, shoes, keyboards, or operating machinery, to assess the stress they place on your body. The most common causes of RSI are overuse or stressful use of computer keyboards or a computer mouse.

To prevent RSI you may need to redesign your work space. For example, your desk and chair should be at a height that is compatible with your particular measurements. You may also need to learn better ways of using instruments and tools — for example, typing with your hands and wrists at the correct angle.

REPETITIVE STRAIN INJURY IN THE FOREARM

The forearm is composed of various muscles, ligaments and tendons. It is particularly prone to RSI in people, such as those who use computer keyboards, who adopt a posture that puts stress on the wrist or who repeatedly use the same posture for prolonged periods without rest.

Muscles and tendons of the forearm

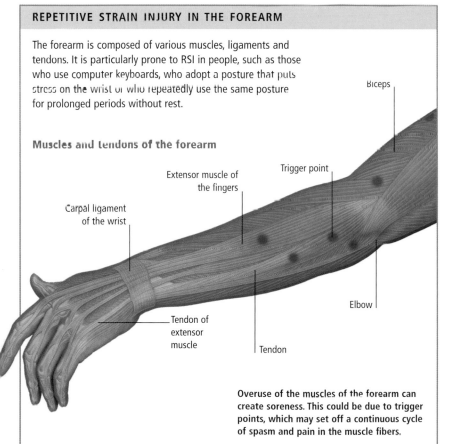

Biceps

Extensor muscle of the fingers

Trigger point

Carpal ligament of the wrist

Tendon of extensor muscle

Elbow

Tendon

Overuse of the muscles of the forearm can create soreness. This could be due to trigger points, which may set off a continuous cycle of spasm and pain in the muscle fibers.

USING A COMPUTER SAFELY

A screen or chair at the wrong height forces users to lean forward and hunch their shoulders. The muscles in the back, shoulders, and neck stay contracted for long periods, which constricts blood flow and in the long term may contribute to RSI.

To avoid this, choose a chair with an adjustable back and seat and use a computer stand if necessary to be sure the screen is at the correct height. Check that overhead lighting does not reflect on the screen and take a short break every hour.

A well-designed workstation

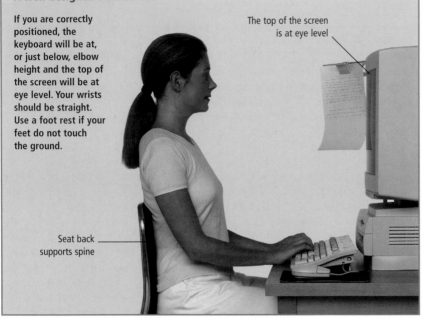

If you are correctly positioned, the keyboard will be at, or just below, elbow height and the top of the screen will be at eye level. Your wrists should be straight. Use a foot rest if your feet do not touch the ground.

The top of the screen is at eye level

Seat back supports spine

Bodywork and Movement Therapies

The most effective approach to reversing the changes to Type 1 and Type 2 muscle fibers (*see p.51*) is learning to perform whatever activities have caused the problem in a less stressful way. At the same time, you need to strengthen the muscles that have become weakened and simultaneously stretch and relax those muscles that have shortened.

THE ALEXANDER TECHNIQUE helps you learn to reuse your body in a better way. A qualified teacher will help you undo your bad postural habits and will show you how to stand, sit, and move with minimal effort. You may only need lessons for a few weeks, although the beneficial effects can last up to a year (*see p.62*).

YOGA THERAPY may help reverse many of the symptoms of RSI. A qualified yoga teacher will show you various exercises that stretch tight muscles and strengthen weak ones. For example, research revealed that the prayer position of the hands (*namaste; see p.153*), which gently extends and stretches the wrists and fingers, can significantly improve your grip strength and reduce pain.

DEACTIVATING TRIGGER POINTS Much RSI pain arises from active trigger points in overused muscles (*see p.55*). These can be treated by injection, acupuncture (using dry needling techniques known as intramuscular stimulation), self-stretching exercises, or by a combination of soft tissue manipulation methods known as neuromuscular techniques (*see p.61*).

FOOT AND ANKLE THERAPY Wearing inappropriate shoes can strain the ligaments and muscles of your ankles. The resulting foot pain, which is a form of RSI, is very common, especially in women. Overuse, repetitive strain, and minor, easily forgotten injuries can lead to chronic foot

and ankle pain. Correct diagnosis and efficient therapy should involve changing the type of footwear (and possibly adding orthotic supports), as well as appropriate physical therapy.

Acupuncture

Clinical experience suggests that acupuncture is of real value in treating RSI. Sometimes, the acupuncturist will use electroacupuncture and, occasionally, ear acupuncture. You usually need six to eight weekly sessions. RSI can be a very persistent and difficult problem, so it is worth continuing treatment for a reasonable period of time.

Mind-Body Therapies

STRESS MANAGEMENT Stress, both at home and in the workplace, can be a contributing factor to RSI. The pain you feel can affect you psychologically in a kind of vicious cycle: pain leads to stress, which leads to more muscle tension and therefore more pain.

Often, there is a period of denial, in which the pain is ignored or not taken seriously. Yet the pain can be restricting and sometimes frightening. The inability to work fully can leave you frustrated and even more stressed. A psychologist, psychiatrist, or clinical social worker may be able to give you guidance and help reduce your levels of stress.

You may find that a stress-management program (*see p.410*) may be helpful, as may be relaxing and practicing meditation regularly (*see p.98*).

PREVENTION PLAN

To prevent RSI from occurring, pay attention to the following:

- Improve the ergonomics of your work space by making simple changes such as adjusting the height of your desk and seating, and using wrist supports for keyboards

- Improve your posture while working

- Take regular breaks from repetitive activities, such as working at a computer keyboard

OSTEOARTHRITIS

Osteoarthritis (OA) is the gradual degeneration of the cartilage that lines the joints, bringing pain, swelling, and restricted movement. It is more common in the large weight-bearing joints, such as the hips and knees, but the joints of the hands, feet, shoulders, neck, and upper back may also be affected. Women are twice as likely to be affected by osteoarthritis as men. The condition sometimes runs in families. Treatments focus on relieving pain and inflammation as well as reducing toxins and maintaining mobility.

WHAT ARE THE SYMPTOMS?

Symptoms are often initially mild and gradually worsen. They include:

- Pain and tenderness in the affected joint
- Swelling around the joint
- Stiffness after periods of inactivity
- Restricted movement in the affected joint
- Crackling of the affected joint (crepitus) when it is moved

WHY MIGHT I HAVE THIS?

PREDISPOSING FACTORS

- Repeated stress on joints
- Repeated injuries to joints
- Excessive weight
- Hereditary factors
- Certain occupations

TRIGGERS

- Solanine-containing foods

TREATMENT PLAN

PRIMARY TREATMENTS

- Lifestyle measures (*see Self-Help*)
- Drugs, such as analgesics, NSAIDs, and corticosteroid injections
- Surgery in severe cases
- Arthritis Self-Management Program

BACKUP TREATMENTS

- Nutritional Therapy
- Glucosamine and chondroitin
- Homeopathy
- Western and Chinese herbal medicine
- Acupuncture
- Bodywork and movement therapies
- Mind–Body therapies

For an explanation of how treatments are rated, see p.111.

WHY DOES IT OCCUR?

In osteoarthritis (OA), the cartilage that covers the ends of the bones in the joints gradually wears away. The bone around the affected joint thickens and bony growths, or osteophytes, form. Osteophytes on the last joint of the fingers are known as Heberden's nodes, while osteophytes on the middle joint of the fingers are called Bouchard's nodes. If the synovial tissue lining a joint capsule becomes inflamed, fluid may accumulate, causing swelling.

Risk factors for OA include repeated stress on joints or repeated minor injuries to joints. Athletes often develop the condition later in life. Certain occupations can also be associated with an increased risk; for example, people with physically demanding jobs tend to develop OA of the hip. Excessive weight also increases the risk of developing OA.

Almost everyone develops OA to a certain degree by the age of 70, although it may not produce any obvious symptoms. However, OA may develop in younger people, usually as a result of joint injuries. Other joint diseases, such as gout (*see p.302*), may predispose a person to OA.

SELF-HELP

The following measures may help reduce the pain of OA:

- Try a heating pad, warm baths, or massage to ease the pain.
- Lose any excess weight.
- Exercise within your limits — don't overdo it.
- Wear shoes with rubber heels for support and use a walking stick to reduce impact on joints.

TREATMENTS IN DETAIL

Conventional Medicine

Your doctor will probably be able to diagnose OA from your symptoms. There are no specific tests for detecting OA, although X-rays may reveal the changes in the body that suggest it.

PRIMARY TREATMENT **LIFESTYLE MEASURES** Your doctor will encourage exercises such as swimming in order to strengthen the muscles around the joints. Try to bring your weight under control if you are overweight.

To help you with everyday activities, ask a physical therapist about specially adapted cutlery and other equipment if OA restricts movement in your hands.

PRIMARY TREATMENT **DRUGS** Analgesics, such as acetaminophen, and NSAIDs may be given for short term pain relief. Occasionally, corticosteroids may be injected into the affected joints to provide a longer period of pain relief.

PRIMARY TREATMENT **SURGERY** For severe OA, joint repair or replacement may be offered. For example, hip replacements are likely to be effective for at least ten years. For very severe pain, some joints such as the wrist can be fused so that they are rigid. This surgical procedure relieves the pain but subsequently you will not be able to move the joint.

CAUTION

NSAIDs can cause side effects; ask your doctor to explain these to you.

Nutritional Therapy

DIETARY CHANGES Avoid foods that contribute to the buildup of acid and other residues. These include acidic fruits and vegetables, such as citrus fruits (except lemons, which have an alkali effect after digestion), strawberries, rhubarb, tomatoes, red meats, and cheese. Wine may make symptoms worse. A diet rich in essential fatty acids, possibly supplemented with fish oils and evening primrose oil, is often beneficial.

ELIMINATING SOLANINE Those with OA may find their symptoms relieved if they avoid foods belonging to the nightshade (Solanaceae) family, such as tomatoes, peppers (capsicum), potatoes, and eggplant. They contain solanine, which may be involved in the processes that cause OA. Eliminating solanine from the diet may bring relief to about 50 percent of people with OA. In practice, it often takes about six months before real benefit is seen.

GLUCOSAMINE AND CHONDROITIN Glucosamine is an essential constituent of cartilage. Reviews of double-blind clinical studies show combination therapy with glucosamine and chondroitin to be effective in reducing the inflammation and pain associated with severe OA, particularly affecting the knee. Two long-term studies show that combination therapy reduces joint space narrowing and thus not only treats the pain of OA but also slows down the disease progression.

The normal recommended dose of glucosamine sulfate or glucosamine hydrochloride is 750mg, 2 times daily. Once your symptoms have improved, you could reduce this dose to once a day. However, glucosamine should be avoided by anyone who has an intolerance or allergy to shellfish or who has diabetes.

Chondroitin sulfate is often taken in conjunction with glucosamine sulfate. It seems to work by attracting fluid into the cartilage of the joint, thereby improving the spongy, shock-absorbing qualities of the cartilage and helping bring essential nutrients to the area.

Many trials have shown that taking chondroitin sulfate supplements can reduce pain, increase joint mobility, and/or bring about healing within the joints of people with OA. The normal recommended dose of chondroitin sulfate is 600mg a day.

NIACINAMIDE (a form of vitamin B_3) is a supplement that may also help people with OA. One 1996 study that compared the effects of taking niacinamide to taking a placebo found that niacinamide improved joint flexibility and reduced inflammation, thus making a reduction in standard anti-inflammatory medications possible. A typical dose of niacinamide is 250mg, taken 4–6 times a day, though larger doses may be needed for individuals with advanced OA. Results can take 12 weeks or more to become apparent.

> **CAUTION**
>
> Consult your doctor before taking vitamin B_3 or niacinamide with HMG-CoA reductase inhibitors or oral diabetic drugs (*see p.46*).

Homeopathy

A systematic review of clinical trials published in 2001 concluded that homeopathy seems to help people with OA, but more research is needed. The trials looked mostly at homeopathic complex medicines, including Zeel®, which contains *Arnica, Dulcamara, Rhus toxicodendron,* and *San-guinaria*; SRL gel, containing *Symphytum, Rhus toxicodendron,* and *Ledum*; and another complex containing *Rhus toxicodendron, Causticum,* and *Lac vaccinum.* In every case, symptoms improved.

Homeopaths most frequently prescribe *Rhus toxicodendron, Calcarea carbonica, Calcarea fluorica, Ledum, Natrum sulphuricum,* and *Causticum,* depending on a person's constitution (*see p.73*). However, for such a common and variable disease, this list is by no means comprehensive.

RHUS TOXICODENDRON One important symptom of people who respond to *Rhus tox.* is the rapid stiffening up of joints. They may say they cannot sit for even short periods of time without becoming stiff and achey; they get up from their seat, limber up, and feel better for a while, only for the feeling to return and the process to be repeated. By the same token, they wake up several times in the night, feeling stiff and restless, and need to limber up before they can get back to sleep.

LEDUM is often appropriate for OA that starts in the feet. Unusually for chronic arthritis, the pain may be relieved by putting the affected joint in or against something cold, such as a cold bath or an ice pack.

CALCAREA FLUORICA is often appropriate when there are many osteophytes, including Heberden's and Bouchard's nodes on the fingers. Those who respond to the remedy often have lax connective tissues and when they were younger they may have had signs of this, such as being double-jointed, having swayback knees, or a tendency to develop hernias.

CALCAREA CARBONICA is given largely on constitutional grounds (*see p.73*). Those who respond to *Calcaraea carbonica* tend to be overweight. Solid both physically and mentally, they are calm, hardworking, and stubborn people. But beneath this solid exterior they may have many fears and anxieties, particularly about their health. They often sweat freely on the head and neck, especially in bed at night, without necessarily feeling hot. They may also suffer from arthritic pain in many regions, but particularly in the lower back.

CAUSTICUM is one of the most commonly indicated medicines for OA of the hips, but it may also be used for other areas. Individuals who respond to it are very sensitive to dampness: they are worse in damp weather, and "feel it in their bones" when it is going to rain.

> Over 50 percent of Americans over the age of 65 have some degree of osteoarthritis.

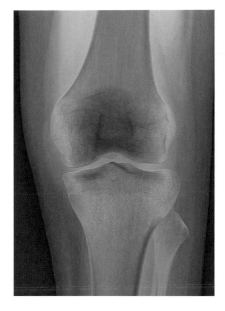
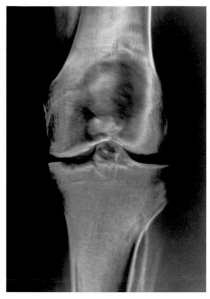

In a normal knee joint *(left)*, the cartilage lining the ends of the femur and tibia prevent bone damage. In an osteoarthritic joint *(right)*, the cartilage is damaged as the degenerative disease takes it course.

Western Herbal Medicine

Traditionally, some Western herbalists see joints as potential bottlenecks in the circulatory flow, where toxins from poor nutrition and waste metabolites can accumulate. Over time, these cause joint stiffness, swelling, and pain.

ANTI-INFLAMMATORIES Certain other antirheumatic remedies, such as meadowsweet (*Filipendula ulmaria*), birch (*Betula alba*) leaves, poplar (*Populus tremuloides*) bark, and willow (*Salix alba*) bark are rich in anti-inflammatory salicylates (the basis of aspirin) that can reduce joint swelling and pain.

Other well-known and researched anti-inflammatory remedies are devil's claw (*Harpogophytum procumbens*), which shows similar effects to NSAIDs in back and knee pain, and two oleo-gum resins used in Ayurvedic medicine — Indian olibanum tree (*Boswellia serrata*) and guggal (*Commiphora mukul*). Make sure you buy a purified extract from a reputable supplier.

TURMERIC (*Curcuma longa*) has been shown to have significant antioxidant and anti-inflammatory activity, as well as some COX-2 inhibition, and is used throughout Asia to treat arthritis. The active ingredient in turmeric is curcumin, which is sometimes isolated; preparations of turmeric should contain not less than 3% curcumin. In Chinese medicine, turmeric is also used to improve blood circulation. This is a useful strategy and if the pulse is faint, practitioners will use other circulatory stimulants, such as prickly ash (*Xanthoylum americanum*) bark and ginger (*Zingiber officinale*), both of which have an anti-inflammatory effect. A clinical trial found that a mixture of two types of ginger (*Zingiber officinale* and *Alpinia galanga*) was superior to placebo. The usual dose of dried ginger is 500 mg four times a day. Boswellia (*Boswellia carterii*) is another plant that has demonstrated anti-inflammatory effects. It is sometimes found in combination products with turmeric and/or ginger.

EXTERNAL TREATMENTS Comfrey (*Symphytum officinale*) root poultices and ointment can be applied to swollen painful joints and Heberden's nodes, as can kelp (seaweed) plasters. Comfrey should not be taken internally due to liver toxicity from its pyrrolizidine alkaloids.

Herbs can be effective at reducing swelling and inflammation and improving joint mobility. Applying capsicum (*Capsicum annuum*) as a cream or roll-on to painful swollen joints (especially when the pain is aggravated by cold, damp weather conditions) invigorates local circulation, thereby imitating the body's natural inflammatory processes that herbalists see as an innate restorative response to disease. In the same way, foot and hand baths made by boiling stinging nettles with celery may also be effective.

Liniments (oily creams that are used for soothing muscle pain) and embrocations (lotions for soothing a sore or pulled muscle) containing menthol, camphor, and plant oils, such as wintergreen (*Gaultheria procumbens*), lavender (*Lavandula angustifolia*), St. John's wort (*Hypericum perforatum*), cinnamon (*Cinnamomum cassia*), pine (*Pinus* spp.), juniper, chamomile (*Matricaria recutita*), and rosemary (*Rosmarinus officinalis*), as well as extracts of calamus (*Acorus calamus*) root and arnica (*Arnica montana*) or daisy (*Bellis perennis*), can be massaged into affected joints and muscles. These invigorate local circulation, but should be avoided if the joints are seriously inflamed.

> **CAUTION**
>
> Considerable care and constant monitoring are needed if herbal and conventional medications are combined. Severe arthritic conditions need expert herbal care and are often unsuitable for self-medication. *(See also p.69.)*

Chinese Herbal Medicine

Traditional Chinese Medicine (TCM) does not specifically differentiate between OA, rheumatoid arthritis (RA; *see p.293*), or gout (*see p.302*), but sees them as varieties of *Bi* (painful blockage) syndrome.

CLIMATIC FACTORS In *Bi* syndrome, two external "factors" (wind–cold–damp and wind–damp–heat) can invade the body, thereby causing the flow of *Qi*, blood and body fluids, to slow down and become blocked. Full movement of the body is lost, as a result, and the joints become inflamed and painful.

AGING *Bi* syndrome is much more common as people age because their fundamental life force — called *Zheng* (upright) *Qi* — weakens, as do the liver and kidneys, which sustain the tendons and bones respectively.

TREATMENT OF BI SYNDROME depends on skillful diagnosis of these variable factors, based on symptoms as well as pulse and tongue diagnosis (*see p.83*).

Acupuncture

Many clinical trials have established that acupuncture can diminish the need for analgesic drugs and, therefore, should be added to conventional treatments of OA. One particularly large clinical trial of 570 patients, comparing acupuncture treatment with placebo (sham acupuncture) over a period of 26 weeks, demonstrated that acupuncture reduces the pain and functional impairment of OA of the knee. Clinical trials have also established that it helps people with OA of the hip, but to a lesser extent. Whether the benefit comes from treating particular acupuncture points, the process of receiving acupuncture, or the specific effect of needling around a joint is unclear.

A series of treatments is probably much better than giving one or two. You will need to persist for at least six, or possibly eight, sessions given on a weekly basis. If

the condition is very acute, treatment may be given every day, or every other day.

When symptoms subside, more long-term constitutional acupuncture may be needed to avoid their recurrence, perhaps received on a monthly basis. This involves identifying the underlying pathogens that trigger *Bi* syndrome (*see Chinese Herbal Medicine, p.291*).

Bodywork and Movement Therapies

It is important to realize that X-ray evidence of osteoarthritic changes in a joint does not necessarily mean that pain is the result of these changes. In fact, many arthritic joints can be virtually pain-free. It is essential to ensure that pain in the affected joint is attributable to osteoarthritis, and not another cause. The joint pain

may arise from neuropathies and/or trigger point activity (*see p.55*).

NONDRUG THERAPIES The objective of manipulation therapy is to treat the symptoms of restriction and the pain. The best results come when nondrug therapies take the lead and analgesics and anti-inflammatory drugs play a secondary role. Nondrug approaches might include postural reeducation (for example, learning proper standing and sitting postures), joint protection (avoiding unnecessary stress), hot and cold treatments (for example, hydrotherapy), and transcutaneous electrical nerve stimulation (TENS) to reduce pain.

The management of OA might also include heat or cold therapy, and often-neglected measures, such as reducing chair height and using an orthotic (shock-absorbing foot support).

REHABILITATION EXERCISES taught by physical therapists focus not only on the local joint problem, such as the knee, but also on the consequences of this problem, such as inactivity and awkward movements. Pain-relieving aids include patellar

> ### Osteoarthritis most commonly affects the knees, finger joints, and the base of the thumb

taping to support the kneecap, shoulder taping, wedged insoles for foot support, and shock-absorbing insoles.

Regular rehabilitation exercises involving strength training can improve functional ability and reduce knee joint pain in people with OA. Indeed, general well-designed exercise programs have been shown to increase the ability of people with OA of the knee to perform everyday tasks.

Therapeutic exercises are of benefit to many patients. Such exercises may include warmup exercises with range-of-motion, muscle strengthening, and various aerobic activities, such as swimming. Exercising by yourself may be as effective as hospital-based physical therapy or supervised hydrotherapy treatment.

MASSAGE Comprehensive treatment of OA joint dysfunction may at times include

appropriate massage therapy and joint mobilization (osteopathic or chiropractic). However, more research is needed to prove the efficacy and safety of these methods for people with OA.

Mind–Body Therapies

PRIMARY TREATMENT **ARTHRITIS SELF-MANAGEMENT PROGRAM (ASMP)** was developed at the Stanford University School of Medicine and is now presented at over 200 facilities worldwide. It has been highly successful and cost-effective in treating arthritis. The Arthritis Foundation now markets this course as the Arthritis Self-Care Program along with education about arthritis, exercise, nutrition, and medication use.

ASMP features relaxation, guided imagery, other cognitive pain management techniques, communication skills, tips on handling the doctor–patient relationship, and group support. Imagery and relaxation exercises play an important part in five of the six ASMP sessions.

Benefits include better health, improved role function and comfort levels, and decreased health resource utilization. Better self-efficacy is considered a likely major contributor to the positive outcomes, which cannot be adequately explained by improved health behaviors.

GUIDED IMAGERY, RELAXATION, AND SELF-HYPNOSIS have proved effective in a number of chronic pain conditions and clinical experience indicates that they are effective for arthritic pain.

As an adjunct therapy, a mind–body practice including relaxation and/or guided imagery can significantly increase self-management skills and the quality of an individual's well-being. It can also decrease excessive dependence on pain-relieving medications.

> ### PREVENTION PLAN
>
> To prevent OA, try the following:
> - Exercise regularly
> - Avoid plants from Solanaceae family (*see Nutritional Therapy, p.290*)

RHEUMATOID ARTHRITIS

Rheumatoid arthritis (RA) is an autoimmune disease in which joints become stiff and painful due to inflammation of the synovial membrane. Rheumatoid arthritis most commonly begins between the ages of 30 and 50 and is three times more common in women than men. The condition sometimes runs in families. Treatment involves relieving inflammation and pain, and maximizing joint function and mobility by eliminating food sensitivities, taking pharmaceutical, homeopathic, or herbal medicines, and keeping environmental hazards to a minimum.

WHAT ARE THE SYMPTOMS?

RA usually develops slowly over weeks or months, although its onset can be abrupt over a few days. The main symptoms are:

- Stiffness and pain in the joints that may be worse in the morning and relieved by movement

Other symptoms may develop, including:

- Swelling of the affected joints
- Small, painless bumps (nodules) on areas of pressure, such as the elbows
- Wasting (thinning) of the muscles around the joints
- Restriction of movement
- Fatigue and depression are common

WHY MIGHT I HAVE THIS?

PREDISPOSING FACTORS

- Family history of the disease
- Smoking

TRIGGERS

- Food sensitivity
- Infection
- Environmental pollutants
- Hormonal changes

WHY DOES IT OCCUR?

Rheumatoid arthritis (RA) is a disease that affects many systems of the body. It most commonly damages joints, causing pain, stiffness, and deformity. RA is an autoimmune disease, which means that for an unknown reason, the body produces antibodies that attack its own tissues — in this case, the synovial membrane of a joint is inflamed. Eventually, the ends of the bones and the cartilage that covers the joint are damaged. Periods of severe pain may be followed by brief relief. In most cases, RA affects several joints and appears in corresponding areas on each side of the body.

AFFECTED AREAS OF THE BODY RA usually appears first in the small joints of the hands and feet, but it may develop in almost any joint. Sometimes, only one joint, in particular the shoulder or knee, is initially affected. Eventually, joint damage may lead to deformities such as "ulnar deviation," in which the fingers deviate (slant) away from the thumb.

Other areas of the body that may be affected include the eyes, kidneys, lungs, heart, and blood vessels. Raynaud's disease (*see p.264*) and carpal tunnel syndrome (*see p.152*) may develop.

COURSE OF THE DISEASE There is no single pattern. For example, it may halt after several years, leaving only slight damage, or progress rapidly over a few years. However, in most cases, RA is a chronic, persistent disease that usually occurs in episodes, lasting for several weeks or months.

A FAMILY HISTORY of RA is a predisposing factor for the disease; genes may be important factors in determining who develops RA and why. However, many people who never develop the disease share the genes thought to be associated with RA, indicating that there are other important factors.

TREATMENT PLAN

PRIMARY TREATMENTS

- Drugs including NSAIDs, analgesics, disease-modifying antirheumatic drugs, and corticosteroids
- Physical therapy and occupational therapy

BACKUP TREATMENTS

- Surgery, including joint replacement
- Food elimination diet
- Homeopathy
- Western and Chinese herbal medicine

WORTH CONSIDERING

- Essential fatty acids
- Environmental health measures
- Acupuncture
- Mind–body therapies

For an explanation of how treatments are rated, see p.111.

SELF-HELP

To reduce discomfort of RA:
- Take acetaminophen or other analgesics.
- Try ointments that contain capsaicin, menthol, eucalyptus, or salicylates (which have an aspirin-like effect).

Conventional Medicine

Your doctor will make a diagnosis mainly from a description of the symptoms and an examination. You will need to undergo tests, such as blood tests for signs of inflammation and X-rays to establish the extent of any damage.

Treatment is designed to control the symptoms and halt or slow the progress of the disease. Your doctor will recommend rest during flare-ups.

PRIMARY TREATMENT **DRUGS** Your doctor may prescribe NSAIDs to relieve pain and stiffness. Analgesics may also provide some relief.

Disease-modifying antirheumatic drugs may be prescribed with the aim of reducing inflammation and helping control symptoms. They may also slow the rate of joint damage. They include:

- *Sulfasalazine* About half of those with RA who are treated with sulfasalazine respond within six months.
- *Methotrexate* This drug can reduce inflammation and slows the damage to joints. It usually improves the symptoms within a few months.
- *Antimalarials* Inflammation can be reduced significantly when antimalarials are taken for up to 12 months.
- *Minocycline* This antibiotic may help control the symptoms of RA.

Oral corticosteroids may be prescribed since they can reduce joint inflammation and help control the symptoms when given in low doses for a few weeks. They may also be given on an occasional basis as an injection into a muscle for particularly severe flare-ups. They may provide relief when injected directly into affected joints, but this will be short-term.

Some new immunosuppressants (drugs that suppress the immune response), such as etanercept and infliximab, may be given by injection. They have been found to improve symptoms and slow or even halt the damage in some cases. These drugs are only used after other disease-modifying, antirheumatic drugs have been tried.

PRIMARY TREATMENT **PHYSICAL THERAPY** is important for maximizing joint movement and maintaining muscle strength. Occupational therapists will help increase upper body strength and advise on methods of dealing with daily activities if mobility or dexterity are limited.

SURGERY can prevent worsening joint damage and relieve pain. It may involve removing the inflamed tissue from a particular joint or fusing the bones together so that there is no movement in the affected joint. Alternatively, the joint may be replaced when damage is severe.

> **CAUTION**
>
> Some of the drugs used for treating RA have a range of serious side effects; ask your doctor to explain these to you.
>
> Some of the drugs should be avoided during pregnancy. Conception should be avoided when either partner is taking methotrexate and for a time afterward.

HOW RHEUMATOID ARTHRITIS AFFECTS JOINTS

When a joint is affected by rheumatoid arthritis, the synovial membranes and the cartilage that lines the bones come under attack. As fluid accumulates, the joint swells and becomes inflamed, causing pain and restricting movement. Antibodies and molecules, such as enzymes and cytokines, damage and deform the membranes and cartilage. Eventually, the bones, ligaments, and tendons are also affected.

A knee damaged by rheumatoid arthritis

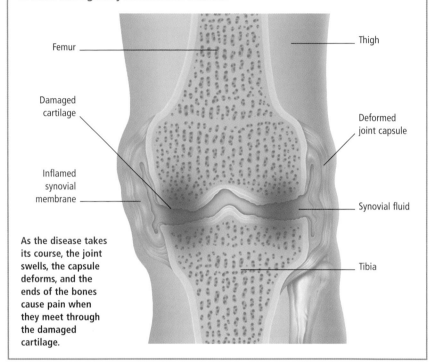

Femur

Damaged cartilage

Inflamed synovial membrane

As the disease takes its course, the joint swells, the capsule deforms, and the ends of the bones cause pain when they meet through the damaged cartilage.

Thigh

Deformed joint capsule

Synovial fluid

Tibia

Nutritional Therapy

FOOD SENSITIVITY Studies show that RA can be related to a food sensitivity, and that avoiding problem foods can improve symptoms. A vegetarian diet and a gluten-free vegan diet have been shown to improve symptoms in patients with RA, and a fasting diet has also proved to be effective. (*For more information about food sensitivities, see p.39.*)

ESSENTIAL FATTY ACIDS People with RA may benefit from eating foods that are rich in essential fatty acids (EFAs). These foods include oily fish (mackerel, trout, sardines, and salmon), extra-virgin olive oil, and walnuts as well as pumpkin, sunflower, and sesame seeds.

There is some evidence that gamma-linolenic acid, an omega-6 fatty acid (in the form of borage oil, blackcurrant seed oil, and evening primrose oil) and omega-

3 fatty acids (in the form of fish oil) can be effective in controlling the symptoms.

The effective daily doses appear to be about 1.5g of gamma-linolenic acid (GLA) and 10g of fish-oil supplements (providing 3g per day of the fatty acids EPA and DHA). Both GLA and the fatty acids EPA and DHA are beneficial because the body uses them to make compounds that have an anti-inflammatory action.

A 2003 study suggests that fish oil is most beneficial as an anti-inflammatory agent in RA if it is taken while eating a diet low in arachidonic acid (an inflammatory omega-6 fatty acid found in eggs and meat, especially beef, liver, and kidney).

Homeopathy

RA is a serious and potentially crippling disease that requires treatment from a qualified and experienced homeopath. Clinical trials suggest that the complex homeopathic medicine *Rheumaselect*, which contains *Bryonia, Rhus toxicodendron, Ledum, Berberis,* and *Nux vomica,* is effective in RA. Meta-analysis of the clinical trials also suggests that homeopathy tailored to the individual is effective.

Among the medicines that are most likely to relieve symptoms when used independently are *Apis mellifica* and *Rhus toxicodendron.* Constitutional medicines, which are prescribed almost entirely on whole-person characteristics rather than on the features of the illness, may act more deeply (*see p.73*). Among the most commonly indicated are *Lycopodium, Pulsatilla, Sepia,* and *Causticum.*

APIS MELLIFICA is useful for hot, swollen, and very tender joints, and also where the pain is relieved by cold, such as an ice pack, but made worse by pressure.

RHUS TOXICODENDRON helps people who are very stiff in the morning, and who become stiff and achey from even short periods of sitting or lying still; hence, they have restless nights. They are worse in cold, wet weather and feel better if given heat treatment, such as from a heating pad or warm bath.

LYCOPODIUM may be an appropriate treatment when the feet are badly affected by the condition. People who respond to

Lycopodium can sometimes be recognized by the way they respond to questions — they will pause, then give a carefully considered reply.

Generally rather reserved, *Lycopodium* types may be socially inept, no good at small talk, and at their best with small groups of old friends. A useful correlative symptom is that they frequently suffer from stomach trouble, particularly gas, and have a sweet tooth.

PULSATILLA A characteristic feature of people who respond to *Pulsatilla* is that the arthritis moves unpredictably from joint to joint. In women, it is often worse in the premenstrual period and may have started a few weeks or months after having a baby.

People who respond to *Pulsatilla* are typically gentle, soft spoken, indecisive, and weepy — for instance, when talking about their illness.

SEPIA People who respond to *Sepia* may experience lower back pain — although RA does not usually affect the back, except for the upper neck — that particularly involves the sacroiliac joints where the spine meets the pelvis. In women, the onset of RA may have developed around the time of menopause (*see p.339*).

Typically, patients are depressed and emotionally flat, although they may appear

lively and vivacious. But this is sometimes a "mask," and they do not like probing questions about how they feel. A common feature, unusual in this context, is that the symptoms are improved by exertion, such as dancing or strenous exercise.

CAUSTICUM People who respond to *Causticum* are often very sensitive to the weather — they are said to "feel it in their bones" well before it rains. Many homeopathic medicines for arthritis and rheumatism are associated with feeling worse in cold or wet weather.

People who respond to *Causticum* may experience the arthritis at unusual sites,

such as the jaw joint, and tend to develop contractures (temporary shortening of ligaments) so that they cannot fully straighten their joints.

A characteristic feature of people who respond to *Causticum* is that they are very sympathetic to the sufferings of others — for example, they may find it too difficult to watch starving children on TV, or to read about the aftermath of a hurricane in the newspaper. They also often have "leakage" of urine when the bladder is full or during a sneeze or cough, as well as recurrent hoarseness.

Western Herbal Medicine

There are many theories to explain why the immune system should be disrupted and cause RA. Some scientists see the trigger as a reaction to a long-term unresolved infection with a slow-acting virus, bacterium, or fungus.

The traditional herbal view is that chronic toxic overload can trigger an attack of RA. As with OA, successful treatment is only possible by analyzing and treating each case individually. There is no standard herbal treatment for arthritis of any type.

ANTI-INFLAMMATORY HERBS During an acute attack of RA, the inflammation can be successfully doused with anti-

> Renoir created about 6,000 paintings despite suffering from severe rheumatoid arthritis

inflammatory herbs. The herbs that can be used for this purpose include willow (*Salix alba*) bark, meadowsweet (*Filipendula ulmaria*), poplar (*Populus tremuloides*) bark, and birch (*Betula alba*) leaves, as well as devil's claw (*Harpogophytum procumbens*), borage (*Borago officinale*), frankincense (*Boswellia* spp.), boswellia (*Boswellia carterii*), guggal (*Commiphora mukul*), sarsaparilla (*Smilax ornata*), ginger (*Zinziber officinale*) and turmeric (*Curcuma longa*) (*see also Osteoarthritis, p.289*).

Other anti-inflammatory remedies that may be effective include barberry (*Berberis vulgaris*) bark, centaury (*Centaurium erythrea*), bogbean (*Menyathes trifoliata*), and feverfew (*Tanacetum parthenium*). Black cohosh (*Cimicifuga racemosa*) has a substantial folk reputation for treating inflammatory arthritis. This herb may be especially appropriate for treating women with RA, especially menopausal women because it appears to have a weak estrogenic action that reduces hot flashes and other menopausal symptoms.

Phytodolor is a German proprietary mixture of European aspen (*Populus tremula*), European ash (*Fraxinus excelsior*), and goldenrod (*Solidago virgaurea*) that appears to be effective against RA.

Licorice (*Glycyrrhiza glabra*) contains

> ## Over two million Americans are sufferers of rheumatoid arthritis.

steroidal saponins that can also rebalance female hormone levels and are anti-inflammatory. Licorice is known to have a mild cortisone-like effect and is especially effective in treating hot and inflamed joints when combined with the unprocessed root of a Chinese herb called rehmannia (*Rehmannia glutinosa*).

IMMUNE-STRENGTHENING HERBS Since RA is a disorder that results from an overactive immune system, you should be careful to avoid any herbs that act by stimulating the immune system. Consequently, herbs such as astragalus (*Astragalus membranaceus*), ginseng (*Panax ginseng*), and Siberian ginseng (*Eleutheroccus senticosus*) should not be used as treatment for RA.

> **CAUTION**
>
> Herbal medication given to people with RA should be closely monitored and regular liver function tests are advisable. Combining herbal medication with conventional drug therapy should be done with considerable care and constant monitoring. Severe arthritic conditions require expert herbal care and are unsuitable for self-medication.

Chinese Herbal Medicine

Traditional Chinese Medicine (TCM) does not specifically distinguish between RA, osteoarthritis, and gout. (*For further information about Chinese herbal treatments of arthritis, see p.291.*)

Environmental Health

There is ample evidence that environmental factors play an important role in the development of RA as well as in other autoimmune disorders. Although studies of identical twins indicate that genetics play some part in the disease development, the larger contribution appears to come from the environment. In fact, one study of over 37,000 twins in Denmark led to the conclusion that family history is of minor importance in the development of rheumatoid arthritis.

AVOID SMOKING Many studies suggest that a link exists between smoking and rheumatoid arthritis. Smokers are twice as likely to develop RA as nonsmokers and this increased risk can persist for up to 20 years after smoking has stopped. There are no controlled studies dealing with second-hand smoke, but if you have RA you should avoid smoky atmospheres.

ORAL CONTRACEPTIVE USE appears to provide some level of protection — women who take oral contraceptives or hormone therapy are less likely to develop RA. Even former users of contraceptives seem to retain a somewhat lower, but still measurable protection, although this effect disappears after several decades. Thus, it appears that the oral contraceptives may simply postpone the development of RA. There has never been a clear explanation for this protective effect, nor are oral contraceptives recommended for this purpose in view of their possible detrimental effects as women age (including cancer, blood clots, and stroke).

AVOID CHEMICAL SUBSTANCES Exposure to several chemical substances may increase the risk of developing RA. In a Swedish study, people who were exposed to organic solvents (including spray painters, lacquer workers, and hairdressers) had a higher risk of developing RA. Farmers were also at higher risk, presumably due to organic dust or pesticide exposures, another potential trigger. Another study revealed that occupational exposure to hydraulic oils doubles the risk of developing RA. Silica dust, frequently encountered among pottery and construction workers, has also been linked to RA.

If exposure to these solvents and chemicals is a cause of your condition, then you should make all possible efforts to minimize exposure, even if the disease process has already begun. Avoid freshly applied paints, thinners, varnishes, and hydraulic oils. If you cannot avoid exposure, be sure to wear respirator masks that are approved for use with organic vapors. Even exposure to common household solvents and chemicals, such as pesticides and fertilizers, should be limited.

INFECTIOUS AGENTS that have been implicated in the development of autoimmune diseases such as RA include the Epstein-Barr virus (the cause of mononucleosis), parvoviruses, and mycoplasma (the cause of "walking pneumonia"). However, results are not consistent between studies. Some environmental health experts, believe it is best to avoid people during the infectious phase of these illnesses. There appears to be no link between vaccinations and the development of RA.

Acupuncture

Acupuncture is often used to treat RA, by following either an anti-inflammatory or a pain-relieving approach. Acupuncture appears to work as well as local steroid injections and many anti-inflammatory medications. Moreover, adverse reactions to acupuncture are less likely than to injections and other medications.

ANTI-INFLAMMATORY EFFECTS This approach uses a Traditional Chinese Medicine (TCM) diagnosis and uses the anti-inflammatory effects of acupuncture and to treat the underlying disease. It has not been adequately evaluated and its benefits are difficult to judge, particularly when

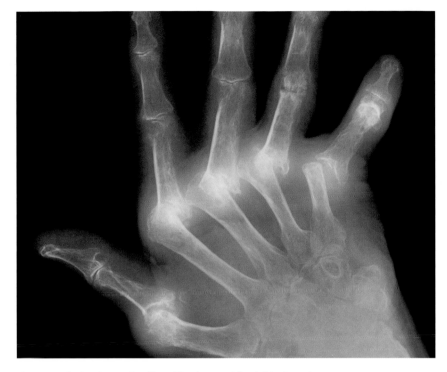

This X-ray of a hand severely affected by rheumatoid arthritis shows how the bones have become affected by the inflammation process. The fingers slant away from the thumb — a deformity known as ulnar deviation.

RA involves relapses and remissions. In general, 10 to 12 weekly sessions of acupuncture will be needed while the disease is relatively stable before it is clear if treatment helps

PAIN RELIEF Acupuncture may be used to relieve pain, an approach supported by a number of clinical trials, which have shown that acupuncture can bring relief to inflamed joints or to joints that are damaged, mechanically disturbed, or suffering from secondary osteoarthritis. This approach is used in the treatment of either acute or chronic muscle and joint pain. Usually, six to eight sessions of acupuncture will be enough to benefit painful knees, hips, or strained muscles. If you do not see an improvement within six to eight sessions, it is unlikely that acupuncture will be of value in treating your pain.

Bodywork and Movement Therapies

BALNEOTHERAPY (hydrotherapy or spa therapy) is one of the oldest forms of therapy for individuals with arthritis. The primary purpose of balneotherapy is to soothe the pain and, as a consequence, to relieve suffering and improve well being.

A 2003 review of the research into balneotherapy concluded that, although there were positive findings, "an answer about the efficacy of balneotherapy cannot be provided at this time." However, it is still worth trying.

AEROBIC EXERCISE is effective in increasing aerobic capacity and muscle strength, without making the disease or the pain worse. It is clear that, as long as you are exercising at a rate you can comfortably

tolerate, active exercise can help maintain body function and well-being.

LOW-LEVEL LASER THERAPY (LLLT) has been used to treat the symptoms of RA for some years. A light source generates "pure" light of a single wavelength. It produces a photochemical reaction in the cells of the affected tissue. LLLT can be considered for short-term relief of pain and morning stiffness, particularly since it has few, if any, side effects. LLLT is available at rheumatology departments, pain clinics, and from physical therapists.

ULTRASOUND is often used as a secondary therapy — in other words, together with another treatment, such as medication. It has anti-inflammatory and pain-relieving properties. Ultrasound alone can be helpful in increasing grip strength. To a lesser extent it can relieve morning stiffness and reduce the number of both swollen and painful joints.

Mind–Body Therapies

Regular practice of mind–body therapies, such as yoga and relaxation, can have a beneficial effect on your pain levels. (*For information about general mind–body treatments of arthritis, see p.292.*)

THE PSYCHOSOCIAL ENVIRONMENT Many studies have linked the development of RA to major life stresses. One study of people with RA found they had marital problems about five years before the onset of RA symptoms and formal diagnosis. By comparison, control populations did not show significant increases in marital discord. If you have RA, you would be wise to reduce conflict and stress in your life, or at least to find a way to avoid the buildup of such emotions.

> Women with RA who become pregnant find that their symptoms are temporarily relieved

PREVENTION PLAN

The following may help prevent the development of RA:

- Avoid problem foods
- Don't smoke
- Avoid exposure to environmental hazards as much as possible

FIBROMYALGIA

Fibromyalgia, also known in the past as fibrositis, is a form of chronic rheumatism (a condition affecting the muscles, ligaments, and other soft tissues). It is characterized by widespread pain, fatigue, and sleep disturbance, and is surprisingly common and debilitating. People with fibromyalgia have tender areas of the connective tissues, particularly in the neck, spine, shoulders, and hips. Fibromyalgia is much more common in women than in men. Treatment focuses on relieving pain, helping with sleep and depression, and reducing stress.

WHAT ARE THE SYMPTOMS?

The symptoms of fibromyalgia usually develop slowly over weeks and may include:

- Persistent connective tissue pain affecting almost any part of the body
- Fatigue, sleep disturbance, and/or unrefreshing sleep
- Fibromyalgia is associated with other conditions, particularly migraine, and irritable bowel syndrome — many people who have fibromyalgia also have these
- Fibromyalgia is also often associated with depression and anxiety
- Tenderness to pressure at 11 or more of 18 tender points (*see illustration, p.299*).

Symptoms may become worse if stress levels increase.

WHY MIGHT I HAVE THIS?

PREDISPOSING FACTORS

- Physical, sexual, or psychological abuse
- Stress
- Sleep deprivation
- Another disorder, such as rheumatoid arthritis, lupus, or hypothyroidism
- Being sensitive to paint solvents and other chemicals
- Being sensitive to cleaning products, heavy metals, silicone

TRIGGERS

- Injury, trauma, or major surgery
- Infection (bacterial or viral)

WHY DOES IT OCCUR?

Stress seems to be a predisposing factor and a number of triggers seem to be able to initiate fibromyalgia (*see left*). One 1997 study showed that a sub-group of fibromyalgia patients (estimated at around 15 percent) have had an obvious traumatic injury — for example, a whiplash injury following a car accident.

People with fibromyalgia display a number of features that may help researchers to discover the underlying cause. One theory centers on the way the brain handles pain signals: reduced levels of serotonin cause an imbalance in the chemical substance P, which makes the brain register pain more readily than normal. Serotonin is also involved in the regulation of sleep and mood. Other studies have shown abnormalities of the metabolism in muscles.

The "tender points" in areas of muscle (*see right*), especially at the base of the skull and near the shoulder blades, are not specific to fibromyalgia. They may also be found in some people with chronic fatigue syndrome (*see p.474*) and other disorders. However, the formal diagnosis of fibromyalgia depends on the presence of large numbers of tender points in particular places.

TREATMENT PLAN

PRIMARY TREATMENTS

- Rehabilitation program
- Homeopathy
- Mind–body therapies

BACK-UP TREATMENTS

- Nutritional therapy
- Acupuncture
- Aerobic exercise
- Breathing retraining
- Bodywork therapies

WORTH CONSIDERING

- Nutritional therapy
- Environmental health

For an explanation of how treatments are rated, see p.111.

SELF-HELP

The following may bring pain relief:
- Analgesics, such as acetaminophen.
- Practicing relaxation and meditation.
- Exercise.

TREATMENTS IN DETAIL

Conventional Medicine

The description of the symptoms and an examination will usually enable a doctor to diagnose fibromyalgia. The doctor may arrange for you to have blood tests to exclude an underlying cause.

PRIMARY TREATMENT | **REHABILITATION PROGRAM** Your doctor will probably recommend a program that involves regular exercise, analgesics to relieve the pain (but not to be used continuously), and certain antidepressants, such as amitriptyline, in low doses to help improve your sleep and reduce pain.

TENDER POINTS

The medical diagnosis of fibromyalgia depends on the presence of tender points at particular locations on the body. The sites of the tender points are located in 9 symmetrical pairs on the body. For someone to have fibromyalgia, according to the strict definition, there should be tenderness to pressure in at least 11 of the 18 tender points. Diagnosis is difficult because tenderness seems to vary from day to day.

Location of the 9 pairs of tender points

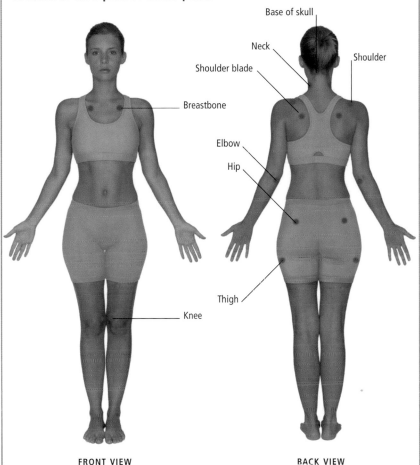

FRONT VIEW

BACK VIEW

Pairs of tender points are located on the breastbone, on the outer edge of the forearms just below the elbow, at the top of the hips and on the fat pad over the knees.

Pairs of tender points are located at the base of the skull, at the base of the neck, over the shoulder blades, on top of the shoulders and on the outside of the hips.

> **CAUTION**
>
> Drugs for fibromyalgia may cause side effects; ask your doctor to explain these to you.

Nutritional Therapy

OMEGA-3 OILS FOR PERSISTENT MUSCLE PAIN Discomfort associated with inflammation may be helped by supplementation with omega-3 fatty acids. Excessive consumption of omega-6 polyunsaturated fatty acids (found in vegetable oils and fast foods) and a relative lack of the omega-3 fatty acids EPA and DHA seem to promote inflammation and pain. Studies show that omega-3 fatty acid supplements reduce inflammatory processes and pain in the body. For example, taking a daily dose of 378mg EPA and 259mg DHA for at least two months may reduce inflammation.

Omega-3 fatty acids can be found in some nuts and seeds, especially walnuts and flaxseeds, and oily fish, such as mackerel, salmon, and sardines. Including these foods in your diet and avoiding foods containing omega-6 fatty acids may help control the pain. Taking 1–3g of concentrated fish oil is likely to help, too.

TRYPTOPHAN is an amino acid that is required for the release of beta-endorphin, one of the body's natural pain-relieving compounds. It is also needed for the production of serotonin, a brain chemical that may reduce a tendency to sense pain. Studies show that tryptophan supplements may be able to increase the body's pain threshold and reduce sensitivity to pain. Tryptophan can be found in foods such as meat, tofu, almonds, peanuts, pumpkin seeds, sesame seeds, and tahini (a paste made from sesame seed).

Tryptophan supplements are not available over the counter in many countries, such as the US. However, 5-hydroxytryptophan (5-HTP), the substance tryptophan is converted into before it is made into serotonin, is a good alternative.

Research suggests that individuals with fibromyalgia may have low serotonin levels in their blood. Studies have shown that supplementation with 300mg per day of 5-HTP relieves some of the symptoms of fibromyalgia. For both persistent muscle pain and fibromyalgia, experts often recommend starting the 5-HTP dosage at 25–100mg a day and increasing to 300mg a day in small increments.

MAGNESIUM There is evidence to suggest that some individuals with fibromyalgia are deficient in magnesium. There is also evidence that the magnesium, in combination with malic acid, can relieve the symptoms of fibromyalgia. A daily intake of 300–600mg of magnesium, together with 1,200–2,400mg of malic acid, can help the production of ATP, the basic fuel source in the body's cells.

> **CAUTION**
>
> Consult your doctor before taking omega-3 fatty acids or fish oils with warfarin, or 5-HTP with zolpidem, venlafaxine, fluoxetine, fluvoxamine, sumatriptan, or paroxetine (see p.46).

Homeopathy

PRIMARY TREATMENT There is quite strong evidence from clinical trials of the effectiveness of homeopathy in treating fibromyalgia. See p.77 for guidelines on how to take the following medicines.

RHUS TOXICODENDRON is the most frequently used medicine. The most important characteristic of syndromes which respond to this medicine is restlessness and rapid stiffening up.

Typically, people who respond to *Rhus toxicodendron* wake up two or three times a night (because they are physically restless, not because they need to go to the toilet), and cannot sit and watch TV, or drive for more than 30–45 minutes without becoming very stiff and achey, and needing to stretch. They may also feel pins and needles and have a tendency to itchy, blistery rashes that may be triggered by contact — for instance, with certain plants or drugs.

IGNATIA is usually thought of as a treatment for emotional shocks, but can be very helpful in fibromyalgia. *Ignatia* is likely to help when the pains are erratic and unpredictable, or when they are severe but short-lived in any one spot. There is often a lot of muscle twitching, and a sensation as if something was stuck in the throat. The problem may have been triggered, or aggravated by, an emotional shock, such as a bereavement or the break-up of a relationship.

CALCAREA CARBONICA is another homeopathic medicine frequently used for fibromyalgia. It is a constitutional medicine, prescribed more for a particular type of person than a disease. Such people may have many of the features of fibromyalgia, including widespread pain, particularly in the low back and knees, and irritable bowel syndrome, often with constipation. Commonly, the cause is a long period of stress, particularly work stress, which has left the person exhausted.

People who respond to *Calcarea carbonica* treatment tend to be solid, well-built, conscientious people, but often with a phobia and anxiety, particularly about their own health. They may conceal these feelings, but if asked will say they are on the verge of breaking down. Their sleep is poor and they have bad dreams and typically sweat a lot on the head, particularly while they are in bed.

CAUSTICUM may also be useful for fibromyalgia. One of its typical symptoms is a great sensitivity to the weather — those who respond to *Causticum* may be able to predict rain (unlike people who respond to *Rhus toxicodendron*, who feel worse when the weather is cold and wet, but cannot predict the weather). The strongest mental characteristic of people who respond to *Causticum* is their great sympathy for the sufferings of others. For example, they cannot bear to watch images of starving children on TV — they have to turn it off or leave the room.

Western Herbal Medicine

CAPSAICIN A placebo-controlled study found that, although topical capsaicin cream decreased tenderness and trigger points in patients with fibromyalgia, it did not have any effect on the pain that is associated with the condition.

Environmental Health

Some of the possible environmental triggers of persistent pain or fibromyalgia include paint solvents and other chemicals, cleaning products, heavy metals, and silicone. The complexities and difficulties in investigating these areas for connections to symptoms underscore the importance of obtaining a detailed environmental and occupational history, perhaps from an environmental health expert who can look for relevant environmental exposures (*to find a therapist, see p.93*). Various prevention strategies are available to decrease overall exposure as much as possible.

Some individuals are particularly sensitive to certain environmental chemicals or have a genetic predisposition that causes them to develop symptoms of fibromyalgia (or other related syndromes) when exposed to chemicals. These reactions can occur at low chemical concentrations that are otherwise considered safe and well below toxic level.

SICK BUILDING SYNDROME An example of a reaction that occurs at a low concentration is what has been termed the "sick building syndrome." This is a set of general symptoms that result from exposure to various compounds in new offices. Although no single cause has been determined, it is thought that some people react to the release of compounds in building materials. The problem is compounded by well-sealed, energy-efficient construction methods.

Sick building syndrome may cause fibromyalgia, in addition to such symptoms as headaches (*see p.114*), asthma (*see p.205*), or skin reactions (dermatitis).

SILICONE BREAST IMPLANTS have been controversially implicated in causing symptoms of fibromyalgia and chronic fatigue syndrome (*see p.474*). Some authors have reviewed the data and conclude that there is no connection between implants and diseases or other conditions. Others point out that some studies seem to indicate that not all women can tolerate breast implants, developing symptoms similar to chronic fatigue syndrome or fibromyalgia. Consult your doctor about the risks and benefits of having breast implants in your specific situation.

DETOXIFICATION Some experts advocate detoxification programs as a way of treating chronic health problems, such as fibromyalgia, especially if a toxic environmental cause is suspected. Removing possible environmental toxins from the body involves a special diet, such as a low allergenic diet, or taking liver-tonifying herbs. Taking supplements, such as vitamin C, vitamin E, selenium, green tea, or mixed carotenoids, can improve the detoxification process in the liver or the function of the intestinal tract.

> Fibromyalgia can affect children, sometimes as young as eight years old

Bodywork Therapies

CHIROPRACTIC, OSTEOPATHY, AND PHY-SICAL THERAPY aim to normalize the spinal areas that may be contributing to pain, to remove associated myofascial trigger points (*see p.55*) and to rehabilitate muscles following disuse.

Many people with fibromyalgia have other pain-inducing conditions, including active trigger points in their muscles and restrictions in spinal and other joints. Many of these conditions can be improved or corrected by a chiropractor, osteopath, physical therapist, or suitably trained massage therapist. Any reduction in the overall amount of pain experienced makes coping with the primary condition less difficult.

HYDROTHERAPY, including the use of sea-water baths in balneotherapy, can benefit some fibromyalgia patients.

> **CAUTION**
>
> Tissue repair is slow in fibromyalgia patients, so any manual therapy must be moderate and gentle to avoid strong reactions, increased pain, and a delayed recovery. Make sure that your therapist is familiar with the manual treatment of fibromyalgia. Overenthusiastic, deep-tissue treatment is inappropriate.

Aerobic Exercise

If you have fibromyalgia, exercise gently (try walking, cycling, or swimming) for 20 minutes a day. Numerous studies show that aerobic exercise helps fibromyalgia in several ways. First, when nonstressful, moderate, aerobic exercise is carried out regularly (for not less than 20 minutes at least three times weekly), it improves both cardiovascular and muscular conditioning. Second, regular exercise reduces pain and other symptoms. Finally, it stimulates the production of growth hormone (the "tissue repair" hormone), which fibromyalgia patients usually have in short supply.

Breathing Retraining

Clinical experience suggests that people with fibromyalgia have breathing patterns that are abnormal. Upper-chest, rapid-rate breathing is common and often linked to feelings of anxiety. Sometimes, anxiety and breathing pattern disorders are a response to the distress of being in pain, and so are not actually a cause. However, they are nevertheless frequent contributors to many of the additional, secondary symptoms of fibromyalgia. (*For more on breathing pattern disorders, see p.57*)

Retraining exercises can help reduce feelings of anxiety and to ease pain, especially when they are accompanied by appropriate manual therapy to relax and normalize the breathing mechanism structures (*see p.62*).

Acupuncture

Two very good clinical trials have examined the application of acupuncture in the treatment of fibromyalgia. The acupuncture was directed toward the tender points (*see illustration, p.299*) and sometimes included the use of intramuscular stimulation, which involves deep and sometimes painful needling (one of the studies used a technique called electroacupuncture). Both studies reported a significant reduction in the amount of pain experienced.

However, it is important to realize that a more traditional Chinese approach to the treatment of fibromyalgia has been largely untested and may ultimately prove to be equally effective to the approaches involving repeated needling of tender points.

Acupuncture may be able to bring about immediate relief from pain, but because fibromyalgia is a chronic illness it requires repeated treatment. If no effect emerges after six treatments, then it is probably not worth continuing. However, if benefit is apparent, then long-term treatment will frequently be required.

Mind–Body Therapies

PRIMARY TREATMENT **PAIN CONTROL** Results strongly indicate that practicing mind–body therapies, combined with regular physical exercise, can help alleviate the pain associated with chronic fibromyalgia. Therapies include meditation or breathing retraining (either at home, with a practitioner or both).

A 1993 study discovered that a stress-reduction program based on meditation can be effective for people with fibromyalgia. Five years later, further research revealed that clinical biofeedback with relaxation, exercise, and a program that combined both all helped people with fibromyalgia to control their experience of pain, cope with their discomfort, and improve their levels of physical activity.

However, in 2000, a review of the studies into the effectiveness of mind–body therapies for fibromyalgia revealed some evidence for improving quality of life, but also showed that there was inconclusive evidence for improving certain aspects of fibromyalgia, such as pain.

Restless legs syndrome (RLS) may occur in 50 per cent of fibromyalgia patients

There is strong evidence that moderate/high intensity exercise (*see Aerobic Exercise, left*) is more effective than most of the mind–body therapies for relieving pain and improving overall, daily functions. Long-term results, however, show that the greatest benefit was obtained by combining mind–body therapies with exercise. The combination of mind-body therapies with exercise and/or antidepressants was most effective at alleviating fibromalgia.

GUIDED IMAGERY Concentrating on pleasant imagery may help relieve the pain of fibromyalgia. A 2002 study explored the effective of amytriptylline and the effectiveness of guided imagery that was either attention-distracting or attention-focusing, on the pain of fibromyalgia. Pleasant imagery reduced the pain, but amitriptyline was no better than a placebo.

> **PREVENTION PLAN**
>
> **The following may help prevent fibromyalgia:**
> - Avoid environmental hazards
> - Take regular exercise

WHAT ARE THE SYMPTOMS?

- Severe pain in the affected joint
- Redness, tenderness, warmth, and swelling in the affected joint
- Fever

WHY MIGHT I HAVE THIS?

PREDISPOSING FACTORS

- Being a middle-aged man or a postmenopausal woman
- Drinking excessive quantities of alcohol, particularly beer
- Eating large amounts of foods containing purines (e.g. red meats and shellfish)
- High-protein diet
- Obesity
- Hereditary factors
- Insulin resistance syndrome
- Long-term use of diuretics

TREATMENT PLAN

PRIMARY TREATMENTS

- Lifestyle measures (*see Self-Help*) including restriction of refined starches and sugars

For acute attacks:
- Nonsteroidal anti-inflammatory drugs (NSAIDs), colchicine, or corticosteroid injections

For recurrent gout:
- Drugs that reduce uric acid levels
- Nutritional therapy

BACKUP TREATMENTS

- Homeopathy
- Western and Chinese Herbal Medicine

For an explanation of how treatments are rated, see p.111.

GOUT

Gout is a metabolic disorder that causes a severely painful type of arthritis. The joint at the base of the big toe is frequently affected, but gout can occur in any joint. The condition is about ten times more common in men than in women and sometimes runs in families, suggesting that genetic factors may be involved. Gout rarely affects women before menopause. Treatment involves reducing pain, swelling, and inflammation, as well as lowering the uric acid levels in the blood by increasing its excretion and inhibiting its production.

WHY DOES IT OCCUR?

People with high blood levels of uric acid are prone to gout. Uric acid is a substance produced in the body when proteins and chemicals called purines are broken down. It can accumulate in the blood when the body produces too much of it and/or the kidneys do not excrete enough.

Uric acid is deposited as sharp crystals in a joint where they accumulate and cause inflammation and severe, sometimes excruciating, pain. The joint at the base of the big toe is most commonly affected. The first attack of gout usually comes without warning and often wakes the individual early in the morning.

People who eat a high-protein diet may have high uric acid levels, as may those who are obese or who drink excessive amounts of alcohol, particularly beer. Uric acid excretion by the kidneys may be impaired for a variety of reasons including long-term use of diuretics.

People who have gout over a long period of time may develop deposits of uric acid crystals in the earlobes and soft tissues of the hands, where they form small lumps known as tophi. People with gout may also develop kidney stones that are composed of uric acid.

SELF-HELP

PRIMARY TREATMENT If you have gout, it is important to make the following changes to your diet:
- Reduce your alcohol intake.
- Follow a weight-reducing diet if needed.
- Avoid purine-rich foods.
- Cut down on refined and starchy foods such as bread.

TREATMENTS IN DETAIL

Conventional Medicine

Your symptoms and an examination will usually enable the doctor to diagnose gout, but the levels of uric acid in the blood may need to be measured. In some cases, fluid is withdrawn from the affected joint and tested for the presence of uric acid crystals.

PRIMARY TREATMENT **DRUGS** Acute attacks of gout tend to subside after a few days without any treatment. However, you may be prescribed nonsteroidal anti-inflammatory drugs (NSAIDs), such as naproxen, to relieve the pain and reduce the swelling. Aspirin is not used to relieve the pain of gout because it slows the elimination of uric acid from the blood.

Alternatively, you may be prescribed colchicine to relieve pain. This traditional remedy has been used for gout since the 18th century and is usually taken at the first sign of symptoms. Corticosteroids may be injected into a muscle or directly into the affected joint.

Recurrent gout may be controlled with uricosuric drugs, which act upon the kidneys to reduce the levels of uric acid in the blood. The uricosuric drug most commonly used is allopurinol, which prevents uric acid production, and rapidly reduces levels of it in the blood. Alternative drugs include probenecid and sulfinpyrazone.

CAUTION

The drugs used for treating gout have a range of side effects; ask your doctor to explain them to you.

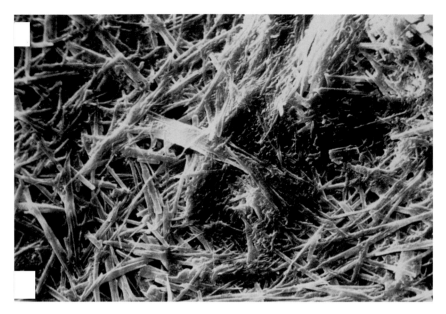

Uric acid crystals are shaped like tiny needles. When the level of uric acid in the bloodstream rises, the crystals may be deposited in certain joints where they accumulate. Their sharpness can cause excruciating pain.

Nutritional Therapy

AVOID PURINE-RICH FOODS Uric acid is one of the end products of the metabolism of dietary elements known as purines. Consumption of large amounts of meat and seafood is associated with an increased risk of gout, whereas a high consumption of dairy products is associated with a decreased risk. Moderate intake of purine-rich vegetables or protein is not associated with an increased risk.

Traditionally, sufferers of gout are advised to limit purine-rich foods. However, this approach is believed to have limited effectiveness, which may relate to the fact that the majority of purines in the bloodstream do not come from the diet, but are made naturally within the body.

ALCOHOL consumption has long been closely associated with high uric acid levels and gout. Limiting alcohol consumption may therefore be effective in the treatment and prevention of gout, although this is far from proven.

FOLIC ACID Although folic acid is an XO inhibior and was once thought to be helpful in treaating gout, a human study found no effect of folic acid in doses up to 1000mcg per day on patients with high uric acid levels. Foods that are rich in folic acid, such as asparagus (*Asparagus officinalis*) and strawberries, may also help relieve the symptoms of gout. Studies show that folic acid is not only an inhibitor of xanthine oxidase but may also be several times more potent than allopurinol.

Other fruits, such as strawberries (*Fragaria* spp.), blackcurrants (*Ribes nigrum*), and cranberries (*Vaccinium macrocarpon*) may be effective for people with gout because of the anti-inflammatory polyphenol flavonoids they contain.

INSULIN RESISTANCE SYNDROME Evidence suggests that high uric acid levels in the blood and gout are often related to a condition known as insulin resistance syndrome (IRS). Believed to be a potential precursor of both heart disease and diabetes, IRS is characterized by a range of factors including excess weight (typically concentrated around the middle of the body), raised levels of total cholesterol and triglycerides, low levels of "healthy" HDL cholesterol, and hypertension (*see p.244*).

IRS is likely to have a number of underlying factors, one of which seems to be the overconsumption of sugar and refined carbohydrates. In one study, the potential benefits of a carbohydrate-restriction diet was tested in a group of middle-aged men with gout. The men were instructed to minimize their intake of bread, potatoes, rice, and pasta and eat plenty of healthy fats in the form of olive oil, nuts, and oily fish such as salmon, trout, and sardines.

Following this diet for 16 weeks brought about significant lowering of uric acid and cholesterol levels, and a reduction in weight and the number of gout attacks. Consequently, restricting carbohydrates, especially refined sugar and starches, may be an effective strategy in combating IRS and gout in the long term.

Homeopathy

Gout is a metabolic disorder whose main manifestation is joint pain and inflammation, but it can affect other organs, especially the kidneys. For this reason, treating the inflamed joint alone may not be sufficient. The homeopathic medicines most frequently suggested for gout are *Benzoic acid*, *Ledum*, and *Lycopodium*.

BENZOIC ACID is appropriate for gout that occurs in the big toe. There may also be pain in the Achilles tendon at the back of the ankle, and small lumps (tophi) elsewhere in the body. However, the most characteristic feature of people who respond to *Benzoic acid* is that their urine smells very strongly, like that of a horse.

> Often referred to as the disease of kings, gout in fact is not always a sign of overindulgence

LEDUM PALUSTRE is appropriate for gout in the base of the big toe which is swollen and tender, yet sometimes unusually pale rather than red. The most characteristic feature of the type of gout that responds to *Ledum* is the great relief that cold brings — putting the affected foot in cold water or walking barefoot on a cold floor eases the pain, although the patient often feels generally chilly. People who respond to

Ledum are sometimes heavy drinkers and their faces tend to be both red and pimply.

LYCOPODIUM is prescribed for gout mostly on constitutional grounds (*see p.73*). One indication that *Lycopodium* may be appropriate is when the gout affects joints on the right side of the body, or has first affected the right foot and then the left. People who respond to *Lycopodium* are often thoughtful and reserved, and may be anxious and depressed. They often have stomach trouble. Their "eyes are bigger than their stomachs"— in other words, they feel hungry when they start eating, but quickly become satisfied. This feature is accompanied by a bloated feeling. They may crave sweet food and they tend to feel at their worst during the late afternoon.

Western Herbal Medicine

The treatment of gout needs to be considered in two phases: during acute attacks and when gout is in remission. Treatment in the acute phase must be fast and effective because an attack of gout is usually very painful. It is sensible to use conventional drugs, such as NSAIDs or colchicine — an alkaloid that is found in the autumn crocus (*Colchicum autumnale*) — which can bring pain relief within a few hours.

Gout is most common in people between the ages of 30 and 60

Once the levels of uric acid have fallen and the pain is gone, herbal medicines have some use. Like conventional drugs, plant medicines can increase the excretion of uric acid or prevent its synthesis. They can also significantly reduce inflammation.

DIURETICS AND ANTI-INFLAMMATORIES
Burdock (*Arctium lappa*) root is a favored gout remedy that is said to have a diuretic and "blood cleansing" action. It may also have anti-inflammatory properties.

Celery (*Apium graveolens*) seed is another well-known gout remedy with anti-inflammatory, diuretic, and anti-arthritic actions. Nettle (*Urtica dioica*) tea is a diuretic and detoxifier; one study

indicated that it enhanced the effect of the NSAID diclofenac in treating rheumatic conditions. Other herbs thought to have anti-inflammatory qualities include sarsaparilla (*Smilax ornata*), yarrow (*Achillea millefolium*), and dandelion (*Taraxacum officinale*) root and leaf.

REDUCING URIC ACID LEVELS Many herbal remedies can reduce uric acid levels in the blood. Cherries have long been a folk remedy for gout, but a research study recently confirmed that cherries are effective because they decrease uric acid levels. Healthy women consumed 9oz (280g) of Bing sweet cherries; this increased urinary excretion of uric acid after three hours and decreased blood levels of uric acid at five hours.

Conventional medicines such as allopurinol inhibit xanthine oxidase, a key enzyme in the synthesis of uric acid in the body. Studies show that several herbs such as milk thistle (*Silibum marianum*), centaury (*Centaurium erythrea*), turmeric (*Curcuma longa*), and licorice (*Glycyrrhiza glabra*) have the same inhibitory effect on xanthine oxidase.

Drinking tea (*Camellia sinensis*) on a regular basis may reduce gout attacks because the polyphenol catechins and flavones in tea are also inhibitors of xanthine oxidase. Studies show that silymarin, which is found in the fruits of milk thistle, is an inhibitor of xanthine oxidase. Similar claims are made for the antioxidant polyphenols in centaury (*Centaurium* spp.), which is the basis of the famous Portland Powder remedy for gout, and for the phenolic constituents of licorice.

Turmeric contains curcumin, which appears to be a powerful inhibitor of xanthine oxidase and COX-2, and also has anti-inflammatory properties.

EXTERNAL TREATMENTS include a poultice of fresh cabbage (*Brassica* spp.*) leaves, a vinegar compress, and a footbath of natrum sulfate or magnesium sulfate with

chopped celery and watercress (*Nasturtium officinale*). These may help reduce swelling and inflammation.

CAUTION

Before taking an herbal remedy for gout see p.69. Some herbalists recommend salicylate-containing remedies such as willow bark, meadowsweet, black cohosh, and birch to treat gout. Until research shows otherwise, avoid these herbs, since doses of moderate to high doses of aspirin can alter blood levels of uric acid.

Chinese Herbal Medicine

Practitioners of Traditional Chinese Medicine (TCM) treat gout as *Bi* syndrome (*see Osteoarthritis, p.291*), rather than as a separate ailment. *Bi* means "painful blockage."

Of the many well-known Chinese herbal medicines for treating arthritic conditions, 122 have been investigated for their xanthine oxidase inhibitory effect. Over half have been extracted in alcohol and shown to have a significant effect. Cinnamon (*Cinnamomum cassia*), wild chrysanthemum (*Chrysanthemum indica*), and shiny bugleweed (*Lycopus lucidum*) were the most effective. The herbal medicines extracted in water showed a somewhat lower rate of inhibiting xanthine oxidase. *Hu zhang* (*Polygonum cuspidatum*) was the most potent.

Studies have shown that purple-leafed perilla (*Perilla fructescens*) is also a potent inhibitor of xanthine oxidase and may prove to be helpful in controlling uric acid levels. One active component discovered in perilla was shown to be as potent as the conventional drug allopurinol.

CAUTION

See p.69 before taking a herbal remedy and, if you are taking a prescribed medication, consult an herbal medicine expert first.

PREVENTION PLAN

Try the following to prevent an increase in blood levels of uric acid:

- Avoid excess alcohol, proteins, and purines in your diet
- Restrict your intake of refined starches and sugars

ANKYLOSING SPONDYLITIS

Ankylosing spondylitis is a chronic, progressive inflammation and stiffness of the joints, usually in the spine and pelvis. The disorder is about three times more common in men than women and mainly affects young white men, usually under the age of 45. The condition may run in families. Treatment involves easing the inflammation with NSAIDs and steroid injections, a diet rich in omega-3 fatty acids, and vitamin D. Exercise, manipulation, and homeopathy can help maintain range of motion and muscle tone and ease the pain.

WHAT ARE THE SYMPTOMS?

- Pain in the lower back, which may radiate into the buttocks and thighs
- Stiffness in the lower back, which is worse in the morning and better with exercise
- Pain in other joints, such as the hips, knees, and shoulders
- Pain in the rib cage and a limited ability to expand the chest
- Without treatment, curvature of the spine and weakening of the back muscles may eventually develop

Other possible features include:
- Uveitis (inflammation of the eye), which may need urgent treatment

WHY MIGHT I HAVE THIS?

PREDISPOSING FACTORS
- Genetic factors, such as having HLA-B27
- Inflammatory diet
- Vitamin D deficiency

WHY DOES IT OCCUR?

The symptoms of ankylosing spondylitis usually appear in late adolescence or early adulthood. They develop gradually over a period of months or years, with symptom-free periods between episodes of inflammation. In addition to the spine and pelvis, the rib cage and other joints around the body may also be affected. Walking and movement become awkward and other, noninflamed joints and muscles become painful and stiff. Eventually, the disease affects joints between the ribs and mid spine, reducing chest expansion.

If left untreated ankylosing spondylitis can result in curvature of the spine. If the spine is severely affected, new bone starts to grow between the vertebrae, which eventually fuse together.

Ankylosing spondylitis is a reactive spondarthropathy, a family of diseases that includes psoriasis (*see p.172*), inflammatory bowel disease, and Reiter's syndrome. Its cause is unknown. However, about 90 percent of people affected share a common factor — they have human leukocyte antigen B27 (HLA-B27). Human leukocyte antigens are proteins present on the surface of most cells in the body. They enable the body's immune system to differentiate body cells from foreign cells, such as bacteria, that it needs to attack. There are many different human leukocyte antigens: individuals inherit their own set from their parents. Not everyone who has HLA-B27 develops ankylosing spondylitis.

What triggers the ankylosing spondylitis in certain individuals is unknown, although some practitioners think that dietary factors and vitamin D deficiency are involved.

TREATMENT PLAN

PRIMARY TREATMENTS
- Exercises
- Drugs such as NSAIDs and steroid injections

BACKUP TREATMENTS
- Nutritional therapy
- Homeopathy
- Bodywork and movement therapies
- Acupuncture

For an explanation of how treatments are rated, see p.111.

IMMEDIATE RELIEF

Acupuncture may bring relief from back and hip pain. The homeopathic medicine *Rhus toxicodendron* may also help relieve the symptoms.

IMPORTANT

Call the doctor immediately if you develop eye pain, redness, blurred vision, or are bothered by bright lights. These symptoms may indicate that uveitis is present.

Conventional Medicine

To help make a diagnosis your doctor will arrange various tests, including X-rays, to look for changes that may occur in ankylosing spondylitis.

PRIMARY TREATMENT **EXERCISES** Early diagnosis of the condition is important so that you can start a regimen of morning physical therapy exercises to maintain mobility and help prevent deformities of the spine.

PRIMARY TREATMENT **DRUGS** During episodes of inflammation, your doctor may prescribe nonsteroidal anti-inflammatory drugs (NSAIDs) to reduce the pain and stiffness and to enable you to continue the physical therapy exercises. A doctor may also inject steroids into inflamed joints.

CAUTION

NSAIDs and steroids may cause side effects; ask your doctor to explain these to you.

Nutritional Therapy

OMEGA-3 FATTY ACIDS Eating foods that are rich in omega-3 fatty acids (*see p.34*) should help reduce inflammation and its associated pain. Omega-3 fatty acids can be found in some nuts and seeds, especially walnuts and flaxseeds, and in oily fish, such as mackerel, salmon, and sardines. One study has shown that taking the omega-3 fatty acids EPA (378mg) and DHA (259mg) each day for at least two months can help reduce inflammation.

Conversely, excessive omega-6 polyunsaturated fatty acids (found in vegetable oils) and a relative lack of omega-3 fatty acids seem to promote inflammation.

VITAMIN D Studies reveal that ankylosing spondylitis patients have very low levels of the various breakdown products of vitamin D metabolism. Research also shows that low levels of vitamin D may accelerate the inflammation process associated with the condition. Consequently, taking 500 IU of vitamin D supplements each day may help reduce inflammation. Osteoporosis (*see p.308*) is often associated with ankylosing spondylitis, so it is very important to take adequate calcium and vitamin D and to have periodic bone density tests.

Homeopathy

RHUS TOXICODENDRON Although there is little formal research, homeopaths often claim that their treatments can help relieve the symptoms of ankylosing spondylitis. One of the treatments most commonly used is *Rhus toxicodendron*, a medicine that is made from poison ivy.

QUAD STRETCH FOR ANKYLOSING SPONDYLITIS

Stretching the major muscle groups every day and putting joints through their range of motion can ease pain. Practice each exercise once or twice a day. Always stretch slowly and gently and stop if it hurts.

1. Stand to the side of a sturdy chair and hold the back with your right hand. Stand tall, keeping your spine as straight as possible.

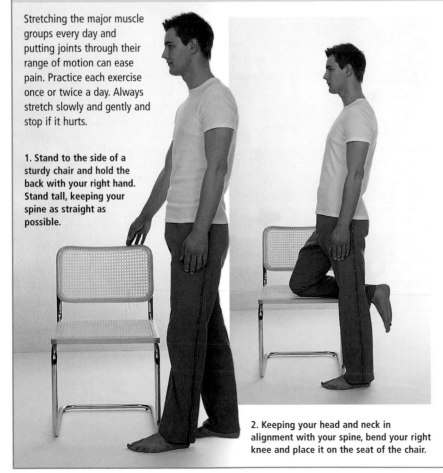

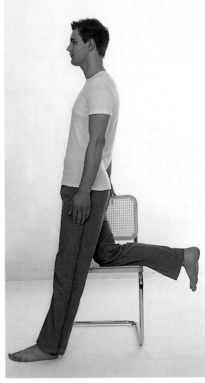

2. Keeping your head and neck in alignment with your spine, bend your right knee and place it on the seat of the chair.

3. Place your left foot as far forward as you can. You should feel a slight stretch in your right thigh.

A key feature of the rheumatic conditions that respond to this medicine is the way a patient's joints rapidly stiffen up. Typically, patients report that pain and stiffness wake them up two or three times every night; after they get out of bed and "limber up" they feel much better and are able to sleep again for a few hours, before the process repeats itself. Similarly, they get stiff and achy from sitting still for 30 minutes. Such symptoms may be masked if the person with ankylosing spondylitis is taking anti-inflammatory drugs.

Other features that suggest *Rhus toxico-dendron* include symptoms that are worse in cold and wet weather, and a tendency to have itchy rashes consisting of fine blisters.

DEEPER-ACTING TREATMENTS If the condition is deep-seated, you will need to consult a well-trained homeopath who may prescribe a remedy, such as bowel nosodes, that acts at a more profound

4. To increase the intensity, bend your left knee, while still keeping your back and neck aligned and relaxed. Hold for 10 seconds. Repeat twice and then turn around to stretch the opposite leg.

level. Bowel nosodes are prepared from bacteria that may be found in human intestines, although they are not part of the healthy intestinal flora.

Bowel nosodes may be helpful when the ankylosing spondylitis seems to be triggered by a "cross-reaction" — the body's immune system attacks invading bacteria and then turns its attention to the body's tissues, because they are of a similar type to the bacteria.

Bodywork and Movement Therapies

As a result of the inflammation that develops in the spinal joints, walking and movement becomes awkward and other, uninflamed, joints and muscles become painful and stiff.

The objective of manipulation therapies and stretching exercises is to help you maintain your range of motion (the normal extent that joints can be moved in certain directions) and the tone of your muscles, and to ease the pain.

PHYSICAL THERAPY, OSTEOPATHY, CHIROPRACTIC, AND THERAPEUTIC MASSAGE may all be able to help you ease the pain and restrictions, as well as assisting the circulation in muscles and joints that are affected by the pain and by altered movement patterns.

EXERCISE Although manipulation needs to be very gentle, try gently stretching and toning, every other day, those muscles and joints that are not actually inflamed, but which are affected by the pain and restriction of the disorder.

Experience has also shown that it is important to put joints through gentle range-of-motion movements every day, even when the inflammation has flared up. Yoga can be an effective way of achieving this.

You may find it easier to perform the exercises in the water rather than out of it because the buoyancy of water allows greater flexibility and ease of movement. Many physical therapy departments have warm-water pools where you can practice exercise sessions under the supervision of physical therapists. These exercises will help you move with greater flexibility.

Research has demonstrated that exercise (whether physical therapy, exercising in water, or exercising at home) brings benefits as long as it is maintained consistently. However, some types of exercises are more effective than others; a controlled trial found that group-based exercises were more effective than home-based ones at reducing impairment.

ANTIAROUSAL BREATHING METHODS may help you cope with chronic pain. For example, pursed-lip breathing exercises improve the mechanics and efficiency of breathing. Breathe in slowly through your nose and then, pursing your lips as if blowing up a balloon, exhale slowly (taking 4–6 seconds) through your mouth. Try practicing these breathing methods for a few minutes each morning after you have finished your exercises.

> **CAUTION**
>
> Manual treatment needs to be extremely gentle when joints are inflamed, to avoid aggravating the tissues.

Acupuncture

There are no direct clinical trials involving acupuncture and ankylosing spondylitis but evidence suggests that it helps relieve the back and hip pain that are features of the condition. Acupuncture does not alter the natural progression of ankylosing spondylitis, but it may provide prolonged periods of pain relief after relatively few acupuncture treatments.

Usually, treatment is given weekly with the expectation that some benefit will begin to emerge after four to six treatments, and treatments should continue until no further clinical improvement occurs.

> **PREVENTION PLAN**
>
> **Try the following to help slow down the progress of the condition:**
>
> - Exercise daily or take up yoga
> - Learn the Alexander method (*see p.62*) to help improve posture

---

OSTEOPOROSIS

Osteoporosis is characterized by a loss of bone tissue that is greater than normal and an increased susceptibility to fractures. Common in men and women over the age of 50, osteoporosis is more prevalent in Caucasian and Asian people. Certain factors act as predispositions to developing osteoporosis, including a family history of the condition, being thin, and not getting enough exercise. The goal of treatment is to slow the rate of bone loss, build up bone density, and reduce the risks of developing the disease.

WHY DOES IT OCCUR?

Bone is a living tissue that is continually broken down and rebuilt by the body. From the age of about 25, when peak bone mass is reached, there is a gradual loss of bone tissue as breakdown occurs more rapidly than formation. However, in many people, bone mass remains within an acceptable range even in old age. When the condition known as osteoporosis occurs, bone mass has fallen below this acceptable range and the risk of fractures is markedly increased.

Although osteoporosis progresses over a period of many years, during which it causes little or no pain or other evidence of the condition, the fractures when they do occur can be very painful, requiring major surgery and prolonged hospitalization. As the body ages, it becomes less able to recover from such major injuries, and they may lead to permanent disabilities.

In both men and women, sex hormones play a part in bone replacement. In women, there is a rapid decrease in bone density in the ten years following menopause. An early menopause (see p.339) increases the risk of osteoporosis, as do other conditions in which there is reduced production of sex hormones, such as anorexia nervosa (see p.441).

People who have certain joint disorders, such as rheumatoid arthritis (see p.293), and hormone disorders, such as an overactive thyroid gland (see p.319), are also more prone to developing osteoporosis. Osteoporosis can develop as a complication of taking certain drugs, including long-term corticosteroids. Other risk factors include poor nutrition during childhood, smoking, and chronic alcohol abuse.

TREATMENTS IN DETAIL

Conventional Medicine

If your doctor suspects osteoporosis, the diagnosis may be confirmed and the severity of the disease measured by bone densitometry of the spinal column or hip. This test uses low-dose X-rays to measure bone density. Further investigations may look for an underlying cause.

PRIMARY TREATMENT **LIFESTYLE MEASURES** For those with a slightly low bone mass, lifestyle factors, such as stopping smoking, will be recommended and a follow-up bone density test done a few years later (see also Prevention Plan, p.311).

WHAT ARE THE SYMPTOMS?

- For many people, the first sign of osteoporosis is a fractured bone following a minor injury

Other symptoms may include:

- A gradual loss of height and rounding of the back, both due to vertebral fractures

WHY MIGHT I HAVE THIS?

PREDISPOSING FACTORS

- Smoking
- Alcoholism
- Genetic factors
- Being thin
- Lack of regular exercise
- Insufficient calcium in the diet, particularly during childhood and adolescence
- Insufficient vitamin D
- Aging
- Early menopause
- Long-term use of corticosteroids
- Joint conditions, such as rheumatoid arthritis
- Hormonal disorders, such as an overactive thyroid gland

TREATMENT PLAN

PRIMARY TREATMENTS

- Lifestyle measures
- Drugs, such as bisphosphonates, calcitonin, estrogen, raloxifene
- Calcium and vitamin D

BACKUP TREATMENTS

- Nutritional therapy
- Weight-bearing exercise and tai chi
- Environmental health measures

WORTH CONSIDERING

- Acupuncture

For an explanation of how treatments are rated, see p.111.

PRIMARY TREATMENT **DRUGS** In more severe cases, drugs may also be prescribed. This is particularly the case when fractures have occurred as a result of minor injuries.

Drug treatments include biphosphonates, such as risedronate, which reduce the rate of bone breakdown and increase bone density, and calcitonin, which can also help prevent and treat osteoporosis

However, the evidence regarding calcium supplementation in later life (especially in postmenopausal women) in order to prevent osteoporosis and fractures is controversial. A 2003 study suggests that the amount of calcium in the diet in later life (including calcium from dairy products) has little or no bearing on bone health and risk of fracture.

One in 3 women and 1 in 12 men over the age of 50 will develop osteoporosis

---

after menopause. Your doctor may recommend calcium supplements (*see Nutritional Therapy, below*).

Hormone therapy (estrogen) reduces bone loss after menopause and also reduces the risk of osteoporosis. It is no longer a primary treatment because of its potential risks but it may be used when other treatments are not effective or tolerated. The drug raloxifene is sometimes used to treat or prevent osteoporosis in postmenopausal women.

While all of these treatments have been shown to increase bone density, some, such as bisphosphonates and hormone therapy, have also been found to reduce the risk of fractures. Regular follow-up is needed to monitor the progress of treatment.

CAUTION

Drugs for osteoporosis may have side effects; ask your doctor to explain these to you.

Nutritional Therapy

PRIMARY TREATMENT **CALCIUM** Most studies show that calcium, either as a regular supplement or as a part of the diet, is important at a young age in order to reach a good peak bone mass (at about the age of 25). This intake of calcium may protect against the development of osteoporosis in later life. A daily dose of 600–1,000mg of calcium before the age of 25 is thought to help obtain optimum bone mass. (*See table, right, and Environmental Health, p.311.*) Bone meal calcium supplements should be avoided because they may contain lead.

Foods that are naturally rich in calcium include green leafy vegetables, dairy products, blackstrap molasses, sesame seeds, and almonds. Calcium is also found, although in smaller amounts, in most other vegetables, such as peas, squash, carrots, broccoli, and celery.

PRIMARY TREATMENT **VITAMIN D** The effect of calcium supplementation on bone health may be more effective if it is combined with vitamin D supplementation. Vitamin D plays an important role in calcium balance in the body by aiding the absorption of calcium from food. It may also help reduce the loss of bone tissue after menopause (*see p.339*).

Many studies show that taking vitamin D in combination with calcium (at about 1,000mg daily) reduces fracture rates and falls in the elderly. One study and a meta-analysis shows that vitamin D alone may be beneficial in reducing fracture risk. The recommended daily dose is 20mcg/800 IU of vitamin D.

FRUITS AND VEGETABLES A number of studies suggest that there is a clear, positive link between fruit and vegetable consumption and bone health. This probably reflects the fact that eating fruits and vegetables helps increase alkalinity in the body, which plays a role in preventing calcium loss from bone. Findings in other studies have demonstrated that women with the lowest intakes of potassium, magnesium, fiber, vitamin C, and beta-carotene had significantly lower bone mineral densities and higher bone loss than other women. Nutrients, such as potassium and

lutein, that are abundant in fruits and vegetables also seem to be associated with higher bone mass in men.

OMEGA-3 FATTY ACIDS There is a certain amount of evidence to suggest that eating a diet that is rich in eicosapentaenoic acid (EPA) and docosahexaenoic acid (DHA) may also be useful in preventing osteoporosis. These omega-3 fatty acids (*see p.334*) can be found in oily fish, such as mackerel, salmon, and sardines. In one study, elderly women with osteoporosis were given 4g of fish oil daily for 16 weeks. Fish-oil supplementation was found to bring about biochemical changes that can be detected in the serum part of blood. These changes include an increase in the

VITAMIN D

This table shows the recommended adequate intakes (AIs) of vitamin D for adults, calculated in 1998 (source: US National Institutes of Health.), and the recommended daily allowance (RDA) of calcium for various ages and for pregnant and breast-feeding women.

VITAMIN D	
Age	**AI**
51–69 over 70	IU 400 IU 600 IU

CALCIUM	
Age	**RDA**
0–6 months 7–12 months	210mg 270mg
19–50 over 50	1,000mg 1,200mg
Pregnant women	
under 18 over 18	1,300mg 1,000mg
Breast-feeding women	
under 18 over 18	1,300mg 1,000mg

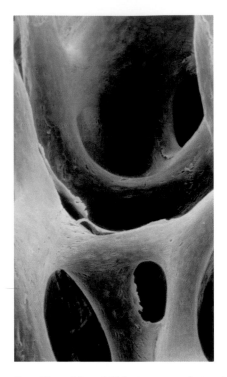
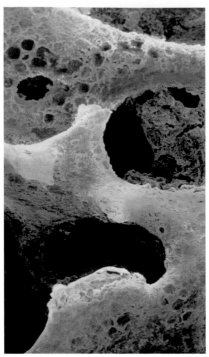

Normal bone (above left) features struts that are both light and strong. In osteoporosis (above right), the fabric of spongy bone tissue becomes thinner, reducing bone mass and making the bones more brittle.

levels of calcium, osteocalcin, and collagen and a reduction in the levels of alkaline phosphatase — all of which are signs of improved bone health.

Eating a diet that is rich in the omega-3 fatty acids EPA and DHA may also reduce the risk of osteoporosis by inhibiting the production of eicosanoids in the body. These inflammatory and hormonelike substances are believed to be involved in the process of bone loss.

PHYTOESTROGENS are plant-derived substances that have an effect on the body similar to that of the hormone estrogen. However, this action is much weaker than that of estrogen. Studies suggest that including soy foods, such as soy milk, tofu, and soy flour, as well as other sources of phytoestrogens, such as beans, lentils, chickpeas, and flaxseeds, in the diet may be beneficial in protecting the bones against osteoporosis, especially in women who have already experienced menopause.

MAGNESIUM appears to be an important nutrient for bone health because it helps encourage the incorporation of calcium

into bone. In one study, eating plenty of magnesium was associated with higher bone mass. Research also shows that taking magnesium supplements and eating a diet that is rich in the mineral can help reduce biochemical signs of bone loss.

In a 1993 study, most of the people who took 250–750mg of magnesium in supplement form over a two-year period stopped losing bone or else increased their bone density. Nuts, seeds, legumes, beans, and whole grains are good sources of magnesium. Taking a supplement that contains 500mg of magnesium each day may also be beneficial to bone health.

> **CAUTION**
>
> Consult your doctor before taking vitamin D with verapamil; omega-3 fatty acids or fish oils with warfarin; magnesium with ciproflaxin, iron, warfarin, or spironolactone; calcium with antibiotics, beta-blockers, or thyroxine (see p.46).

MULTIVITAMIN/MINERAL SUPPLEMENT Research suggests that zinc, copper, potassium, vitamin K, vitamin C, silicon, and manganese may be important to bone

health. Taking a multivitamin/mineral supplement regularly may also help.

AVOID CAFFEINE AND CARBONATED DRINKS A high intake of caffeine and carbonated drinks has been linked to reduced bone mass and an increased risk of fracture. These drinks contain phosphoric acid, which leaches (removes) calcium from the bones. Try to limit your intake of these foodstuffs in your diet.

Exercise

The objectives of exercise and movement techniques, such as tai chi, are to reduce bone loss, increase bone density, improve strength, balance, and coordination, and reduce the chances of falling and fracturing fragile bones.

PHYSICAL EXERCISE increases bone mineral density (BMD) in healthy young adults and slows the rate of bone loss in later life. One study also shows that progressive low-impact exercise is a potentially effective method of increasing BMD in people with Crohn's disease (see p.216). These people absorb nutrients poorly as a result of intestinal inflammation; therefore, bone loss is a very real risk. If the exercise is sustained, the increases in bone mass should reduce the risk of osteoporotic fracture.

WEIGHT TRAINING AND WEIGHT-BEARING EXERCISE The objectives of an exercise program change with age. One study found that structured weight training and weight-bearing exercise in the middle adult years may generate small increases in bone mass. The goal in older adults, particularly those who have osteoporosis, is to combine physical therapy and exercise to conserve bone mass, improve mobility and function, encourage correct posture, and reduce pain. Walking is a recommended weight-bearing exercise.

Italian research has shown that physical exercise combined with thermal mud packs increases bone density and is more effective than exercise alone.

REDUCING THE RISK OF FALLING is important for people with osteoporosis, not least because they become unsteady with age and more likely to fracture a bone, most commonly the hip. About 95 percent of hip fractures result from falls. Suggestions for strategies to reduce falls include wearing footwear that promotes stability, and protective hip pads that reduce the risk of fracture if and when falls do occur.

TAI CHI A number of studies confirm that movement techniques, such as tai chi, can help restore some sense of balance. A three-month study of older women living in a retirement community who attended twice-weekly, 30-minute tai chi classes found that they had made significant improvements in balance and mobility, so they were less likely to experience a fall.

Another study showed that elderly people who regularly practiced tai chi developed a postural stability in challenging conditions, such as maintaining balance on an unstable surface when they had their eyes closed. Tai chi has also been shown to retard bone loss.

Acupuncture

Acupuncture cannot treat the bone demineralization that occurs in osteoporosis but it can relieve the pain, particularly

enough vitamin D, or getting enough calcium in your diet (*see also Nutritional Therapy, p.309*).

It is important to make sure that you consume enough, but not too much, calcium in order to build strong bones (*see table in Nutritional Therapy, p.309*). Beware, however, of the source of your calcium supplement, since bone meal and other sources of medical or supplemental calcium can be laden with toxic heavy metals, especially lead.

Cod liver oil is an easy way to supplement your diet with vitamin D but take it in moderation to prevent consuming too much of another fat-soluble vitamin — vitamin A — which can weaken bones. Recent research warns that the retinol form of vitamin A (not the carotene form) is associated with frail bones and clinical fractures.

In addition to consuming enough vitamin D, you need sunlight to transform the inactive dietary form of vitamin D into the bioactive vitamin D necessary for calcium absorption and bone formation. If possible, try to receive at least 10–15 minutes a day of unfiltered sunlight — this is sunlight that is not filtered through clouds,

cadmium in the air or in the soil near sites where cadmium pollution is produced.

Most foods have small amounts of cadmium, but certain vegetables, shellfish (but not regular fish), liver, and kidney tend to have higher concentrations.

Chelation therapy is a treatment that attempts to reduce cadmium in the body by chemically binding and filtering it from the bloodstream. Unfortunately, there is no compelling clinical evidence that supports the use of this treatment.

PSYCHOLOGICAL STRESS that increases your body's production of the stress hormone cortisol can contribute to worsening osteoporosis. This is because cortisol and the related steroid, cortisone, are notorious for inducing and exacerbating osteoporosis.

DRUGS AND OTHER SUBSTANCES that seem to be detrimental to bone health include blood thinners, anticonvulsants, antacids containing aluminum, chemotherapy, lithium, and certain antibiotics.

FLUORIDE is commonly added to public supplies of drinking water to help reduce dental decay. Fluoride has also been used as a treatment for osteoporosis because it encourages osteoblasts to generate new bone tissue and increase the bone mineral density. Although fluoride may make bones thicker, it also makes them more brittle and more vulnerable to fractures.

> ## The most common sites of fractures due to osteoporosis are in the spine, wrists, and hip

in the stress fractures that may occur in the spine. Acupuncture will probably need to be provided on a weekly basis until the pain subsides. Benefit from the treatment should be apparent within the first six to eight sessions.

Environmental Health

VITAMINS AND MINERALS Osteoporosis prevention and treatment depend upon environmental factors to a large extent. If you live in northern latitudes, or your access to sunlight is otherwise impeded (due to air pollution or style of dress, or because you wear sunscreen that is SPF 8 or greater), you may also be putting yourself at risk for osteoporosis. This is because you may not be receiving enough sunlight on your skin and therefore not producing

pollution, sunscreens, clothing, and glass windows — to ensure that your skin is exposed to enough UV radiation to transform your vitamin D into the form necessary to combat osteoporosis.

CADMIUM Studies have shown that the more cadmium is present in the body the less dense the bones are likely to be. Since cadmium can persist in your tissues for several decades, make sure your children also limit their cadmium exposure.

Your intake of cadmium is markedly elevated by smoking cigarettes or by working in zinc-refining areas (or in a nickel/cadmium battery manufacturing plant or with metal soldering). If you have osteoporosis or are at risk for developing it, you need to stop smoking and avoid exposure to occupational sources of

PREVENTION PLAN

The following may help prevent the development of osteoporosis:

- Eat plenty of calcium-containing foods, particularly in childhood and adolescence, to help achieve good bone mass
- Avoid becoming too thin
- Take vitamin D supplements to help you absorb calcium
- Engage in regular weight-bearing exercise, such as walking
- Do not smoke and avoid caffeine and carbonated drinks
- Stay within the recommended limits for alcohol consumption (14 units weekly for women and 21 for men)

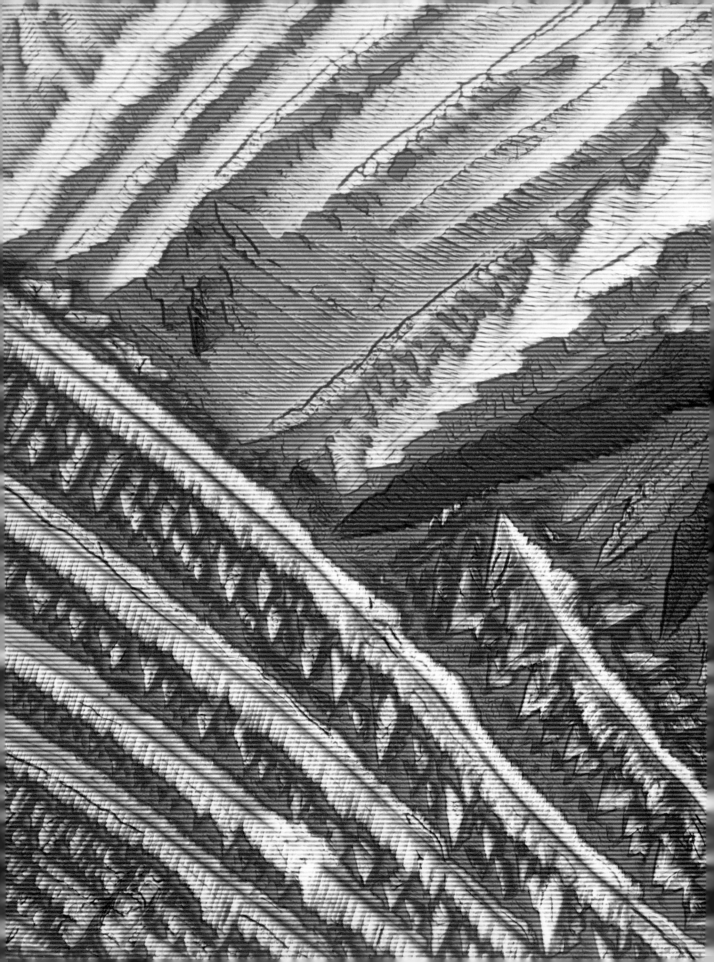

Hormonal System

A complex chemical communication system flows via the bloodstream and modifies the way we function on every level. Drug treatments are often effective in hormonal disorders, and nutritional controls are vital in diabetes. However, using herbs and other more subtle therapies can also enhance the function of these delicate systems.

DIABETES MELLITUS

In diabetes mellitus, the pancreas does not produce sufficient amounts of insulin, or body cells become resistant to its effects. In some cases, both abnormalities are present. The hormone insulin enables the body to absorb the sugar glucose from the bloodstream, which provides the cells with energy. Treatment aims to keep the amount of glucose in the blood within normal levels. This may be achieved through dietary measures, drug treatment, or insulin injections, depending on individual circumstances. Exercise and relaxation also help.

WHAT ARE THE SYMPTOMS?

- Excessive urination
- Thirst and a dry mouth
- Weight loss
- Blurred vision

WHY MIGHT I HAVE THIS?

PREDISPOSING FACTORS

For type 1 diabetes:

- Early exposure to cow's milk
- Exposure to viruses and environmental toxins
- Genetic tendency

For type 2 diabetes:

- Blood-sugar instability
- Overweight and obesity
- Stress
- Exposure to environmental toxins
- Genetic tendency

IMPORTANT

If someone with type 1 diabetes develops ketoacidosis (excessive thirst and urination, weakness, hyperventilation, nausea and vomiting, and breath that smells like nail polish remover), seek medical help at once. If someone with either type 1 or type 2 diabetes develops hypoglycemia (sweating, tremor, and drowsiness), give a sugary drink followed by a high-carbohydrate snack and monitor them. If they become unconscious, call 911 for an ambulance. Relatives of diabetics should familiarize themselves with the symptoms.

WHY DOES IT OCCUR?

TYPES There are two types of diabetes mellitus. In type 1, the pancreas produces little or no insulin. The disorder usually develops suddenly in childhood or adolescence, and a genetic tendency to diabetes is thought to be involved. In type 2 diabetes, which is much more common than type 1, the body cells become resistant to the effects of insulin, and there may also be a lack of insulin (but to a much lesser degree than occurs in type 1 diabetes). Type 2 develops slowly and may go unnoticed for many years. Like type 1 diabetes, type 2 may be due in part to a genetic tendency.

CAUSES Type 1 diabetes is usually caused by an autoimmune response in which the body produces antibodies against its own tissues, in this case the insulin-secreting cells of the pancreas. Although genes are thought to contribute to the development of type 1 diabetes, the actual triggers of the abnormal immune reaction are unknown. Viruses may also play a role.

Why type 2 diabetes develops is also not fully understood, but genes and obesity are important factors. Type 2 diabetes is a growing problem in affluent societies where food intake is excessive and increasing numbers of people, including children, are very overweight. The sedentary lifestyle led by many is also thought to be a major factor. Type 2 diabetes, which was once considered a disease of middle and old age, is now occurring in adolescents.

Diabetes mellitus sometimes develops temporarily during pregnancy, when it is known as gestational diabetes. Urine tests are done regularly at prenatal visits to check for the development of this kind of diabetes, which can usually be treated with dietary measures alone. Gestational diabetes usually resolves after the baby is born.

In a few cases, diabetes mellitus results from another disorder, such as cirrhosis (in which the liver becomes damaged, often as a result of chronic alcohol abuse) or long-term inflammation of the pancreas.

KETOACIDOSIS If individuals with type 1 diabetes miss their insulin or have another illness, such as an infection, that disrupts their blood-sugar control, unused glucose

TREATMENT PLAN

PRIMARY TREATMENTS

- Monitoring blood sugar
- Dietary changes
- Insulin (for type 1 diabetes)
- Antidiabetic drugs

BACKUP TREATMENTS

- Fish oil, vitamins, and minerals
- Exercise
- Acupuncture
- Relaxation and guided imagery

OTHER OPTIONS

- Homeopathy
- Massage
- Avoiding environmental toxins

For an explanation of how treatments are rated, see p.111.

NORMAL REGULATION OF BLOOD GLUCOSE

The amount of glucose (a simple sugar) in the blood is kept within a fairly narrow range by the body. The mechanism for keeping blood-glucose within these relatively narrow limits is complex and involves the liver and the pancreas. If blood-glucose levels are high, the pancreas produces insulin to enable the transport of glucose into body cells. If blood-glucose levels are low, the pancreas produces the hormone glucagon, which enables release of glucose reserves from the liver into the bloodstream.

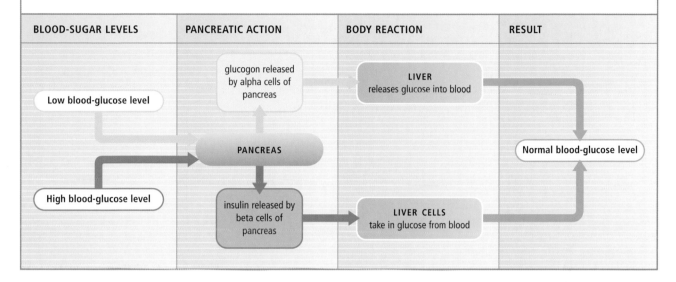

builds up in the blood and a condition known as diabetic ketoacidosis may arise. In this condition, the body begins to use its fat cells for energy, causing ketones (toxic substances) to be released into the blood. Ketoacidosis may lead to coma within a few hours without medical attention.

HYPOGLYCEMIA Hypoglycemia is a condition in which the level of blood sugar falls too low in a person with diabetes. The usual cause of hypoglycemia is too much insulin in the bloodstream, which may be caused by too high a dose or an incorrect diet. Hypoglycemia may also result from certain medications taken for type 2 diabetes (*see p.316*). Symptoms include sweating, tremor, and later drowsiness. If blood-sugar levels continue to fall, the person may lose consciousness or have a seizure.

LONG-TERM COMPLICATIONS The possible long-term complications of diabetes include coronary artery disease (*see p.252*), peripheral vascular disease (in which the blood supply to the limbs, hands, and feet is impaired) and stroke (*see p.148*). In addition, the retina (the light-sensitive layer at the back of the eye) may be damaged, kidney damage may occur, and neuropathy (*see p.127*) may develop,

symptoms of which may include tingling, numbness of the feet, and erectile dysfunction. These complications come about because diabetes damages blood vessels throughout the body, especially when it is poorly controlled. Why this damage occurs is not fully understood.

TREATMENTS IN DETAIL

Conventional Medicine

PRIMARY TREATMENT **MONITORING** Diabetes mellitus is usually diagnosed by measuring blood-glucose levels. People with diabetes must monitor their blood-sugar levels carefully and regularly.

In both type 1 and type 2 diabetes, regular checkups are necessary, not only to check blood-glucose control but also to look for evidence of any complications; for example the eyes are examined to look for damage to the retina. Peripheral vascular disease in diabetes mellitus makes the feet vulnerable to disease. It is very important to look after your feet carefully and to check them daily for signs of injury. Loss of sensation may prevent individuals from noticing damage to their feet and minor injuries may become serious without appropriate care.

PRIMARY TREATMENT **LIFESTYLE MODIFICATIONS** will be recommended for people with both types of diabetes mellitus, including a diabetic diet, exercising regularly, moderating alcohol intake, and refraining from smoking. The latter is important because smoking causes atherosclerosis (accumulation of fatty deposits in the arteries; *see p.252*) and can cause complications to occur earlier and to be more serious.

PRIMARY TREATMENT **INSULIN** People with type 1 diabetes need insulin injections to moderate the amount of glucose in their bloodstream. There are various types of insulin preparations available, some of which act more quickly than others.

The types of insulin given and the frequency of injections vary from person to person. The dose may need to be changed according to the blood-glucose levels.

Insulin is injected under the skin; common sites for injection are the wall of the abdomen and the outer thighs. The drug may be delivered by a needle and syringe or a pen device. Less commonly, pumps are used that can deliver insulin as a continuous trickle under the skin. The site of insulin injections should be changed regularly to avoid the development of fatty lumps in the area, which can affect insulin absorption.

PRIMARY TREATMENT **ANTIDIABETIC DRUGS** For type 2 diabetes the doctor may prescribe one or more drugs. These might include sulfonylurea drugs, such as tolbutamide and gliclazide, which stimulate the pancreas to produce insulin. These tend to be associated with weight increase and are therefore not usually given to people who are overweight. There is a small risk of hypoglycemia with these drugs.

The drug biguanide metformin may also be prescribed. It tends to be used less now due to its possible side effects (which include a small risk of hypoglycemia); however, unlike the sulfonylurea drugs, it is not associated with weight increase. It is thought to work by increasing the sensitivity of the tissues to insulin, which promotes glucose uptake.

Thiazolidinediones (also known as glitazones), such as rosiglitazone, are newer drugs that also increase the sensitivity of the tissues to insulin. They are used in combination with sulfonylureas or metformin. They may also be associated with weight gain and there is a small risk of hypoglycemia.

Other newer drugs known as meglitinides, such as repaglinide, may also be prescribed. These stimulate insulin production and are taken before meals. Side effects are relatively uncommon with these drugs but there is a small risk of hypoglycemia.

Finally, a group of drugs known as alpha-glucosidase inhibitors, such as acarbose, may be prescribed. These drugs delay the absorption of glucose in the small intestine, and help regulate blood-glucose levels.

CAUTION

Drugs for diabetes mellitus can cause a range of possible side effects; ask your doctor to explain these to you.

Nutritional Therapy

PRIMARY TREATMENT **DIETARY CHANGES** There is no substitute for good control of blood sugar in treating diabetes. Whatever the precise nature and cause of diabetes, eating a diet that helps keep blood-sugar levels steady is important. Eating regular meals with an emphasis on low-glycemic-index (GI) foods is the cornerstone of this approach. See p.44 for more details about how to do this.

Most people who have type 2 diabetes are overweight or obese. Excess weight around the middle of the body (abdominal fat) is believed to increase the risk of the body becoming resistant to the effects of insulin, which is a central feature in type 2 diabetes. Many studies show that type 2 diabetes improves with weight loss.

FISH OIL People who have type 2 diabetes may benefit from eating more oily fish (such as salmon, trout, mackerel, herring, and sardines). Those who eat fish regularly seem to be protected against the development of blood-sugar related problems, and some studies have demonstrated that fish-oil supplements can improve blood-sugar control in type 2 diabetes. If you have been diagnosed with type 2 diabetes, try taking 1g of concentrated fish oil, once or twice a day, and eat more oily fish.

ANTIOXIDANT studies in people with diabetes have not been impressive. A large study was conducted with 20,536 adults (aged 40–80) who had coronary artery disease, other occlusive arterial disease, or diabetes, and were given antioxidant therapy (600mg vitamin E, 250mg vitamin C, and 20mg beta-carotene daily) or a placebo. Over the five-year study period, there was no advantage to the antioxidant group in preventing heart attacks, strokes, or death, or by any other measure

VITAMIN E Studies indicate that taking vitamin E supplements improves blood-sugar control in people with type 2 diabetes, although benefits may not become apparent for three or more months. Vitamin E has also been shown to reduce a process known as glycosylation in diabetes. Glycosylation, when sugar binds to and damages protein molecules in the body, is thought to be an important cause of many of the complications of diabetes. If you have type 2 diabetes, it might be worth taking 400–800 IU vitamin E each day.

A recent trial of vitamin E supplements failed to show any benefit in preventing cardiovascular disease in people with diabetes. However, the supplemental dose used was quite low at 400mg per day.

VITAMIN C Studies on vitamin C for cardiovascular health in diabetics are mixed. One study in people with type 2 diabetes found that 500mg/day of vitamin C for a month effective for reducing blood pressure and arterial stiffness (a risk factor for cardiovascular disease). However, another study found that 1500mg/day had no effect on blood pressure or arterial function.

NICOTINAMIDE, a form of niacin, has been thought to delay loss of pancreatic function in children with type 1 diabetes, but a recent large, five-year long trial found no benefit of nicotinamide over placebo. The addition of vitamin E 15mg/kg to niacinamide helped preserve pancreatic function in children who were over 9 years old when they were diagnosed; there was no difference in children who were younger at diagnosis.

B VITAMINS Many people with diabetes have low blood levels of vitamin B_6. Vitamin B_6 supplementation may improve blood-sugar control. If you have diabetes, try taking 50–100mg of vitamin B_6 per day.

The B vitamin niacinamide (vitamin B_3) at a dose of 500mg daily for one month, followed by 250mg daily, has been shown to help some individuals with type 2 diabetes by reducing blood-sugar levels. If you have type 2 diabetes, try taking a supplement of niacinamide at these doses.

CHROMIUM Many clinical trials have been performed on the potential benefits of chromium for people with diabetes. A review of studies in people with type 2 diabetes found that 13 of 16 trials showed improved glucose levels, insulin levels, or lipids. Almost all positive studies involved doses of 400mg a day or more; all five studies with chromium picolinate, which is more bioavailable than other forms, had positive results with 1000mg a day. Chromium also appears to help impaired

The effect of diet on diabetes was first noticed during the siege of Paris in the early 1870s

glucose tolerance, a risk factor for diabetes. A review of controlled studies of chromium compounds found that 12 of 15 studies showed a benefit for the chromium-treated group.

MAGNESIUM Levels of magnesium are often low in people with diabetes and research shows that taking magnesium supplements can improve insulin production in type 2 diabetes. Some research suggests that insulin requirements are lower in people with type 1 diabetes who supplement with magnesium. If you have diabetes, take 300–400mg of magnesium daily.

Homeopathy

Although there is no substitute for good control of blood sugar, homeopathy can help in borderline type 2 diabetes and with certain complications. An individualized diagnosis from a skilled practitioner is essential. Medicines that may be helpful for diabetes and its complications include *Phosphoric acid*, *Phosphorus*, *Lycopodium*, *Secale*, and *Arsenicum album*.

PHOSPHORIC ACID may be useful in the early stages of the illness, particularly if the diabetes was precipitated by an acute illness or emotional upset. Typically the patient feels exhausted, especially mentally, with a very weak memory and poor concentration. There is profuse urination and there may also be diarrhea.

PHOSPHORUS People who respond to *Phosphorus* typically feel run down and tired but are briefly better from rest, and so feel better first thing in the morning. There is a general tendency toward easy bleeding, including nosebleeds and easy bruising of the skin. Other associated symptoms include recurrent laryngitis and vertigo, especially in older people. There may be pancreas or liver problems, such as pancreatitis. People who respond to *Phosphorus* tend to be slim and sensitive both to the human and physical environment. They may be phobic of things such as storms or being alone in the dark.

LYCOPODIUM will usually be prescribed on "constitutional" grounds (*see p.73*). It is typically appropriate for reserved, intellectual people with digestive problems. This medicine is indicated when there is right-sided pain or pain that starts on the right, before moving to the left. These people tend to feel worse between 4:00 PM and 8:00 PM.

ARSENICUM ALBUM AND SECALE may be indicated for the circulatory problems associated with diabetes. These medicines are indicated if the person's extremities are usually very cold. *Arsenicum album* is often helpful for skin ulcers associated with severe, burning pain.

Western Herbal Medicine

GINSENG reduces high blood sugar. A double-blind, placebo-controlled trial of ginseng extract *(Panax ginseng)* (200 mg daily for 8 weeks) reduced blood glucose levels and increased physical activity in patients recently diagnosed with type 2 diabetes. Three small placebo-controlled studies found that American ginseng (1–3g) reduced blood sugar in both healthy subjects and people with diabetes. Higher doses were not more effective.

Environmental Health

BREAST-FEEDING Many studies strongly indicate that early exposure to cow's milk may increase the likelihood of developing type 1 diabetes. Breast fed babies may have a lower risk of diabetes later in life.

TOXINS Possible environmental triggers for diabetes include nitrosamines, dioxins, and dioxin-like compounds (DLCs), nitrates, arsenic, and smoking.

NITROSAMINE compounds, most prevalent in cured and smoked meats, have been proven to cause damage to the pancreas and hasten the onset of diabetes. You should try to avoid these products, especially if you have other risk factors for diabetes.

DIOXINS AND DLCS are highly toxic environmental contaminants and by-products of certain industries. They may be implicated in diabetes because they compete for receptors with the body's natural hormones. It is estimated that 90 percent of human exposure to dioxins occurs through the food supply. Although the relationship between dioxin exposure and diabetes is speculative, you can decrease your dioxin exposure by trimming fat from meat, consuming low-fat dairy products, and cooking food as simply as possible. Avoid eating predatory fish from rivers or lakes known to be contaminated with dioxins or close to industrial centers.

NITRATES AND ARSENIC are both threats to the water supply and have been associated with increased prevalence of diabetes. Nitrates are toxic to the pancreas, while arsenic disrupts the insulin receptor and glucose transport mechanisms in the body.

The primary sources of nitrates include human sewage and livestock manure and fertilizers. Arsenic, a naturally occurring element, is a component of many pesticides. To reduce the risk of nitrate and arsenic exposure, you should be aware of your community's water quality and have your water checked.

VACOR A final example of a toxin that may lead to diabetes is the rodenticide Vacor. This N-nitroso compound was clearly shown to induce diabetes because of its toxic effects on the beta cells of the pancreas. Although Vacor was removed from the commercial market in the late 1970s, if it was used to treat your home or workplace environment, traces of it may still be present. Check with your local environmental protection agency if you are concerned.

Acupuncture

The overall control of diabetes lies firmly within the sphere of diet, exercise, and appropriate medication to normalize blood-sugar levels. However, frequently people with diabetes develop neurological and circulatory disorders associated with the slow degeneration of the blood supply to various organs and tissues. Acupuncture may help stave off these complications by directly improving local microcirculation. Studies indicate that long-term acupuncture may help diabetic neuropathy and improve digestive function. There is also some evidence that acupuncture may affect the autonomic nervous sytem and create vasodilation, which can maximize blood flow to organs that are potentially affected by diabetes. While not definitely proven, this is probably the mechanism through which acupuncture may be of assistance in conditions such as diabetic retinopathy and intermittent claudication.

Massage

Stress levels seem to strongly influence both the progression and seriousness of type 2 diabetes. Stress appears to affect blood-sugar levels, causing them to rise, and may also make individuals more susceptible to unhealthy habits, such as smoking. Massage has been shown to reduce stress levels and

to allow better control of blood-sugar levels. Research was done on the effect of parents giving massages regularly to children with type 1 diabetes. Twenty-four children, between ages five and eight, either were taught to use progressive muscular relaxation methods (which were carried out under supervision by a parent just before bedtime) or were given a daily 15-minute massage by a parent just before bedtime.

Both groups improved, but both parents and children in the massage group showed greater reduction in stress and anxiety. The children showed behavioral improvements as well. Most importantly, the outcome at the end of the month was that blood-glucose levels decreased significantly toward the normal range in the massage group.

Exercise

Regular exercise has a positive effect on many aspects of type 2 diabetes, including better functioning of insulin and improved metabolism of glucose and fats. Exercise can also be a powerful preventive measure for those likely to develope type 2 diabetes.

The best type of exercise for people with diabetes is aerobic exercise, although yoga (see right) can be beneficial for reducing stress levels. Brisk walking, done for 20–30 minutes at least five times a week, is a good way to begin. Begin any exercise regimen gradually and, if you have diabetes, check with your doctor first.

If you have type 1 diabetes, you may need to monitor your blood-glucose levels before, during, and after any strenuous exercise to determine how the activity affects your need for insulin and food.

Yoga

Practicing yoga regularly can help lower stress levels, which affect blood-sugar levels (see Mind–Body Therapies, below). The slower, gentler forms of yoga are the most suitable for this purpose. Yoga that emphasizes slow, abdominal breathing is particularly good for reducing stress.

Type 2 diabetes is becoming increasingly common in children and adolescents

Mind–Body Therapies

STRESS AND BLOOD SUGAR Stress affects blood sugar directly and indirectly. It can cause chronic overproduction of stress hormones, such as epinephrine and cortisol, making blood-sugar levels rise. Also, people under stress tend to adopt unhealthy habits, such as a poor diet, not exercising, smoking, and drinking alcohol, all of which can have a negative impact on blood-sugar levels.

Studies demonstrate a strong physiological relationship between stress and blood-sugar levels in people with diabetes. For example, researchers in Japan studied the health effects of the 1995 Kobe earthquake. Compared to diabetics in the city of Osaka, where little earthquake damage occurred, Kobe residents with diabetes found it harder to manage their blood sugar. Research also suggests that stress can increase insulin resistance.

IMPROVING COMPLIANCE Many people with diabetes find their dietary restrictions and medication programs burdensome and frustrating. Anxiety and depression may develop, leading some people with diabetes to ignore dietary restrictions and neglect drug treatment some or all of the time.

Failure of patients to comply with dietary measures and drug treatment to control diabetes is the biggest cause of diabetic complications, which include kidney failure, blindness (due to diabetic retinopathy), amputation (due to peripheral vascular problems), and heart disease.

However, when depression and anxiety can be alleviated using mind–body techniques, compliance with diet and drug

treatment regimens tends to improve, leading to a better quality of life for people with diabetes, as well as fewer short- and long-term complications from the condition.

SELF-HELP TECHNIQUES Practicing mind–body techniques such as relaxation and guided imagery regularly (see p.99) may be especially beneficial if you have type 2 diabetes. These techniques may enable you to manage stress more effectively and thereby have better control over your blood-glucose levels and your diabetes in general.

RELAXATION AND SELF-HYPNOSIS Mood improvement techniques are a vital component of diabetes management, especially in type 2 diabetes, where they appear to lower blood-glucose levels directly. Researchers at the Medical College of Ohio found that depression and anxiety were partially relieved through relaxation and self-hypnosis.

GUIDED IMAGERY Researchers at the University of Wisconsin-Green Bay also found that diabetes patients who listened to guided imagery tapes took better care of themselves in general and also complied more closely with their care regimens.

STRESS-MANAGEMENT PROGRAMS In a randomized trial at Duke University Medical Center, patients with type 2 diabetes who participated in a five-session stress-management program (including training in relaxation, imagery, and other techniques) showed significant reductions in blood-glucose levels. Laughter was also found to lower the increase in blood glucose that follows a meal.

PREVENTION PLAN

The following may help prevent the onset of diabetes:

- Breast-feeding
- Lose weight if you are overweight
- Follow a blood-sugar stabilizing diet
- Exercise regularly
- Avoid environmental toxins
- Do relaxation and guided imagery exercises to reduce stress levels

THYROID PROBLEMS

The thyroid gland, located in the neck, produces two types of hormones, both of which help control the body's metabolism (the rate at which it burns fuel). The most common thyroid disorders are hyperthyroidism, in which excessive amounts of thyroid hormones are produced, and hypothyroidism, in which insufficient amounts are produced. Since 1960, newborns have been tested for hypothyroidism. The aim of treatment is to restore the normal balance of thyroid hormones. Hormonal and other drugs are usually tried first, before surgery.

WHAT ARE THE SYMPTOMS?

Symptoms of hyperthyroidism:
- Weight loss, despite increased appetite
- Palpitations
- Trembling of the hands (tremors)
- Lowered tolerance to heat
- Excessive sweating
- Anxiety and insomnia
- Swelling in the neck
- Frequent bowel movements
- Muscle weakness
- Irregular menstruation
- Protruding eyes (exophthalmos) in Graves' disease

Symptoms of hypothyroidism:
- Fatigue
- Poor memory
- Weight gain
- Constipation
- Deepened voice
- Swelling in the neck
- Lowered tolerance to cold
- Puffy eyes and dry, thickened skin
- Generalized thinning of the hair
- Heavy or less frequent menstrual periods
- Weakness and aching of muscles
- Joint pains

WHY MIGHT I HAVE THIS?

PREDISPOSING FACTORS

For hyperthyroidism:
- Genetic predisposition

For hypothyroidism:
- Previous radioiodine treatment or surgery for hyperthyroidism

IMPORTANT

Rarely, hyperthyroidism gets worse very rapidly. Symptoms may include a high fever and agitation. If this happens, seek medical help immediately.

WHY DOES IT OCCUR?

Hyperthyroidism (an overactive thyroid gland) may have several causes, the most common of which is Graves' disease, an autoimmune disorder in which antibodies attack the thyroid gland, causing it to produce excess hormones. Graves' disease appears to have a genetic component. Hypothyroidism (an underactive thyroid) may also have a variety of causes, the most common being atrophic thyroiditis, in which antibodies are produced that result in shrinkage of and damage to thyroid tissue. Radioactive iodine or surgery to treat hyperthyroidism (by destroying or removing part of the thyroid gland) can also result in permanent hypothyroidism, for which thyroid hormone supplements must be taken. Insufficient iodine in the diet can cause hypothyroidism, but this is rare in developed countries. Only a minute quantity of iodine is required each day and it is normally obtained through vegetables, drinking water, and seafood.

Thyroid disorders are common, but onset is usually gradual and they may not be diagnosed for months or even years. In both hyper- and hypothyroidism, an enlarged thyroid gland (goiter) may cause swelling in the neck. Both conditions are more common in women. Children born with hypothyroidism may develop the small stature and subnormal intelligence of cretinism if the condition is not treated.

TREATMENT PLAN

PRIMARY TREATMENTS

For hyperthyroidism:
- Antithyroid drugs
- Radioiodine

For hypothyroidism:
- Thyroid hormone replacement

BACKUP TREATMENTS
- Surgery to remove part of the thyroid gland (for hyperthyroidism)
- Iodine and other nutritional supplements

WORTH CONSIDERING
- Thyroid glandulars
- Spa treatment
- Avoiding toxic chemicals
- Acupuncture
- Manual lymphatic drainage (after surgery)

For an explanation of how treatments are rated, see p.111.

TREATMENTS IN DETAIL

Conventional Medicine

Your doctor will arrange for blood tests to check the levels of thyroid hormones and the level of thyroid stimulating hormone (TSH), which is produced by the pituitary gland and controls the production of thyroid hormones. He will also look at your neck to see if the thyroid is enlarged.

PRIMARY TREATMENT **TREATMENT FOR HYPERTHYROIDISM** If hyperthyroidism is diagnosed, there are three treatment options: drugs, radioiodine, and surgery.

THYROID FUNCTION

The body has a complex system for regulating the function of the thyroid gland, which is situated in the neck just below the Adam's apple. The hypothalamus secretes thyrotropin-releasing hormone (TRH), which causes the pituitary gland to release thyroid-stimulating hormone (TSH).

This hormone causes the thyroid gland to produce thyroid hormones T_3 and T_4. When levels of thyroid hormones in the blood reach a certain level, the pituitary gland produces less TSH. If the levels of thyroid hormones drop too low, the pituitary gland produces more TSH.

Thyroid hormone feedback mechanism

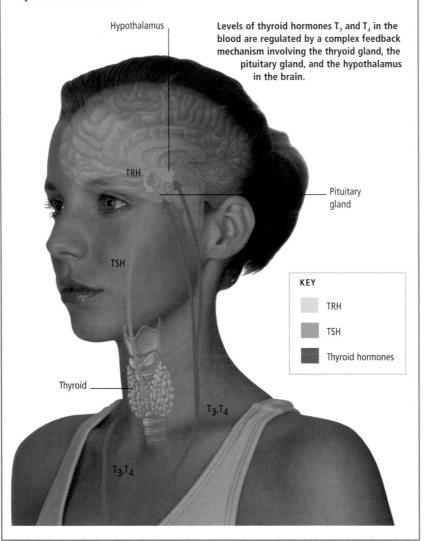

Hypothalamus

Levels of thyroid hormones T_3 and T_4 in the blood are regulated by a complex feedback mechanism involving the thryoid gland, the pituitary gland, and the hypothalamus in the brain.

TRH

Pituitary gland

TSH

KEY

TRH

TSH

Thyroid hormones

Thyroid

T_3, T_4

T_3, T_4

The first option is antithyroid drugs, such as methimazole and propylthiouracil, used to prevent production of thyroid hormones. Symptoms may take up to three weeks to improve with these drugs, and beta-blockers may be used in the interim. In some cases, antithyroid drugs may be needed for two years or more. Hyperthyroidism recurs in about half of all people treated.

The second option is treatment with radioiodine to destroy some of the thyroid tissue. This involves taking a capsule containing radioactive iodine, which accumulates in the thyroid. Thyroid hormone levels usually take up to three months to return to normal following treatment. There is a risk of developing hypothyroidism after this treatment.

The third treatment option is surgery to remove part of the thyroid gland. Possible side effects include damage to the nerves supplying the voice box, resulting in hoarseness, and hypothyroidism.

PRIMARY TREATMENT **TREATMENT FOR HYPOTHY-ROIDISM** requires thyroid hormone replacement; the drug is taken in tablet form. The levels of thyroid hormones are monitored by blood tests and the dose may be increased or decreased as necessary. It may take up to six months for symptoms to be brought under control and treatment is likely to be lifelong.

> **CAUTION**
>
> Drugs for hyperthyroidism and hypothyroidism can cause a range of possible side effects; ask your doctor to explain these to you.

Nutritional Therapy

The thyroid is essentially the body's thermostat, which determines its temperature as well as the speed at which it burns fuel. If, for any reason, thyroid function is disrupted, none of the cells in the body tend to function as well as they should. There are many tests to measure how efficiently the thyroid gland is working and whether it is over- or underproducing hormones (*see p.319 and p.43*).

SUPPLEMENTS If mild hypothyroidism is the problem, several herbs and nutrients may help, including iodine, selenium, vitamin A, and the amino acid L-tyrosine. Some practitioners recommend supplements containing actual thyroid tissue. These extracts, often referred to as "thyroid glandulars," are usually made from cow or pig thyroid and should only be taken under the supervision of a doctor experienced in their use (*see p.43*).

FOODS TO AVOID Brassica vegetables (such as broccoli, cabbage, brussels sprouts, and cauliflower) contain glucosinolates, which can impair the uptake of iodine into the thyroid and thereby affect thyroid function. For this reason, vegetables from the brassica family are best avoided by anyone with thyroid problems.

Homeopathy

Homeopathy may be useful alongside conventional drugs in alleviating symptoms when the thyroid has become overactive. The most useful medicines are *Iodum*, *Lachesis*, *Lycopus*, and *Natrum muriaticum*.

IODUM This medicine is useful if exophthalmos (protruding eyes), caused by hyperthyroidism, is present. The patient may be very thin but with a good appetite.

He or she may feel hot most of the time and want to be in the open air. These patients feel worse in a warm room and better after eating and strenuous exercise.

OTHER MEDICINES, such as *Lachesis*, *Lycopus*, and *Natrum muriaticum*, should be used only under the supervision of an experienced homeopath in collaboration with your doctor. Under- or overactive thyroid problems always require conventional investigation and, unless mild, conventional treatment.

Environmental Health

Thyroid function can be altered by many substances in the environment, such as herbicides, pesticides, fungicides, organohalogen compounds (for example, polyhalogenated aromatic hydrocarbons (PHAHs), polychlorinated biphenyls (PCBs), and chemicals in cigarette smoke. These agents can all disrupt the distribution and action of hormones, including those involved in thyroid function.

HERBICIDES AND PESTICIDES You should limit the use of these products around your work and home environments, especially when there are small children present. Any substances that affect thyroid function can be particularly disruptive for children, given the importance of thyroid hormones in fetal and childhood development. Try to choose organic foods as much as possible. These foods, when certified organic by a reputable regulatory body, are free of herbicides, pesticides, fungicides, fertilizers, and other contaminants.

PCBS AND PHAHS Polychlorinated biphenyl compounds (PCBs) and polyhalogenated aromatic hydrocarbons (PHAHs) are human-made compounds used in plastics and other industries that can disrupt the body's hormonal system.

The two PHAHs most commonly implicated in thyroid problems are polychlorinated biphenyl compounds (PCBs) and dioxins. They share a similar structure with natural thyroid hormones and may interfere with thyroid function by imitating the natural hormones, rendering actual thyroid hormones inactive.

PCBs and PHAHs are common environmental contaminants, despite recent efforts to remove them. The production of PCBs was banned in the US in 1977, but people can still be exposed to them through contact with old transformers, capacitors, fluorescent lighting fixtures, and old electrical devices and appliances. The most common source of exposure for people is from contaminated food, such as predatory fish caught in contaminated waterways.

Dioxins are found everywhere in the environment, and most people are exposed to very small background levels of dioxins from the air, food, or milk, or have skin contact with dioxin-contaminated materials. For the general population, more than 90 percent of the daily intake of dioxins comes from food, mainly meat, dairy products, and fish.

PHAHs require a long time to degrade in the environment and become concentrated in higher levels of the food chain (bioaccumulation), especially in the fatty tissues of animals. Bioaccumulation occurs when PHAHs first enter the soil or water and then contaminated plants are eaten by animals, until even the largest predators are affected. To reduce your exposure to PHAHs, you should choose low-fat meat products and trim excess fat off the meat. Limit or avoid consumption of predatory fish or fish from sources that are known to be contaminated with PHAHs.

Acupuncture

Thyroid disease, whether due to an under- or overactive thyroid, always needs conventional diagnosis and treatment. Acupuncture may occasionally be used for the treatment of some of the symptoms but is not a treatment for thyroid disease itself.

Acupuncture may be able to help generalized aches and pains, lack of energy in people receiving conventional thyroid treatment, and sometimes the relief of symptoms that may be caused by thyroid eye disease.

Depending on the severity and acuteness of the thyroid problem, acupuncture should show benefits in four to six weekly treatment sessions, based on a traditional Chinese approach. Talk with your acupuncturist if no benefit is apparent.

Bodywork Therapies

Evidence suggests spa therapies and massage may help in the treatment of thyroid conditions. Russian research, for example, suggests that spa treatment (involving mud and electrotherapy) for children with cardiac conditions produced general health benefits including a positive trend in thyroid conditions.

MANUAL LYMPHATIC DRAINAGE Surgery for thyroid problems sometimes results in local swelling and fluid retention (edema). A study evaluated the benefits of massage to encourage normal circulation and drainage in such situations. A type of gentle massage known as manual lymphatic drainage was found to eliminate swelling and edema completely in approximately half of cases after 10 days of daily massage. The researchers concluded that massage therapy of the neck is necessary in all patients who have had surgery to the thyroid gland.

> **CAUTION**
>
> Do not have neck massage or manipulation if you have an enlarged thyroid (goiter).

The Dublin physician Dr. Robert Graves first described hyperthyroidism with goitre in 1835

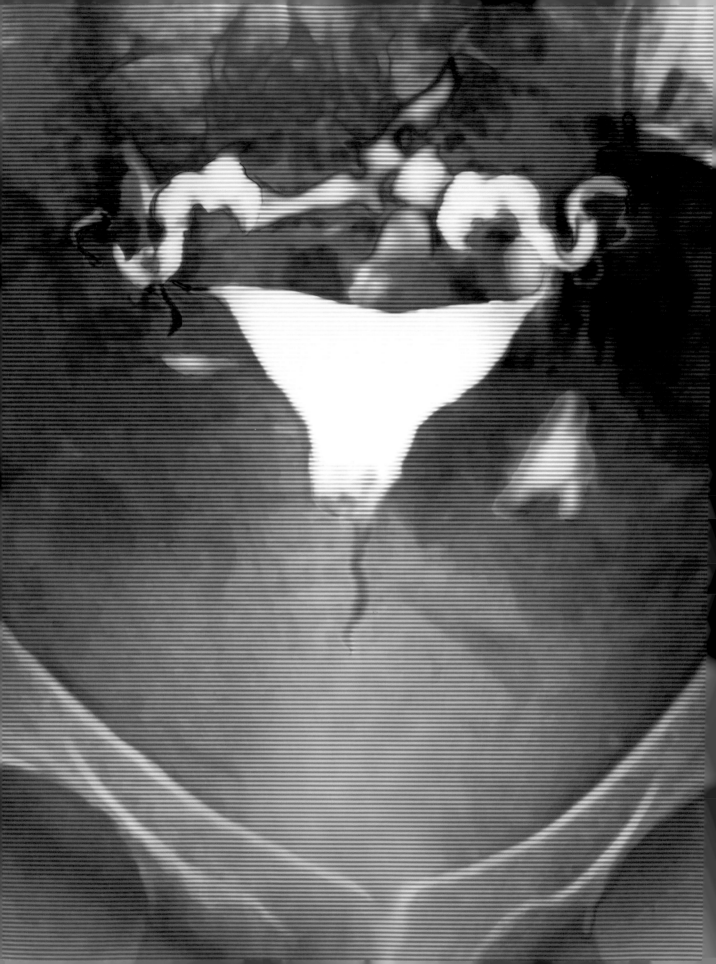

Women's Health

Many women's health issues are linked to monthly changes in hormones. Common problems respond well to drugs, and dietary changes or supplements. Talking therapies can be useful in managing emotional fluctuations and their effects, while the gentle influence of herbs and other complementary therapies also helps keep hormones in balance.

WHAT ARE THE SYMPTOMS?

- Tenderness and/or lumpiness of the breasts
- A feeling of being bloated, caused by fluid retention
- Mood changes, including irritability, depression, and anxiety
- Feeling tired
- Difficulty concentrating and making decisions
- Headaches, including migraines
- Backache and muscle stiffness
- Disrupted sleep
- Unusual food cravings

WHY MIGHT I HAVE THIS?

PREDISPOSING FACTORS

- High-sugar diet
- Caffeine
- Genetic tendency

PREMENSTRUAL SYNDROME

The term premenstrual syndrome (PMS) is used to describe a varying combination of symptoms that begin in the two weeks before menstruation and stop by the end of the period. The condition affects as many as one woman in three, and in one woman in 20 it is severe enough to disrupt her life. Treatment for PMS usually depends on the symptoms and their severity, but might involve hormonal and other drugs and dietary changes. Manipulation therapy, exercise, acupuncture, and relaxation can also be beneficial.

WHY DOES IT OCCUR?

The cause of PMS is not known, but it is thought that the symptoms are triggered by the action of the female sex hormones, particularly progesterone, in the weeks or days before menstruation.

Sugar, caffeine, and stress may all make the symptoms worse, and women are more likely to experience the condition if close female relatives have had similar problems, suggesting that genetic factors may be involved.

SELF-HELP

In the weeks before menstruation:
- Reduce or eliminate caffeinated beverages, including coffee, tea, and cola
- Avoid sugary foods and snacks, such as chocolate, and try to keep your blood-sugar levels stable (*see p.42*).
- Do regular, moderate exercise.
- Practice relaxation exercises, yoga, or meditation.

TREATMENTS IN DETAIL

Conventional Medicine

There are many possible treatments for premenstrual syndrome, ranging from dietary supplements and exercise to hormonal drugs. Vitamin B$_6$ supplements may help relieve the symptoms, as may regular aerobic exercise. Relaxation techniques may be helpful and may also be recommended (*see p.327*).

TREATMENT PLAN

PRIMARY TREATMENTS
- Combined oral contraceptive pill
- Nonsteroidal anti-inflammatory drugs for headaches and backache
- Chaste-tree berry

BACKUP TREATMENTS
- Other hormonal medicines
- Diuretics for fluid retention
- Magnesium
- Elimination of caffeine and sugar
- Antidepressants

WORTH CONSIDERING
- Vitamin B$_6$ and other supplements
- Evening primrose oil and other herbal medicines
- Individualized homeopathy
- Massage and relaxation
- Reflexology
- Exercise
- Acupuncture

For an explanation of how treatments are rated, see p.111.

PRIMARY TREATMENT **FIRST-LINE TREATMENTS** The combined oral contraceptive pill can help relieve PMS symptoms. Nonsteroidal anti-inflammatory drugs (NSAIDs) such as ibuprofen can help with headaches and backaches.

PRIMARY TREATMENT **TREATMENTS FOR SEVERE SYMPTOMS** If symptoms are persistent and troublesome, certain other drugs may be suggested.

The antidepressants known as SSRIs (selective serotonin reuptake inhibitors), such as fluoxetine, have been shown to relieve premenstrual symptoms.

Danazol prevents ovulation and reduces PMS symptoms. However, due to side effects associated with long-term use, such as hirsutism (increased body hair), acne, and voice deepening, it is given for only short periods.

Certain drugs known as gonadotropin-releasing hormone (GnRH) analogs inhibit the release of the sex hormones estrogen and progesterone and reduce PMS symptoms. However, they cannot be used for more than six months because they may cause osteoporosis (*see p.308*).

DRUGS FOR SPECIFIC SYMPTOMS Studies have shown that the diuretic spironolactone improves symptoms of PMS associated with fluid retention, such as breast tenderness and bloating. Bromocriptine is a drug that acts on the pituitary gland (the tiny gland at the base of the brain); it also relieves breast tenderness

> **CAUTION**
>
> Drugs for PMS can cause a range of possible side effects; ask your doctor to explain these to you.

Nutritional Therapy

CAFFEINE AND SUGAR In clinical practice, both caffeine and sugar seem to increase the risk of PMS. In a number of studies, women who ate more sugary foods appeared to have an increased risk of PMS. Research also showed that consumption of caffeine-containing beverages is associated with increases in prevalence and severity of PMS.

MULTIVITAMIN SUPPLEMENTS A daily multivitamin and mineral supplement may be one of the simplest ways to help reduce PMS symptoms. There is evidence that this can bring positive benefits.

VITAMIN B$_6$ A number of studies support taking vitamin B$_6$ for PMS. It can help relieve a variety of premenstrual symptoms, including depression, irritability, tension, violence, coordination, breast tenderness, bloating, headache, and acne. The effective dose for most women seems to be 100mg vitamin B$_6$ per day.

VITAMIN E$_6$ Various double-blind studies have demonstrated that vitamin E can cause a reduction in PMS symptoms. The recommended dosage is 400 IU per day.

MAGNESIUM Studies show that women who are commonly affected by PMS are often deficient in magnesium and that supplementation of this mineral may reduce symptoms. In a double-blind trial, a daily supplement of 200mg of magnesium over a two-month period produced significant improvement in women with PMS, resulting in reduced fluid retention, breast tenderness, and abdominal bloating. Magnesium supplements may also relieve menstrual migraine. A reasonable dose to try would be 200–400mg per day for two to three months.

CALCIUM Taking calcium supplements appears to relieve PMS symptoms. Women who include a lot of calcium in their diets experience less PMS, and, when they do have it, the symptoms are less severe. In a large, double-blind trial over the course of three menstrual cycles, women who took 1200mg of calcium per day had a 48 percent reduction in PMS symptoms, compared to a 30 percent reduction in the placebo (sham treatment) group. Other double-blind trials have also shown that taking 1000mg of calcium per day relieves PMS symptoms.

ZINC It is possible that some women who experience PMS have lower levels of zinc in their bodies, particularly during certain times in their ovulatory cycle. Taking 50mg of zinc per day may be useful for women who are affected by PMS. If you take zinc supplements, you should also take 1mg of copper for every 15mg of supplemental zinc because zinc supplements can induce copper deficiency.

> **CAUTION**
>
> Zinc, magnesium, and calcium can reduce the effectiveness of certain drugs, including some antibiotics, beta-blockers, and blood-thinning drugs, such as warfarin. Ask your doctor for advice. (*For more information, see p.46.*) People with kidney problems should not take calcium supplements.

Homeopathy

A clinical trial showed that individualized homeopathy is effective in PMS. Five homeopathic medicines were used: *Lachesis*, *Natrum muriaticum*, *Nux vomica*, *Pulsatilla*, and *Sepia*.

LACHESIS is useful for women whose PMS symptoms improve soon after bleeding begins. These women cannot tolerate tight clothes and collars and may have a sensation of constriction at the throat. They may have hot flashes and find it difficult to breathe lying down. They tend to sleep on their right side and most of their menstrual pain is on the left side of the body. There may be dark clots in the menstrual blood. These women tend to have a jealous or suspicious disposition, and this may become much worse during the premenstrual period.

NATRUM MURIATICUM is prescribed when women with PMS have a taste for salty things. They often have headaches, which tend to start in the morning and are caused or made worse by exposure to the sun. These women tend to be sad and averse to consolation; they are reserved, closed, and prefer to be alone.

> ## Women who have had more children tend to get more severe PMS symptoms

NUX VOMICA may be useful for women who have constipation as part of their PMS symptoms. These women are generally tense and irritable and are very sensitive to cold, noise, and smells and may drink a lot of coffee.

> **CAUTION**
>
> Avoid coffee if taking *Nux vomica*.

PULSATILLA is useful for women whose periods stop at night and in whom the menstrual flow is generally intermittent. These women tend to feel worse in closed rooms. They weep easily, but their moods change rapidly. They dislike being alone. During the night, their feet become hot.

SEPIA may be used when women have much vaginal discharge that is greenish in color. Their sexual drive is low or diminished and they may feel pressure or heaviness in the lower abdomen. In these women menstruation usually starts in the morning. They feel detached, indifferent, or irritable, especially toward their families.

Western Herbal Medicine

An herbalist selects a range of plant medicines to relieve PMS symptoms. For example, cramp bark (*Viburnum opulus*) and wild yam (*Dioscorea villosa*) can pro-

chosen. These help to correct imbalances in hormone release by the pituitary gland. For example, chaste-tree berry (*Vitex agnus-castus*) inhibits secretion of several hormones including prolactin. Chaste-tree berry is the most frequently used herb for PMS, helping regulate the menstrual cycle and improve hormone balance. Clinical studies involving over 5,000 women have found it has positive benefits in PMS (and to a lesser extent in relieving breast pain).

There are other herbs with a hormonal action. For example, helonias (*Chamaelirium lutea*) improves ovarian function.

RELAXING HERBS In addition to advising women to exercise and rest, an herbalist will, when appropriate, prescribe relaxant and adaptogenic herbs (which help the body adapt to stress), such as withania (*Withania somnifera*). If there is nervous irritablity or other emotional disturbance, sedative, relaxant, or stimulant herbs such as St. John's wort (*Hypericum perforatum*) will be given. Other herbs commonly used to treat emotional disturbance, especially irritability, include skullcap (*Scutellaria laterifolia*), vervain (*Verbena officinalis*), and linden flowers (*Tilia cordata*).

EVENING PRIMROSE OIL Research results are contradictory of the value of taking evening primrose (*Oenothera biennis*) oil. However, the oil is rich in gamma-linolenic

Acuncture

Acupuncture

There are several small and limited studies of a Traditional Chinese Medicine-based approach to treating premenstrual syndrome, and all the evidence suggests that acupuncture is an effective treatment for the symptoms of PMS.

Clinical experience suggests that acupuncture has a long-term effect on PMS; it prevents symptoms from recurring in menstrual cycles after treatment has been completed. Ideally, women should have several treatment sessions over two to three months.

Bodywork Therapies

A review of pooled research to examine the benefits of manual therapies such as massage, reflexology, and chiropractic in the treatment of PMS concluded: "Despite some positive findings, the evidence was not compelling for any of these therapies, with most trials suffering from various methodological limitations. On the basis of current evidence, no complementary/alternative therapy can be recommended as a treatment for premenstrual syndrome."

However, among the "positive findings" discounted in this overview are some studies that seem to strongly suggest that there are indeed benefits to be gained in using methods such as massage, reflexology, chiropractic, aerobic exercise, and acupressure in treating PMS.

> Premenstrual syndrome was first recognised as a medical disorder by Dr T. Frank in 1931

vide relief from period cramps and, in the longer term, help restore menstrual regularity and hormonal balance.

DETOXIFICATION Herbs such as dandelion root (*Taraxacum officinale*) may be given to stimulate liver and colon function. They promote detoxification and elimination, clearing toxins from the body. Improved liver metabolism also leads to a reduced load on the kidneys.

PRIMARY TREATMENT **CHASTE-TREE BERRY** Hormone-balancing herbs, which act on the pituitary gland, will be

acid (GLA), and there is some evidence that women with PMS have trouble metabolizing linoleic acid, which is converted in the body to GLA. Therefore, extra GLA should theoretically be helpful in PMS. If you want to try evening primrose oil, take 3–4g per day for several menstrual cycles. It may be particularly helpful if you have breast tenderness or fibrocystic disease.

> **CAUTION**
>
> See p.69 before taking a herbal remedy and, if you are already taking prescribed medication, consult a medical herbalist first.

MASSAGE AND RELAXATION In one study, 24 women with a history of severe PMS were divided into two groups, one received massage (twice weekly for 30 minutes for five weeks) while the other group was instructed in the use of progressive muscle relaxation methods, to be followed for 30 minutes, twice weekly for five weeks. The results showed that those women in the massage group had significantly reduced anxiety levels and improved mood, along with reduction in pain and fluid retention levels, when compared with the women in the relaxation group.

REFLEXOLOGY may also be beneficial for women who regularly experience PMS. In a study of 32 women with PMS, half had treatment to specific reflexology points on the feet, hands, and ears and the other half

REFLEXOLOGY FOR PREMENSTRUAL SYNDROME

Reflexology, in which points on the feet (and sometimes on the hands and ears) are pressed to influence health in corresponding parts of the body, may be effective in relieving both the physical and psychological symptoms of PMS. You can visit a reflexologist, or you can perform reflexology for yourself. The most relevant point on the feet for relieving PMS and menstrual pain is shown in the picture below. For PMS, you should work the uterus reflex area every day throughout the month. For menstrual pain, work the uterus reflex area three or four times a day until the pain subsides. Do one foot at a time, giving each foot equal treatment.

Using your thumb, press firmly on the uterus reflex area just above the inside of the heel (*shown below*). You can also press on this area while rotating the ankle, first clockwise, then counterclockwise.

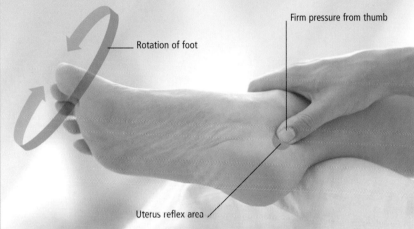

Rotation of foot

Firm pressure from thumb

Uterus reflex area

had "placebo" reflexology (i.e. gentle massage to these general areas). Symptom records were kept daily for the week prior to the next period. The results are described in the study as follows: "At the end of the study the reflexology group reported a 45 percent decrease in both somatic (bodily) and psychological symptoms, compared with a 20 percent reduction in the placebo group."

Exercise

The effects of aerobic exercise and strength training on premenstrual symptoms were evaluated in 23 women. Results showed that while participation in both forms of exercise was associated with an improvement of many premenstrual symptoms, the symptoms of those women in the aerobic group (especially their premenstrual depression) improved more markedly.

If you experience PMS on a regular basis, you could try doing some mild aerobic exercise, such as fast walking, for at least 20 minutes, three times a week. Try to exercise in the open air if possible.

Regular exercise of the abdomen and pelvis, such as occurs in Egyptian belly dancing, is also worthwhile. It can be particularly helpful in relieving PMS and menstrual cramps.

Yoga

Practicing yoga may help reduce stress in the weeks leading up to menstruation. Some practitioners also believe that practicing yoga on a regular basis can help regulate hormone levels in the body. In this way, doing yoga may help reduce the severity of PMS symptoms.

Yoga for easing PMS symptoms should be gentle, incorporating plenty of floor poses. Poses that work the low back, such as the bridge and the cobra, may influence the kidneys and adrenal glands and relieve fatigue. These poses have the added advantage of easing any muscle tension and stiffness in the low back.

Yoga that incorporates side stretches helps tone the muscles as well as improve overall flexibility. Poses that open the chest, such as the fish, can also help reduce stress levels and, done on a regular basis, may promote calmness and clarity.

If you have not done yoga or stretching exercises before or have not done them for some time and would like to try yoga, be sure to start gradually. Make sure you listen to your body and do not try to do too much too soon.

Mind-Body Therapies

RELAXATION AND GUIDED IMAGERY If you experience PMS regularly, you could try doing 20 to 30 minutes of relaxation exercises or meditation daily throughout the month. (*For a sequence of relaxation exercises, see p.99.*) You could also try using a relaxation or guided imagery tape, or a tape of soothing music or sounds.

Regular relaxation has proven effective in dealing with both the physical and emotional symptoms of PMS, according to a number of studies. One study looking at biofeedback, for example, found "a significant positive correlation" between frontal muscle tension (which is felt in the forehead) and the psychological symptoms of PMS. If the tension can be relieved, the psychological symptoms may also be eased. In another study, women who participated in a regular relaxation program reported a significant improvement of 58 percent in their premenstrual symptoms.

Using relaxation therapies and guided imagery to reduce the severity of PMS can lead to lowered stress, increased comfort, and decreased absenteeism, without the cost and potential undesirable side effects of some medications.

PREVENTION PLAN

The following may help if you are prone to PMS:

- Avoid caffeine and sugar, at least in the weeks leading up to menstruation.

- Take a multivitamin daily.

- Eat nutritious snacks regularly to help keep your blood-sugar level stable.

- Exercise regularly.

- Practice relaxation exercises on a regular basis throughout the month.

MENSTRUAL CRAMPS

Menstrual cramps, or dysmenorrhea, affects around 75 percent of women at some time. Doctors identify two types: primary dysmenorrhea, for which no cause can be found; and secondary dysmenorrhea, which has an identifiable cause. Around 15 percent of women have menstrual cramps severe enough to disrupt normal life. Treatment depends to some extent on severity of symptoms and might include analgesics and other drugs. Dietary changes, homeopathy, manipulation therapy, acupuncture, and relaxation may all bring relief.

WHAT ARE THE SYMPTOMS?

- Cramping lower abdominal pain that comes in waves and may radiate to the lower back and down the legs
- Dragging sensation in the pelvis

The pain may be accompanied by other symptoms, such as bloating and headache.

WHY MIGHT I HAVE THIS?

PREDISPOSING FACTORS

- Stress
- Genetic tendency
- Endometriosis or fibroids
- Pelvic inflammatory disease

IMPORTANT

Consult a doctor if you are experiencing menstrual cramps for the first time or if they become severe.

WHY DOES IT OCCUR?

Primary dysmenorrhea is thought to result from excessive production of prostaglandins, hormonelike substances that make the uterine wall contract before and during menstruation. It is not known why it occurs but women with close female relatives who have had primary dysmenorrhea are more likely to experience it, suggesting genetic factors may be involved. Primary dysmenorrhea often begins soon after the onset of menstruation. Unlike primary dysmenorrhea, secondary dysmenorrhea usually starts later in a woman's reproductive life. Secondary dysmenorrhea has various identifiable causes, including endometriosis (*see p.334*), in which fragments of the tissue that normally lines the uterus are found elsewhere in the pelvis. It may also be caused by fibroids, benign tumors that grow in the wall of the uterus, and pelvic inflammatory disease, in which the female reproductive organs become inflamed as the result of a bacterial infection.

TREATMENT PLAN

PRIMARY TREATMENTS

- Analgesics and NSAIDs
- Drugs that suppress ovulation
- Treatment of underlying cause (secondary dysmenorrhea)
- Magnesium and calcium supplements

BACKUP TREATMENTS

- Niacin, vitamin E, and fish-oil supplements
- Osteopathy and chiropractic
- Trigger point deactivation

WORTH CONSIDERING

- Massage and yoga
- Acupuncture
- Homeopathy
- Relaxation and guided imagery

For an explanation of how treatments are rated, see p.111.

IMMEDIATE RELIEF

- Take an over-the-counter analgesic, such as acetaminophen.
- Relax with a hot-water bottle or take a warm bath.
- Try the homeopathic remedies *Magnesia phosphoricum*, *Chamomilla*, or *Nux vomica*.

TREATMENTS IN DETAIL

Conventional Medicine

Your doctor may order tests, such as an ultrasound scanning of the pelvis, to look for an underlying cause.

PRIMARY TREATMENT **PRIMARY DYSMENORRHEA** The pain of primary dysmenorrhea may be relieved by simple analgesics, such as acetaminophen, or by certain nonsteroidal anti-inflammatory drugs (NSAIDs), including ibuprofen. Suppressing ovulation, often by using the combined oral contraceptive pill, may be recommended if pain persists.

PRIMARY TREATMENT **SECONDARY DYSMENORRHEA** is relieved by treating the underlying cause whenever possible. For endometriosis, this may involve drug treatments, such as the oral contraceptive pill. Alternatively, endometriosis may be treated with surgery, or gonadotropin-releasing hormone (GnRH) analogs to destroy the abnormal patches of uterus lining.

> **CAUTION**
>
> Drugs used to treat primary and secondary dysmenorrhea can cause a range of possible side effects; ask your doctor to explain these to you.

Nutritional Therapy

PRIMARY TREATMENT **CALCIUM AND MAGNESIUM** Calcium and magnesium are essential to muscle function and supplements can be very effective in reducing menstrual cramps. Clinical experience suggests that 1000mg of calcium and 500mg of magnesium should be taken each day. During the menstrual period itself, taking about 250mg of calcium and 100mg of magnesium every four hours can often help relieve symptoms.

NIACIN Fifty years ago, a research study showed that niacin (a form of vitamin B_3) may have the ability to relieve menstrual cramps. In one study, 40 women were given 200mg of niacin per day and up to 100mg every two or three hours on the days when they experienced cramping. Eighty-seven percent of the women reported relief on this regimen in the uncontrolled trial. No research appears to have been done since.

VITAMIN E also seems to be effective in relieving menstrual cramps. In one study, taking 150mg of vitamin E per day improved the condition of 68 percent of dysmenorrhea patients. In another study, 350mg of vitamin E per day, given two days before the beginning of menstruation and for the first three days of bleeding, was effective in relieving pain.

If you experience dysmenorrhea regularly, try adding these supplements together to your diet at the doses recommended above.

FISH OILS There is growing evidence to suggest a role for fish-oil supplementation (omega-3 fatty acids) in relieving menstrual cramps. One study found that supplementation with fish oil providing 1,080mg EPA and 720mg DHA for two months caused a significant reduction in menstrual cramps. In addition to including oily fish (such as salmon, trout, mackerel, herring, and sardines) in the diet, taking supplements of concentrated fish oils (2–3g per day) may help control period-related pain.

> **CAUTION**
>
> See p.46 before taking vitamins B_3 and E, magnesium, and calcium. Fish-oil supplements can enhance the action of blood-thinning drugs such as warfarin; ask your doctor for advice.

Homeopathy

As is often the case with homeopathy, menstrual cramps can be tackled on different levels. There are several medicines that you could try for yourself, based on your symptoms. If they do not help or only partly relieve the problem, it may be worth trying "constitutional" homeopathic treatment (see p.73), but for this you will need to consult a trained homeopath.

> Prostaglandins, which make the uterus contract, may be responsible for menstrual cramps

Chamomilla, Magnesia phosphoricum, and *Nux vomica* are some of the most common medicines for menstrual cramps.

CHAMOMILLA AND NUX VOMICA have some similarities: women who respond to these medicines tend to be irritable with the pain of menstruation. Women who respond to *Chamomilla* tend to get relief from vigorous activity (such as brisk walking), while women who respond to *Nux vomica* can be bad-tempered and impatient, particularly over minor frustrations or inefficiency. Symptoms tend to be worst first thing in the morning.

MAGNESIA PHOSPHORICA Women who respond to this medicine have a quite different character. Their pains are severe and cramping, but they feel exhausted and washed out rather than bad-tempered. They may find relief from heat over the lower abdomen using a hot-water bottle or a heating pad.

OTHER MEDICINES For more complicated problems and especially for secondary dysmenorrhea, other homeopathic medicines may help. These include *Viburnum opulus.* Women who respond to this medicine have light periods and, perhaps paradoxically, the pains seem worst when the bleeding is at its lightest. By contrast, women who respond to *Cactus grandiflorus* have pain that is associated with passing clots of blood.

In women who respond to *Kalium carbonicum*, the pains are felt particularly in the lower back and patients usually feel weak and run-down, also tending to perspire easily. They are often prone to chest trouble and bronchitis that is typically slow to clear up. An unusual but common feature of this medicine is that those who respond to it are worse around 3–4 AM, when they may be awakened by period pains or coughing.

Of the major "constitutional" medicines, the most commonly indicated is *Pulsatilla*. In women who respond to it, periods are irregular and unpredictable, as are their pains. These women are typically gentle, soft-spoken, and indecisive. They may weep easily, but respond to human warmth and quickly cheer up.

Acupuncture

The evidence from clinical trials is limited, but acupuncture and acupressure are frequently used to treat menstrual cramps. There are many reports of cases in which they have helped in both the short- and long-term, with possibly some preventive effect in subsequent cycles after the end of treatment. A traditional Chinese diagnosis is usually required before embarking on treatment. A traditional Chinese diagnosis is usually required before embarking on treatment, and several treatments are likely to be needed over two to three months. Commonly, a diagnosis of blockage and blood stagnation is made and the spleen channel (which runs down the inside of the leg) may be needled.

Bodywork Therapies

OSTEOPATHY AND CHIROPRACTIC Clinical experience suggests that the painful symptoms of primary dysmenorrhea are often significantly reduced following either osteopathic or chiropractic manipulation to those regions of the spine from which the nerve supply to the pelvic region emerges.

Spinal manipulation has recently been shown, in a full-scale clinical trial, to reduce pain as well as the levels of prostaglandins, the hormonelike substances that induce the uterine contractions. In osteopathic research, tests following manipulation showed a marked reduction in prostaglandins. This finding coincided with reports from the 12 patients being studied that menstrual cramping was much reduced, as was lower back discomfort. In one chiropractic study, close to 90 percent of women with menstrual cramps reported that their symptoms were significantly relieved following treatment of the lower back.

MASSAGE Massage therapy, during and before menstruation, that specifically relaxes the spinal and abdominal muscles (as well as providing general relaxation) has produced marked relief from both the symptoms of premenstrual syndrome (*see p.324*) and the pain of menstruation itself.

TRIGGER POINT DEACTIVATION Research into the effects of trigger points (sensitive areas in muscles) on chronic pain report that trigger points in the abdominal muscles (lower rectus abdominis) can initiate spasms and dysmenorrhea. Earlier research suggested that menstrual cramps may involve nerve entrapment in the lower abdominal muscles, which might be improved by appropriate manual therapy such as physical therapy (*see p.55*).

YOGA FOR MENSTRUAL PAIN

Gentle bending and stretching exercises can often help to ease menstrual pain. Some yoga positions, such as the Cat pose (shown below), are especially beneficial because they gently stretch the abdominal area and the low back. These areas are often the sites of pain and cramping during menstruation. Gentle exercise increases blood flow to these areas and helps to loosen muscles that may have become tense due to pain. (Avoid this exercise if you have severe back problems.)

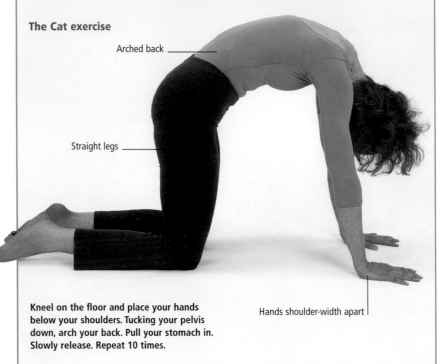

The Cat exercise

Arched back

Straight legs

Hands shoulder-width apart

Kneel on the floor and place your hands below your shoulders. Tucking your pelvis down, arch your back. Pull your stomach in. Slowly release. Repeat 10 times.

Yoga

Certain yoga positions that gently stretch the muscles of the abdomen and lower back can help ease menstrual aches and cramping (*see above*). Try to practice some gentle yoga positions daily throughout your menstrual period.

Mind-Body Therapies

RELAXATION AND GUIDED IMAGERY If you experience dysmenorrhea on a regular basis, try doing a series of relaxation exercises for 20 minutes to half an hour each day. Alternatively, try meditation or listen to a guided imagery tape for the same amount of time.

Studies support the use of psychological therapies, such as relaxation and guided imagery, for menstrual cramps. One study demonstrated that relaxation training, either alone or combined with imagery,

was effective in reducing the amount of time women with spasmodic dysmenorrhea needed to rest.

Relaxation not only helps with menstrual cramps and discomfort but is also effective in reducing absenteeism due to both. These effects have been shown to last as long as 18 months. While psychological strategies can relieve menstrual distress, they can also affect the length of the menstrual cycle; women in a guided imagery study were able to lengthen their cycles.

PREVENTION PLAN

To prevent painful periods:

- Eat a balanced diet that is high in calcium, magnesium, and B vitamins
- Do relaxation exercises every day

HEAVY PERIODS

The amount of menstrual flow varies from woman to woman and may also vary from period to period. Unusually heavy bleeding on a regular basis, known as menorrhagia, may lead to iron-deficiency anemia, which in turn can cause faintness and fatigue. About one woman in 20 has heavy periods. The condition is more common in overweight women and in those approaching menopause. Treatment which aims to reduce blood loss might involve drugs or surgery. Homeopathy, supplements, and acupuncture may also help relieve symptoms.

WHAT ARE THE SYMPTOMS?

- Unusually heavy and often prolonged bleeding during menstruation

WHY MIGHT I HAVE THIS?

PREDISPOSING FACTORS

- Fibroids
- Uterine polyps
- Endometriosis (*see p.334*)
- Underactive thyroid (*see p.319*)
- IUD use
- Being overweight
- Approaching menopause

TREATMENT PLAN

PRIMARY TREATMENTS

- Treatment for any underlying cause
- Hormonal and nonhormonal drugs

BACKUP TREATMENTS

- Surgery

WORTH CONSIDERING

- Iron therapy; vitamins A and D; flavonoids
- Homeopathy
- Herbal treatment
- Acupuncture
- Exercise

For an explanation of how treatments are rated, see p.111.

WHY DOES IT OCCUR?

Heavy menstrual bleeding may be a symptom of certain disorders of the uterus, including fibroids (benign swellings that arise from the muscle of the uterine wall; *see p.332*) or uterine polyps (noncancerous swellings in the uterus). Both of these disorders increase the surface area of the endometrium (the lining of the uterus) and can therefore cause increased blood loss during menstruation. Cancer of the endometrium can also cause heavy periods. Endometriosis (*see p.334*) and persistent pelvic infections are other possible causes. A single late, heavy period may be an early miscarriage.

Heavy periods may also occur as a side-effect of using an intrauterine contraceptive device (the coil or IUD). They may also be due to a more general medical disorder, such as hypothyroidism (*see Thyroid Problems, p.319*). Heavy periods sometimes occur in women who are approaching menopause, when the uterine lining becomes thicker than normal.

In some cases, there is no apparent cause, and if a woman's periods have always been heavy, there may be no cause for concern. However, it is always best to consult a doctor in order to rule out any underlying disorder.

IMPORTANT

If you begin to experience menstrual periods that are heavier or more prolonged than usual, see your doctor without delay. In some cases heavy periods may have a serious underlying cause.

TREATMENTS IN DETAIL

Conventional Medicine

The doctor will make a diagnosis from a description of the symptoms. Investigations may include blood tests to look for anemia and sometimes for an underactive thyroid (hypothyroidism). Other tests to look for an underlying cause may include an endometrial biopsy (taking a sample of the lining of the uterus for analysis). This is particularly likely to be necessary in women over the age of 40. It may be performed during a hysteroscopy, in which a thin, flexible viewing instrument is passed into the uterus through the vagina. Pelvic ultrasound scanning may be arranged. This procedure can detect certain conditions such as fibroids. A laparoscopy, in which a small viewing instrument is inserted into the abdomen, may be done to look for evidence of endometriosis or of a pelvic infection.

The underlying cause will be treated when possible; for example, fibroids may be removed surgically (myomectomy). However, often no cause for heavy bleeding can be found, in which case it may be treated with nonhormonal or hormonal drugs and, in some cases, surgery.

PRIMARY TREATMENT **NONHORMONAL DRUGS** Nonhormonal treatments include the drug tranexamic acid, which is taken during menstrual periods. It prevents the breakdown of blood clots and has been shown to reduce the blood loss of menorrhagia. Studies have also shown that nonsteroidal anti-inflammatory drugs (NSAIDs), such as mefenamic acid, can reduce bood loss.

DEVELOPMENT OF FIBROIDS

Fibroids, which are a very common cause of heavy periods, affect about one woman in five over the age of 35. They are non-cancerous tumors that grow in the uterus and can be as small as a pea or as large as a grapefruit. The most common variety are intramural fibroids which grow within the muscular wall of the uterus. Subserosal fibroids grow just under the surface of the outer uterine wall and submucosal fibroids grow under the endometrium. A penduncu-lated fibroid protrudes into the cervix.

Types of fibroid

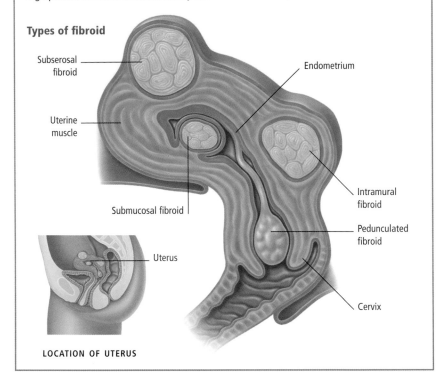

Subserosal fibroid

Uterine muscle

Submucosal fibroid

Endometrium

Intramural fibroid

Pedunculated fibroid

Uterus

Cervix

LOCATION OF UTERUS

PRIMARY TREATMENT **HORMONAL DRUGS** Hormonal treatments include combined oral contraceptives, which suppresses ovulation and can reduce bleeding. Progestogen tablets, such as norethindrone, are sometimes prescribed. An intrauterine device containing progesterone often makes periods light or even absent, although there may be initial spotting or prolonged periods. The drug danazol may reduce bleeding and in higher doses it stops bleeding altogether. However, it is only used in very severe cases and then only for short periods due to the side effects associated with its long-term use, including hirsutism, acne, and deepening of the voice. You must use contraception while taking danazol because it can adversely affect a developing fetus.

SURGERY Surgical options for treating heavy periods include endometrial ablation, in which laser or diathermy (heat treatment) may be used to destroy most of the tissue lining the uterus. This may result in lighter or even absent periods. Possible complications include perforation of the uterus. Hysterectomy (removal of the uterus) may be performed in severe cases when a woman does not want to conceive.

CAUTION

Drugs and surgery for heavy periods can cause a range of possible side effects; ask your doctor to explain these to you.

HYPOTHYROIDISM Clinical experience suggests that low thyroid function (hypothyroidism) is a common cause of heavy periods. (*For details about the diagnosis and treatment of low thyroid function, see p.319.*)

Nutritional Medicine

VITAMIN A seems to be very effective in treating heavy periods. A study showed that 25,000 IU of vitamin A taken twice a day for 15 days brought about a significant reduction of menstrual flow in more than 90 percent of women. You can also try eating foods rich in vitamin A, including oily fish, butter, apricots, and carrots, to help relieve heavy periods.

IRON is another nutrient used for treating heavy periods. Iron deficiency is a common result of heavy periods. It is less well known that iron can treat the problem. It appears to help blood vessels contract, which is important for the body to bring an end to bleeding from the uterus. The best way to have iron levels checked is with a blood test that determines the amount of ferritin in the blood. If iron levels are low, iron supplements may help improve heavy periods.

VITAMIN C AND BIOFLAVANOIDS Vitamin C and bioflavanoids, which are both found in citrus fruits, may be useful in the treatment of heavy periods. Both help protect capillary (small blood vessels) damage and may therefore help protect against the excessive blood loss during menstruation. One study found that taking 200mg of vitamin C and 200mg of bioflavonoids three times per day was useful in reducing symptoms of heavy periods.

CAUTION

Vitamin A should not be taken in doses exceeding 10,000 IU per day by women who are pregnant or trying to conceive. Vitamin C can affect the action of blood-thinning drugs such as warfarin; ask your doctor for advice. (*For more information, see p.46.*)

Homeopathy

A number of homeopathic medicines may help with heavy periods. These include the *Phosphorus* family, particularly *Phosphorus* and *Calcarea phosphoricum*; the *Carbonica* family, especially *Calcarea carbonica* and *Kali carbonica*; and others, including *Natrum muriaticum* and *Sabina*. (*For dosages, see p.77.*)

PHOSPHORUS AND CALCAREA PHOSPHO-RICUM Women who respond to medicines of the *Phosphorus* group tend to be slim and sensitive. They tire quickly and may have a general tendency to bleeding and easy bruising. *Calcarea phosphoricum* is often useful for treating heavy periods in teenage girls who have just had a growth spurt and complain of joint aches and pains. (*For the constitutional features of* Phosphorus *itself, see p.73.*)

CARBON REMEDIES People who respond to medicines of the *Carbonica* group are more stocky and solid but feel "worn out," have frequent backaches, and a tendency to sweat. *Kali carbonica* patients are often "chesty" and they get bronchitis at least once every winter.

NATRUM MURIATICUM The clue to *Natrum muriaticum* patients is their mental makeup: they are "copers" who take care of everybody else but they never discuss their own feelings and they may

have a very strong flavor that does not appeal to everyone. You can include seaweed in your cooking by adding it to soups, salads, and casseroles.

TRADITIONAL REMEDIES Cinnamon (*Cinnamomum cassia*) is a traditional remedy for various menstrual problems, including heavy periods. You can either include cinnamon in your cooking or add it to beverages.

The herb black horehound (*Ballota nigra*) is another traditional remedy for heavy periods, but its effectiveness has not been studied scientifically. There is some research on the antihemorrhagic effect of avens (*Geum urbanum*). Many Western herbalists use the aerial part of the plant, but existing research only examines the root (known as burnet). Burnet is also widely used in Traditional Chinese Medicine (TCM) to treat heavy periods.

Astringent herbs, such as cranesbill (*Geranium maculatum*), witch hazel (*Hamamelis virginia*), and periwinkle

The loss of blood during persistent heavy periods may lead to anemia and fatigue

be depressed. There are other constitutional features that also suggest this medicine (*see p.73*).

SABINA This homeopathic remedy is useful for women whose periods are heavy with clotting and with pain that passes around the pelvis to the back; the pain may resemble labor pains. A peculiar characteristic of this medicine is that women who respond to it may be irritated by hearing music.

Western Herbal Medicine

SEAWEED Trace minerals, such as iodine, can be important in curbing heavy periods. They improve the health of the thyroid gland, which plays a major role in regulating menstrual flow. These trace minerals are found in abundance in seaweed of all types.

Try a milder-tasting seaweed, such as hizike or dulse. Kelp, while beneficial, can

(*Vinca minor*), contain tannin, which decreases menstrual discharge. Raspberry (*Rubus idaeus*), alfalfa (*Meticago sativa*), nettle (*Urtica dioica*) leaves, and yarrow (*Achillea millefolium*) have the same effect.

You can make a tea using two parts raspberry leaf, two parts nettle leaf, one part alfalfa leaf, and one-half part yarrow leaf. Put four to six tablespoons of the mixed herbs in a pitcher and add a quart of boiling water. Cover the pitcher and let the herbs steep for 20 minutes. Strain the tea and drink two or three cups of it every day. You can keep the leftover tea and drink it either at room temperature or chilled in the refrigerator.

CAUTION

The iodine content in seaweed may interfere with treatment for thyroid problems; ask your doctor for advice. Do not take herbal remedies with prescription drugs without consulting an herbal medicine expert first.

Acupuncture

The effectiveness of acupuncture for heavy periods is unproven by randomized controlled trials, but its usefulness has been demonstrated by many acupuncturists. It can also help with problems associated with polycystic ovary syndrome (*see p.337*) and its associated hormone imbalance.

In order to treat heavy periods effectively, a traditional Chinese diagnosis is always required. The usual diagnoses include *Qi* deficiency, which leads to an inability to keep blood in vessels; excess heat, which leads to heavy bleeding; deficiency of heat, which may be due to long-term emotional stress or excessive sexual activity; or blood stasis, which may be due to depression.

Ideally, the acupuncture should be given over three to four cycles, perhaps involving six to nine treatments. If this fails to prove effective, then acupuncture is unlikely to be helpful in the longer term.

Exercise

Being overweight can be a factor that contributes to heavy periods. In women who are overweight, regular exercise, such as walking, cycling, or swimming, aids weight loss and also helps keep weight down once a goal weight is reached. Brisk walking for 30 minutes five times a week is a good way to start, gradually working up to more strenuous activity.

If you have not exercised for some time, make sure to begin slowly and avoid doing too much too soon. If you have any preexisting medical conditions, check with your doctor before beginning an exercise program.

PREVENTION PLAN

The following measures can help prevent heavy periods:

- Maintain a normal weight
- Choose a different method of contraception than the IUD (coil), which can cause heavy periods
- If you have an underactive thyroid, follow your treatment plan carefully

WHAT ARE THE SYMPTOMS?

- Pain in the lower abdomen, which is often most severe before and during menstruation
- Irregular periods
- Heavy periods
- Pain during sexual intercourse

WHY MIGHT I HAVE THIS?

PREDISPOSING FACTORS

- Not having children

TREATMENT PLAN

PRIMARY TREATMENTS

- Hormonal drugs (e.g. oral contraceptives)

BACKUP TREATMENTS

- Surgery (if symptoms are severe)

WORTH CONSIDERING

- Identifying possible food intolerances
- Improving liver function
- Fish oil
- Herbal treatments and homeopathy
- Deactivating trigger points, acupuncture

For an explanation of how treatments are rated, see p.111.

ENDOMETRIOSIS

In endometriosis, pieces of the tissue that lines the inner uterus (known as the endometrium) are found attached to other areas within the pelvis, such as the ovaries. These pieces of tissue respond to the hormones of the menstrual cycle and bleed during menstruation. The blood, which cannot escape, irritates the surrounding tissues, causing pain and eventually scarring and cysts. Treatment depends on the severity of the symptoms and usually involves drugs or, less commonly, surgery. Dietary changes, homeopathy, and other therapies can also help.

WHY DOES IT OCCUR?

The exact cause of endometriosis is not known, but there are many theories as to why it occurs. One theory is that fragments of the uterine lining shed during menstruation do not leave the body through the vagina as normal, but travel along the fallopian tubes and into the pelvis, where they attach themselves to nearby organs. These patches of endometrial tissue are usually found in the pelvic cavity, but in rare instances pieces of endometrial tissue are found in other parts of the body, such as the lungs and the kidneys. Tissue may arrive at such sites via the circulatory or lymphatic systems. The condition only affects women of childbearing age and is found particularly in women in their 30s and early 40s.

Endometriosis may not produce any symptoms. If severe symptoms are present, they do not necessarily indicate severe endometriosis, and conversely a woman who has severe endometriosis may have few symptoms or none at all.

If symptoms do develop, they vary depending on which organs are affected. The most common symptom is pain during menstruation. Occasionally, a cyst formed from blood released by the misplaced endometrial tissue bursts, leaking its contents and causing severe pain. Rarely, there may be blood in the urine or stools if the bladder or rectum is affected. Endometriosis may also cause fertility problems (*see p.346*).

The symptoms abate during pregnancy and cease at menopause because it is menstruation that causes the symptoms and complications. Women who do not have children are more at risk of developing the condition, probably because they do not experience the hormonal changes that take place during pregnancy.

TREATMENTS IN DETAIL

Conventional Medicine

Your doctor may suspect endometriosis from your description of your symptoms, and will refer you to a gynecologist for further examination. Endometriosis is present in many women, and may or may not be associated with pelvic pain. Many doctors recommend laparoscopy surgery, in which a viewing instrument is inserted through small incisions in the abdomen under general anesthesia. If endometriosis is detected, it can be removed during the procedure. However, in actuality laparoscopy is of limited use because the procedure may not pick up endometriosis if it is hidden within tissue or in tiny, scattered amounts that are difficult to see. It may make sense to avoid the risks of surgery in favor of trying a drug treatment when endometriosis is suspected.

All drugs used for endometriosis are likely to reduce pain associated with the condition. However, symptoms tend to return once the drugs are stopped. Also, if infertility is a problem, drug treatment is unlikely to improve it. The options include the drugs described below.

PRIMARY TREATMENT **ORAL CONTRACEPTIVES** Combined oral contraceptives may be prescribed because they induce a pregnancy-like state. In other cases, progestogens, such as medroxyprogesterone, may be prescribed. These drugs also induce a pregnancy-like state.

ORGANS COMMONLY AFFECTED BY ENDOMETRIOSIS

The abdominal organs are most often affected by endometriosis, in which fragments of endometrial tissue travel from the uterus and attach themselves to other organs. The most commonly affected organs include the ovaries, fallopian tubes, ileum (lower part of the small bowel), large bowel, rectum, appendix, and bladder. Symptoms of endometriosis may depend on which organs are affected. However, some women with endometriosis experience few symptoms or none at all.

Endometriosis in the abdominal cavity

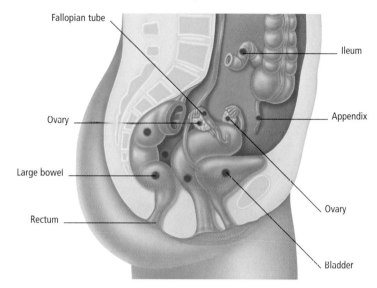

This side view of a woman's abdominal cavity shows the organs that are most frequently affected by endometriosis. Fragments of endometrium (the lining of the uterus) may sometimes travel via the blood and lymph to more distant parts of the body.

DANAZOL The drug danazol is another treatment option for endometriosis. It has similar effects to the hormone testosterone (an androgenic effect) and also counteracts the effects of estrogens. You must use contraception while taking danazol — in general, it is recommended that you use two types just to be sure — because it can have adverse effects on a developing fetus.

GNRH ANALOGS Gonadotropin-releasing hormone (GnRH) analogs may be prescribed. They mimic the hormones that trigger the pituitary gland (the tiny gland located at the base of the brain) to release follicle-stimulating hormone (FSH) and luteinizing hormone (LH). These two gonadotropin hormones act with estrogens and progesterone to regulate the menstrual cycle. The drugs prevent the ovaries from producing estrogens and thereby induce a state that is similar to menopause.

CAUTION

Drugs for endometriosis can cause a range of possible side effects; ask your doctor to explain these to you.

SURGERY If surgical treatment is appropriate, laser treatment or diathermy (heat treatment) that is performed during a laparoscopy may be used to destroy the patches of endometrial tissue. Alternatively, adhesions (fibrous tissue that forms between tissues and organs due to inflammation) may be cut and cysts removed. These methods may provide a longer-lasting improvement in the symptoms than drug treatments and may improve fertility. Occasionally, for very severe pain and in cases when a woman does not wish to be able to conceive, the uterus, ovaries, and fallopian tubes are removed, inducing menopause.

Nutritional Therapy

DIETARY CHANGES There is some evidence that endometriosis is related to an excess of, or extra sensitivity to, the female hormone estrogen. Improving liver function can help reduce estrogen levels by enhancing its breakdown in the liver. More details about improving liver function can be found on p.32.

NUTRITIONAL SUPPLEMENTS Fish oils (omega-3 fatty acids) may help in the management of endometriosis. These oils appear to increase the production of substances called eicosanoids, which may reduce the inflammation and pain that are associated with the condition. In addition to eating plenty of foods that are rich in omega-3 fatty acids (for example, oily fish), taking supplements of concentrated fish oils at a dose of 1g, once or twice a day, may also be helpful.

CAUTION

Consult your doctor before taking fish-oil supplements with anticoagulant drugs, such as warfarin; ask your doctor for advice. (*For more information, see p.46.*)

Homeopathy

Successful homeopathic treatment of endometriosis is likely to require a consultation, and probably a course of treatment, with a skilled homeopathic practitioner.

A case series has suggested that the condition responds well to homeopathy. In the studies, several medicines were often required, with some being given to relieve pain and other being appropriate on "constitutional" grounds (*see p.73*). The homeopathic medicine *Lachesis* was the most frequently helpful; other helpful medicines included *Graphites, Nux vomica,* and *Oophorinum.*

LACHESIS is useful for endometriosis, particularly affecting the left side. In women who respond to this, the symptoms are worsened by pressure (as caused by tight clothes and so forth) and heat and are worst in the premenstrual period.

GRAPHITES Women who respond to *Graphites* often have bowel problems, particularly constipation before or during their period. They may also have skin problems, especially eczema that tends to crack and ooze. This eczema often appears behind the ears or on the nipples or genitalia.

NUX VOMICA is useful when great irritability is part of the picture. Women who respond to this medicine may also have bowel or bladder problems, especially tenesmus (the urge to empty the bowel or bladder again just after doing so).

OOPHORINUM (which is made from healthy ovary tissue) was used in the studies as a general supportive medicine, particularly when infertility was also part of the problem.

OTHER REMEDIES including *Pulsatilla, Sepia,* and *Sulphur,* may also be helpful for some patients when prescribed on an individual basis (*see p.73*).

Western Herbal Medicine

Whatever the initial cause for endometriosis, estrogen affects its growth. Reducing estrogen levels in the body and regulating hormonal production are both key aims of herbal treatment.

The liver is the organ that is responsible for turning estrogen into a substance known as estriol. This is a particular form of estrogen that does not cause endometrial tissue to proliferate. For this reason, improving liver function can be an important factor in treating endometriosis. By improving liver function and thereby increasing the ratio of estriol to estrogen in the body, the growth of endometrial tis-

> ## In most women with endometriosis, the condition is mild and does not impair fertility

sue may be limited and, therefore, the symptoms of endometriosis may be lessened, although the condition may not disappear completely.

HERBS FOR ENDOMETRIOSIS The most important herbs for treating endometriosis are chasteberry (*Vitex agnus-castus*), dong quai (*Angelica sinensis*), wild yam

(*Dioscorea villosa*), dandelion (*Taraxacum officinale*), milk thistle (*Silibum marianum*), and burdock (*Arctium lappa*). Drinking tea made using 3 parts dandelion root, 3 parts wild yam root, 1 part chaste berry, 2 parts burdock, and half a part dong quai three or four times a day may be helpful in easing endometriosis symptoms.

> **CAUTION**
>
> See p.69 before taking a herbal remedy.

Chinese Herbal Medicine

In Traditional Chinese Medicine (TCM), the mechanism that causes endometriosis is known as Blood Stasis. The objective of treatment is to invigorate the blood and remove stasis, and to this end both acupuncture (*see below*) and Chinese herbal medicine are used.

HERBS FOR BLOOD STASIS The herbs most often prescribed for dispersing blood stasis are *Dan Shen* (salvia), *Chi Shao* (red peony root), *Tao Ren* (persica seed), *Hong Hua* (safflower), and *San Leng* (bur-reed rhizome). Endometriosis may also involve Cold, Heat, Deficiency, or Excess patterns, which are determined from a patient's signs and symptoms. Various decoctions may be prescribed based on the diagnosis.

> **CAUTION**
>
> Do not attempt to self-treat for endometriosis using traditional Chinese herbs. Seek advice from a qualified Chinese herbalist. (*See also p.69.*)

Acupuncture

Acupuncture is widely used to treat pelvic pain, such as occurs in endometriosis. Usually, a traditional Chinese diagnosis (*see above*) is required. There have been one or two series of case studies published in the acupuncture literature suggesting

that acupuncture may be effective in managing the pain of endometriosis. The clinical experience of many acupuncturists, however, is that acupuncture does appear to be very successful in the treatment of this particular condition.

Further research into the use of acupuncture for endometriosis is required. More detailed clinical trials are particularly important for us to understand exactly how effective acupuncture actually is and what its mechanisms might be.

If you would like to try acupuncture for your condition, treatment should initially be given on a weekly basis, which will usually trigger a positive response in the first four to six treatments. If acupuncture is beneficial, treatment should continue until no further benefit is apparent. After this, maintenance treatments should be considered on a monthly or three-monthly basis.

Bodywork Therapies

A significant number of women with chronic pelvic pain have been shown to have myofascial trigger points (sensitive points in the muscles) in the structures of the lower abdomen and pelvis, close to surgical incision scar-tissue sites, following hysterectomy to remove endometrial tissues or as a result of endometrial adhesions. These trigger points are partially or totally responsible for their pain. They may be deactivated by acupuncture, or, in some cases, by manual pressure and stretching techniques, as used by osteopaths, massage therapists (particularly those with a neuromuscular therapy training), and some physical therapists and chiropractors. Self-treatment (massage) of tense tissues has been found to be a useful addition to treatment of endometriosis.

Psychological Therapy

GROUP THERAPY Preliminary reports suggest that support groups for women with endometriosis may help them cope better with the psychological and emotional issues associated with this condition, which may include depression and anxiety.

A pilot study showed that simply discussing treatments and problems with other women added to women's satisfaction with their overall care.

POLYCYSTIC OVARY SYNDROME

In polycystic ovary syndrome (PCOS), multiple, small, fluid-filled cysts on the ovaries are accompanied by an imbalance of sex hormones, including higher than normal levels of the male sex hormone testosterone. In some cases multiple cysts are present but there is no hormonal imbalance, in which case the women are simply said to have polycystic ovaries. Various measures, such as weight loss and drug treatment, may promote improvement. Dietary changes, homeopathy, and acupuncture may also help.

WHAT ARE THE SYMPTOMS?

The symptoms of PCOS vary from woman to woman. In some cases there are no symptoms. Typical symptoms include:

- Infrequent or absent menstrual periods
- Obesity
- Acne
- Excessive hair growth (hirsutism)

WHY MIGHT I HAVE THIS?

PREDISPOSING FACTORS

- Blood-sugar instability
- Genetic tendency

TREATMENT PLAN

PRIMARY TREATMENTS

- Weight loss (if necessary)
- Blood-sugar stabilizing diet
- Antidiabetic drugs
- Combined oral contraceptive pill
- Ovulation-inducing drugs and/or assisted conception techniques (for women who wish to conceive)

BACKUP TREATMENTS

- Surgery
- Acupuncture

WORTH CONSIDERING

- Nutritional supplements
- Individualized homeopathy
- Western herbal medicine

For an explanation of how treatments are rated, see p.111.

WHY DOES IT OCCUR?

How polycystic ovary syndrome develops is not fully understood but tissue resistance to insulin, a hormone produced by the pancreas that enables cells to absorb the sugar glucose from the bloodstream, is thought to play a key role. To compensate for this resistance, the pancreas produces large amounts of insulin, which is thought to cause excess production of male sex hormones (androgens), such as testosterone. These male hormones disrupt the normal functioning of the ovaries and, as a result, ovulation may be absent or irregular. It is not known why some women develop PCOS, but genetic factors are thought to be involved.

About five percent of women of childbearing age are affected by PCOS. The condition is associated with infertility if ovulation does not occur, but this can often be successfully treated.

Women who have PCOS are at increased risk of developing diabetes mellitus (*see p.314*) because their tissues are resistant to insulin. They may also be at increased risk of developing high blood pressure (*see p.244*), coronary artery disease (*see p.252*), and cancer of the endometrium (uterine lining).

TREATMENTS IN DETAIL

Conventional Medicine

If your doctor suspects that you have PCOS, he will arrange investigations, such as blood tests to check hormone levels and ultrasound scans, which may show cysts on the ovaries. If PCOS is diagnosed, various treatment options are available.

PRIMARY TREATMENT **WEIGHT LOSS** Your doctor will suggest losing weight if you are overweight or obese. This may reduce insulin resistance and also correct the hormonal imbalance, restoring ovulation, and regulating periods.

PRIMARY TREATMENT **DRUGS** Drugs that induce ovulation, such as clomiphene, may be prescribed if fertility is affected and a woman wishes to become pregnant. Clomiphene is taken at the beginning of the menstrual cycle and can be taken for up to six months. If clomiphene does not induce ovulation, gonadotropins may be tried. With any of these drugs there is a risk of multiple pregnancy.

Women who do not wish to conceive may take the combined oral contraceptive pill to regulate menstrual periods and reduce the risk of endometrial cancer. A pill containing an antiandrogen drug may be prescribed if acne and hirsutism are particular problems. However, this treatment may make menstrual periods irregular and the symptoms will return after the treatment is stopped.

Recent evidence suggests that certain antidiabetic drugs (such as metformin) that increase the sensitivity of the tissues to insulin, may be beneficial for PCOS in terms of reducing insulin levels in the blood and reducing excess androgen levels. Such drugs may consequently restore ovulation and regulate menstruation.

SURGERY If drugs are unsuccessful, the ovaries may be treated surgically using a technique known as laparoscopic ovarian diathermy (LOD), often called "ovarian drilling." In this procedure, diathermy (a form of heat treatment) is used to make several small holes in each ovary during laparoscopy (in which a viewing instrument is introduced through a small incision in the abdominal wall under a general anesthetic). The surgery is usually done on an out-patient basis.

Ovarian drilling can restore regular ovulation or make the ovaries more sensitive to ovulation-stimulating drugs, such as clomiphene, if a woman wishes to conceive. It is not known why it has this effect. Multiple pregnancy rates tend to be lower in women who receive ovarian drilling when compared with those who receive treatment with gonadotropins.

ASSISTED CONCEPTION If the drugs and surgery described above are unsuccessful in inducing ovulation, assisted conception methods, such as in vitro fertilization or gamete intrafallopian transfer (GIFT), may be considered (*see p.346*).

> **CAUTION**
>
> Drugs to treat PCOS can cause a range of possible side effects; ask your doctor to explain these to you.

Nutritional Therapy

PRIMARY TREATMENT **BLOOD-SUGAR STABLIZING DIET** There is evidence that some women with PCOS have a problem with blood-sugar regulation. Surges of sugar into the bloodstream tend to stimulate the secretion of relatively large amounts of the hormone insulin, which may in turn stimulate the secretion of male hormones (androgens).

High insulin levels also make weight gain more likely. Women with PCOS tend to carry excess weight around the middle of their bodies. High levels of insulin are also associated with insulin resistance, which is strongly implicated in PCOS. Women with PCOS seem to be at greater risk of having problems tolerating sugar in their systems (impaired glucose tolerance), especially if they are overweight.

The best diet for women with PCOS seems to be one that ensures stable levels

The exact relationship between insulin resistance and PCOS has yet to be established

of blood sugar and lower insulin levels. See p.32 for more details and the specific nutrients that help this condition (such as chromium, magnesium, and vitamin B_3). A diet low in refined carbohydrates is essential, with attention to eating foods low on the glycemic index (*see p.43*).

Homeopathy

In one study, 40 women were treated with individualized homeopathy for ovarian cysts, of whom 14 had PCOS. When ultrasound examination of the ovaries was repeated after nine months of homeopathic treatment, the cysts had resolved in all but three women.

The homeopathic medicines that were most frequently associated with good results in this study were *Calcarea carbonica*, *Sepia*, and *Pulsatilla*.

CALCAREA CARBONICA In women who respond to *Calcarea carbonica*, menstrual periods are irregular, although when they do occur they are often heavy and prolonged. These women tend to be stout and phlegmatic, although they may have many anxieties and fear that they are suffering from a severe or incurable condition. They feel run down and may experience other problems, including polyps at various sites (such as the uterus), urticaria (hives), and lower back pain. A particularly characteristic feature is sweating easily.

SEPIA Women who respond to *Sepia* have lower back and pelvic pain, typically of a dragging character, and usually loss of sex drive. They may also have hemorrhoids and be constipated. These women may be depressed, "flat," and uninterested in their families or partners. Symptoms may improve with vigorous exertion.

PULSATILLA In women who respond to *Pulsatilla* treatment, menstrual periods are completely irregular and unpredictable; often, they are completely absent. Breast swelling and tenderness may accompany the other symptoms.

Western Herbal Medicine

Several key remedies are available for PCOS that promote hormonal balance and ovarian function, while reducing the severity and frequency of symptoms.

CHASTE-TREE BERRY (*Vitex agnus castus*) is almost invariably used to treat PCOS, as it inhibits androgen release and raises progesterone levels.

OTHER HERBS for PCOS include saw palmetto (*Serenoa repens*) and nettle root (*Urtica dioica*). Licorice (*Glycyrrihiza glabra*) and white peony (*Paeonia laciflora*) may also be used. A Japanese study showed that these herbs can help lower androgen levels and normalize pituitary hormone balance.

> **CAUTION**
>
> Consult an herbal medicine expert for treatment for PCOS and see p.69 before taking an herbal remedy.

Acupuncture

Acupuncture has well-documented and fundamental effects on the hormonal system in PCOS. In one study, women with PCOS who were receiving acupuncture showed a decrease in male hormone levels combined with a more normal pattern of ovulation. PCOS is a chronic condition that usually requires weekly treatment over a period of a few months before any sustained benefit begins to emerge. If you are planning to try acupuncture to treat PCOS, you should be prepared to continue treatment for a reasonably long period of time to see if it works for you.

MENOPAUSAL PROBLEMS

The end of a woman's childbearing years is known as menopause. During this period, the ovaries stop releasing eggs and produce less of the female sex hormones estrogen and progesterone. Menopause is complete when a woman has not had a menstrual period for a year but it may last as long as five years. Many women feel well throughout the menopausal transition, but some have distressing symptoms, such as hot flashes and mood swings, which may be eased with drugs, dietary measures, homeopathy, relaxation exercises, and other treatments.

WHY DOES IT OCCUR?

Most women experience menopause between the ages of 45 and 55, although a tendency to have an early or a late menopause may run in families, suggesting that genetic factors play a part. Smoking may also increase the likelihood of entering menopause at a young age.

As women approach menopause, ovarian production of the sex hormones estrogen and progesterone becomes erratic. During the menopausal transition, hormone levels may bounce around, sometimes being higher or lower than than the normal variation experienced over the course of a normal menstrual cycle of their premenopausal years. When levels drop, the pituitary gland in the brain attemps to stimulate the failing ovaries by secreting more follicle-stimulating hormone (FSH).

Eventually the hormones stabilize at a new lower level. Symptoms that result from elevated hormone levels, including heavy periods and breast tenderness, are always cured by menopause. However, symptoms that are associated with lower estrogen levels, such as hot flashes and vaginal dryness, may persist for months or even years after menopause. Most of the symptoms of menopause result from the increased levels of FSH as levels of estrogen drop.

Many women experience no bothersome symptoms during menopause and most of the symptoms that do occur will disappear after menopause. However, menopausal symptoms tend to be more severe when menopause takes place either prematurely or abruptly, for instance if the ovaries are removed surgically during a hysterectomy or if they are damaged by chemotherapy or radiation therapy.

The menopausal transition usually lasts between one and five years, during which time the symptoms do not require treatment unless they are troublesome.

The decline in estrogen levels affects the body in other ways than simply preventing ovulation and menstruation. The gradual loss of bone tissue that occurs with age is accelerated during the ten years after menopause as a result of the lack of estrogen, increasing a woman's risk of developing osteoporosis (see p.308), in which the bones become brittle and prone to fracture.

The risk of a woman developing heart disease also increases as the levels of estrogen in her body drop. This is because estrogen has a preventive effect against hypertension (see p.244) and coronary artery disease (see p.252), which accounts for the lower incidence of coronary artery disease among premenopausal women than men. This protective effect wears off at about the age of 60, after which the risk of developing heart disease is the same for women as it is for men.

SELF-HELP

PRIMARY TREATMENT You can reduce the discomfort of menopausal symptoms with the following self-help measures:

- Maintain a healthy weight (making sure that you are neither underweight nor overweight) and include flaxseeds and plenty of soy-rich foods, such as tofu, in your diet.
- Don't smoke.
- Use yoga, relaxation, deep breathing (see p.99), and other techniques to deal with underlying stress.

COMPLEMENTARY THERAPIES FOR MENOPAUSE

Many of the problems that arise during the menopausal years can be addressed successfully with complementary therapies. While some of these therapies carry a lower risk of side effects than many of the drug treatments that are available to treat menopausal problems, many of them have not been subjected to rigorous or long-term testing. Approaches that incorporate yoga and meditation are likely to benefit well-being on the whole and can be combined with conventional treatments.

SYMPTOMS	CAUSE	TRY THE FOLLOWING
Hot flashes, night sweats	Sudden drop in estrogen	• Soy, black cohosh, evening primrose, dong quai, vitamin E, homeopathy • Avoid caffeine, alcohol, stress, spicy foods, hot environments
Mood disturbances, depression, anxiety	Less estrogen	• St. John's wort, valerian, ginseng, counseling, exercise, acupuncture • Avoid tea, coffee, sugar
Loss of libido, vaginal dryness	Low hormone levels making vaginal walls thinner. Less natural lubrication	• Water-soluble lubricant, homeopathy, soy, chasteberry, ginseng
Menstrual disorders, heavy periods	Fluctuating hormones	• Wild yam
Increased coronary artery disease risk	Less estrogen (which protects the heart)	• Soy, flax seeds and oil, fish oil
Increased osteoporosis risk	Less estrogen (which aids calcium uptake)	• Ipriflavone (a soy extract), calcium, magnesium, vitamin C, weight-bearing exercise • Avoid carbonated drinks, which contain phosphoric acid that depletes the body of calcium

- Get regular daily exercise.
- If you have hot flashes, avoid alcohol, caffeine, and spicy foods and wear layers that you can easily remove.
- Maintain regular sexual activity.

TREATMENTS IN DETAIL

Conventional Medicine

HORMONE THERAPY Hormone therapy (HT) may be prescribed for the short-term relief of menopausal symptoms such as hot flashes, vaginal dryness, pain during intercourse, and thinning of vaginal walls. It may also be taken long-term for the prevention of osteoporosis, but the risks of long-term therapy (*see right*) are often thought to outweigh this benefit.

HT usually comprises both estrogens and progestins. If estrogen is given alone, there is an increased risk of cancer of the endometrium (uterine lining), but this risk is eliminated if progestins are also given. Women who have had hysterectomies, and are therefore not at risk for developing endometrial cancer, may take estrogen alone. Progestins taken alone have no known side effects and may decrease the severity of hot flashes and night sweats.

HT is available in various forms, most commonly as a pill, However, the most effective dosage and schedules for taking HT are different for every woman. Combination pills are available that contain both estrogen and progestin, or these hormones can be taken as separate pills that contain only estrogen (which is usually taken in the morning) and only progestin (usually taken at night). Estrogen is also available as a patch, which is usually accompanied by progestin pills.

Estrogen is also available as rings and creams that can be placed in the vagina on a short-term basis to improve lubrication and help eliminate painful intercourse. Once a ring is inserted, it cannot be felt and usually does not interfere with intercourse. The ring must be replaced every three months and may be preferred by women who find creams too messy.

LONG-TERM USE OF HT Few women have taken HT for more than 10 years and information regarding its long-term use is limited. It is associated with an increased risk of breast and, possibly, ovarian cancer. HT may increase the risk of a heart attack or stroke, or of a blood clot forming in a vein. However, HT has been shown to offer some protection against bowel cancer

It is important that you discuss the benefits and risks of HT with your doctor before deciding to use it. He or she can work with you to find the smallest dose possible that will relieve your symptoms while minimizing the risk of side effects.

OTHER MEASURES The effects of estrogens and progestins can be achieved by the single drog tibolone, which also has a mild testosterone-like effect. It not only reduces hot flashes and night sweats, but may improve libido.

Other drugs may be prescribed for specific problems, such as antibiotics for urinary tract infections.

EMOTIONAL ASPECTS For some women during menopause, anxiety and depression may be a problem. As depression may be related to coming to terms with the end of the fertile phase of life, emotional support and counseling may be beneficial (*see p.104*). In some cases, antidepressants may also be appropriate for the treatment of women in this position.

Nutritional Therapy

ISOFLAVONE-RICH FOODS Women from Eastern countries, such as Japan, seem to have relatively few problems with menopause. The low rate of menopausal symptoms, especially hot flashes, may be related to the consumption of significant quantities of soy-based foods, including tofu and soy milk.

Soy and flaxseed contain substances called isoflavones (also known as phytoestrogens), which can mimic the effect of estrogen in the body. They are thought to "lock-on" to estrogenic receptor sites and compensate for the drop in estrogen levels that occurs naturally during menopause. In one double-blind study of menopausal women receiving either soy protein or placebo, the soy protein was found to be significantly superior compared with the placebo in reducing the number of hot flashes after four, eight, and 12 weeks of treatment.

Other double-blind research has also reported a reduction in the number of hot flashes menopausal women experience with soy-product supplementation.

ANTIOXIDANTS Phytoestrogenic foods also have antioxidant and anti-inflammatory actions and are thought to help prevent osteoporosis and coronary disease. Flaxseed (the ground seed taken fresh) is particularly useful because it contains unusually high levels of omega-3 oils. If you are experiencing menopausal symptoms, include flaxseed and soy products (such as tofu, soy milk, and soy flour) in your diet.

VITAMIN E Several studies done in the 1940s showed that vitamin E supplements can also be very effective in relieving hot flashes and vaginal dryness. Unfortunately, there are no recent studies on the effect of vitamin E supplements on these and other menopausal symptoms.

However, recent research does suggest that a diet rich in vitamin E can decrease the increased risk of cardiovascular disease that normally follows menopause. A recent six-day study of 54 women discovered that vitamin E absorbed from food acts as an antioxidant, reducing the effect on blood vessels of LDL cholesterol, which can lead to atherosclerosis (*see p.252*). It did not, however, have the same effect when taken as supplements. Good food sources of vitamin E include nuts, vegetable oils, and cereals, in particular wheat germ.

About 75 percent of women experience noticeable symptoms during menopause

Homeopathy

Menopausal symptoms, especially hot flashes, tend to respond quite well to homeopathic treatment. It is best to consult a homeopath who can prescribe the most suitable medicine for you. The homeopathic medicines that most frequently give good results are *Amylenum nitrosum*, *Calcarea carbonica*, *Lachesis*, *Natrum muriaticum*, *Pulsatilla*, and *Sepia*

REMEDIES FOR HOT FLASHES *Amylenum nitrosum* is specified for hot flashes when there is a sensation of blood surging to the head, sometimes with a throbbing headache, followed by profuse sweating and chilliness. The other medicines mentioned below are more deep acting and may help with a number of menopausal problems as well as hot flashes.

LACHESIS is the most frequently prescribed medicine for menopause. It is appropriate when there are frequent hot flashes and the woman feels too hot most of the time. Other features that suggest this medicine are migraines (particularly left-sided), intolerance of tight clothes (particularly collars, but also tight belts and bras), and easy bruising.

CALCAREA CARBONICA may be useful for those who sweat heavily on the head and neck at night. Women whom it helps are often anxious and tend to obsess over little things. They may be woken by bad dreams. They are tired and run down, and may suffer from problems, such as urticaria, nasal polyps, and lower back pain.

NATRUM MURIATICUM AND SEPIA *Natrum muriaticum* may be prescribed for women who are depressed but keep their condition well hidden. They often have vaginal dryness and recurrent cold sores on the lips. Women who respond to *Sepia* may also have these. However, *Sepia* women may have become bad-tempered and less affectionate since menopausal symptoms began.

PULSATILLA may be given to women who show great changeability, both in mood and in symptoms. These women are typically soft spoken and easily moved to tears.

GRAPHITES may also help with menopausal symptoms. It has similarities with *Pulsatilla*, but the woman who responds to *Graphites* is typically weepy over sentimental films and sad music, rather than as a result of depression. Strangely, women who respond to *Graphites* may become pale during a hot flash. They may also have skin trouble, particularly cracked eczema, which easily exudes a sticky fluid. Constipation is also quite common in these women.

Western Herbal Medicine

An herbal approach to menopausal problems seeks to look beyond the narrow focus of hormone levels. Menopausal symptoms can result from long-term stress and chronic ill health, and these are factors that make it harder for the body to adapt and establish a new (postmenopausal) hormonal balance. Advice on diet, exercise, and relaxation is central, but practitioners will prescribe herbs to support hormonal function, relieve menopausal symptoms, and promote emotional balance.

PRIMARY TREATMENT **BLACK COHOSH** (*Cimicifuga racemosa* or *Actaea racemosa,*) is a traditional Native American remedy for women's health problems. A 1998 review of eight clinical trials concluded that black cohosh extract might be a safe and effective alternative when HT was contraindicated or rejected. Black cohosh is especially useful for hot flashes, sweating, sleep disorders, and nervous irritability. When nervous exhaustion or depression is also a feature, it combines well with St. John's wort (*Hypericum perforatum*).

Most research has been conducted on extracts of black cohosh standardized to the triterpene glycosides and doses of 20–80mg twice daily. Studies have not shown significant effects on hormone levels nor demonstrated that black cohosh stimulates breast cancer cells.

Extrapolating from Japanese research into other herbs related to black cohosh, it has been proposed that this herb might inhibit the loss of calcium from bone and protect menopausal women against osteoporosis.

SAGE AND ALFA-ALFA may also be useful for menopausal symptoms. A small clinical trial investigated the efficacy of a sage (*Salvia officinalis*) and alfa-alfa (*Medicago sativa*) combination in relieving hot flashes and night sweats. It found significant improvement in symptoms, with all the women experiencing reduced symptoms and most finding that hot flashes and night sweats completely disappeared.

RED CLOVER A systematic review published in the journal *Menopause* suggested red clover (*Trifolium pratense*) might help women with severe menopausal problems.

OTHER HERBS Many other herbal medicines have long been used to treat menopausal symptoms. Licorice (*Glycyrrhiza glabra*) and fenugreek (*Trigonella foenum-graecum*) are both valuable for treating dry skin, vaginal dryness, and lowered libido. Chaste tree berry (*Vitex agnus-castus*), which has a progesterogenic action, is most often used for problems in the phase of a woman's life leading up to menopause.

CAUTION

See p.69 before taking a herbal remedy.

Acupuncture

Acupuncture can be used to treat certain symptoms, such as hot flashes. There is some evidence that a course of four to six acupuncture treatments will have a beneficial effect on hot flashes for three months or longer. Other menopausal symptoms, such as fatigue, muscular aches, and joint pains, may also be improved by treatment with acupuncture.

A traditional Chinese diagnosis is required and treatment may need to be carried out intermittently throughout the menopausal period. Usually treatment focuses on the prevailing symptoms at the time, so the traditional Chinese diagnosis may vary depending on the exact symptoms. If symptoms are acute (sudden and short-lived), weekly treatment is recommended, and if it appears to be effective, then it is probably worthwhile having acupuncture every month or two as a preventive measure.

Bodywork Therapies

Manual therapies such as massage may promote restful sleep and relieve symptoms. A survey of 886 women aged 45–65 years was carried out in Washington state. Of the women surveyed, 31.6 percent had consulted a chiropractor, while 29.5 percent had received massage therapy. More than 89 percent of the women who had participated in the study reported that they had found the treatment helpful, particularly in improving sleep.

The study participants had used a wide range of alternative therapies to treat their menopausal symptoms, including homeopathy and herbal medicine as well as various bodywork therapies. Up to 75 percent of the participants found the therapy they had chosen to be helpful. The most popular alternative therapies were chiropractic, acupuncture, massage therapy, and stress management.

CHIROPRACTIC Chiropractic manipulation of the upper back and neck has been shown in one study to decrease the frequency of hot flashes by up to 90 percent.

REFLEXOLOGY AND FOOT MASSAGE When the benefits of treating specific reflexology points on the foot were compared with the

T'AI CHI

The slow, gentle, focused movements of t'ai chi can help you relax, which may help you better with menopausal changes. As a form of exercise, tai chi does not put undue stress on the joints and promotes flexibility and suppleness. As a form of meditation, tai chi may help lessen anxiety, especially if it is done regularly.

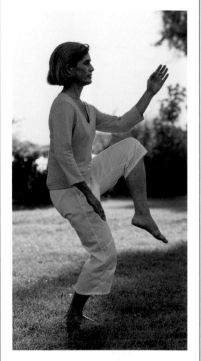

T'ai chi is an easy and inexpensive way to take gentle exercise. It can be done outdoors and does not require special clothing or equipment.

effects of general foot massage in easing some symptoms of menopause, it was found that both methods were equally effective. Symptoms that improved with these treatments included anxiety, depression, hot flashes, and night sweats.

Since the reduction in symptoms associated with menopause after foot massage seems to derive from reduced feelings of anxiety, it is worth considering trying other treatments (such as general massage, yoga, tai chi, and regular breathing exercises; *see left and opposite*), which also have calming effects, as treatments for menopause. (*See also Anxiety and Panic Disorder, p.414.*)

Exercise

AEROBIC EXERCISE Physical exercise can reduce anxiety levels and hot flashes and maintain bone density. For these reasons, women should be sure to exercise regularly in the years around menopause. The use of exercise programs during these years has been shown to increase bone density by a significant amount. Many experts say that doing some aerobic, weight-bearing exercise, such as fast walking or slow jogging, for about 30 minutes every other day can be very beneficial.

However, while there is evidence that mild but regular exercise, such as walking, can slow down bone loss, there is little evidence showing that exercise comes close to replicating the effects of HT in preventing bone loss during menopause. (*See also Osteoporosis, p.308.*)

TAI CHI Performing tai chi (*see opposite*) can help improve mood and preserve flexibility and physical strength during menopause. The gentle, flowing movements of tai chi do not put stress on joints, while the stretching and deep breathing it incorporates help maintain suppleness and encourage relaxation. Since tai chi demands focus, it is also a form of meditation, which can help relieve anxiety and bring about a sense of calm.

Breathing Retraining

BREATHING FOR PANIC ATTACKS Learning to control the breath and avoiding shallow, rapid breathing can be very helpful in controlling stress, anxiety, and panic attacks, which some women find accompany menopause. (*See p.62 for more information on how to do this.*)

BREATHING FOR HOT FLASHES Abdominal breathing has been found to help relieve menopausal hot flashes. Studies show that the frequency of hot flashes can be reduced by about 50 percent by regularly using slow, abdominal breathing. Robert Freeman, a professor of psychiatry and behavioral neurosciences at Wayne State University in Detroit, says that women can prevent or shorten the duration of hot flashes by slowing their breathing to a rate of seven or eight breaths a minute.

If you are experiencing hot flashes, try doing abdominal breathing (*see p.62*) regularly, and try to avoid shallow breathing, especially if you are feeling tense or stressed.

Yoga

Practicing yoga can help during the period around menopause. Yoga can reduce stress and foster a positive attitude to the changes that menopause involves.

Some practitioners believe that yoga can also help regulate hormone levels in the body. In this way, doing yoga regularly may help reduce the frequency of menopausal symptoms such as hot flashes and mood swings.

The best yoga for menopause is slow and gentle, with an emphasis on floor poses. Poses that work the lower back, such as the bridge and the cobra, may influence the kidneys and adrenal glands as well as relieving fatigue. These poses have the added advantage of easing muscle tension and stiffness in the lower back.

Side stretches can help tone the muscles and improve flexibility. Poses that open the chest, such as the fish, can help reduce stress and induce a state of calmness and clarity.

If you have never done yoga or stretching exercises before or if you have not done them for some time and would like to try yoga, be sure to start gradually. Make sure you listen to your body and do not try to do too much too soon.

Mind–Body Therapies

RELAXATION Regular relaxation has been found to be effective in reducing the frequency and intensity of hot flashes, decreasing tension and anxiety, as well as improving mood in women going through menopause. Researchers in Detroit found that women who were taught to slow their breathing rate had fewer hot flashes than thos who did not (*see Breathing Retraining, left*).

GUIDED IMAGERY Sitting quietly and listening to a guided imagery tape, which helps you imagine that you are in a soothing and pleasant place, may help you relax and may also relieve anxiety during menopause.

BIOFEEDBACK Learning to control your body's responses to certain signals using biofeedback (*see p.94*) can also help you relax during menopause. Once you have learned to relax your body at will, you can also use the technique to help cope with

> During menopause, production of estrogen drops by as much as 90 percent in a few years

anxiety and panic attacks, if these have been troublesome for you

If you are experiencing symptoms of menopause, try a program of daily relaxation exercises (*see p.99*), which may increase your ability to cope with this stage of your life. You could also try guided imagery or learn biofeedback. Following a relaxation program may mean that you have less need of medication for your menopausal symptoms.

SOCIAL SUPPORT Social support is very important in the menopausal period, since women may feel isolated and may experience "empty nest syndrome" as grown children leave home. Women at this stage of life may need help in redefining their roles, and counseling may provide this.

PREVENTION PLAN

As menopause approaches, try the following to minimize problems:

- Eat a balanced diet
- Avoid having too much caffeine or alcohol
- Get regular, weight-bearing exercise
- Do relaxation exercises regularly
- If you smoke, stop

VAGINAL YEAST

Vaginal yeast infections occur when there is increased growth of the yeast *Candida albicans*, which is often present naturally in the vagina. The condition is not serious but can cause uncomfortable symptoms. Yeast infections affect many women at some point in their lives, often during their childbearing years, and once one occurs they may recur regularly. There are several ways to treat yeast infections and prevent recurrence, including antifungal drugs, dietary changes and supplements, homeopathic medicines, and stress-relieving techniques.

WHAT ARE THE SYMPTOMS?

- Intense irritation and itchiness in the area around the opening of the vagina (the vulva) and inside the vagina
- Vaginal discharge, which may be thick and white, cheesy, or watery in appearance
- Redness of the vulva

WHY MIGHT I HAVE THIS?

PREDISPOSING FACTORS
- Pregnancy
- Diabetes mellitus
- Oral contraceptives
- Menstruation

TRIGGERS
- Perfumed bath products
- Spermicides
- Antibiotics
- Stress

TREATMENT PLAN

PRIMARY TREATMENTS
- Vaginal or oral antifungal preparations

BACKUP TREATMENTS
- Anti-candida diet
- Probiotics and probiotic suppositories

OTHER OPTIONS
- Homeopathy
- Stress relief

For an explanation of how treatments are rated, see p.111.

WHY DOES IT OCCUR?

The candida fungus is naturally present in the vagina of many women and does not usually cause problems because its growth is suppressed by the immune system and by bacteria that normally live in the vagina. If these harmless bacteria are destroyed, for example by certain antibiotics or spermicides, the candida fungus may multiply. Changes in the levels of a woman's sex hormones, which can occur as a result of pregnancy, menstruation, or oral contraceptives, can also result in fewer protective bacteria and allow the condition to become established.

Stress may trigger the condition, as may perfumed bath products and spermicides, all of which can interfere with the body's natural defenses against candida. Infection with *C. albicans* can also occur in other areas of the body, such as the mouth (*see Oral Yeast, p.383*).

Male sexual partners can catch yeast infections; symptoms of infection in men include redness, itchiness, and soreness of the foreskin and the head of the penis. If these symptoms are present, men should see their doctor for treatment.

SELF-HELP

If you have had yeast infections before and are confident that your symptoms are due to a recurrence, you can ask your pharmacist for over-the-counter antifungal drugs and suppositories. You can also:
- Use probiotic supplement capsules as suppositories.
- Eat plain yogurt every day.
- Follow an anti-candida diet (*see p.40*).

TREATMENTS IN DETAIL

Conventional Medicine

The doctor will likely take a sampling that will be tested for the fungus. If a vaginal yeast infection is diagnosed, he or she may then prescribe the following treatments and will also be able to advise you on self-help measures.

PRIMARY TREATMENT **SUPPOSITORIES AND CREAMS** Studies have shown that vaginal suppositories or creams containing imidazole antifungal drugs, such as clotrimazole, are helpful in relieving the symptoms of yeast infections. The antifungal drug nystatin used vaginally may also help. These vaginal treatments can be used during pregnancy.

PRIMARY TREATMENT **ORAL DRUGS** Alternatively, oral treatment with a triazole antifungal drug, such as itraconazole, may be preferred as more convenient. You may also be given oral drugs to take at the same time that you are using suppositories or creams. If yeast infections are recurring, they may be treated with long-term antifungal therapy.

Some vaginal and oral treatments for vaginal yeast infections are now available without a prescription; ask your pharmacist for advice.

CAUTION

Drugs to treat vaginal thrush can cause a range of possible side effects; ask your doctor or pharmacist to explain these to you.

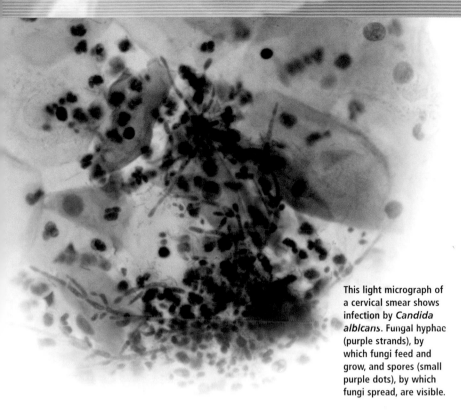

This light micrograph of a cervical smear shows infection by *Candida albicans*. Fungal hyphae (purple strands), by which fungi feed and grow, and spores (small purple dots), by which fungi spread, are visible.

Nutritional Therapy

The source of *C. albicans* in the body is the digestive tract, which is why treating only the vaginal source of the infection with suppositories and creams often fails to bring lasting relief. The candida fungus may be transferred from the anal area to the vagina when wiping after going to the bathroom. Therefore, it is important to wipe from front to back to help prevent this from occurring.

To treat vaginal yeast infections efficiently, it is usually necessary to combat the overgrowth of *C. albicans* in the digestive tract. (*See p.40 for details of how to follow an anti-candida diet.*)

PRIMARY TREATMENT | **PROBIOTICS** If you have recurrent vaginal yeast infections, try eating 8oz (225ml) of unsweetened live yogurt every day. This approach is supported by research.

A study assessed whether daily ingestion of probiotic yogurt containing the bacterium *Lactobacillus acidophilus* could prevent vaginal candida infection. A group of women who had recurrent vaginal candida infection ate a yogurt-free diet for six months and a diet containing yogurt for six months. A threefold decrease in vaginal candida infections was seen when they ate yogurt containing *Lactobacillus acidophilus*. Eating 8oz (225ml) of yogurt containing *Lactobacillus acidophilus* decreased both candidal colonization of the bowel and infection of the vagina.

PROBIOTIC SUPPOSITORIES The use of probiotic supplement capsules inserted vaginally (as a suppository) can often be helpful too. Increasing the number of healthy bacteria in and around the vagina seems to help keep yeast infections at bay.

Homeopathy

ISOPATHY A clinical trial indicated that isopathy (treatment of a disease with a homeopathic preparation of the agent that causes the disease) may be effective in alleviating vaginal yeast infections. Several US manufacturers sell homeopathic preparations containing *Candida*, available as suppositories. These preparations are widely available in pharmacies, health food stores, and nutrition centers.

HELONIAS Although *Helonias* is not a widely used homeopathic remedy, it is important for vaginal yeast infections when the discharge is lumpy, like curdled milk. The discharge may be accompanied by lower back pain.

KREOSOTUM The remedy *Kreosotum* may help if vaginal yeast infections are accompanied by irritation and soreness of the vulva and if the discharge seems to burn and smells foul.

TREATMENT FOR RECURRENT YEAST INFECTIONS Individualized constitutional treatment by a qualified homeopath may be necessary if yeast is chronic or recurrent. Important medicines that may be used include *Pulsatilla*, *Sepia*, and *Thuja*; deciding which to use is based on a woman's constitutional features (*see p.73*).

Mind-Body Therapies

RELAXATION AND MEDITATION Most women experience at least one episode of vaginal yeast infection at some time in their adult lives. Since stress is known to be a trigger for attacks of vaginal yeast infections, it stands to reason that taking steps to reduce stress may help reduce the frequency of attacks. Chronic stress lowers immunity and makes the body more vulnerable to infection.

If you have recurrent episodes of vaginal yeast infections, it may be worth keeping a diary recording them to see whether they coincide with periods of stress. If they do, you could try practicing a sequence of relaxation exercises every day (*see p.99*). Alternatively, you could try meditating for 20 minutes daily or taking up a mind-body therapy such as yoga.

PREVENTION PLAN

Try the following if you are prone to vaginal yeast infections:

- Avoid perfumed bath products and soaps when bathing
- Do not use vaginal deodorants or scented tampons
- Wear cotton underwear, or underwear with a cotton gusset
- Avoid tight jeans or pants
- Wipe from front to back when going to the bathroom
- Include yogurt in your daily diet

INFERTILITY IN WOMEN

Many couples begin to feel anxious if they have been trying to conceive for several months without success. If they are under 35, doctors will advise them to keep trying for a year before seeking medical treatment. On average, 80 percent of couples trying to conceive will be successful within a year, and 90 percent will be successful within two years. If conception does not occur naturally, there are several measures that may help, ranging from dietary changes and psychological therapies, to drugs and assisted conception techniques.

WHAT ARE THE SYMPTOMS?

- Inability to become pregnant after approximately one year of regular intercourse

WHY MIGHT I HAVE THIS?

PREDISPOSING FACTORS

- Low thyroid function
- Caffeine
- Smoking
- Nutritional deficiency
- Stress and anxiety
- Being significantly underweight or overweight
- Polycystic ovary syndrome (see p.337)
- Endometriosis (see p.334)
- Previous pelvic infection
- Previous abdominal surgery
- Fibroids

TREATMENT PLAN

PRIMARY TREATMENTS

- Treatment of underlying cause (e.g. low thyroid function) where possible

BACKUP TREATMENTS

- Stimulation of ovulation
- Assisted conception techniques

WORTH CONSIDERING

- Caffeine elimination
- Nutritional supplements
- Herbal treatments
- Homeopathy
- Avoiding toxic chemicals
- Acupuncture
- Breathing retraining
- Relaxation and group counseling

For an explanation of how treatments are rated, see p.111.

WHY DOES IT OCCUR?

For conception to occur naturally, at least one of a woman's two ovaries must be capable of releasing a mature egg; if fertilization occurs, the fertilized egg must be able to travel down the fallopian tube and implant in the uterine lining. If any stage in the process is interrupted, natural conception cannot take place. Conception also relies on production of enough healthy sperm by the man to make fertilization possible, and delivery of this sperm into the vagina. Problems with male fertility and treatment options are described on p.373.

There are various factors that can cause infertility in women.

PROBLEMS WITH OVULATION (the release of a mature egg by an ovary) are a common cause of infertility. Ovulation is controlled by a complex hormonal interaction in the body, and if there is a hormonal imbalance ovulation may not take place regularly or at all. Polycystic ovary syndrome (see p.337) is a common cause of hormonal imbalance. Underactivity of the thyroid gland (see p.319) may also disrupt hormonal balance and affect fertility. In some cases, if women have been taking oral contraceptives for many years or have used contraceptive implants, it may take time to reestablish a normal hormonal cycle and pattern of ovulation. Other factors that can disrupt hormone levels and affect fertility include stress, excessive exercise, and being significantly underweight or overweight.

PROBLEMS WITH SPERM DELIVERY can also cause infertility. In some women, it may not be possible for the man's sperm to reach the egg because the cervix produces mucus which contains antibodies that destroy sperm.

DAMAGED FALLOPIAN TUBES may prevent conception. Once an egg has been fertilized, it needs to travel down one of the fallopian tubes to reach the uterus. Damage to the fallopian tubes may prevent this and is a common cause of infertility. The fallopian tubes may be damaged by pelvic infections, endometriosis (see p.334), or previous abdominal surgery.

PROBLEMS WITH THE UTERUS may prevent a fertilized egg from implanting and result in infertility. Damage to the uterine lining by an infection, is one such problem. Fibroids (benign swellings in the muscle of the uterine wall; see p.332) are another. In rare cases, structural abnormalities of the uterus can cause problems with implantation.

AGE may be a factor in some cases. Fertility in women decreases with age and is usually lower in women over 35. This is partly due to lower egg quality in older women and partly due to hormonal changes. Fertility also tends to decrease in men as they age, since sperm tend to become less mobile and less robust.

IMPORTANT

If you have been trying to conceive for several months unsuccessfully and are concerned, go as a couple to see your doctor. This is especially important if one or both partners are over 35.

To increase the chances of conceiving both partners should do the following:

- Avoid smoking or drinking alcohol.
- Eliminate caffeine from the diet.
- Get enough rest and relaxation.
- Eat well and keep to a healthy weight.
- Get adequate, but not excessive, exercise.
- Have sex regularly — particularly halfway through the menstrual cycle (a woman's most fertile time).

TREATMENTS IN DETAIL

Conventional Medicine

TESTS Various tests may be arranged to look for underlying causes of fertility problems. If investigations are needed to discover whether there is a problem conceiving, it is important that both the man and the woman are examined. In about half of all cases, the problem lies with the woman and in about a third of all cases, the problem lies with the man. In some couples, no problem can be found, and their infertility is unexplained.

Preliminary investigations are likely to include blood tests for the woman, to assess hormone levels and whether ovulation is likely to be taking place, as well as semen analysis for the man. If the results of these are normal, a couple may decide to continue trying to conceive for an agreed period of time. Otherwise, further tests may be arranged. For example, ultrasound scanning may be used to check a woman's pelvic organs. The fallopian tubes may be assessed using a procedure known as hydrosonography, in which radiopaque dye is introduced into the uterus through the cervix and a series of X-rays is taken as the dye passes along the tubes. Alternatively, the passage of dye along the tubes may be monitored during a laparoscopy, in which a viewing instrument is passed through a small incision in the wall of the abdomen under a general anesthetic.

PRIMARY TREATMENT **UNDERLYING CAUSES** If an underlying cause is identified, it will be treated where possible. For example, the thyroid hormone supplement levothyroxine may be prescribed for an underactive thyroid gland (hypothyroidism).

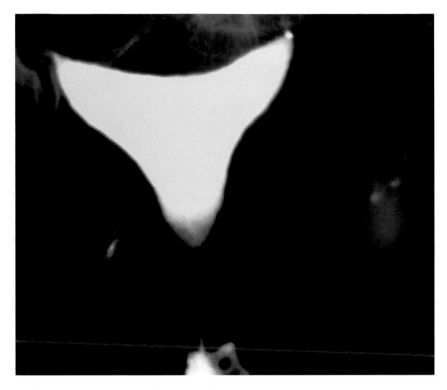

In this hydrosonogram (reproductive contrast X-ray), the woman's right fallopian tube (left on image) cannot be seen because a blockage near the uterus has prevented the contrast medium from reaching it.

In certain cases, it may be possible to repair damaged fallopian tubes with keyhole surgery.

STIMULATING OVULATION Impaired ovulation, as occurs in polycystic ovary syndrome (*see p.337*), may be treated with the drug clomiphene, which stimulates ovulation. There is a risk of multiple pregnancy with this treatment. Clomiphene is taken at the beginning of the cycle and can be continued for up to six months.

ASSISTED CONCEPTION TECHNIQUES If infertility cannot be explained or, alternatively, the cause cannot be treated, techniques that aim to improve the chances of conception may be considered.

Intrauterine insemination (IUI) may be tried, in which sperm are introduced into the uterus through the cervix via a thin, soft tube. This may be used in cases of unexplained infertility and is only suitable if the fallopian tubes are normal. Drugs are sometimes prescribed to ensure that ovulation takes place.

In vitro fertilization (IVF) involves removing eggs from the ovaries, adding sperm outside the body, and then, if fertilization occurs, introducing the eggs into the uterus. It is sometimes used for women who have damaged fallopian tubes, as well as in cases of unexplained infertility.

Gamete intrafallopian transfer (GIFT) involves removing eggs from the ovaries and introducing them and the sperm into the outer end of the fallopian tube through a fine tube. The egg and sperm can then mix and fertilization may occur. This may be used for unexplained infertility.

Both IVF and GIFT require a number of fertility drugs to stimulate the ovaries to produce eggs. The ovaries are monitored regularly with ultrasound scans until the eggs are ready to be removed and prepared for the procedure.

Other methods, such as intracytoplasmic sperm injection (ICSI), are used when there is a problem with the sperm (*see p.373*). Success rates for all treatments depend on the individual couple as well as the clinic they attend.

COUNSELING Having fertility treatment can affect couples emotionally as well as, in some cases, financially. Support and understanding is needed for both partners during what, for most couples, is a very difficult time. Fertility clinics offer counseling to couples undergoing treatment. Other psychological treatments, such as group therapy, may also help.

> **CAUTION**
>
> Drugs given to treat infertility can cause a range of possible side effects; ask your doctor to explain these to you.

Nutritional Therapy

Infertility in women may be related to low thyroid function (hypothyroidism). For more details about the diagnosis and treatment of low thyroid function, see p.319.

ELIMINATING CAFFEINE Caffeine consumption appears to reduce fertility and to increase the length of time it takes to conceive. Just one to one and a half cups of coffee per day is associated with delayed

> Infertility affects about 10 percent of the population who are of reproductive age

conception and may reduce fertility by half. If you are trying to conceive, you may benefit from giving up coffee, tea, and cola.

NUTRITIONAL SUPPLEMENTS Infertility may be related to nutrient deficiencies. One study found that taking a general multivitamin and mineral supplement increased fertility. The multivitamin-mineral supplement appeared to make female ovulatory cycles more regular. A healthy, balanced diet based on fruits, vegetables, nuts, fish, whole grains, and unprocessed/unrefined foods is very important, but additional supplementation with a multivitamin and mineral preparation may also help.

Homeopathy

Although there is no published research, many homeopaths report success in treating infertility and repeated miscarriage in

the first three months of pregnancy, especially when no organic cause can be shown by medical tests.

SEPIA The most commonly used homeopathic medicine for infertility in women is *Sepia*, which has been found particularly helpful in "post-pill" infertility (that is, women who have trouble conceiving after they have been on oral contraceptives). However, it may also be effective in other circumstances. Women who respond to *Sepia* are said to be depressed, emotionally "flat," and lacking sex drive; they suffer from lower back pain and are often chilly. Yet some women who respond to *Sepia* are, or at least appear to be, happy and vivacious. This is sometimes a mask: women who respond to *Sepia* don't easily "open-up" and discuss their feelings. They feel better temporarily from exercise, especially when it is done to music. The normal dose would be *Sepia* 30C, two pills weekly for two or three menstrual cycles.

OTHER MEDICINES Other medicines that may be helpful include *Aristolochia*, when menstrual periods are light, irregular, or even completely absent. Some doctors use the homeopathic medicines *Oophorinum* and *Folliculinum* (made from human ovary and ovarian follicle respectively) at particular points in the menstrual cycle to stimulate ovulation. This treatment requires specialist advice.

Some women can conceive but suffer recurrent early miscarriage in the first three months of pregnancy. Many early miscarriages are due to fetal abnormalities, and it is best to let nature take its course. This problem should not be treated unless it has happened repeatedly. Among the medicines recommended for recurrent miscarriage are *Sepia* and *Kalium carbonicum*, which is, in some ways, similar to *Sepia*. *Caulophyllum* and *Helonias* may also be appropriate when there is lack of cervical tone. (*See p.77 for guidelines on how to take these medicines.*)

Western Herbal Medicine

Within certain boundaries, herbal medicine can prove very effective in increasing fertility and the chances of conception. It may be useful when the woman is in moderate to good general health, particularly if she is over 35.

However, herbal medicine will not overcome physical factors that impair fertility, such as a blocked fallopian tube, which should be excluded before herbal treatment is undertaken. In addition, herbal treatment cannot compensate for very disordered pituitary and ovarian hormone levels. These should be within normal range or only moderately imbalanced before considering herbal treatment.

OBJECTIVES OF TREATMENT Establishing regular ovulation and menstruation is often the first objective of treatment and may involve treatment of an underlying hormonal imbalance. Relevant hormone levels should be monitored to provide feedback on treatment. Other factors that may require treatment and are amenable to herbal medicine include heavy menstrual blood loss and anemia (*see p.331*), endometriosis (*see p.334*), anxiety and stress (*see p.414*), mild thyroid dysfunction (*see p.319*), and problems in which the woman's mucus contains antibodies that attack the sperm.

POSSIBLE HERBS An herbal medicine expert may prescribe a combination of herbs, selecting from hormonally active remedies, such as the chaste-tree berry (*Vitex agnus castus*), black cohosh (*Cimicifuga racemosa*), and helonias (*Chamaelirium lutea*). Circulatory stimulants — for example, cayenne pepper (*Capsicum anuum*) and prickly ash (*Xanthoylum americanum*) — and menstrual tonics, such as dong quai (*Angelica sinensis*) and motherwort (*Leonarus cardiaca*), which improve blood flow to the pelvis, may also be chosen. Bitters and liver tonics may be given as well to improve nutritional status.

> **CAUTION**
>
> See p.69 before taking an herbal remedy and, if already taking prescribed medication, consult an herbal medicine expert first.

Environmental Health

Exposure to compounds that may be toxic to egg development or parts of the reproductive tract may affect fertility in women. Women who have problems with fertility or menstruation should consider possible exposure to chemicals at home or work and take measures to decrease it. It may be useful to speak to an environmental health expert to assist with this.

LEAD AND SOLVENTS Lead exposure at high levels may cause spontaneous abortions. Exposure to solvents, such as those used in laboratory work, or paints, increased spontaneous abortions two- to four-fold in one study, and led to infertility and menstrual disorders in other studies.

SMOKING Research has shown that exposure to cigarette smoke may cause infertility or increase the time it takes to conceive. Women should not smoke during pregnancy because exposing a female fetus to cigarette smoke can affect the baby's egg development and future fertility.

CHEMICALS AND ALCOHOL Compounds such as perchloroethylene (used in the dry-cleaning industry), chlorinated hydrocarbons (for example the pesticide DDT or PCBs), and ethylene oxide (a chemical used in medical and dental clinics) may increase the possibility of spontaneous abortion. Exposure to toluene (used in some color printing businesses) may increase the time it takes for a woman to conceive. Regular alcohol consumption may have a similar effect.

XENOHORMONES These compounds have a hormonal effect on the human body. Examples include pesticides (such as DDT), dyes and paints, and bisphenol A, which is a common lining in food and drink cans as well as a component of dental sealants. Controversial studies have shown that these compounds may increase spontaneous abortion.

Acupuncture

Many women who are infertile visit acupuncturists. The main aim of the acupuncturist in this situation is to make a clear diagnosis of the underlying energy imbalances that a woman may be experiencing, and then to treat the appropriate organs and pathogens. The aim, within a traditional Chinese context, is to maximize appropriate energy flow around the body and improve the chances of conception.

While there are no hard data, many women report that apparently unexplained infertility disappears after a period of acupuncture. This usually involves two to four treatments a month over a three- or four-month period.

Some preliminary work has been carried out in conditions such as polycystic ovary disease (*see p.337*) suggesting that acupuncture may normalize hormone levels. This may help explain the effectiveness of acupuncture in treating infertility.

Breathing Retraining

Anxiety is widely considered to contribute to infertility in some instances. It is certainly a common reaction to intensive, high-technology infertility treatments. Anxiety symptoms can usually be eased by regularly practicing antianxiety breathing exercises. For a description of suitable breathing methods, see p.62.

Mind-Body Therapies

There is increasing evidence that psychological approaches may be effective in treating the emotional aspects of infertility and may lead to higher conception rates.

RELAXATION TRAINING One study looked at the "relaxation response" in a group of women trying to conceive. The women who practiced this well-documented psychological technique showed significant decreases in anxiety, depression, and fatigue, and increased energy levels. In addition, 34 percent of these women became pregnant within six months of completing the program. The study further suggested that behavioral treatment should be considered for couples with

infertility before and/or in conjunction with reproductive technologies such as intrauterine insemination (IUI), in vitro fertilization (IVF), and gamete intrafallopian transfer (GIFT).

PSYCHOTHERAPY In a different study, the same research team found infertile women had much higher levels of distress than fertile women and became most distressed between the second and third years of infertility. The researchers looked at whether group psychological therapy could prevent this surge of distress. When compared with a control group, partici-

> Many couples with one to three years of unexplained infertility conceive spontaneously

pants in the study showed significant psychological improvement after both six and 12 months. Generally, the women who received cognitive behavioral therapy experienced the greatest positive change. Another study was performed to determine the effectiveness of two different group psychological interventions on conception rates in women with infertility of less than two years' duration. The women joined a ten-session cognitive behavioral group, a standard support group, or a control group that received no therapy. The research team concluded that group therapies appear to lead to increased pregnancy rates in women with infertility.

If you are having difficulty conceiving, you might try cognitive behavioral or group therapy. In one study, hypnosis improved the success rate of IVF by 20 percent.

PREVENTION PLAN

Keeping to the following guidelines may help maintain fertility:

- Avoid smoking, caffeine, and alcohol
- Maintain a healthy weight
- Avoid toxic chemicals
- Make time to relax every day

WHAT ARE THE SYMPTOMS?

- Lack of interest in sex
- Inability to enjoy sex
- Pain during sex

WHY MIGHT I HAVE THIS?

PREDISPOSING FACTORS

- Anxiety and stress
- Depression
- Relationship difficulties
- Fatigue
- Hormonal changes
- Certain drugs, including oral contraceptives and some antidepressants
- Previous traumatic sexual experience
- Sexual inhibitions
- Poor sexual technique with partner
- Poor communication between partners
- Pregnancy, postpartum, or menopause

TREATMENT PLAN

PRIMARY TREATMENTS

- Treatment of any underlying physical cause
- Couple therapy and/or psychotherapy

BACKUP TREATMENTS

- Arginine and vitamin B$_6$
- Western and Chinese herbal medicine

WORTH CONSIDERING

- Homeopathy
- Manipulation therapies
- Acupuncture

For an explanation of how treatments are rated, see p.111.

SEXUAL PROBLEMS IN WOMEN

Many women experience a sexual problem of some kind during their lives. Some of the most common include a lack of or decrease in sex drive, failure to achieve orgasm, and painful intercourse. If an underlying physical cause can be identified, it will usually be treated as a first course of action. Since many sexual problems involve mental as well as physical factors, psychological therapies are often an important part of treatment. Nutritional supplements, homeopathy, herbal treatments, acupuncture, and manipulation therapy may also help.

WHY DOES IT OCCUR?

Sexual difficulties are usually the result of psychological or physical problems, or may be a combination of the two. Upbringing and attitudes to sex may also play a role.

PROBLEMS WITH SEX DRIVE A decrease in sex drive is more common with increasing age and may be seen as part of the aging process. Since sex drive varies among individuals, a woman's sex drive should be judged only in comparison with her own usual behavior, not in comparison to the claims of other people. Many women find that their interest in sex declines after childbirth, and some women lose interest in sex during pregnancy. Many women report a temporary decline in interest in sex around and after menopause. In all of these cases, hormonal changes are likely to play a role. Low thyroid function (see p.319) and low adrenal gland function can also be responsible.

Psychological conditions, such as anxiety disorders, depression, and stress, can also have an adverse effect on a woman's sex drive. Fatigue is a common factor. Relationship difficulties are also likely to reduce sexual desire and arousal, perhaps more in a woman than a man. Some drugs, including oral contraceptives and certain selective serotonin reuptake inhibitor (SSRI) antidepressants, can also cause a decrease in sex drive.

PROBLEMS WITH ORGASM Failure to achieve orgasm is a common problem in women and is usually due to psychological factors, including anxiety about sexual performance, a previous unpleasant sexual experience, or sexual inhibitions. The latter may be due to a strict upbringing regarding sex, or physical, emotional, or sexual abuse in childhood.

Poor sexual technique is also a common contributing factor in failure to achieve orgasm; often insufficient time is allowed for a woman to become fully aroused. Sexual inexperience or lack of communication between partners can also make orgasm difficult. Certain physical disorders, such as chronic constipation, can in rare cases affect a woman's ability to reach orgasm. Direct or indirect clitoral stimulation is almost always needed for female orgasm. Manual stimulation of the clitoris during intercourse may be successful.

PAINFUL INTERCOURSE Painful intercourse (dyspareunia) may have either a psychological or physical cause. Superficial dyspareunia, felt around the entrance to the vagina and in the lower part of the vagina, may be due to an infection, vulvodynia, or psychological factors, such as anxiety, guilt, or fear of sexual penetration. Physical causes of painful intercourse include vaginal atrophy (thinning of the vaginal tissue), which can occur after

IMPORTANT

If you experience persistent pelvic pain or painful intercourse, see your doctor as soon as possible to rule out any serious underlying causes, such as pelvic inflammatory disease.

menopause; genital tract infections; and poor vaginal lubrication, which may be related either to psychological factors or insufficient foreplay, or it may accompany vaginal atrophy.

Pain that is felt higher in the vagina and deep within the pelvis during intercourse (which is known as deep pareunia) may be due to a disorder of the pelvic cavity, such as a persistent pelvic infection or endometriosis (see p.334).

VAGINISMUS This rare condition, in which the pelvic floor muscles go into spasm before or during intercourse, is usually due to psychological factors and often occurs in women who believe that penetration will be painful. This belief may be due to a previous traumatic sexual experience, sexual abuse, or painful vaginal examination. Another cause of vaginismus is fear of pregnancy. Anxiety and guilt about sex can also be contributing factors.

TREATMENTS IN DETAIL

Conventional Medicine

A doctor will compile a careful history to look for evidence of physical and psychological causes. He or she will aim to treat the underlying cause when possible.

PRIMARY TREATMENT **PHYSICAL CAUSES** Management of physical causes for sexual problems may include changing prescribed medication, laxatives for chronic constipation, or antibiotics for genital tract infections. Vaginal atrophy may be relieved either by a lubricant or by a hormonal cream, which are placed in the vagina (see Menopausal Problems, p.339). Poor lubrication may be improved by allowing time to achieve adequate arousal during foreplay and using sexual lubricants if needed.

PRIMARY TREATMENT **PSYCHOLOGICAL FACTORS** Various options are available to address psychological factors. For example, relaxation techniques may help with stress. Depression may be treated with drugs and psychotherapy as appropriate. Psychotherapy may also be used to help with anxiety and sex therapy may be needed to address attitudes to sex, which may be deeply entrenched. Your doctor

may refer you to a specialist for this. Sex therapy can also focus on key issues such as communication between partners and sexual technique (see Psychological Therapies, p.353).

Nutritional Therapy

ARGININE Sexual function and responsiveness, in both men and women, is to a degree dependent on the supply of blood to the genital organs. Dilation of blood vessels, allowing increased blood flow, depends on a substance called nitric oxide. The amino acid arginine is essential for the formation of nitric oxide in the body and many studies have shown that it improves male sexual function (see p.376).

One study assessed the effect of a supplement called ArginMax (which contains arginine in combination with herbs, vitamins, and minerals) in a group of women. After four weeks, more than 70 percent of the ArginMax group reported greater satisfaction with their sex lives, compared with only 33 percent of women taking a placebo. Notable improvements were observed in sexual desire, increased vaginal lubrication, frequency of sexual intercourse and orgasm, and clitoral sensation.

VITAMIN B Women taking oral contraceptives may have low levels of vitamin B$_6$, which is linked with decreased sex drive. Vitamin B$_6$ is needed in the formation of many brain chemicals involved in pleasure, sensation, and mood (such as dopamine, serotonin, and acetylcholine). Supplements may improve sex drive in women who are deficient in vitamin B$_6$. Taking 25–50mg of vitamin B$_6$ every day may help restore sexual desire in some women.

CAUTION

Vitamin B$_6$ supplements may interact with certain drugs, such as levodopa and phenobarbital, and reduce their effectiveness; ask your doctor for advice.

Homeopathy

For decreased sex drive, perhaps relating to depression or age, the most commonly used medicines are Causticum and Sepia.

A number of studies have looked at homeopathic treatment of childhood sexual abuse and its consequences. Several homeopathic medicines are reported to be helpful where sexual problems in adult life are a result of childhood abuse. Among these are Sepia, Platina, Phosphoric acid, and Staphysagria.

CAUSTICUM Women likely to respond to Causticum are often quite depressed as a result of a long period of stress, which manifests itself in strong feelings of injustice. These women are often campaigners for human or animal rights. A very characteristic feature is that they find it too painful to watch images of human suffering in the news. Other features include urge or stress incontinence (leakage of urine when the bladder is full or if they sneeze or cough), recurrent hoarseness or a tickling cough coming from the throat, and localized paralysis, for instance of the face (Bell's palsy).

Causticum and Staphysagria are medicines that are often used together, with Causticum often being used after Staphysagria as a follow-up treatment.

> Up to 70 percent of couples experience problems with sex at some time

STAPHYSAGRIA In the context of sexual problems, Staphysagria is an important medicine; its keynote is said to be suppressed indignation.

Women who respond to Staphysagria may have suffered sexual assault or an abusive relationship as an adult and are tremendously angry about what has been done to them. However, this anger may be suppressed and expressed through physical symptoms, particularly recurrent bladder problems (see p.238) that have no identifiable cause. Sometimes the anger is expressed, in which case these patients can be prickly, sensitive, and generally difficult to deal with.

SEPIA Women who respond to *Sepia* are flat and indifferent to others. They are depressed and irritable, particularly with their families, and they have no interest in sex. They often suffer from lower back pain and a range of menstrual or menopausal problems.

PLATINA Women who respond to *Platina* often have either a sensation of numbness or the opposite, with excessive sensitivity or itching of the genitalia that is made worse by sexual activity and prevents intercourse. They may "put on airs" and appear haughty, but this may be a defensive mechanism to hide their sense of shame. They may be very depressed and fear violence, especially from their partners. *Platina* patients (and *Staphysagria* patients, *see p.351*) may have other psychosexual problems, apart from loss of sex drive. These may include such things as promiscuity and sexual perversion.

PHOSPHORIC ACID Patients who respond to *Phosphoric acid* are quite similar to *Sepia* patients, being emotionally flat and worn out, with no interest in sex. Symptoms that suggest *Phosphoric acid* might be suitable, rather than *Sepia*, include weak memory and poor concentration, along with diarrhea or loose bowels.

Western Herbal Medicine

Western herbal medicine can be used to treat sexual problems when they are related to problems with circulation, mild hormonal imbalances, or depression and anxiety. If problems are longstanding, it is probably best to consult a trained herbal practitioner for help with treatment.

HERBS TO IMPROVE CIRCULATION Ginkgo (*Ginkgo biloba*) helps increase peripheral circulation and may therefore improve circulation to the sexual organs. This herb should be taken at a dose of 50–100g per day to see whether sexual responsiveness improves.

Other herbs that may be used to stimulate the circulation include hawthorn (*Crataegus monogyna*), ginger root (*Zingiber officinalis*), rosemary (*Rosmarinus officinalis*), and prickly ash (*Xanthoxylum clavaherculis*). These herbs may be used alone or in combination. Three cups of tea

per day, or 20–30 drops of tincture taken three times each day, is the usual dose.

IMPROVING HORMONAL BALANCE Mild hormonal imbalances may be treated with various herbs, of which the most important is probably chaste-tree berry (*Vitex agnus castus*). However, this herb must be taken over a relatively long period of time (12–18 months) before its effects are seen.

Damiana (*Turnera diffusa*) appears to support testosterone levels, which may be too low in women with reduced or absent sex drive. Milk thistle (*Silybum marianum*), vervain (*Verbena officinalis*), and dandelion root (*Taraxacum officinale*) are all valuable for supporting the liver and

Women between the ages of 35 and 65 are more likely to experience problems with sex

restoring hormonal balance. They may be used in combination to make a tea (or a tincture), of which one cup (or 15–20 drops) should be taken before each meal. Saw palmetto (*Serenoa repens*) may also help restore hormonal balance.

HERBS FOR DEPRESSION-RELATED PROBLEMS St. John's wort (*Hypericum perforatum*) may be used to alleviate depression, as may kava kava (*Piper methysticum*), lemon balm (*Melissa officinalis*), gotu kola (*Centella asiatica*), skullcap (*Scutellaria lateriflora*), and passion flower (*Passiflora incarnata*). They may be combined equally to make a tea (or a tincture), which should be taken one cup (or 20–30 drops) two times each day. It may take up to two months before results are apparent.

> **CAUTION**
>
> See p.69 before taking an herbal remedy and, if you are taking prescribed medication, consult an herbal medicine expert first.

Chinese Herbal Medicine

Traditional Chinese herbalists may treat sexual problems using herbs that strengthen the adrenal glands and improve

muscle strength. These herbs may be combined with blood-strengthening and moistening herbs, which act to reduce stress and increase sexual fluids.

ADRENAL TONICS Herbs that act on the adrenal glands are especially important for women, whose sexual problems are often related to fatigue and/or hormonal imbalances. Nettle (*Urtica dioica*) is important for women who have long-term exhaustion, which may be coupled with autoimmune problems and allergies. Other important adrenal tonics include clove (*Syzygium aromaticum*), sage (*Salvia officinalis*), and fenugreek (*Trigonella foenum-graecum*).

GINSENG Traditional Chinese herbalists have used ginseng (*Panax ginseng*) to treat sexual problems for centuries. Ginseng is believed to improve hormonal function. A study at Yale University School of Medicine showed that ginseng stimulates nitric oxide, which assists the body in a number of circulatory functions, improving blood vessel dilation and blood pressure regulation. Ginseng may be combined with solomon's seal (*Polygonum multiflorum*) to balance its stimulating effects.

> **CAUTION**
>
> Do not take ginseng if you have high blood pressure. See also p.69.

Acupuncture

Acupuncture can be a very useful therapy in treating sexual problems, particularly when it is combined with other therapies such as herbal treatments, psychological therapies, and massage or manipulation therapies. Case studies have shown that women with loss of libido and a history of prior sexual abuse have responded well to acupuncture treatment, although it was recommended that they persist with follow-up psychological therapies to help

CHIROPRACTIC TREATMENT FOR SEXUAL PROBLEMS

Chiropractic can help some problems, particularly painful intercourse or chronic pelvic pain. The chiropractor may manipulate the low back to deactivate trigger points, sensitive areas in muscles that cause pain. Distractive decompressive manipulation is good for this.

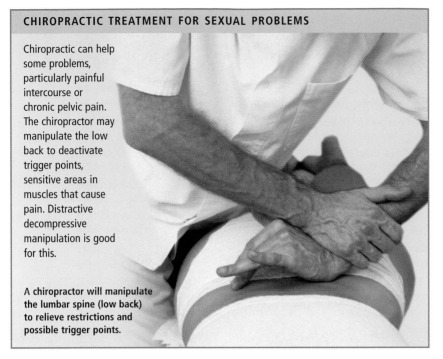

A chiropractor will manipulate the lumbar spine (low back) to relieve restrictions and possible trigger points.

them come to terms with their past trauma. An initial course of 3–4 treatments is likely to be given. If the response is good, treatment may be given once or twice weekly for two months, with maintenance treatment twice yearly after that.

Bodywork Therapies

Sexual dysfunction that develops because of painful intercourse or chronic pelvic pain can sometimes be treated by appropriate chiropractic or osteopathic manipulation, or by deactivation of active trigger points that produce pain in the pelvic organs. Trigger points can be deactivated by acupuncture, as well as by manual pressure and stretching techniques as used by osteopaths and chiropractors.

A particular form of chiropractic treatment, using a technique that is known as distractive decompressive manipulation of the lumbar spine (the lower back, from where the nerves that supply the pelvic organs emerge), has been shown to be especially effective in relieving the cause (commonly pain) of some women's sexual dysfunction.

Psychological Therapies

Female sexual disorders can been divided into four main categories: low sexual desire, difficulties in sexual arousal, difficulties in achievement of orgasm, and pain associated with sexual activity.

PRIMARY TREATMENT **COUPLE THERAPY** is used to treat sexual dysfunction and is perhaps the most eclectic of the talking therapies, in that it combines a variety of approaches, including cognitive behavioral therapy (CBT) and psychodynamic ideas. A woman with sexual problems is usually treated with her partner on the assumption that their relationship is stable enough to enable clear communication to take place. If the relationship is not stable, couple or marital therapy may be more appropriate, because some of the sexual difficulties may be an expression of a troubled relationship.

PRIMARY TREATMENT **SEX THERAPY** Pioneered by Masters and Johnson in 1970, sex therapy normally follows a series of stages. An initial assessment is followed by a formulation or plan of therapy. This is usually followed by counseling, which may have psychodynamic and CBT components. This stage is usually accompanied by "homework" tasks and simple sex education. The couple may be asked to examine their attitudes to sex and how these ideas were formed earlier in their life. Then they may be asked to try out new ways of

touching each other without focusing on each other's genitals (known as nongenital sensate focus) before moving into more overt genital contact (genital sensate focus). Masturbation exercises may also be encouraged, particularly for women who have difficulty in achieving orgasm. Other methods such as gradual introduction of the penis into the vagina with the woman in control can be used for problems such as vaginismus.

RESEARCH A number of studies support the use of sex therapy. For low sexual desire, researchers worked with 32 couples and found that nearly 70 percent of the women reported they had totally or partially regained their interest in sex. Another study examined the effect of working with couple and women-only treatment. They found that both methods achieved significant results. Researchers also examined the use of CBT for both women and men and found effective in increasing positive attitudes toward sex, including sexual arousal.

The treatment of women who have difficulty in achieving orgasm has been studied by a number of researchers. They found that the Masters and Johnson method was effective in helping women achieve orgasm, although in one study this was achieved mainly through masturbation.

The treatment of vaginismus has also shown positive results. In a study of 30 couples in whom the women had vaginismus, researchers found that the problem was totally or largely resolved in 80 percent of the women.

PREVENTION PLAN

The following measures can help prevent sexual problems:

- Get adequate rest so that you do not become overtired. This is especially important after the birth of a baby, or if you have young children

- Practice relaxation exercises or yoga regularly to reduce levels of stress and anxiety

- Do Kegel exercises regularly, and every day if possible

- Eat a healthy, balanced diet and maintain a normal weight

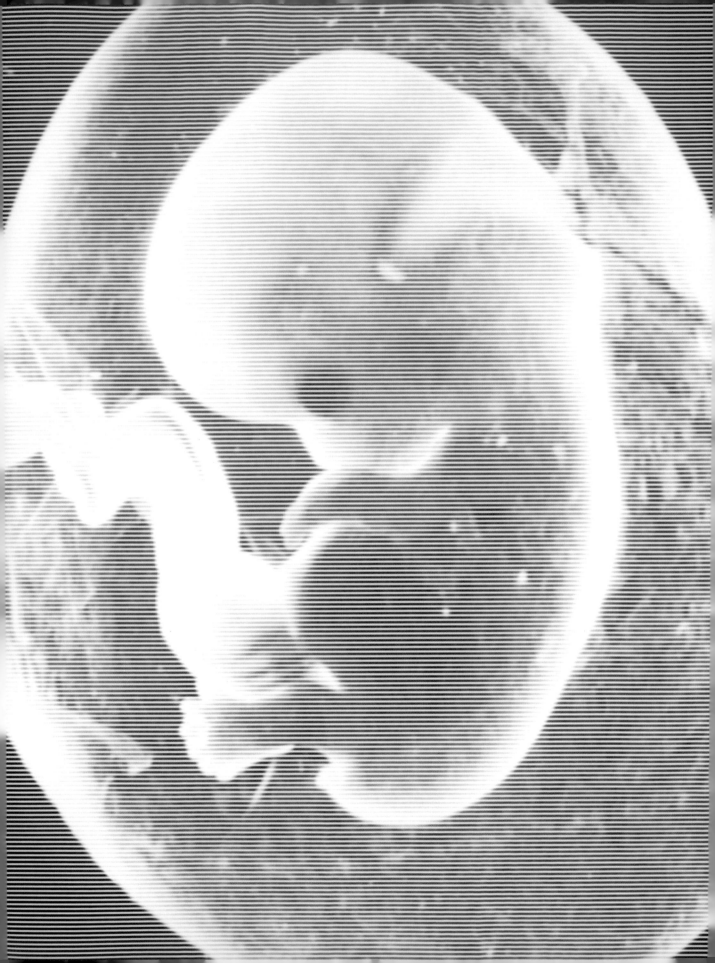

Pregnancy
& Childbirth

During pregnancy and childbirth the mother's
body undergoes immense changes, which can
be both physically and emotionally stressful.
Conventional medicine plays a vital role in
protecting the health of mother and child, but
supportive complementary therapies should not
be underestimated, particularly since pregnancy
is a time when many drugs should be avoided.

MORNING SICKNESS

The nausea known as morning sickness is one of the most common complaints of early pregnancy. Its name is misleading because it is not always confined to the morning but may also be present during the day and the evening. However, it usually clears up by the 14th to 16th week of pregnancy and although it is unpleasant it is not usually dangerous. Dietary changes and other measures such as acupressure can relieve morning sickness, but a pregnant woman should not take any remedies for nausea without first consulting her doctor.

WHAT ARE THE SYMPTOMS?

- A feeling of nausea, which may be worse on awakening
- Vomiting
- Sensitivity to strong smells, such as garlic

WHY MIGHT I HAVE THIS?

TRIGGERS

- Exposure to strong smells
- Fatty foods
- Large infrequent meals

TREATMENT PLAN

PRIMARY TREATMENTS

- Small, frequent meals
- Ginger
- Pressing P6 acupressure point
- Acupuncture

BACKUP TREATMENTS

- Intravenous fluids, antihistamines, and antinausea drugs (for hyperemesis gravidarum)
- Nutritional therapy
- Homeopathy
- Chamomile and slippery elm
- Reflexology and osteopathy

For an explanation of how treatments are rated, see p.111.

WHY DOES IT OCCUR?

It is not known why morning sickness occurs. Some women do not develop it at all, while others may feel nauseous throughout their pregnancies. It is thought that the rapidly increasing levels of certain hormones, perhaps human chorionic gonadotropin (a hormone produced by the placenta), during early pregnancy are at least partially responsible for the condition. Although a woman with morning sickness may not feel well for much of the time, she should continue to eat. Morning sickness is not dangerous for either the mother or the baby unless the vomiting becomes so severe that fluids or food cannot be kept down. This condition is known as hyperemesis gravidarum and may cause dehydration, chemical imbalances, and weight loss. Antihistamines or antivomiting drugs may be necessary as well as hospital admission for intravenous fluids.

SELF-HELP

- Eat small, frequent, protein-filled meals.
- Nibble dry biscuits and crackers.
- Sip chamomile tea.
- Include ginger in the diet.
- Drink plenty of water.
- Press the P6 point (see Acupressure, p.357).

IMPORTANT

Consult your doctor before taking any remedies (conventional or herbal) for morning sickness. If vomiting becomes severe and you are unable to keep down any fluid or food, see your doctor immediately.

TREATMENTS IN DETAIL

Conventional Medicine

No medical treatment is usually required for mild nausea and occasional vomiting in pregnancy. More persistent vomiting may require tests to look for a possible underlying cause, such as a urinary tract infection, and hospital admission may be necessary, where intravenous fluids can be given.

In hyperemesis gravidarum, antihistamines such as promethazine or the antiemetic metoclopramide may be prescribed; or the antihistamine doxylamine is available over the counter. However, these treatments are only rarely needed. Although there is no evidence to suggest that they cause harm in pregnancy, they are used only when absolutely necessary. If vomiting is persistent, vitamin supplements such as vitamin B_6, may be used (see p.357).

CAUTION

Drugs for hyperemesis gravidarum can cause a range of possible side effects; ask your doctor to explain these to you.

Nutritional Therapy

PRIMARY TREATMENT **DIETARY CHANGES** Nausea in pregnancy has been associated with a poor diet and with eating large, infrequent meals. In practice, morning sickness appears to be worse on an empty stomach. Symptoms may be relieved by eating small, frequent meals, to help keep blood-sugar levels stable. Foods that are are low in fat are particularly important, since fatty foods, such as red meat, dairy products, and fried foods, tend to make nausea worse. Taking steps to improve digestion, such as chewing food thoroughly and not drinking too much fluid with meals, can also help.

NUTRITIONAL SUPPLEMENTS Vitamin B_6 (pyroxidine) may help relieve nausea and vomiting in pregnancy. One study found that vitamin B_6 at 30mg per day was effective in relieving the severity of nausea in early pregnancy. Vitamin C taken with vitamin K may help relieve the symptoms of morning sickness. In one study, women who received 5mg of vitamin K and 25mg of vitamin C per day reported the complete disappearance of morning sickness within three days. Taking a multivitamin and mineral supplement containing vitamins B_6, C, and K may help control morning sickness.

> **CAUTION**
>
> Women who are pregnant, trying to conceive, or breast-feeding should not take supplements containing more than 2,000 IU of vitamin A without their doctor's advice.

Homeopathy

IPECACUANHA (also known as *Ipecac*) is the most commonly used homeopathic medicine for morning sickness. Women who respond to it have severe and constant nausea, retching, and vomiting, and vomiting does not relieve their nausea. Vomiting may be accompanied by nosebleeds and/or bouts of coughing. Ipecac should be taken in the 12C strength, two pills four times daily, or more frequently if required.

NUX VOMICA Other commonly suggested medicines for morning sickness include *Nux vomica*. It is indicated for women who have nausea that is much worse in the morning, often waking them early. There is often severe nausea and a lot of retching, but relatively little vomiting. All the senses seem oversensitive, with every smell making the nausea worse, noises seeming too loud, and bright lights hurting the eyes.

COCCULUS AND SEPIA Women who respond to *Cocculus* have dizziness and are sensitive to movement. Traveling makes the nausea much worse. Those who respond to *Sepia* have nausea that is made much worse by the smell of food, especially frying food. These women may crave sharp, acidic foods (such as pickles or lemons), which may temporarily relieve the sickness. There is often heavy lower back pain; these women may feel very tired and emotionally flat.

Western Herbalism

SAFETY ISSUES As a rule, herbal remedies (as with almost all medicines) should not be taken during the first three months of pregnancy, and some herbs should be avoided throughout pregnancy. That said, appropriate herbal treatment may be a safe and effective option for pregnancy problems such as morning sickness. There are some foods, such as ginger, that have medicinal properties and in general this category of herbal medicines can be safely recommended for use during pregnancy.

Several herbs are traditional remedies for morning sickness. These include ginger, chamomile, and slippery elm. With the exception of ginger, little research has been done.

PRIMARY TREATMENT **GINGER** Over the last 20 years, research interest into ginger (*Zinziber officinalis*) has increased, and has established that the dried root has powerful anti-inflammatory and antiemetic activity. A number of clinical trials have shown ginger to be as effective as conventional treatments in preventing motion sickness, and in preventing postoperative nausea in patients undergoing surgery. In one 1990 double-blind, randomized, crossover trial, 30 pregnant women with morning sickness took four 250mg capsules of dried ginger a day It significantly helped relieve symptoms.

CHAMOMILE AND SLIPPERY ELM Chamomile tea (*Matricari recituta*) is a useful, safe treatment for morning sickness: its ability to soothe and relieve nausea and indigestion is well established. Slippery elm (*Ulnus fulva*) capsules can help settle the digestion — the powder may also be taken mixed with water, although the sticky consistency is often off-putting.

PROFESSIONAL ADVICE There is a wide range of other herbs, some with hormonal activity, which are commonly prescribed by practitioners. If self-medication with ginger, chamomile, or slippery elm is unsuccessful, consult an herbal medicine expert.

Acupuncture

PRIMARY TREATMENT Acupuncture is particularly useful for morning sickness because ailments that occur in early pregnancy are problematic to treat with medicines due to the risk of side effects. There is no doubt that acupuncture provides a safe treatment. A number of clinical trials have examined applying pressure to the P6 acupuncture point (*see below*), which helps even severe morning sickness. Vickers produced a systematic review of a large number of clinical trials looking at acupuncture and nausea. Clinical trials carried out subsequently to 1966 served to confirm this positive effect. Some of the studies reviewed by Vickers include using acupressure on the P6 acupuncture point.

Bodywork Therapies

ACUPRESSURE AND REFLEXOLOGY A **PRIMARY TREATMENT** number of research studies have confirmed that pressure applied to the Pericardium acupoint 6 on the forearm (known in Chinese medicine as *Neiguan*), can significantly reduce morning sickness and nausea. This point lies about two thumb-widths above the front wrist crease, in line with the ring finger (*see p.154*). Find a tender area on one wrist, by careful probing, and then press this firmly for five to 10 minutes. Treat yourself in this way as often as needed. You can also buy special wrist straps ("C-bands") that produce a constant pressure on this point.

Reflexology has also been shown useful in treating some cases of morning sickness.

OSTEOPATHY Experience suggests that osteopathic treatment that alleviates spinal imbalances and restrictions can improve the symptoms of morning sickness, but no research as yet confirms this.

> **PREVENTION PLAN**
>
> **Try the following:**
>
> - Eat little and often
> - Avoid fried, fatty, or spicy foods
> - Eat something bland, such as crackers, before getting up in the morning

LABOR

The process of childbirth, known as labor, usually begins around the 40th week of pregnancy. Labor has three distinct stages: the first, when the uterus contracts and the cervix widens; the second, when the baby passes through the birth canal; and the third, when the placenta is delivered. Many things can be done to make labor a more comfortable process, including taking pain-relieving drugs and having a birthing partner present to give psychological support. Techniques such as massage, acupuncture, relaxation, and self-hypnosis can also help.

TREATMENT PLAN

PRIMARY TREATMENTS

For pain relief:
- Abdominal breathing techniques
- Relaxation and self-hypnosis
- Drug-free methods, e.g. TENS
- Pethidine and other drugs for pain
- Epidural analgesia

To accelerate labor:
- Oxytocin injections

BACKUP TREATMENTS
- Active labor
- Massage and birthing pool
- Forceps or vacuum extraction
- Cesarean section

WORTH CONSIDERING
- Homeopathy
- Intradermal water blocks
- Acupuncture
- Mind–body therapies

For an explanation of how treatments are rated, see p.111.

HOW DOES IT OCCUR?

STAGE ONE The trigger for labor to begin is not known, but it may be a surge of the hormone oxytocin, which causes the uterus to contract. The usual first signs of labor are strong and mildly painful contractions of the uterus. The plug of mucus that has been blocking the cervix during pregnancy usually comes away at this time but may appear as many as ten days before labor. When this happens, a small amount of blood and mucus, known as the "show," is passed from the vagina but many women are unaware of it. Additionally, the amniotic sac that surrounds the baby usually ruptures either shortly before or during the first stage of labor and is often referred to as the water breaking. A woman usually notices if her water breaks before labor is established but it may go unnoticed if it happens during the first stage of labor. Contractions become stronger and more painful as labor progresses and the cervix becomes wider (dilates).

STAGE TWO The second stage of labor begins when the cervix is fully dilated to 4in (10cm). At this stage the baby passes from the uterus through the vagina and is born. The second stage is much quicker than the first stage and usually lasts between one and two hours. The baby's head presses on the pelvic floor, causing an overwhelming urge in the mother to bear down, or push. When the baby's head is visible at the opening of the vagina, the birth is imminent.

STAGE THREE The third stage of labor takes place shortly after the baby is born. The placenta, which has been nourishing the baby during pregnancy, separates from the inner surface of the uterus, which resumes contracting to expel it. Blood vessels in the uterus also contract to stop the bleeding.

DIFFERENT EXPERIENCES OF LABOR The length of each stage of labor varies and may depend on the number of times a woman has given birth previously — second and subsequent labors tend to be shorter than the first.

The contractions women experience during labor are painful, and the birth of the baby is also painful and may be exhausting if it takes a long time. Many pregnant women are understandably concerned about the length of labor and pain. However, women differ in their tolerance to pain, so the experience of labor and birth is not the same for everyone. Becoming familiar with the process of labor can help women know what to expect at each stage and to approach the birth and pain relief with an open mind.

SELF-HELP

The following suggestions may help make your labor more comfortable:
- Attend prenatal classes regularly and discuss any concerns with your obstetrician or midwife.
- Make sure your birth partner supports the type of birth you want.
- Practice guided imagery and relaxation during pregnancy (*see p.99*).
- Make a birth plan beforehand but be prepared to change it during labor.
- Get regular, gentle exercise during pregnancy — your midwife or doctor can advise you about what is appropriate.

Conventional Medicine

CHOICES IN LABOR There are various options for pain relief during labor. Some women choose to avoid medication and rely on breathing techniques and relaxation methods instead (*see* p.361). Many women choose a combination of natural methods and drugs. The help and encouragement of a supportive birthing partner can be invaluable. Attending prenatal classes can also be helpful in making prospective mothers and their partners aware of what may happen and the many options available to help cope with labor.

PRIMARY TREATMENT **DRUG-FREE METHODS** The simplest way for a woman to relieve discomfort during labor is to move into different positions, from standing and squatting to lying down. Another method of pain relief is transcutaneous electrical nerve stimulation (TENS), which is helpful particularly during the early stages of labor. TENS helps relieve pain by deliver-

USING TENS IN LABOR

A transcutaneous electrical nerve stimulation (TENS) machine is a pain-relieving device that delivers small electrical impulses through electrodes on the skin. The wearer can control the intensity and timing of the impulses.

ing tiny electrical impulses through electrodes on the back. It may also be used for lower back pain. However, the exact reasons why this method is effective are not yet fully understood.

PRIMARY TREATMENT **DRUGS FOR PAIN RELIEF** Terbutaline may be given as an injection to relax uterine muscles. Other

> ## The length of a full-term pregnancy may be anywhere between 37 and 43 weeks

drugs used for pain relief during labor include the opiates meperidine and morphine. Morphine may cause women to feel drowsy and confused. Medication for nausea is usually given with morphine to counter some of the side effects. Morphine may also cause sedation in newborns, which is reversed by the drug naloxone.

Some women choose to have an epidural, which is an injection of local anesthetic into the epidural space (the space surrounding the membranes that envelop the spinal cord) in the lower back. The anesthetic can either be given continuously or individual doses can be given intermittently as needed. An epidural can give complete pain relief; in fact all sensation from the top of the abdomen down is usually lost, although women can still feel pressure. Once the epidural is set up, movement is limited and regular monitoring of pulse rate and blood pressure is required. Troublesome side effects are relatively uncommon, but may include severe headaches.

PRIMARY TREATMENT **SPEEDING UP LABOR** Measures may be taken to speed up the first and second stages. In the first stage, if the cervix is dilating too slowly, and the woman's water has not broken, a doctor or midwife may perform an amniotomy (AROM). In this procedure the membranes of the amniotic sac are artificially ruptured, releasing further prostaglandins that may help establish regular uterine contractions. Another way to increase the frequency, strength, and duration of contractions in the first stage of labor is to administer the drug oxytocin by intravenous infusion. Careful monitoring

is needed and the dose is adjusted accordingly, because oxytocin may cause various side effects. Eventually a cesarean section may be recommended if there has been little or no progress and the baby's well-being is at risk.

Oxytocin may also be given during a prolonged second stage. If the baby is still not delivered, an assisted delivery using forceps or vacuum extraction may be advised. These tools may cause a slight deformation to the baby's head, because the bones of a baby's skull are not yet fused, but this is not harmful and will disappear soon.

Oxytocin, ergonovine, or methyl-ergonovine maleate are routinely given to stimulate the muscles of the uterus to contract, in preparation for the third stage of labor. These drugs help the uterus expel the placenta and reduce bleeding from the uterine surface.

> **CAUTION**
>
> Drugs and procedures to assist labour have a range of possible side effects; ask your midwife or doctor to explain these to you.

Homeopathy

CAULOPHYLLUM There is evidence from clinical trials in the 1990s that homeopathic treatment decreased the duration of labor and reduced the number of cesarean sections required.

The main medicine used in the trials was *Caulophyllum*. It is given for delay in labor, when the cervix is rigid, preventing it from fully dilating. It can also be used in preparation for labor, when it should be taken in the 6C strength twice every day, starting between the 34th and 36th weeks of pregnancy. When labor starts, an additional three doses at half-hourly intervals should be taken.

OTHER MEDICINES A number of other homeopathic medicines help with labor

MASSAGE FOR BACK PAIN IN LABOR

Many women experience pain in the lower back during labor. This can be greatly relieved by simple massage techniques, which can be done by a caregiver or a birthing partner. Diluted essential oils of lavender and/or rose help the hands glide over the skin and may also heighten the relaxing effect of massage for the mother.

Massaging the lower back during labor can help relieve pain in this area, which may be caused by the baby's head pressing on nerves as it passes through the pelvis.

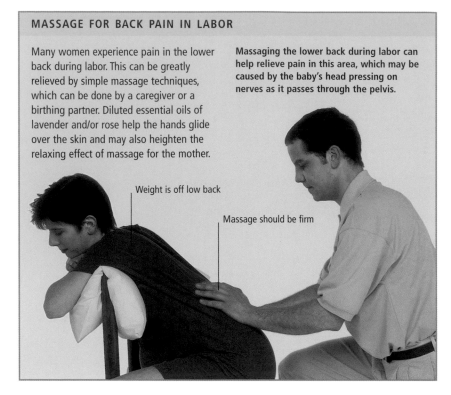

Weight is off low back

Massage should be firm

problems, but these should be used only with the advice of a midwife or other health professional trained in homeopathy. One of the most frequently suggested is *Actea racemosa* (also known as *Cimicifuga racemosa*). It is appropriate when the contractions are weak and irregular, although the pain may be very severe. The woman may become almost hysterical, as well as very loquacious.

Other homeopathic medicines that your practitioner may use include *Pulsatilla*, when the contractions are irregular and the woman feels faint with them. A cool breeze typically makes her feel better. She may be weepy and emotional.

Chamomilla and *Magnesia phosphoricum* have a reputation for helping with labor pains. Women who respond to *Chamomilla* are typically very angry, responding to the pain by shouting and swearing. Strangely perhaps, the only thing that seems to help these women is moving around quite vigorously.

Women who respond to *Magnesia phosphoricum* have a very different character. They are exhausted rather than bad-tempered from the pain, which is severe and cramping. Warmth placed on the lower abdomen (from a hot water bottle or heating pad) provides some pain relief.

Acupuncture

ACUPUNCTURE TO INDUCE LABOR
Acupuncture has commonly been used to induce ripening of the cervix and indeed full normal labor. However, a review of the research available in 2003 failed to show that this is true. It is quite possible that acupuncture will induce cervical ripening and consequent labor, but better-designed randomized controlled trials are needed to evaluate the role of this treatment.

Usually two or three daily sessions of acupuncture are required and needles are applied to specific points. It is common to give electroacupuncture, which involves electrical stimulation of the needles.

ACUPUNCTURE FOR BREECH PRESENTATION Traditional Chinese Medicine (TCM) uses moxibustion (smoldering herbs to stimulate acupuncture points) of acupoint BL67 to promote turning of babies in breech presentation. The BL67 point is located beside the outer corner of the fifth toenail and stimulation of this acupoint may increase the baby's activity in the uterus, which frequently causes them to turn. A randomized controlled trial evaluated this therapy for breech presentations and found it effective. The

technique can be taught by an acupuncture practitioner and can be administered at home, preferably by someone other than the pregnant woman.

ACUPUNCTURE FOR PAIN RELIEF
Acupuncture has been used extensively to alleviate pain during labor, and there are several clinical trials indicating that it has a substantial and immediate effect.

A study involving 46 women in labor compared the pain intensity, degree of relaxation, and delivery outcomes of those who had acupuncture with those who did not. Acupuncture that was administered during labor signficantly reduced the need for epidural pain relief and allowed the women who had it a greater degree of relaxation than the women who did not receive acupuncture.

Acupuncture had no negative effects, so it could be a good alternative for women seeking an alternative to drugs for pain relief during childbirth. Further trials with a large number of women are needed to clarify whether the main effect of acupuncture during labor is pain relief or relaxation.

Both body and ear acupuncture have been used to alleviate labor pain: the advantage of the latter technique is that it can be controlled by the mother during labor and delivery.

Bodywork Therapies

The value of five drug-free methods for relieving pain in labor — continuous labor support, baths, touch and massage, maternal movement and positioning, and intradermal water blocks — were evaluated in a review of research evidence. All five methods were researched in controlled studies and were found to be effective in reducing labor pain and improving other obstetric outcomes. They are all considered safe when used appropriately.

LABOR SUPPORT A birth partner is essential to provide physical comforting, touch and massage, assistance with positioning, bathing and grooming, hot-water bottles or ice packs as required, and emotional support and information. The latter includes nonmedical advice and acting as a mediator between the woman and her medical staff.

LABORING IN WATER Simple baths are an effective and safe method of delivery, as long as submersion in the bath occurs after dilation has reached 5cm. The water temperature should not exceed body temperature. Research published in 2004 involved 99 first-time mothers in spontaneous, active labor and at low risk of result in more effective contractions and shorter labors with less distress to the baby. It was also found that fewer medical interventions were required.

INTRADERMAL WATER BLOCKS may help relieve severe, continuous back pain, which is experienced by up to one third of

> ## Women with support from a birth partner are less likely to require medical interventions

complications who were making slow progress during childbirth. Laboring in water under midwifery care may be an effective option for treating slow progress in labor, because it reduced the need for obstetric intervention and was an alternative to giving drugs.

TOUCH AND MASSAGE The power of a reassuring touch should not be underestimated. According to touch and massage research, providing caring physical contact to a mother in labor may relieve pain, reduce anxiety, and allow for a quicker delivery. Touch may come from a birth partner or a nurse, in forms such as hand-holding, stroking, embracing, and massage.

MOVEMENT AND POSITIONING Encouraging the soon-to-be mother to change positions during labor can make her more comfortable, as well as speed up the process. She may feel most at ease when upright in stage one and squatting during stage two.

ACTIVE LABOR Recent research proposes that movement is a central aspect of normal labor. Given the choice, women change position an average of seven times in the course of normal labor. Yet bed-bound labors and birth with women semi-lying is still the norm in many hospitals despite the benefits of "active birth" being recognized since the 1970s.

In active birthing, women are encouraged to move and position themselves freely throughout labor and to give birth in more upright positions.

Active birth centers teach prenatal yoga classes to help build stamina and flexibility. A review of 18 randomized controlled trials determined that active birth tends to

women during labor. Intradermal water blocks entail injections of only 0.1ml of sterile water into the skin of the lower back in four different locations (corresponding approximately to the borders of the sacrum). The reason why these blocks relieve back pain in labor is not known but numerous research studies confirm that women receiving the sterile water blocks experience increased pain relief when compared with women who have had placebo (sham) injections.

CRANIAL MANIPULATION AND OSTEOPATHY Clinical experience suggests that the use of very gentle cranial manipulation (such as cranial osteopathy, craniosacral therapy, and sacro-occipital technique), as well as osteopathic treatment of the pelvic structures, can enhance the efficiency of the delivery process.

Mind–Body Therapies

PRIMARY TREATMENT **SELF-HYPNOSIS** Although the programs of Lamaze are the most widely used forms of childbirth preparation in the US, psychological and educational preparation with self-hypnosis (also known as guided imagery) has proven effective in several studies. Developed from the pioneering work of Dr. Dick-Read in the 1930s and 1940s, modern day self-hypnosis combines deep relaxation with positive suggestion. It addresses the physical fear response that many women experience during labor.

In a recent study of pregnant teenagers in Florida, 22 women who had learned self-hypnosis before labor had shorter hospital stays and fewer surgical interventions than other women.

In another study, half of a group of 60 pregnant women received hypnotic suggestions for an enjoyable childbirth. in the form of deep relaxation or glove anesthesia. Their first stages of labor progressed more quickly than those of the other women, they reported less pain during the birth, they needed less medication, and their babies had higher Apgar scores (in "scores" the baby from one to ten on breathing, movement, and color) at one and five minutes after birth.

PRIMARY TREATMENT **RELAXATION** Relaxation techniques, imagery, and self-hypnosis are also effective in reducing complications. For example, one researcher taught guided imagery to 100 women with a baby in breech (feet first) position, comparing them to another group of women who also had breech babies. In the hypnosis group, 81 percent of the breech babies spontaneously converted to a normal (head first) presentation, compared to 48 percent of the babies who were in the comparison group.

TYPES OF PROGRAMS In some preparation programs for labor using hypnosis, few mothers use the techniques once labor starts, making the programs less effective.

More effective programs use continuous play tapes that mothers can listen to all the way through labor, for optimum relaxation and comfort. The use of taped lessons, instead of live therapists, makes the program less costly and much more flexible. Supplementary workbooks also provide valuable educational material about the childbirth process.

MIND–BODY PRACTICES From these and other studies, as well as clinical experience, it is clear that relaxation and/or guided imagery incorporating childbirth education can increase pregnant women's feelings of control and confidence in the labor process.

Pregnant women should seek their doctors' or midwives' advice in finding a suitable program that teaches self-hypnosis and relaxation for labor. Such techniques can also significantly reduce perception of pain and help women handle any complications that might arise; overall they might help reduce the likelihood of a lengthy hospital stay or a major surgical intervention, such as a cesarean section.

POSTPARTUM DEPRESSION

Many mothers experience mild depression and mood swings in the weeks following the birth of their baby. These "baby blues" usually disappear on their own within a few weeks. However, if depression persists or if symptoms are severe, a new mother may have postpartum depression, which requires medical attention. Treatment for postpartum depression involves emotional support, and counseling usually plays a central role. Antidepressant drugs are necessary in some cases. Dietary changes, relaxation, and acupuncture may also help.

WHAT ARE THE SYMPTOMS?

The symptoms of postpartum depression may develop up to six months after the birth of a baby and may include:

- Sadness
- Feeling constantly exhausted
- Having little or no interest in the new baby
- Feeling inadequate and overwhelmed by responsibilities
- Feeling guilty
- Having difficulty sleeping
- Loss of appetite

WHY MIGHT I HAVE THIS?

PREDISPOSING FACTORS

- Isolation
- Lack of emotional support
- Difficult labor
- Problems with partner
- Single motherhood
- Past history of depression
- Family history of postpartum depression

TREATMENT PLAN

PRIMARY TREATMENTS

- Emotional support and, if depression is severe, psychiatric support
- Counseling and other psychological therapies
- Antidepressants if appropriate

BACKUP TREATMENTS

- Nutritional therapy
- Acupuncture
- Mind-body therapies

WORTH CONSIDERING

- Homeopathy

For an explanation of how treatments are rated, see p.111.

WHY DOES IT OCCUR?

Hormonal changes following the birth of a baby may be partially responsible for postpartum depression. Fatigue and lifestyle changes associated with having a new baby may also be contributory factors. Some women have been depressed previously in their lives, and it seems to run in families.

Certain other factors, such as isolation, feelings of inadequacy, and doubts about being able to cope with motherhood, can all contribute to feelings of depression. Women who have had difficult labors may be at greater risk, and women who are having relationship difficulties with their partners or who are on their own as single mothers may also be more at risk.

TREATMENTS IN DETAIL

Conventional Medicine

PRIMARY TREATMENT **PSYCHOTHERAPY AND ANTI-DEPRESSANTS** Women with postpartum depression need emotional and

IMPORTANT

If you are a new mother and experience depression or mood swings that are extreme or last beyond the first few weeks after the birth, see your doctor.

Pregnant or breast-feeding women should not take any over-the-counter drugs, herbal remedies, or nutritional supplements without consulting their doctor first.

practical support from friends and family as well as care from their doctor. Psychological therapies are likely to be recommended (*see p.364*) and antidepressants may also be prescribed (*see Depression, p.436*).

Nutritional Therapy

ESSENTIAL FATTY ACIDS The omega-3 fatty acids such as eicosapentaenoic acid (EPA) and docosahexaenoic acid (DHA) seem to play an important role in mood maintenance (*see Depression, p.436*). During pregnancy, mothers transfer DHA to the fetus to support development of the fetal brain. Low levels of DHA in the mother's diet increase the risk of the mother becoming depleted of this nutrient, which may increase the risk of postpartum depression.

One study found that higher concentrations of DHA in mothers' milk (a sign that DHA had not been depleted during pregnancy) and greater seafood consumption (during and after pregnancy) were associated with lower risk of postpartum depression. These findings suggest that having an adequate intake of omega-3 fatty acids before, during, and after pregnancy might help prevent postpartum depression. Pregnant mothers should consume at least two portions of oily fish a week. Some species of oily fish (such as tuna, marlin, and swordfish) tend to be contaminated with mercury, and there is some thought that this might interfere with the neurological development of the fetus. Oily fish that tend not to be contaminated with mercury include salmon, trout, mackerel, herring, and sardine. It considered safer for women

THE "BABY BLUES" AND POSTPARTUM DEPRESSION

Postpartum depression is not the same as the "baby blues," the short period of sadness or moodiness that many women experience a few days after giving birth. The baby blues are not serious and are probably due to fatigue and fluctuating hormone levels. Most women recover from them within a few weeks. Postpartum depression is a more serious condition in which a woman may feel a prolonged sense of inadequacy and despondency. It may require professional treatment.

BABY BLUES	POSTPARTUM DEPRESSION
• Mood swings, from happy to weepy	• Sadness that persists for weeks on end
• More irritable than usual on occasion	• Lack of interest in outside world
• Difficulty concentrating	• Profound fatigue and lethargy that persists
• Difficulty resting when baby is asleep	• Feelings of guilt and inadequacy
• Diminished appetite	• Insomnia
• Feeling overwhelmed by responsibility	• Anxiety and panic attacks

to consume these types of oily fish during pregnancy and breast-feeding. However, recent US research showed that farmed Scottish salmon may be contaminated with high concentrations of certain chemicals. Pregnant and breast-feeding women might also take a supplement of 1–2g of concentrated fish oils each day.

FOLIC ACID Low levels of folic acid have also been found to be associated with depression, and there is some evidence that they may play a part in postpartum depression. Pregnancy tends to deplete the body of folic acid. Also, women with postpartum depression tend to have lower levels of folic acid compared to postpartum women who are not depressed. Supplements of 400mcg of folic acid per day is often advised for women with postpartum depression.

5-HYDROXYTRYPTOPHAN Women with postpartum depression also seem to have low tryptophan levels. Tryptophan is an amino acid found in foods such as meat, tofu, almonds, peanuts, pumpkin seeds, sesame seeds, and tahini. It is an essential building block for serotonin, a brain chemical that helps maintain mood.

Tryptophan is not available over the counter in many countries, including the US. However, 5-hydroxytryptophan (5-HTP), the substance that tryptophan is converted into before it is made into serotonin, is an alternative and available in the US. The normal recommended dose is 50mg of 5-HTP, taken two or three times a day.

> **CAUTION**
> Ask your doctor for advice before taking fish-oil supplements with anticoagulant drugs such as warfarin. (*See also p.46.*)

Homeopathy

Homeopathy can be used to treat depression following childbirth, but if symptoms are severe or persistent (lasting more than two to three weeks), a woman should consult her doctor without delay.

IGNATIA This medicine is appropriate if the woman feels upset and tense; grief may be a component of her emotions, sometimes due to a difficult birth or one that did not go as she had planned.

ARSENICUM ALBUM Women who respond to this medicine feel insecure; they may be very restless, yet seem incapable.

CIMICIFUGA This medicine is indicated when the woman feels anxious and may perceive, probably falsely, that everything in her life is going wrong. Significantly in terms of postpartum depression, she may also doubt her capabilities as a mother.

CALCAREA CARBONICA Women who respond to this medicine may feel weak and be very tired in general. They are easily fatigued by exercise and may also have anxiety, insomnia, and nightmares.

AURUM METALLICUM Women who respond to this medicine may feel worthless. Dark days and bad weather make them worse, and they may feel worse at nighttime. Women who had depression before childbirth often respond well.

NATRUM MURIATICUM This medicine is appropriate when a woman feels sensitive and emotional; she may cry frequently. She may have trouble getting along with other members of the family and doubt her ability to cope with the baby.

SEPIA Women who respond to *Sepia* may feel exhausted to the point of indifference. They may feel resentful. Physical symptoms may include a weak pelvic floor.

PULSATILLA Women who respond to *Pulsatilla* are extremely insecure and may require almost constant emotional reassurance. They feel better in the open air and worse in warm, stuffy rooms.

Acupuncture

Acupuncture has been used to treat depression that has many different causes, including postpartum depression. There is some clear evidence that acupuncture can help with depression. Two clinical trials were done comparing electroacupuncture with conventional antidepressants in the treatment of depression (*see p.436*). It is probable that acupuncture has an effect on the chemical messengers within the brain and may act to "balance" processes and reactions. Although there are no clinical trials done to look at postpartum depression specifically, it is very likely that acupuncture can help with this condition.

Deciding whether acupuncture treatment is appropriate in a particular case depends on the severity of the depression. If it is very severe, verging on psychotic or suicidal, it is unwise to use a relatively untested treatment such as acupuncture. However, for mild depression, acupuncture could offer a very safe and effective treatment, perhaps alongside counseling or mind–body therapy. This is especially true for breast-feeding mothers, since there is no possibility of unwanted, or potentially dangerous, chemicals emerging in the mother's breast milk.

A traditional Chinese diagnosis and treatment would probably be the best approach for postpartum depression. Treatment should usually be given two or three times a week, and you would usually expect to see a response within four to six treatments. If there is a response, continue with treatment, but if not, abandon this approach after six to eight sessions.

Mind–Body Therapies

RELAXATION AND GUIDED IMAGERY Results from a study on the effects of these therapies showed that women who used them had less anxiety and greater self-esteem than women who did not.

Between 10 and 15 percent of women develop postpartum depression lasting over two weeks

OTHER TREATMENTS Approximately 13 percent of women experience postpartum depression. In 2001 a meta-analysis updated the findings of an earlier meta-analysis of postpartum depression risk factors. Thirteen significant predictors or predisposing factors were revealed, which ranged from prenatal depression and low self-esteem to a lack of family support, difficult family relationships, history of previous depression, being a single mother, and an unplanned pregnancy. Although there is little actual research into mind–body treatments for postpartum depression, many of these predisposing factors may be helped by therapies such as yoga, guided imagery, or relaxation. If you have any of the risk factors, a mind-body therapy during pregnancy may help prevent depression after birth.

Psychological Therapies

A number of studies indicate that talking therapies can be effective, significantly reducing depressive symptoms in women

diagnosed with postpartum depression. There are a variety of approaches that are effective. Methods from the supportive/experiential group, from the CBT group, interpersonal psychotherapy, group therapy, and couple therapy have all been researched.

Most of these therapies can be used either by the mother alone or with the participation of the mother's partner as well. One study suggests that participation by the partner can help with parenting skills and increase support for the mother. This study reported a reduction in the couples' depressive symptoms and a general improvement in their health.

SUPPORTIVE AND EXPERIENTIAL GROUP THERAPY Using this method, the practitioner gives the woman an opportunity to explore ways of becoming more self-reliant, which can help with well-being. Sometimes this allows women to focus on ways to address and resolve specific problems. It may also enable them to make decisions and to improve their ways of coping with crises, working through conflict, or improving relationships with others.

PRIMARY TREATMENT | SUPPORTIVE TALKING THERAPIES Other studies have shown the benefit of supportive talking therapies when provided by health professionals who have been trained in the method. The treatment is brief, around six to eight sessions, and has been shown to be effective in reducing postpartum depression.

PRIMARY TREATMENT | COGNITIVE BEHAVIORAL APPROACHES Several studies support the use of CBT for postpartum depression. Women with postpartum depression are encouraged to become more aware of unhelpful thoughts and their consequent behavior as a result of them. They are then encouraged to generate alternative thoughts and problem-solving techniques.

CBT is often a brief course of treatment, involving eight to twelve sessions, and studies have shown that it is effective in reducing depressive symptoms in women during the

postpartum period. These brief types of treatment can be as effective as antidepressants in treating mild to moderate depression in new mothers.

Unlike antidepressants, CBT also leaves clients with reusable skills should they become depressed again in the future. CBT has been done successfully over the telephone, which is particularly useful when the mother is in an isolated position.

PRIMARY TREATMENT | INTERPERSONAL THERAPY The interpersonal therapy approach focuses on how the mother relates to others, such as her partner, her relatives, and her baby. It also focuses on how she might relate to herself. An important aspect of this form of therapy is the focus on her relationship with her own mother to examine how parenting skills have been learned and passed down. This form of "talking therapy" helps her relate problematic aspects of these relationships to her current depression. Using these techniques, interpersonal therapy has been shown to significantly reduce symptoms of postpartum depression.

PRIMARY TREATMENT | INTERACTION-FOCUSED TREATMENTS The way in which a mother relates to her new baby may also affect the level of her depression. Women who have not bonded well with their babies may feel less satisfaction with motherhood and be less effective as mothers than women who have bonded well with their babies. Some studies have focused on teaching the mother different ways of relating to her baby and have found that an improved mother-baby bond has helped relieve the mother's depression.

PREVENTION PLAN

The following may help:

- Avoid becoming isolated
- Make sure you get adequate rest and some time to yourself every day
- Let relatives and friends know when you feel you need help or support
- Practice yoga or relaxation during pregnancy

BREAST-FEEDING PROBLEMS

Although breast-feeding is a natural process, it isn't always an easy one. Problems can arise before and even after feeding is established. These include engorged breasts, cracked nipples, and mastitis, which is an infection of the milk ducts in a breast. Treatment for breast-feeding problems depends on what is wrong, but might include expressing milk and using creams to soothe cracked nipples. Homeopathy, hot and cold cloths, and manual therapies can all help ease engorgement and related pain. If mastitis develops, antibiotics may be necessary.

WHAT ARE THE SYMPTOMS?

Symptoms of engorgement include:
- Hard, swollen, painful breasts

Symptoms of cracked nipples include:
- Red, sore patches on the nipples
- Fine cracks on the nipples

Symptoms of mastitis include:
- A red, sore patch on the breast that may feel hot
- Sometimes, flu-like symptoms such as muscle aches and fever

WHY MIGHT I HAVE THIS?

PREDISPOSING FACTORS

For engorgement:
- Not feeding regularly

For cracked nipples:
- Not positioning the baby correctly on the nipple during feeding
- Not drying the nipples after feeding

For mastitis:
- Cracked nipples
- Engorgement

IMPORTANT

Untreated mastitis may develop into a breast abscess (a collection of pus in the breast tissue), which requires urgent treatment. If you think you are developing mastitis, see your doctor.

WHY DOES IT OCCUR?

Breast engorgement may occur when a mother's milk first comes in during the days following child birth, or it may occur if a baby's feeding routine is interrupted for some reason, such as illness.

Cracked nipples are usually caused by a baby not "latching on" properly to the mother's breast during feeding. To feed correctly, a baby must take the whole nipple and most of the areola (the darker area around the nipple) into his or her mouth so that the lips form an air-tight seal on the breast (*see p.366*).

TREATMENT PLAN

PRIMARY TREATMENTS
- Positioning the baby correctly and other self-help measures (*see p.366*)
- Express excess milk (for engorgement)

BACKUP TREATMENTS
- Antibiotics (for mastitis)

OTHER OPTIONS
- Homeopathy
- Trigger point deactivation
- Lymphatic drainage
- Mind-body therapies

For an explanation of how treatments are rated, see p.111.

Mastitis is the result of a milk duct infected with a bacterium, usually *Staphylococcus aureus*. The bacterium may enter the skin through a cracked nipple. Mastitis tends to occur when the breasts are engorged as a result of not being adequately drained.

SELF-HELP

PRIMARY TREATMENT The following will help you avoid problems:
- Wear a firm, supportive bra.
- Make sure the baby is positioned on the nipple correctly (*see p.366*).
- Dry the nipples after each feeding.
- Try to relax as much as possible.
- Drink plenty of fluids.
- Take an analgesic (such as acetaminophen if breast-feeding) for any discomfort.
- Saturate a piece of woolen material (a towel will do, but is not as effective) in hot water, wring it out, and place it on the breasts. After five minutes, remove and replace with a cool, damp cloth for a few seconds, while the hot material is rewarmed, wrung out, and replaced. Repeat this process two or three times.

TREATMENTS IN DETAIL

Conventional Medicine

PRIMARY TREATMENT **AVOIDING ENGORGEMENT** Women who are not intending to breast-feed should avoid expressing milk, since this is likely to stimulate further milk production. The engorgement should settle within a few days. Acetaminophen may be

CORRECT BREAST-FEEDING TECHNIQUE

In order to feed properly, a baby must be correctly "latched on" to her mother's breast. When this happens, the baby's mouth forms an airtight seal around the nipple and most or all of the areola, the darker area of skin around the nipple. If a baby is not latched on correctly, the mother's nipple will soon become irritated

and sore; in time, it may even crack and bleed. To remove a baby from the breast once she has finished feeding, or to switch to the other breast, gently insert a finger between the baby's mouth and the breast to break the seal. Pulling the baby away from the breast without doing this first will also irritate the nipple.

Latching on

Removing the baby from the breast

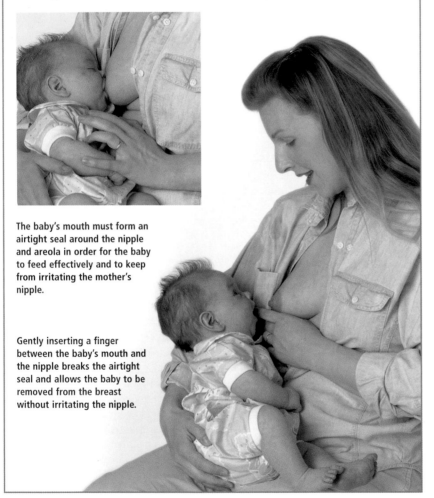

The baby's mouth must form an airtight seal around the nipple and areola in order for the baby to feed effectively and to keep from irritating the mother's nipple.

Gently inserting a finger between the baby's mouth and the nipple breaks the airtight seal and allows the baby to be removed from the breast without irritating the nipple.

taken to help relieve the discomfort. Occasionally, drugs such as bromocriptine are prescribed. Bromocriptine stops the pituitary gland (a tiny gland at the base of the brain) from releasing the hormone prolactin, which stimulates milk production by the breasts.

A woman who wishes to breast-feed and whose breasts become engorged may gently express the excess milk until the baby's feeding pattern has become established

and the breasts are producing the correct amount of milk to meet the baby's needs. When women decide to stop breast-feeding, they should gradually replace one feeding session at a time with formula in order to avoid engorgement.

PRIMARY TREATMENT **AVOIDING CRACKED NIPPLES** Carefully drying the nipples after feeding should help prevent cracked nipples. Women should also seek advice on

the positioning of the baby from their midwife or breast-feeding counselor. If you do develop cracked nipples, the problem should settle over a few days. Creams to treat cracked nipples can be bought over the counter, but seek medical advice if the problem persists. An infection may be present that requires treatment with antibiotics.

PRIMARY TREATMENT **HELP FOR MASTITIS** If you develop mastitis you should continue breast-feeding and express any milk left after feeding if possible. Acetaminophen may help relieve the pain, as may warmth applied to the affected area. This may also help the milk flow. (*See Self-Help, p.365.*) It is important to keep drinking plenty of fluids.

See your doctor if you develop mastitis, since antibiotics might be necessary to prevent an abscess from developing. The doctor may send a sample of your milk for analysis to identify the infection and ensure that the appropriate antibiotic is prescribed.

If an abscess develops, you should not feed from the affected side but you should express the milk. Like mastitis, an abscess is treated with antibiotics, but the pus may need to be drained with a needle and syringe under local anesthetic.

> **CAUTION**
>
> Drugs to treat breast-feeding problems can cause a range of possible side effects; ask your doctor to explain these to you.

Homeopathy

Homeopathy can help with a number of breast-feeding problems. The homeopathic medicine *Graphites* may be used to treat cracked nipples, while a number of homeopathic medicines may be used for mastitis. The three most common are *Belladonna*, *Bryonia*, and *Phytolacca*.

GRAPHITES The remedy *Graphites* (made from graphite, a form of carbon) taken by mouth is the classical homeopathic treatment for cracked nipples. Suck two *Graphites* pills, in the 6C strength, three or four times daily. This medicine is available from many chemists and health food shops and can be used in conjunction with creams to help soothe and heal the nipples.

BELLADONNA The sort of mastitis that responds to *Belladonna* is usually of sudden onset and the breast is hot, red, and very tender, with throbbing pain. The woman herself may be flushed and feverish and the pupils of her eyes may be dilated.

BRYONIA The type of condition that responds to *Bryonia* is also usually quite acute. The breast is hard and the pain is typically stitching in character and is made worse by any movement or jarring. The support of a well-fitting bra is helpful. The woman's mouth is often dry and she may be thirsty; she also may have sharp pains elsewhere, including in the neck and head.

PHYTOLACCA When *Phytolacca* is indicated, the breast is hard and there may be excessive milk flow, with pains that seem to shoot from the breast to locations all over

the body. This type of mastitis may be associated with a sore throat and rheumatic aches and pains in the back, legs, and the rest of the body.

Bodywork Therapies

TRIGGER POINT DEACTIVATION Trigger points (sensitive spots) in the pectoral and serratus anterior muscles in the chest can cause extreme discomfort and pain in the breasts and nipples (these symptoms have been reported in both men and women). These symptoms may be accompanied by a sense of engorgement of the breast tissue, related to sluggish lymphatic drainage. If this occurs during breast-feeding, the woman may find it impossible to continue breast-feeding.

It has been reported that deactivation of trigger points, particularly those found in the pectoralis major muscle (near the armpit) rapidly eases symptoms of pain and congestion. Trigger points can usually be deactivated by acupuncture, or by injections of procaine. Manual pressure and stretching techniques, as used by osteopaths, massage therapists (particularly those with neuro-

muscular therapy training), and some physical therapists and chiropractors can also deactivate trigger points.

LYMPHATIC DRAINAGE Because some of the main lymph drainage channels pass through, in front of, and around the pectoralis major muscles, if these tissues are tense and shortened (or contain trigger points) lymph will not be able to flow as easily and congestion in the breast tissues becomes likely. Lymphatic drainage massage (or, if appropriate, trigger point deactivation) can usually ease this restriction, and thereby, the congestion.

Mind-Body Therapies

STRESS AND BREAST-FEEDING Although the precise connection between emotional stress and breast-feeding difficulties is not

> Virtually all women can breast-feed if given the proper instruction and support

clear, experimental studies of breast-feeding women have shown that acute physical and mental stress can impair the milk ejection reflex by reducing the release of the hormone oxytocin during a feed. If this occurs repeatedly, it can reduce milk production by preventing proper emptying of the breast.

Having a stressful labor and delivery may be a factor in many breast-feeding difficulties. Studies indicate that emergency cesarean sections or long duration of labor in vaginal deliveries are associated with delayed onset of breast-feeding. Mothers who experience high levels of stress during and after childbirth should receive additional breast-feeding guidance from their midwife or breast-feeding counselor.

DELAYED ONSET OF LACTATION Usually milk comes into the breast during the first few days after child birth. If there is a delay beyond these few days, it can affect a woman's confidence and therefore her ability to breast-feed.

One recent study examined the onset of lactation in a group of 136 Guatemalan women. Researchers found that the breast milk of the women who had experienced a

stressful pregnancy and/or labor and delivery took longer to arrive than breast milk in other women.

If you feel anxious that your milk is not coming in a quickly as it should, try practicing relaxation techniques (*see p.99*) and make sure you are getting adequate rest.

MIND–BODY TECHNIQUES Despite the importance of this problem and the clear indication that stress interferes with lactation and breast-feeding, there are few studies to date of the potential effectiveness of mind-body methods. However, it is believed that these techniques can relieve stress and promote healthy, timely lactation for the benefit of the mother and baby.

One study looked at mothers separated from premature babies in intensive care units. Understandably, these mothers often find it difficult to keep up production of breast milk, despite expressing milk using a pump. Research showed that periods of holding their babies skin-to-skin increased the milk supply.

Breast-feeding mothers obviously need rest and time to establish the relationship with their babies needed to make milk flow, and experience certainly suggests that a protected rest day spent in intimate, quiet contact with the new baby will encourage more frequent feedings and therefore greater milk production.

Stress and fatigue tend to turn off the letdown reflex, which causes milk to flow. In a research trial, mothers whose babies were in a premature care unit listened to a relaxation and guided imagery tape. They showed a 60 percent increase in milk production afterward.

It seems very likely that relaxation techniques could play an effective part in helping women to overcome breast-feeding difficulties, in conjunction with good breast-feeding education and support.

PREVENTION PLAN

Try the following:

- Get advice on positioning and technique early from a breast-feeding counselor (lactation consultant)

- Use stress-reduction techniques if you feel tense

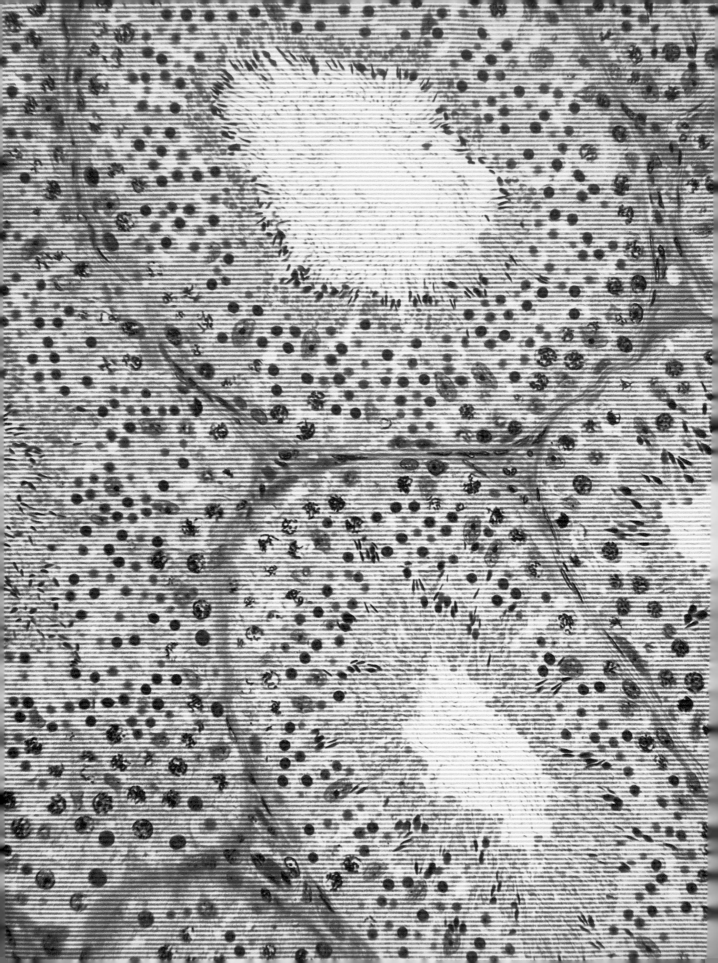

Men's Health

An integrated approach to resolving male reproductive issues acknowledges that sexual function is closely linked to emotions. Relaxation techniques, stress reduction, and talking therapies may all be appropriate, as well as conventional drugs. Herbal medicine and homeopathy can also be effective treatments.

WHAT ARE THE SYMPTOMS?

- Frequent urination, during both the day and night
- Delay in beginning to urinate, especially at night or when the bladder is full
- Weak and intermittent urine flow
- Dribbling of urine at the end of urination
- A feeling that the bladder has not emptied completely

WHY MIGHT I HAVE THIS?

PREDISPOSING FACTORS

- Being male and over 50

TREATMENT PLAN

PRIMARY TREATMENTS

- Restricting fluid intake in the evening (for mild symptoms)
- Drugs
- Surgery (for severe symptoms)
- Saw palmetto

BACKUP TREATMENTS

- Essential fatty acids
- Zinc supplements and pumpkin seeds
- Isoflavones
- Herbs containing beta-sitosterol

WORTH CONSIDERING

- Lycopene
- Chinese herbal medicine
- Exercise
- Acupuncture

For an explanation of how treatments are rated, see p.111.

BENIGN PROSTATIC HYPERTROPHY

Benign prostatic hypertrophy (BPH) is an enlargement of the prostate gland. The majority of men over the age of 50 have some degree of prostate enlargement. Among older men the disease is practically universal; it is found in approximately 90 percent of men over 85 years old. It is not cancerous and is different from prostate cancer. Treatment aims to shrink the prostate tissue and control the flow of urine.

WHY DOES IT OCCUR?

The cause of benign prostatic hypertrophy (BPH) is not known, but the male hormone testosterone plays a role. If the prostate gland is only slightly enlarged in a middle-aged man, it may be seen as a normal part of the aging process. It becomes a problem only if the gland encroaches on the urethra, the tube that carries urine from the bladder to the outside.

This encroachment can restrict urination, which may lead to various complications. For example, if the bladder is not fully emptied, it may enlarge and cause the abdomen to become distended. Urine may also collect in the bladder and stagnate, which may increase the likelihood of urinary tract infections and the risk of bladder stone formation. Rarely, backward pressure from retained urine in the bladder causes kidney damage. If an enlarged prostate gland suddenly blocks the flow of urine completely, emergency medical treatment is required.

BPH symptoms may be worse in cold weather or after drinking large amounts of fluid, especially alcoholic beverages. Drugs, such as diuretics that increase urine production, can also make symptoms worse.

IMPORTANT

- If you cannot urinate despite having the urge to do so, seek medical help at once.
- Prostate cancer can cause similar symptoms to BPH (although it is much less common).
- Men with symptoms of BPH should consult their doctor as soon as possible so that prostate cancer can be excluded.

TREATMENTS IN DETAIL

Conventional Medicine

The doctor will give you a digital rectal examination and may recommend tests to find out whether your prostate gland is significantly enlarged. These include monitoring the rate of urine flow and ultrasound scanning to measure the amount of urine that is left in the bladder after urination.

Particular treatments are recommended on the basis of several factors, including general health, the severity of the symptoms, and the size of the prostate gland.

PRIMARY TREATMENT **RESTRICTING FLUID INTAKE** If your symptoms are mild, you may not need treatment. Your doctor may simply recommend restricting fluid intake in the evening and may change your existing medication.

PRIMARY TREATMENT **DRUGS** If your symptoms are more severe, your doctor may prescribe an alpha-blocker drug, for example alfuzosin, which relaxes the smooth muscle around the urethra, thereby improving the flow of urine and helping reduce the symptoms.

Alternatively, your doctor may prescribe antiandrogen drugs, such as finasteride, which prevent the activation of testosterone in the prostate gland with the aim of shrinking the swollen tissue. This may have the effect of improving the symptoms and reducing complications.

PRIMARY TREATMENT **SURGERY** Prostatic gland tissue that reduces the flow of urine may be removed with an instrument

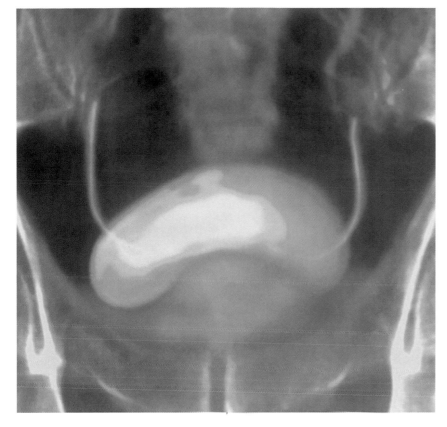

The walnut-sized prostate gland surrounds, and secretes fluid into, the urethra during ejaculation. In BPH, excessive cell division in the center of the gland causes it to expand and press on the urethra.

inserted along the urethra. In transurethral resection, the instrument cuts the tissue. In transurethral microwave thermotherapy, the instrument applies heat to the tissue without needing an incision. If the gland is very large, the surgeon may remove the tissue through an incision made in the lower abdomen.

> **CAUTION**
>
> Alpha-blockers and antiandrogens have side effects and surgery may involve certain risks; ask your doctor to explain these to you.

Nutritional Therapy

DIET Studies show that eating more fruit and vegetables appears to protect the prostate gland and may reduce the risk of prostate enlargement. Studies conversely reveal that consumption of butter, milk, margarine, and meat are associated with an increased risk of prostate enlargement.

ESSENTIAL FATTY ACIDS (EFAs) seem to play an important role in maintaining the health of the prostate gland. Research shows that they can improve the symptoms of prostatic enlargement. EFAs, such as omega-3 fatty acids, can be found in raw nuts and seeds, oily fish such as salmon, trout, mackerel, and herring, and extra-virgin olive oil. Eating an abundance of these foods, together with plenty of fruit and vegetables, is likely to help maintain the health of the prostate gland and may possibly reduce the risk of enlargement.

LINSEED OIL In addition, take one tablespoon of linseed oil, which is rich in omega-3 fatty acids, each day for several months. Then reduce the dose to 1–2 teaspoons a day. Take 200 IU of vitamin E daily with the linseed oil to protect the oil from oxidation damage in the body.

PUMPKIN SEEDS Try to include pumpkin seeds in your diet. They are rich in zinc and vitamin E, known to be important for

the health of the prostate gland. Pumpkin seeds also contain beta-sitosterol (*see Western Herbal Medicine, below*). In one German study, pumpkin seed extract was tested on over 2,000 men with mild to moderate BPH and over 40 percent improved significantly.

ZINC SUPPLEMENTS The prostate gland contains a very high concentration of zinc. Supplementation with zinc, often in conjunction with linseed oil, may help reduce prostatic enlargement. Zinc can be found in fish, seafood (especially oysters), and seeds. In practice, taking 30–60mg of zinc supplements a day is often useful. Long-term consumption of zinc supplements can deplete the body of copper, so take 1mg of copper for every 15mg of zinc.

LYCOPENE Regular intake of lycopene, which is present in tomatoes, watermelon, pink grapefruit, and chilies, appears to confer protection against prostate cancer. Researchers suggest that lycopene might also have a general therapeutic effect on the prostate gland. Eating cooked tomatoes and olive oil, as in the Mediterranean diet, is recommended because the absorption of lycopene by the body requires the presence of fats or oils.

> **CAUTION**
>
> Consult your doctor before taking zinc with antibiotics (see p.46).

Western Herbal Medicine

As men age, the blood level of testosterone falls as the level of dihydrotesterone (DHT), a derivative of testosterone, increases. Under normal circumstances, the enzyme 5-alpha-reductase converts testosterone to DHT and stimulates growth of the prostate gland. There is evidence that 5-alpha-reductase activity is higher in cells affected by BPH than in normal prostate gland tissue.

Herbal medicines are usually effective in preventing and treating mild to moderate BPH. Plant medicines have been used to treat BPH in Germany, France, and Italy for the last 20 years. Several have been shown to inhibit 5-alpha-reductase, and consequently reduce the size of an enlarged prostate. They also have an anti-inflammatory effect on the gland.

PRIMARY TREATMENT **SAW PALMETTO** (*Seronoa serrulata* and *S. repens*) is an effective treatment for the early stages of BPH. In the 1960s, researchers discovered that saw palmetto berries contained fatty acids (liposterols) that inhibit 5-alpha-reductase. One study revealed that the plant also relaxed smooth muscle within the urethral wall, thereby increasing urinary output. It also reduces swelling and inflammation of the prostate gland. You can safely take saw palmetto — try 2–4g of berries a day, or 160mg of a standardized extract, twice a day.

BETA-SITOSTEROL Meta-analyses showed that beta-sitosterol displayed significant improvements in relieving the symptoms of BPH and in increasing urine flow.

The bark of the evergreeen pygeum tree (*Pygeum africanum*) is rich in beta-sitosterol, which also inhibits 5-alpha-reductase. However, in a double-blind study that compared pygeum with saw palmetto, the latter produced a greater reduction in BPH symptoms. Pygeum has been widely used in Germany and France, but its increasing use has endangered the plant in its native African habitat. Other plants containing beta-sitosterol include the African potato (*Hypoxis hemerocallidea*), as well as species of pine (*Pinus* spp.) and spruce (*Picea* spp.), and these plants are an effective option for the treatment of BPH.

ISOFLAVONES Plants containing isoflavones can help patients with BPH. Evidence suggests that the isoflavones in legumes are related to lower rates of BPH and prostate cancer among Asian men. Men concerned about their prostate health should consider incorporating soy (*Glycine max*) into their diet.

Red clover (*Trifolium pratense*), available in tablet form, is another rich source of isoflavones. An Australian study showed that isoflavones derived from red clover had a significant effect on prostatic growth by acting as an antiandrogenic agent.

OTHER PLANTS that show promise for the treatment of BPH include willowherb (*Epilobium* spp.) and golden rod (*Solidago virgaurea*). Nettle (*Urtica dioica*) root con-tains phytosterols that can relieve the symptoms of BPH and is often combined with saw palmetto for greater effect.

> **CAUTION**
>
> See p.69 before taking an herbal remedy and, if you are taking prescribed medication, consult an herbal medicine expert first.

Chinese Herbal Medicine

BPH occurs in older men and in Traditional Chinese Medicine (TCM) is commonly thought to be due to a waning of kidney *Qi*, often complicated with "damp heat" and "stagnation of the blood." TCM practitioners generally recognize four main syndromes.

DEFICIENCY OF KIDNEY YIN BPH may occur against a background of "deficient kidney *Yin*." The patient complains of an aching back, weak legs and knees, insomnia, and dream-disturbed sleep. Urine flow is unsteady, dark, and possibly burning. The principle of treatment is to nourish kidney *Yin* and clear damp heat from the bladder. Treatment is based on Anemarrhena and Phellodendron Rehmannia Six Ingredient Pill (*Zhi Bai Di Huang Wan*).

DEFICIENCY OF KIDNEY YANG is another common pattern of BPH. The patient has frequent urination and/or retention of urine, is tired and cold, especially in the lower back, legs, and knees. Treatment is based on The Golden Chest Kidney Pill (*Jin Gui Shen Qi Wan*). Aconite (*Aconitum carmichaeli*) may be replaced with either red ginseng (*Panax ginseng*) or dried ginger (*Zingiber officinale*).

DAMP HEAT A "damp-heat" presentation of BPH occurs when the man's urination is hesitant, dribbling yet burning, and the urine is dark with a strong smell. The prescription is usually based on a variation of the Eight Herb Powder for Rectification (*Ba Zheng San*). *Mu Tong* and rhubarb root may be replaced by juncus (*Juncus effuses*), seven-lobed yam (*Dioscorea hypoglauca*) and the rhizome of sweet flag (*Acorus gramineus*).

BLOOD STAGNATION The fourth pattern appears because of "blood stagnation." Urinating is difficult and may even cease in severe cases. There is distending pain in the low back, loin perineum, and lower abdomen. There may be blood in the urine. The prescription is based on Resolve Resistance Decoction (*Dai Di Dang Tang*). Nonplant products may be replaced with vaccaria (*Vaccaria segetalis*) seed, zedoary (*Curcuma zedoaria*) and burreed (*Sparganium stolonifarum*) tuber.

> **CAUTION**
>
> Do not take Chinese herbal remedies with prescribed drugs without first consulting a health-care practitioner.

Exercise

Get regular exercise 3–4 times a week. A 1998 research study revealed that exercise and physical activity reduce the chances of a man developing prostate problems.

Acupuncture

Acupuncture may help with some BPH symptoms, although it offers no proven cure. Symptom relief may be only transitory if the underlying enlarged prostate is not managed appropriately with conventional and nutritional treatments.

Acupuncture should begin on a weekly basis and improvement noticed within six treatments. If there is improvement, continue treatment until no further benefit is apparent. Maintenance treatments every one to three months may be required, particularly if symptoms tend to recur.

> **PREVENTION PLAN**
>
> **The following may help prevent the development of BPH:**
>
> - Eat plenty of oily fish, soy, fruit and vegetables, extra-virgin olive oil, and pumpkin seeds
> - Avoid butter, milk, margarine, and meat
> - Take zinc supplements
> - Take flaxseed oil each day
> - Get regular exercise

MALE INFERTILITY

Many couples feel anxious if they have been trying to conceive for several months without success. Statistically, 80 percent of couples trying to conceive will be successful within a year, and 90 percent will be successful within two years. Older couples may be advised to start having investigations earlier as fertility declines with age, particularly in women. Treatment focuses on resolving any underlying cause, boosting sperm viability and function, assisted conception, relieving anxiety, and avoiding exposure to potentially harmful environmental toxins.

WHAT ARE THE SYMPTOMS?

- Nonconception after about a year of regular intercourse

WHY MIGHT I HAVE THIS?

PREDISPOSING FACTORS

- Low sperm count
- Production of abnormal sperm
- Poor sperm mobility
- Smoking
- Higher than normal scrotal temperature
- Long-term illnesses
- Certain infections, such as mumps
- Treatments, such as chemotherapy and radiation, for testicular cancer
- Disorder of the pituitary gland
- Chromosome disorder
- Excess alcohol
- Sexually tranmsitted disease
- Erectile dysfunction
- Prostate surgery
- Exposure to xenestrogens
- Exposure to environmental toxins, such as lead, phthalates, and glycol ethers

IMPORTANT

If you have been trying to conceive for several months unsuccessfully and you are concerned, go as a couple to see your doctor. This is especially important if one or both partners are over 35.

WHY DOES IT OCCUR?

In men, fertility depends partly on producing enough normal sperm to fertilize an egg, and in part on the ability to deliver the sperm into the vagina during intercourse. If there are problems with either of these, fertilization of an egg may not be possible.

The cause of infertility is identifiable in only about a third of the men investigated. In about half of all couples with fertility problems, the problem lies with the woman (*see Infertility in Women, p.346*) and in about a third, the problem lies with the man. In some couples, no problem can be found.

TREATMENT PLAN

PRIMARY TREATMENTS

- Treatment for underlying cause wherever possible

BACKUP TREATMENTS

- Assisted conception techniques
- Supplements, such as vitamins C and E, selenium, and zinc
- Homeopathic medicines
- Avoid toxic exposures
- Avoid xenestrogens
- Stop smoking

WORTH CONSIDERING

- Stress management
- Western herbal medicine

For an explanation of how treatments are rated, see p.111.

LOW SPERM COUNT Semen analysis is one of the first tests and it requires various measurements. There should be more than 20 million sperm per milliliter of semen and more than 50 percent should have good motility (ability to swim). At least 30 percent should be a normal shape.

An abnormal sperm count may have various causes. Because of their position in the scrotum, the testes have a lower temperature than the rest of the body by about 3.6°F (2°C). Anything that raises this temperature, such as tight underwear, may have an adverse effect on sperm production.

Sperm production can also be affected by long-term illnesses, such as chronic renal failure, by mumps if it occurs after puberty (*see p.395*), and by medical treatments, including surgery, chemotherapy, and radiation therapy for disorders such as testicular cancer.

Occasionally, a low sperm count may be due to low levels of testosterone, sometimes caused by a disorder of the pituitary gland (the tiny gland at the base of the brain which controls testosterone production by the testes) or, rarely, by a chromosomal abnormality. Lifestyle factors, such as drinking excessive alcohol, smoking, and using certain prescription or recreational drugs, may also affect sperm production.

In most cases, the cause of a low sperm count cannot be identified, and the condition is known as idiopathic oligospermia.

POOR SPERM DELIVERY Many factors can cause problems with delivery of sperm into the vagina. The most easily identified is erectile dysfunction (*see p.376*). Other less obvious factors are damage to the epididymides (the tightly coiled tubes that lie above and behind each testis where sperm

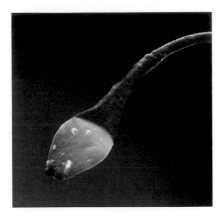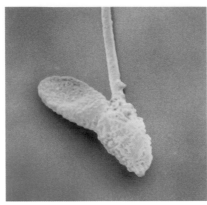

A healthy human sperm cell (*above left*) is composed of a rounded head, which contains the male DNA, and a tail that enables the cell to swim. An abnormal sperm cell (*above right*) would be infertile.

are stored and mature) and the vas deferentia (the tubes that transport sperm away from the epididymides toward the urethra). Damage is often due to a sexually transmitted disease, such as gonorrhea.

Sperm delivery is also affected by retrograde ejaculation, when semen flows back into the bladder from the urethra. This occurs if the valves at the outlet of the bladder fail to close properly and may be caused by prostate surgery.

SELF-HELP

The following measures may improve your chances of producing normal sperm:
- Have sex regularly.
- Don't smoke or take recreational drugs.
- Don't drink alcohol excessively.
- Eat organic food and drink filtered water to reduce exposure to toxins.
- Avoid hot baths.
- Avoid wearing tight underpants. If you sit for long periods, stand up and stretch or walk briefly on a regular basis.
- Avoid carrying a cell phone near your genital area.

TREATMENTS IN DETAIL

Conventional Medicine

PRIMARY TREATMENT **UNDERLYING CAUSES** A doctor will give you a physical examination, ask about your sex life, and recommend tests to assess your sperm count and sperm motility. If these are low, the underlying cause is treated whenever possible. For example, hormone injections may be given if testosterone levels are low. Erectile dysfunction may be treated with the drug sildenafil or various other options and psychological therapies may be recommended, including sex therapy (*see p.379*).

ASSISTED CONCEPTION If it is not possible to identify or to treat the cause of male infertility, measures may be taken to try to increase a couple's chances of conceiving.

If there are few or no sperm in the ejaculate, some couples choose to use donor sperm. If the sperm count is very low or sperm motility is poor, a single sperm selected from a semen sample may be injected into an egg removed from the ovaries (this process is called intracytoplasmic sperm injection, or ICSI). If an embryo starts to develop, it is introduced into the uterus, where it may become embedded in the wall and grow. ICSI may still be possible even if the ejaculate contains no sperm. In such cases, sperm may be removed directly from the testes or epididymides. Sperm removed in this way may also be introduced into the uterus through a soft plastic tube passed through the cervix (intrauterine insemination).

If the sperm count is only slightly low, in-vitro fertilization (IVF) may be an option. In this technique, a sample of sperm is added to eggs collected from the ovaries in the hope that fertilization will occur.

Nutritional Therapy

VITAMIN C SUPPLEMENTS Low or deficient vitamin C levels have been associated with low sperm count, increased numbers of abnormal sperm, reduced motility, and agglutination (when sperm stick together). In one study examining the effect of vitamin C on smokers, as much as 1,000mg of vitamin C per day improved sperm viability, motility, and agglutination, and reduced the percentage of abnormal sperm. The authors of the study concluded that taking 500mg twice a day of vitamin C is reasonable for any infertile man.

VITAMIN E SUPPLEMENTS Vitamin E also seems to be important to maintain sperm function. In one study, when sperm samples were taken from infertile men, the more motile sperm contained greater vitamin E concentrations. The authors suggest that vitamin E may help protect sperm against free radical damage. Other studies show that supplementation with vitamin E increases the quality of sperm and fertilization rates. The recommended dose is 200–400 IU of vitamin E each day.

SELENIUM SUPPLEMENTS Selenium seems to be important for normal sperm structure and function. In one study, selenium supplementation in subfertile men lacking the mineral improved sperm motility and the chance of successful conception. The recommended dose is 100–200mcg per day.

ZINC SUPPLEMENTS Zinc plays an important role in normal testicular development, sperm production, and sperm motility. In one study, infertile men had significantly lower serum and semen zinc levels than fertile men. In another, it was found that zinc deficiency decreased testosterone levels and semen volume. The recommended dose is 50mg per day for several months. Long-term consumption of zinc supplements can deplete the body of copper, so take 1mg of copper for every 15mg of zinc.

Folic acid and zinc were tested separately and together in men with low sperm counts. The combination (folic acid at 5mp per day with zinc sulfate at 66mg per day for six months) significantly increased the sperm count.

CAUTION

Consult your doctor before taking vitamin E with blood thinners, vitamin C with antibiotics or warfarin, Coenzyme 10 with warfarin, or zinc with antibiotics (*see p.46*).

Homeopathy

In a 2002 clinical study of men with fertility problems, individualized homeopathy helped improve sperm count and sperm motility, and in some cases led to pregnancy. The most commonly used homeopathic medicines are *Sulphur*, *Natrum muriaticum*, *Lycopodium*, and *Calcarea carbonica*.

SULPHUR Men who respond to *Sulphur* are often "larger than life" characters: sociable, outgoing, flamboyant, and untidy. They are generally strong-willed to the point, sometimes, of being argumentative or garrulous. Their feet are especially hot and may be smelly — they kick off their shoes at every opportunity and may stick their feet out of the bed at night. They often have skin trouble, with a rash that is often very itchy. They are very thirsty and enjoy rich and spicy food.

NATRUM MURIATICUM The type of man who responds to *Natrum muriaticum* often has a masked depression — he is very depressed, but does not like to talk about it. He may have had an upsetting experience, such as a bereavement or break up, that he has never discussed. These men may have other problems, such as migraines, various skin problems, including dry, crusty skin rashes, urticaria (*see p.176*), and recurrent cold sores on the lips. They often crave salty food, such as savory snacks.

LYCOPODIUM men are often serious people in responsible, demanding jobs, yet they may lack self-confidence. They may be socially rather inept, no good at small talk, yet they do not like being alone; they are at their best with small groups of old friends. They often have stomach trouble because their "eyes are bigger than their stomach." *Lycopodium* men feel hungry when they sit down to eat, but quickly become full. They suffer from an excess of gas and bloating, and their favorite flavor is sweet. Their worst time of day is 4–8pm, or after lunch, when they feel very drowsy.

CALCAREA CARBONICA The type of man who responds to *Calcarea carbonica* is stocky and solidly built, with a tendency to be overweight. He is phlegmatic — solid, stubborn, and hard working. His calm exterior may conceal many anxieties and fears and he may have bad dreams. He tends to sweat a great deal, especially on the head and neck.

Western Herbal Medicine

Herbal treatment for infertility may be useful when a man is in general good health. Low sperm count or low sperm motility can sometimes be successfully treated with remedies such as ginseng (*Panax ginseng*), ashwaganda (*Withania somnifera*), and ginger (*Zingiber officinale*).

> **CAUTION**
>
> See p.46 before taking a herbal remedy and, if you are taking prescribed medication, consult an herbal medicine expert first.

Environmental Health

Environmental medicine aims to help men avoid exposure to compounds that may be toxic to sperm development or to parts of the reproductive tract. A lack of convincing scientific evidence, combined with problems applying animal studies to humans, makes it difficult to establish beyond doubt that a chemical or toxic exposure leads to infertility. Nonetheless, there are many compounds that seem to have negative effects on male fertility.

If you have problems with libido, sperm counts, sperm quality, or overall fertility, look for possible exposures in the home or workplace. If there are offending chemicals, make changes to reduce your exposure.

AVOID TOXIC EXPOSURES A high level of lead exposure may lower sperm counts, increase the proportion of abnormal sperm, and decrease overall fertility. Glycol ethers, which are solvents used in the manufacture of paints, dyes, inks, cleaners, and soaps, seem to damage testicular function, lower sperm counts, and possibly cause infertility.

Researchers who examine the decline in sperm quality over the past few decades indicate that environmental agents, even in low concentrations, might be involved. For example, exposure to phthalates may be related to the decline in semen quality. Phthalates are extremely common compounds, found in food, consumer products (plasticisers or spreading agents), and medical devices. Certain phthalates may be more toxic to sperm than others.

Exposure to different types of solvents cause sperm to be abnormal and decrease libido. Research has shown that exposure to manganese, in steel manufacturing, mining, and dry-alkaline battery production plants, can cause erectile dysfunction, reduced fertility, and decreased libido.

STOP SMOKING Some studies have found a connection between boys born to women who smoked during pregnancy and low sperm counts years later, perhaps through an adverse effect on sperm development. Other studies have demonstrated that exposure to cigarette smoke decreases semen volume and overall male fertility.

XENESTROGENS may play a part in falling sperm counts by mimicking the action of female hormones and/or blocking the effect of androgens (male hormones). Agrochemicals, plastic bottles, food wrappings, and tap water are thought to be the main sources. Examples are DDT and other pesticides, dyes and paints (such as phenol red), or bisphenol A, which comes from the degradation of plastics.

Avoiding xenestrogens altogether is probably unrealistic, although eating organically as much as possible and drinking mineral water from glass bottles will help reduce exposure. Animal studies and some human studies show an effect of these compounds on male libido, sperm counts, and sperm quality, although the exact association is unclear.

Stress Management

Anxiety contributes to infertility in some instances and its symptoms can usually be eased by regularly practicing antianxiety breathing exercises (*see Anxiety, p.414*).

> **PREVENTION PLAN**
>
> The following may improve fertility:
>
> - Avoid alcohol and give up smoking.
> - Ensure your diet is rich in zinc, selenium, vitamins C and E
> - Avoid exposure to environmental hazards

ERECTILE DYSFUNCTION

Erectile dysfunction (ED), previously referred to as impotence, is the inability to achieve or sustain an erection. Occasional occurrence is normal and affects most men at some time, becoming more common with increasing age. Persistent, long-term occurrence may cause distress, both to a man and to his partner. Despite this, only about 10 percent of men experiencing long-term erectile dysfunction seek help for it. Treatment is aimed at relieving the underlying cause, increasing blood flow to the penis, and helping men relax and feel less anxious.

WHAT ARE THE SYMPTOMS?

- The inability to achieve or sustain an erection

WHY MIGHT I HAVE THIS?

PREDISPOSING FACTORS

- Stress at work
- Anxiety about sex
- Depression
- Relationship problems
- Overwork
- Fatigue
- Drinking alcohol excessively
- Smoking
- Drugs, such as certain antidepressants and antihypertensives
- Surgery
- Vascular disease
- Poorly controlled diabetes
- Chronic illness

WHY DOES IT OCCUR?

Erectile dysfunction can be caused by either psychological or physical factors. Sometimes, it is due to a combination of the two. In general, if ED is intermittent it is usually the result of a psychological cause, such as anxiety disorders (*see p.414*) or depression (*see p.436*). Other psychological factors may include stress (*see p.408*), relationship difficulties, or anxiety about sexual performance. The condition may be prolonged by the fact that many men are reluctant to discuss it, even in private with their doctor.

If the condition develops gradually and is persistent, it tends to be due to physical causes. These include drugs, such as certain antidepressants and antihypertensives (drugs used to treat high blood pressure), poorly controlled diabetes, surgery that may affect the nerves supplying the penis, and chronic illness.

In middle-aged and older men, ED is often due to vascular disease (disease of the blood vessels), commonly caused by atherosclerosis (a disease in which fatty deposits on the lining of arteries cause progressive narrowing) that reduces the blood supply to the penis. Lifestyle factors, such as heavy drinking, smoking, or overwork, can also increase the risk of ED.

TREATMENT PLAN

PRIMARY TREATMENTS

- Treatment of any underlying cause
- Lifestyle changes, such as avoiding heavy drinking and overwork
- Better communication (*see Self-Help, right*)
- Counseling and sex therapy
- Drugs, such as sildenafil (Viagra)
- Ginseng

BACKUP TREATMENTS

- Other drugs
- Devices and prostheses
- Arginine supplements
- Homeopathic medicines
- Western herbal medicine
- Osteopathy and chiropractic

WORTH CONSIDERING

- Chinese herbal medicine
- Breathing retraining
- Acupuncture
- Vitamin B_{12} supplements

For an explanation of how treatments are rated, see p.111.

SELF-HELP

PRIMARY TREATMENT You can reduce your anxiety about sex and improve your relationship with your partner through communicating. When you discuss your problem with your partner, remember to:
- Choose your words and timing carefully — you need to be positive and open, not hostile and critical.
- Make practical suggestions about what you would like to do and how you would like to improve your sex life.
- Listen carefully to your partner's replies.
- Devise a plan that suits both your needs.

TREATMENTS IN DETAIL

Conventional Medicine

PRIMARY TREATMENT **UNDERLYING CAUSE** The doctor will discuss lifestyle, medical, and psychological factors with you to look for an underlying cause. In some cases, treatment may involve replacing a medication that is causing the condition and sometimes psychological therapy may be recommended.

PRIMARY TREATMENT **DRUGS** Some approaches aim to treat the erectile dysfunction directly. For example, the drug sildenafil relaxes the muscles in the penis and in the walls of the blood vessels that supply it, thereby increasing the flow of blood. While sildenafil is taken orally, alprostadil may be either injected into the penis or introduced into the urethra.

> **CAUTION**
>
> The drugs sildenafil (Viagra) and alprostadil may have side effects; ask your doctor to explain these to you.

DEVICES AND PROSTHESES In some circumstances, a vacuum device may be suggested to draw blood into the penis to make it erect. A special rubber band is then placed around the base of the penis to maintain the erection.

Alternatively, a prosthesis can be inserted into the penis to keep it stiff. The position of the penis can be altered. Other implants can be inflated by a pump to erect and deflate the penis as required.

Nutritional Therapy

ARGININE SUPPLEMENTS A man's ability to attain and maintain an erection is, to a certain degree, dependent on the blood supply to the penis. The dilation of the blood vessels (allowing increased blood flow) that are necessary to achieve an erection depends on the presence of a substance called nitric oxide. The amino acid arginine is essential for the formation of nitric oxide.

A 1994 study found that some men with erectile dysfunction, after taking 2800mg of arginine every day for two weeks,

experienced improved erections and were able to achieve better vaginal penetration.

In 1999, a larger, double-blind, placebo-controlled study showed that a third of men with confirmed erectile dysfunction benefited from taking 5,000mg of arginine each day for six weeks. They reported improvement and satisfaction in their sexual performance.

In a 1998 study of men with mild to moderate erectile dysfunction, a formulation with a principal constituent of 2,800mg of arginine helped many of the participants. It improved their ability to maintain an erection during sexual intercourse and enhanced their satisfaction in their sex lives.

In general, at least some men with erectile dysfunction may be helped by taking 2,800–5,000mg of arginine each day.

VITAMIN B$_{12}$ SUPPLEMENTS There is some evidence to suggest that erectile dysfunction can sometimes be the result of vitamin B$_{12}$ deficiency and that taking 1,500mcg per day of the methylcobalamin form of vitamin B$_{12}$ may help.

> **CAUTION**
>
> Consult your doctor before taking arginine if you have a herpes infection (see p.46).

Homeopathy

PHOSPHORIC ACID In case reports in which the homeopathic treatment of erectile dysfunction was successful, the medicine that is most frequently suggested is *Phosphoric acid*.

AGNUS CASTUS is another important medicine that may be recommended by a homeopath when a man's erectile dysfunction is accompanied by depression, with itching, particularly of the eyes, and anxiety about health.

CONIUM may be appropriate for older men whose erectile dysfunction accompanies the start of a new relationship after a long period without sex. The man may experience a dizziness that is made worse by lying down.

LYCOPODIUM is a constitutional medicine *(see p.73)*, which is prescribed more for the person than the complaint. Men who respond to *Lycopodium* are typically rather reserved; they dislike large gatherings. They are often conscientious people who worry in advance of important occasions and may be quite depressed, because they take their responsibilities very seriously. They often have stomach trouble, especially gas, and tend to be at their worst in the afternoon.

Western Herbal Medicine

Various plants have the reputation of being able to treat erectile dysfunction, but some only have a placebo effect. Not only is reliable evidence scarce, but some remedies, such as yohimbe (*Pausinystalia yohimbe*), may have significant and dangerous side effects or interact with conventional medicines.

TRADITIONAL HERBS The following herbs have traditionally been used to treat erectile dysfunction: ashwaganda (*Witha-*

About 10 percent of men experience erectile dysfunction on a recurring basis

It is appropriate for men who have lost their libido (sex drive) and it often helps when the problem has started after a prolonged period of emotional stress or, sometimes, an acute illness. There is accompanying weakness of memory and loss of concentration; there may be diarrhea or looseness of the bowels.

nia somnifera), catuaba (*Erythroxylum catuaba*), cowhage (*Macuna pruriens*), red kwao krua (*Butea superba*), damiana (*Turnera diffusa*), ginseng (*Panax ginseng*), garlic (*Allium sativum*), ginkgo (*Ginkgo biloba*), and maca (*Lepidium meyenii*).

Other traditional herbs include muira puama (*Ptchopetalum olacoides*), and its close relative with the same Brazilian common name (*Liriosma ovata*), sarsaparilla (*Smilax officinalis*), suma (*Pfaffia paniculata*), tribulus (*Tribulus terrestis*), saw palmetto (*Seronoa serrulata*), and Siberian ginseng (*Eleutherococcus senticosus*).

Only a few of these remedies have reliable research data to justify this traditional use and safety data is scanty in many cases. For this reason, it is unwise to attempt self-medication for erectile dysfunction. Herbal medicine experts will be able to assess the cause of erectile dysfunction in each case before recommending treatment. There is no one magic formula to remedy this condition.

Plant medicines are at their best when they are prescribed by a practitioner who can take health problems as a whole into account rather than focusing narrowly on the mechanisms of erection.

PRIMARY TREATMENT **GINSENG** is perhaps the best-known herb for treating erectile dysfunction. Famed throughout China as a *Qi* (energy) tonic, accumulated research has confirmed its adaptogenic (restoring balance within the body) and tonic properties.

The root of ginseng contains steroidal saponins called ginsenosides, which are generally thought to enhance the action of the adrenal hormones through an indirect effect on the pituitary gland.

Taking ginseng on a long-term basis can increase overall well-being, and feeling

GINKGO leaves may be effective in treating erectile dysfunction that is due to a lack of blood flow to erectile tissue. This may be due to ginkgo's ability to increase blood flow through arteries and veins without a rise in blood pressure. However, ginkgo probably needs to be used for several months before results can be expected.

RED KWAO KRUA The tubers of red kwao krua constitute a traditional Thai plant medicine that has a long history of treating male sexual dysfunction. In a three-month, randomized, double-blind clinical trial on volunteers with erectile dysfunction, the results revealed that 82 percent improved significantly and, in addition, did not experience side effects.

SAW PALMETTO is a treatment for benign prostatic hypertrophy and may play a part in treating erectile dysfunction that is the result of enlargement of the prostate (*see p.370*).

> **CAUTION**
>
> ● See p.69 before taking a herbal remedy and, if you are taking prescribed medication, consult an herbal medicine expert first.
>
> ● Consult an herbal medicine expert before taking one of the traditional herbal remedies for erectile dysfunction since many are potentially toxic.
>
> ● Do not take ginseng for more than six weeks without a break.

At least 20 percent of men in their 70s have persistent erectile dysfunction

more relaxed and energetic can lead to an increase in libido.

Research indicates that red Korean ginseng has constituents that can specifically improve sexual function in men with erectile dysfunction.

Siberian ginseng (*Eleutherococcus senticosus*) also contains steroidal saponins and has demonstrated a range of effects (antifatigue, antistress, antidepressant, and an ability to enhance the immune system), which may also help men overcome erectile dysfunction.

Chinese Herbal Medicine

Traditional Chinese Medicine (TCM) practitioners believe that a man's ability to achieve and maintain an erection is primarily dependent on the proper functioning of his kidneys and his liver. A review summarizing the TCM approach to male infertility and erectile dysfunction was published in 2001.

Kidney *Yang* and the fire of the kidneys (*Ming Men*: "the Fire of Life Gate") govern the functional aspects of an erection and

sperm motility. Kidney *Jing* and *Yin* are largely responsible for the health of the sperm and fertility. Male sexual function also depends on a sound psychological state. Severe shock or fright can directly disorder kidney function.

KIDNEY YANG DEFICIENCY can lead to loss of libido (sex drive) and erectile dysfunction. The man is cold, listless, and pale. He may have to get up several times during the night to urinate. Typically, his back and knees are weak and sore. For this condition, a Chinese herbalist may prescribe a combination of Restore the Right Kidney Pill (*You Gui Wan*) and Special Pill to Aid Fertility (*Zan Yu Dan*).

KIDNEY YIN DEFICIENCY generates "false heat" that can excite the kidneys and briefly fire up the libido, but sexual activity cannot be sustained. A man with kidney *yin* deficiency may be treated with a modified and combined version of the Six-Flavor Rehmannia Formula (*Liu Wei Di Huang Wan*) and Restore the Left Decoction (*Zuo Gui Yin*).

LIVER QI STAGNATION Since the liver meridian passes through the external genitals, liver *Qi* stagnation can also be a cause of erectile dysfunction. The flow of liver *Qi* can be obstructed by mental stress, resentment, or anger. Liver *Qi* stagnation is typically found in men who are stressed by work or home circumstances, leading to a loss of libido and erectile dysfunction. The main prescription is Rambling Powder (*Xiao Yao San*).

QI AND BLOOD DEFICIENCY In TCM, anxiety, shock, and emotional highs and lows are thought to affect the function of the heart, which governs blood flow. Overwork, poor diet, irregular eating patterns, worry, and anxiety can damage the spleen so that it fails to make sufficient *Qi* and blood, thereby undermining sexual performance. Prolonged or severe illness can also cause *Qi* and blood deficiency.

Heart-blood and spleen-*Qi* deficiency can be a cause of erectile dysfunction, since lack of *Qi* and blood cannot sustain an erection. This type of erectile dysfunction is made worse by fatigue. The man may be treated with a modified Return the Spleen Decoction (*Gui Pi Tang*).

DAMP HEAT that can settle in the genital area and disrupt sexual function can be brought on by an overly rich diet, too much hot and spicy food, drinking alcohol, or smoking. Overwork or excessive lifting, standing, or sexual activity can damage kidney *Qi*, *Yin*, and *Yang*. The main treatment is a modified version of Two Marvel Powder (*Er Miao San*), with other damp-removing herbs and a tonic herb to boost the liver and kidneys.

> **CAUTION**
>
> See p.69 before taking a herbal remedy and, if you are already taking prescribed medication, consult a herbalist first.

Bodywork Therapies

OSTEOPATHY AND CHIROPRACTIC If a man is experiencing pelvic pain as well as erectile dysfunction, the nerve supply to the pelvic organs from the lower back may be irritated. Specialized prostatic massage by an osteopath or chiropractor may be able to resolve both problems.

Breathing Retraining

Learning to breathe properly (*see p.62*) may help relieve the anxiety that accompanies erectile dysfunction, and which may often be part of the cause. This is particularly true if fatigue is an associated symptom, since men who hyperventilate are often too tired to have sex. (*See Anxiety, p.414, for suitable breathing methods.*) Kegel exercises may also alleviate the condition.

Acupuncture

Acupuncture is one of many traditional Chinese remedies for erectile dysfunction, which is thought of as "withered *yang*." Although there are few controlled trials in this somewhat controversial area, acupuncture is worth a try — it is safe and relatively free of side effects, but there is certainly no guarantee of cure.

A preliminary trial of men with erectile dysfunction gave them two electroacupuncture treatments a week for one month. The results showed that 15 percent of the participants had better erections and in 31 percent of the men sexual activity

was improved. Another preliminary trial achieved good results in more than half the men treated. However, in the only controlled trial of electroacupuncture for erectile dysfunction, a placebo produced as good an improvement in sexual function as acupuncture. So, in everyday terms, there is a one in two chance that electroacupuncture would be useful treatment for erectile dysfunction.

Acupuncture should generally be given weekly for six to eight sessions; if there is no response it should be discontinued. If it is beneficial then consider maintenance treatments on a monthly basis until no further treatment is required.

Psychological Therapies

PRIMARY TREATMENT **COUNSELING AND SEX THERAPY** Sexual dysfunction in men occurs in several categories. At the sexual arousal stage, men sometimes find themselves unable to achieve an erection (erectile failure). At the orgasm stage, ejaculation may be too soon (premature ejaculation) or may be delayed or absent (male orgasmic disorder). Some men experience pain during intercourse (dyspareunia). Erectile dysfunction may be treated by sex therapy (*see below*).

ERECTILE FAILURE is treated by a form of graded exposure. A sex therapist will ask the couple to caress each other, but to avoid the penis (nongenital sensate focus) until they become relaxed with each other. The man's partner stimulates the penis gently until an erection is achieved and then stops until the penis subsides. The couple repeat this process two or three times so that the man is not only able to experience an erection — indeed, he comes to expect one.

PREMATURE EJACULATION is readily treatable and high success rates have been reported. The therapist helps the man relax and become less anxious through cognitive therapy and relaxation training. The man's

partner then employs the "squeeze technique," which was developed by the well-known sex researchers W.H. Masters and V.E. Johnson.

In this technique, the partner stimulates the man until he almost reaches orgasm, and then squeezes the tip of the penis until the urge for orgasm dissipates. This procedure is repeated several times until the man begins to gain more control.

Some research suggests that it is important for the couple to maintain this technique and use it on a regular basis, as longer term follow-up studies have shown that some men relapse and experience erectile dysfunction again.

> Anxiety is the most common cause of temporary erectile dysfunction

Mind-Body Therapies

Although there is virtually no research into the use of mind–body therapies in the treatment of erectile dysfunction, stress and anxiety can have an impact on the condition and mind–body therapies may help relieve it. Try practicing stress management techniques, such as guided imagery, relaxation, and breathing on a regular basis. Concentrate on communicating and enjoying sensual and affectionate experiences with your partner.

HYPNOTHERAPY In one trial, in which men underwent three hypnosis sessions a week (reducing to one per month over a six-month period), 75 percent of men showed improvement.

> **PREVENTION PLAN**
>
> The following may help prevent erectile dysfunction:
> - Practice relaxation
> - Communicate well with your partner
> - If you are a smoker, stop
> - If you are a heavy drinker, reduce your alcohol intake

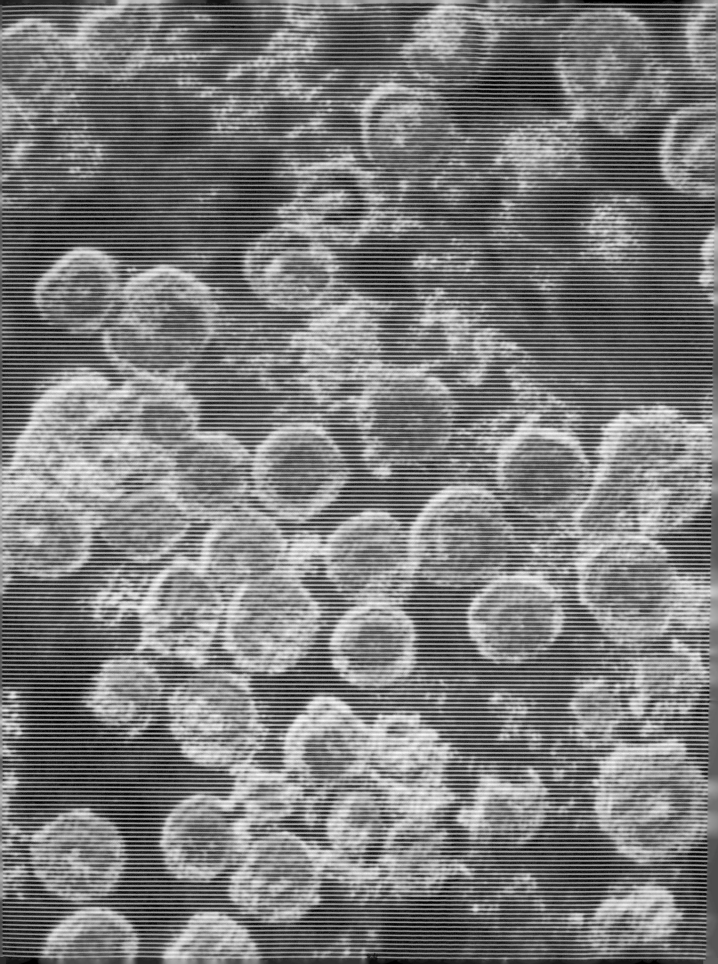

Children's Health

A child's immune system is constantly being exposed to new, potentially harmful organisms. In most cases, a healthy diet and plenty of exercise give enough resilience to combat most common illnesses. When children become ill, their self-healing systems can be supported by rest and attention, coupled with the occasional supplement, antibiotic, or homeopathic remedy.

DIAPER RASH

Diaper rash, in which the area of skin covered by the diaper becomes sore and inflamed, is a common problem in babies. It affects nearly all babies at some point and can make them irritable. If possible, the best way to deal with diaper rash is to prevent it in the first place by cleaning and drying the area thoroughly, changing diapers frequently and applying a barrier cream at the first sign of redness. Diaper rash may be treated with emollient and antifungal creams and simple self-help measures, as well as with probiotics and homeopathic remedies.

WHAT ARE THE SYMPTOMS?

- Redness in the diaper area (but not in the skin folds and creases)
- Sometimes, a scaly rash similar to cradle cap in the diaper area

WHY MIGHT MY BABY HAVE THIS?

PREDISPOSING FACTORS

- Insufficient diaper changing

TRIGGERS

- Food sensitivity
- Candida overgrowth

TREATMENT PLAN

PRIMARY TREATMENTS

- Self-help measures, including emollient creams (*see Helping your child, right*)
- Antifungal creams (if there is *Candida* infection)

BACKUP TREATMENTS

- Eliminate food sensitivities
- Probiotic supplements
- Homeopathic medicines

For an explanation of how treatments are rated, see p.111.

WHY DOES IT OCCUR?

Diaper rash usually begins when ammonia in the urine or stools irritates the delicate skin of the diaper area. It becomes worse if the diaper is not changed frequently, or if the diaper area is not cleaned thoroughly at each change. Perfumed baby care products or certain laundry detergents may irritate a baby's skin and cause or worsen diaper rash. If the rash is present in areas not directly in contact with a soiled diaper, such as the creases between the legs and groin, it may be due to an infection, such as candidiasis (*see Oral Yeast, p.383*).

HELPING YOUR CHILD

PRIMARY TREATMENT The following measures can prevent and treat the rash:
- Change your baby's diaper frequently.
- Cleanse the diaper area thoroughly with water and make sure it is completely dry before putting on a new diaper.
- Use an emollient cream, such as zinc oxide or vitamin A and D, at the first sign of redness to protect the affected area.
- Let your child be diaper-free as much as possible. Exposing the affected skin for a short while to sunlight may also help.

TREATMENTS IN DETAIL

Conventional Medicine

PRIMARY TREATMENT If your baby's rash does not clear up in a few days, take him or her to your doctor. If there is an associated candidiasis infection, the doctor might prescribe an antifungal cream. Occasionally, a mild corticosteroid cream is prescribed for a few days to reduce inflammation.

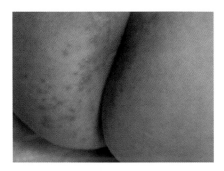

Diaper rash inflames the skin, making it red, sore, and uncomfortable. Occasionally, the skin may become blistery and infected.

Nutritional Therapy

FOOD SENSITIVITY may sometimes give rise to diaper rash, perhaps during the weaning period when you introduce your child to new foods. Some babies may be intolerant to cow's milk. (*For more details about food sensitivity, see p.39.*)

CANDIDA ALBICANS If a breast-feeding mother takes probiotics, or gives them to her baby, a diaper rash caused by *Candida* may be alleviated. (*See also p.40.*)

Homeopathy

The same medicines recommended for other types of dermatitis (*see Eczema, p.167*) are often effective for diaper rash. These include *Rhus toxicodendron*, *Sulphur*, *Calcarea carbonica*, and *Croton tiglium*. They should be given in the 6C strength. Crush one tablet or two pills between two teaspoons and give a small amount, dry on the tongue, three times a day at least ten minutes before or after feeding. The medicines are not available as creams.

ORAL YEAST

Oral yeast is a fungal infection caused by an overgrowth of *Candida albicans* in the mouth. White patches are visible on the tongue and on the lining of the baby's mouth. Common in babies under one year old, oral yeast can cause the baby's mouth to feel sore and make it reluctant to feed. The condition is sometimes associated with diaper rash that is caused by the same fungus. Treatments include antifungal creams, a *Candida*-elimination diet (if the mother is breast-feeding), probiotics, and the homeopathic remedy *Borax*.

WHY DOES IT OCCUR?

Candida albicans is a yeast organism that is naturally present in the mouth and gut. An overgrowth of the yeast in the mouth results in oral yeast if the bacteria that keep it in check are disturbed by certain antibiotics. Some complementary practitioners say that a dietary imbalance may also disturb the bacteria. Oral yeast can also affect the elderly and people with impaired immunity.

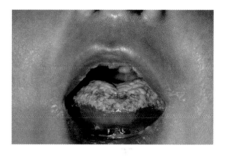

The white or creamy-yellow spots of oral thrush affect a baby's mouth, gums, soft palate, and tongue. They form a distinctive coating that is hard to wipe away.

SELF-HELP

- If you bottle-feed your baby, be sure to thoroughly clean all equipment.

TREATMENTS IN DETAIL

Conventional Medicine

PRIMARY TREATMENT **ANTIFUNGAL CREAMS** The doctor will examine your baby's mouth and may take a mouth swab to check for *Candida*. If oral yeast is confirmed, the doctor may prescribe an antifungal treatments, such as nystatin, to be applied to the baby's mouth. Oral yeast usually improves shortly after starting the treatment and should clear up within a week, but it may recur.

Nutritional Therapy

PRIMARY TREATMENT **CANDIDA ALBICANS,** the yeast responsible for oral yeast, thrives on sugar. Eliminating or reducing sugar and refined carbohydrates, such as white flour products, can help starve yeast out of the system. To help clear oral yeast in a breast-fed baby, the mother can cut back on her intake of sugar and refined carbohydrates, and take probiotics.

PROBIOTICS (healthy gut bacteria supplements) may be very useful in treating oral yeast. You can give probiotics to babies by adding the contents of a capsule or a powder to water or another drink. (*For more details about the treatment of* Candida *in the body, see p. 40*).

Homeopathy

BORAX is the homeopathic medicine routinely given to treat oral yeast. Babies who respond to *Borax* may be nervous and jumpy, particularly from loud or unexpected noises. They may be very frightened of falling, and scream and cling to their mothers when being carried downstairs or when lowered into a cradle or onto a changing mat. Give *Borax* in the 6C strength. Crush one tablet or two pills between two teaspoons and give a small amount, dry on the tongue. Administer three times a day at least ten minutes before or after feeding.

TEETHING

Teething is the eruption of primary (milk) teeth in babies and small children. The eruption of a new tooth through the gum can be uncomfortable; babies may cry and be difficult to soothe as a result. A teething baby also may be less willing to eat and may not sleep well at night. Treatments include rubbing a teething gel onto the baby's gums, and giving liquid acetaminophen or homeopathic *Chamomilla*. Letting a baby gnaw on a chilled teething ring or other suitably hard object can also help bring relief.

WHAT ARE THE SYMPTOMS?

In babies and small children:

- Drooling
- Crying
- Flushed cheeks
- Red, swollen gums where the tooth is emerging
- Reluctance to eat

IMPORTANT

Fever, vomiting, and diarrhea are not symptoms of teething, although they may occur during teething. See your doctor if your baby develops any of these symptoms as they may indicate an infection.

TREATMENT PLAN

PRIMARY TREATMENTS

- Pain relief (*see Helping your child, right*)
- Homeopathic remedy *Chamomilla*

For an explanation of how treatments are rated, see p.111.

WHY DOES IT OCCUR?

A child's first tooth usually emerges at about six months of age and the remaining primary (milk) teeth by the age of three. The process of teething continues until the mid-teens, as the secondary teeth replace the primary teeth. As the root of a tooth grows, the tooth breaks through the skin of the gums, causing pain — more so from the canines and molars than the incisors.

HELPING YOUR CHILD

PRIMARY TREATMENT Help relieve the pain and discomfort of teething with the following measures:

- Let your baby gnaw on a cold, hard object, such as a teething ring. To chill, put the ring in the refrigerator, not in the freezer. You could also try vegetables such as celery sticks or carrots.
- Rub an over-the-counter teething gel containing anesthestic onto the baby's gums. Rubbing the gum without the gel may help too.
- Consider giving liquid acetaminophen to babies over three months (do not give aspirin to children under 12 because of the risk of Reye syndrome).
- Keep the baby's face dry because drooling can cause a face rash. Give the baby plenty of water to replace fluids.
- Give the baby diluted chamomile tea.
- Bathe the baby in a bath with lavender.

Homeopathy

PRIMARY TREATMENT **CHAMOMILLA** is the standard homeopathic treatment. When prepared as fine granules, it is called homeopathic teething granule. *Chamomilla* pills in the 6C strength contain the same homeopathic medicine. Both the pills and granules are made of lactose (milk sugar) which tastes slightly sweet, so getting the baby to take them is not a problem. Hyland's Teething Tablets, available in the US, contain *Calcarea phosphorica*, *Chamomilla*, *Coffea cruda*, and *Belladonna*.

Chamomilla is likely to help when the baby gets very cross and can only be soothed by vigorous movement: the baby quiets when rocked, picked up, or walked around, only to start crying again as soon as the movement stops.

Give *Chamomilla* in the 6C strength. Crush one tablet or two pills between two teaspoons and give a small amount, dry on the tongue, three times a day at least ten minutes before or after feeding.

ORDER OF PRIMARY TEETH

A baby's primary, or "milk," teeth are already developing at the time of birth. The first teeth to come through, either the top or bottom jaw, are usually the incisors, which often cause no pain. The rest of the primary teeth come through in no particular order. The canines and molars are often the most painful.

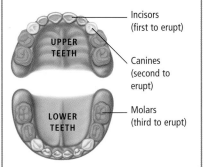

UPPER TEETH

LOWER TEETH

Incisors (first to erupt)

Canines (second to erupt)

Molars (third to erupt)

HEAD LICE

Head lice are tiny, almost transparent, wingless insects that infest the scalp, where they suck blood and cause irritation and itching. Their eggs, known as nits, are laid close to the scalp and can be seen as tiny white specks attached to the hair shafts. Infestations of head lice are common in school-age children, especially in girls, who tend to have long hair. Treatments include the use of products containing insecticides, wet combing with conditioner, and applying neem, turmeric, and other herbal remedies to the scalp.

WHAT ARE THE SYMPTOMS?

- Itchiness of the scalp, which may be intense
- Small, white specks (nits) at the base of the hair shafts near the scalp
- The presence of lice themselves (tiny, almost transparent, wingless insects)

WHY MIGHT MY CHILD HAVE THESE?

TRIGGERS

- Close head to head contact with someone who has head lice
- Sharing a hat or comb that is infested with lice

WHY DOES IT OCCUR?

Head lice (*Pediculus capitis*) are adapted to live on the scalp and neck hairs of humans. Children are more commonly infested than adults and the lice are usually transmitted by close head-to-head contact and by sharing items, such as hair accessories, hats, and combs. Their presence on your child's scalp is not an indication of poor hygiene or sanitation.

Adult head lice live by sucking blood from the scalp and cannot live for more than a day without food. The females can lay about six eggs a day and are able to lay about 100 eggs in total. The female has to be inseminated by a male for the eggs to hatch. In general, an infested scalp may have ten or so adults, but hundreds of eggs that are either dead, hatched, or viable.

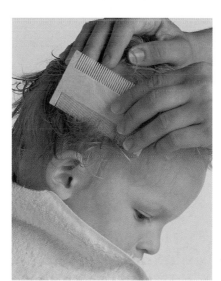

After applying conditioner to your child's head, use a fine-toothed comb to carefully remove the lice and eggs from the hair shafts.

TREATMENTS IN DETAIL

Conventional Medicine

Once you have confirmed that your child has lice, check the rest of the family and tell your child's school.

PRIMARY TREATMENT **INSECTICIDAL SHAMPOOS** Over-the-counter products containing insecticides, such as malathion and permethrin, are effective, although there may be some skin irritation. The particular chemical recommended may vary depending on the resistance patterns of the lice. You usually need to apply the products twice, with a week between treatments (*see p.386*). Always follow the directions carefully.

> **CAUTION**
>
> Lindane can cause seizures or other neurotoxic effects. All insecticides can have side effects; consult your doctor before using.

PRIMARY TREATMENT **WET COMBING** To avoid using chemicals, thoroughly wet your child's scalp and hair and use a fine-toothed comb to remove the lice and nits. The best way is to apply plenty of conditioner before painstakingly combing for up to half an hour. Wipe the comb on a piece of tissue after every stroke. Rinse the hair thoroughly and dispose of the tissue. Repeat every 2–4 days for two weeks or more.

> **CAUTION**
>
> Consult your doctor before treating a child under the age of two or a child with allergies, eczema, or asthma.

TREATMENT PLAN

PRIMARY TREATMENTS

- Insecticidal shampoos
- Wet combing
- Herbal shampoos, such as neem, turmeric, and quassia

For an explanation of how treatments are rated, see p.111.

THE LIFE CYCLE OF HEAD LICE

The eggs of a head louse hatch after 7–10 days. The nymphs mature after 10–14 days when they, too, can lay eggs. In order to synchronize the shampooing of your child's hair with the life cycle of the lice, you need to do three weekly insecticidal shampoo treatments from the time you discover the lice. The first kills any live lice. A week later, the second would kill those that had hatched between days one and seven. The third kills those that had hatched on day 10 — the last day that an egg could hatch.

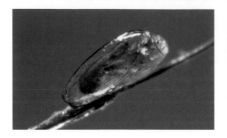

A nymph spends about eight days developing inside an egg case, which becomes almost transparent at the time of hatching.

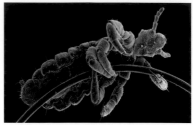

Evolution has endowed the six legs of the adult head louse with the ability to grasp the shaft of a human hair.

When to shampoo your child's hair

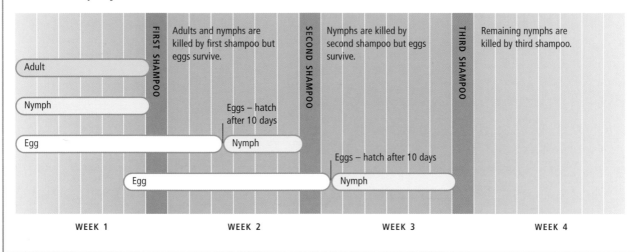

FIRST SHAMPOO

Adults and nymphs are killed by first shampoo but eggs survive.

SECOND SHAMPOO

Nymphs are killed by second shampoo but eggs survive.

THIRD SHAMPOO

Remaining nymphs are killed by third shampoo.

Adult

Nymph

Egg

Eggs – hatch after 10 days

Nymph

Egg

Eggs – hatch after 10 days

Nymph

WEEK 1   WEEK 2   WEEK 3   WEEK 4

Western Herbal Medicine

There are many traditional approaches to treating head lice, some of which are effective. Apply one of the herbal remedies to wet hair and comb through. A water-based remedy can be left in, but an oil-based remedy must be washed out. The eggs (nits) are not destroyed, the application needs to be repeated regularly for two weeks, by which time all the eggs will have hatched and the newly emerged head lice can be killed.

PRIMARY TREATMENT **NEEM**, a tree found in much of tropical Asia, is a safe and generally effective insecticide, antimalarial, and insect repellant. It is strongly bitter and its main active constituents (liminoids) are toxic to many parasites, including lice. An infusion made from the leaf or seed oil are the most common preparations and are used topically.

PRIMARY TREATMENT **TURMERIC** powder or decoction is commonly mixed with neem to treat head lice. A study involving 814 people with lice found the combination 98 percent effective. Treatment also included boiling clothing and bedding.

PRIMARY TREATMENT **QUASSIA** is used for head lice in many parts of the world. An infusion of the powdered wood, or a tincture, is applied to the hair and scalp. Clinical studies have found it effective for head lice and other infestations.

ESSENTIAL OILS Use various combinations (with neem seed oil as the carrier oil), allowing them to soak into the scalp, then rinse. Good essential oils include aniseed (*Pimpinella anisum*), eucalyptus (*Eucalyptus globulus*), geranium (*Pelargonium* spp.), clove (*Syzygium aromaticum*), rosemary (*Rosmarinus officinalis*), tea tree (*Melaleuca alternifolia*), lemon (*Citrus limonum*), and lavender (*Lavandula angustifolia*). A controlled study found that a topical herbal preparation containing the oils of coconut (*Cocos nucifera*), aniseed, and ylang-ylang (*Cananga odorata*) was as effective as a topical insecticide. The appropriate dosage levels are important, particularly with children, so purchase a prepared product or see an herbal medicine expert.

PREVENTION PLAN

The following may help prevent your child from having head lice:

- Teach your child not to share hats or combs with other children, who may have head lice
- Check your child's hair regularly so that any problem that develops can be treated early

CROUP

Croup is a common complaint characterized by noisy breathing and a barking cough. It particularly affects children between the ages of six months and three years, and occurs mainly in the fall and winter. Boys seem more susceptible to croup than girls, but the reason for this is not known. Treatment for croup includes putting the child in a steamy atmosphere as well as giving doses of vitamin C, gentle massage, and homeopathy. Severe cases are treated with corticosteroids.

WHAT ARE THE SYMPTOMS?

- Barking cough, which may be worse at night
- Noisy breathing, especially when inhaling
- Hoarseness, often noticed when the child is crying
- Symptoms of croup are usually mild, but occasionally breathing may be severely affected

WHY MIGHT MY CHILD HAVE THIS?

PREDISPOSING FACTORS

- Upper respiratory tract infections

TREATMENT PLAN

PRIMARY TREATMENTS

- Increase the humidity (*see Helping your child, right*)
- Corticosteroids (for severe cases)

BACKUP TREATMENTS

- Vitamin C supplements
- Massage
- *Aconite* and other homeopathic medicines

For an explanation of how treatments are rated, see p.111.

WHY DOES IT OCCUR?

Croup often follows the symptoms of a common cold, such as a runny nose, by one or two days. In an attack, the trachea narrows, restricting the flow of air to the lungs and causing noisy breathing and a characteristic barking cough.

Most children recover from croup completely within a week, but the condition may recur until they reach about the age of five. At this age, the airways are wider and less likely to become significantly narrowed in response to a viral infection.

HELPING YOUR CHILD

PRIMARY TREATMENT The following measures may help relieve the symptoms:
- Give your child plenty of fluids to drink.
- Increase the humidity of your child's room with a humidifier, a boiling kettle, or a bowl of steaming water (make sure the child doesn't touch it), or sit together in a steamy bathroom. The moist air may help ease congestion and discomfort, reducing the intensity and frequency of coughing bouts.
- Give your child a chest rub with eucalyptus and lavender oils.
- Sometimes, breathing the cool air outside for a few minutes is helpful.

IMPORTANT

In a severe case of croup, breathing may become difficult and rapid or labored. A child's lips and tongue may take on a bluish color due to lack of oxygen (cyanosis). If your child is having difficulty breathing or if cyanosis develops, call an ambulance.

TREATMENTS IN DETAIL

Conventional Medicine

PRIMARY TREATMENT **CORTICOSTEROIDS** Oral or inhaled corticosteroids may be prescribed to help relieve inflammation. Children with severe symptoms will need to be treated in a hospital.

Nutritional Therapy

VITAMIN C SUPPLEMENTS Several studies show that vitamin C can reduce the symptoms and duration of viral infections. For children aged two years or more, give 1g of vitamin C a day, divided into three or four doses and administered as a powder dissolved in a drink. If the vitamin C loosens the child's bowels, reduce the dose until normal bowel movements resume.

Bodywork Therapy

MASSAGE Gently massaging a sick, coughing, and wheezing child can relax the tense muscles of the upper chest and throat and also ease breathing.

Homeopathy

ACONITE, HEPAR SULPHURIS, AND SPONGIA For over 150 years, homeopaths have treated croup with a sequence of these three medicines. Preferably, each should be given in the 30C potency. Place two pills on the child's tongue (crush them between two teaspoons if necessary for very young children). As with all homeopathic medicines, the pills should be chewed or sucked, not swallowed whole. Give half-hourly for the *Aconite* and hourly for the *Hepar sulphuricum* and *Spongia*.

OTITIS MEDIA WITH EFFUSION

Also known as glue ear, the thick, sticky fluid that fills the middle ear can cause partial hearing loss. Since the condition develops while the child is acquiring language, it may delay development of speech and language. It is more common in boys and may run in families. Eliminating food sensitivities, manipulation, and homeopathy are usual treatments but grommet insertion or autoinflation may be necessary.

WHAT ARE THE SYMPTOMS?

Symptoms of otitis media with effusion develop gradually and may not be noticed at first. The symptoms may seem less severe at times but are usually worse in winter. They may include:

- Partial deafness
- Speech or pronunciation that is immature for a child's age
- Behavioral problems due to frustration at not being able to hear and therefore understand properly
- Slowed progress at school

WHY MIGHT MY CHILD HAVE THIS?

PREDISPOSING FACTORS

- Middle ear infection
- Food sensitivity
- Parents who smoke
- Genetic tendency
- Having Down syndrome or a cleft palate
- Allergic rhinitis and other allergic conditions

TREATMENT PLAN

PRIMARY TREATMENTS

- Food elimination diet

BACKUP TREATMENTS

- Grommet insertion
- Autoinflation

WORTH CONSIDERING

- Reduce sugar intake
- Nutritional supplements
- Homeopathy

For an explanation of how treatments are rated, see p.111.

WHY DOES IT OCCUR?

The middle ear must be full of air so that the normal vibrations of the eardrum can be transmitted via the ossicles (the tiny bones of the middle ear) to the inner ear. The air comes from the throat to the middle ear via the eustachian tube.

If one or both of the eustachian tubes become blocked, as sometimes happens following middle ear infections, air cannot reach the middle ear and fluid is secreted from the lining of the tube. This fluid thickens and prevents the normal vibrations of both the eardrum and the ossicles. In some cases, the reason for the blockage of the tube is unknown.

One indication of glue is a child showing signs of impaired hearing. This becomes evident if he or she turns the volume of the television up high or sits very close to it.

Otitis media with effusion is more common in children whose parents smoke and in children with allergic conditions, such as allergic rhinitis. Children who have Down syndrome or who are born with a cleft palate are also at greater risk of developing it.

In most cases, the condition will subside with time, but sometimes it persists and may result in permanent impairment of hearing. It is rare in children over the age of eight because, as a child grows, the eustachian tubes widen and are less likely to become blocked.

IMPORTANT

If you think your child has a hearing problem, consult your doctor as soon as possible.

TREATMENTS IN DETAIL

Conventional Medicine

If you suspect your child has otitis media with effusion, consult your doctor, who will examine your child's ear with a viewing instrument called an otoscope. Often, the doctor will recommend waiting to see whether the condition disappears.

If the child continues to have difficulties, or has hearing problems, the child will be referred to an ear, nose, and throat (ENT) specialist. The specialist will reexamine the ears and may refer the child for hearing tests and tympanometry, in which the movements of the eardrum are assessed.

GROMMET INSERTION In some cases, the specialist may recommend the insertion of a grommet for persistent otitis media with effusion associated with hearing loss. This procedure, which is carried out under a general anesthetic, involves making a small hole in the eardrum to allow the fluid to drain away. A tiny tube (a grommet) is then inserted to allow air to enter and circulate in the middle ear. These tubes often fall out within a year and the eardrum heals. In some cases, the procedure is repeated. Occasionally, during the same operation, the child's adenoids are removed, which may reduce the risk of further episodes of otitis media with effusion.

AUTOINFLATION may be recommended as a means of relieving otitis media with effusion. This maneuver is designed to open up the eustachian tube by raising the pressure in the nose — for example, the child tries to blow up a balloon through a small plastic tube inserted into the nostril.

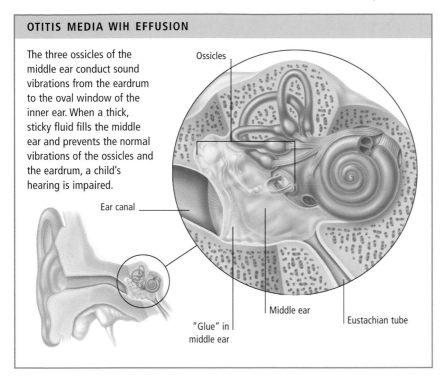

OTITIS MEDIA WIH EFFUSION

The three ossicles of the middle ear conduct sound vibrations from the eardrum to the oval window of the inner ear. When a thick, sticky fluid fills the middle ear and prevents the normal vibrations of the ossicles and the eardrum, a child's hearing is impaired.

Ossicles

Ear canal

"Glue" in middle ear

Middle ear

Eustachian tube

Nutritional Therapy

PRIMARY TREATMENT **FOOD ELIMINATION DIET** Evidence suggests that food sensitivity is a common factor in recurrent otitis media with effusion and ear infections. A 2001 study found that milk, eggs, beans, citrus fruit, and tomatoes were the most likely culprits. Eliminating the suspect food led to a significant reduction of symptoms in most patients. Reintroducing suspect foods into the diet tended to provoke a recurrence of the condition. (*For more details about food sensitivity, see p.39.*)

REDUCE SUGAR INTAKE Try restricting the child's sugar intake if ear infections are recurrent. Although sugar intake has not been studied in direct relation to ear problems, it is known that sugar consumption can impair immune function.

SUPPLEMENTS A 2002 study of children showed that a daily multivitamin and mineral tablet, along with cod liver oil, may help prevent ear infections and reduce the need for antibiotics. Give half a teaspoon of cod liver oil each day.

PROBIOTICS Antibiotics given to a child with recurrent ear infections can disturb the normal balance of beneficial bacteria in the gut. In the long term, this can lead to problems with irritable bowel syndrome (*see p.222*), yeast overgrowth (*see p.40*), and food sensitivity (*see p.39*). To avoid this, try giving the child probiotic supplements in capsule form for 1–2 months. If necessary, you can open the capsule and add the contents to a drink.

N-ACETYLCYSTEINE Evidence suggests that taking 200mg of the amino acid supplement N-acetylcysteine (NAC) twice a day may help treat otitis media with effusion. It is anti-inflammatory and helps break down mucus. In a 2000 study, NAC significantly reduced the recurrence, the need for reinserting grommets, the number of episodes of ear problems, and the frequency of visits to an ear, nose, and throat specialist.

XYLITOL Studies suggest that xylitol, a natural sugar found in some fruits, can interfere and prevent the growth of some bacteria, thereby protecting against recurrent ear infections.

Bodywork Therapies

Studies reveal that otitis media with effusion usually gets better on its own, whatever treatment is used. This makes it difficult to verify the claims of parents and practitioners that massage, cranial osteopathy, and chiropractic can improve a child's problem by draining the middle ear.

Homeopathy

This is one of the pediatric conditions most frequently treated by homeopathy. The many success stories are backed up by a clinical trial in 1999, which suggested that homeopathy might be more effective than routine medical care. However, more research is needed.

The chronic secretions are commonly triggered by acute otitis media and they appear to be more likely if the infection is treated with antibiotics. Clinical trials and studies of the outcome of treatment suggest that homeopathy is an effective treatment for acute otitis media.

The following medicines should be given as two pills or tablets of the 6C strength, three times a day.

KALIUM SULPHURICUM is the most commonly used medicine for otitis media with effusion. Children who respond to *Kali. sulph.* experience deafness with clicking in the ears when they swallow. They tend to have thick and lumpy discharge that may extend down the back of the nose.

PULSATILLA Children who respond to *Pulsatilla* have similar symptoms to those who respond to *Kalium sulphuricum*, but they also tend to be weepy, whiney, and clingy, but quickly cheer up after being cuddled.

OTHER REMEDIES If these medicines do not work or seem inappropriate, consult a homeopath for other remedies.

PREVENTION PLAN

The following may help prevent your child from developing otitis media with effusion:

- Chewing gum sweetened with xylitol
- Don't use a pacifier
- Breast-feed for the first few years when possible and include fresh fruit and vegetables in the child's diet
- If you are a smoker, stop

COLIC

Colic is a condition in which an otherwise healthy baby has regular episodes of prolonged, vigorous crying, often for up to three hours. Colic can be distressing for parents, who may think their baby is in pain. Colic clears up on its own and does no harm, but may be helped if cow's milk is avoided and if the baby is allowed to eat on demand. Some babies have been helped with homeopathy or cranial osteopathy.

WHAT ARE THE SYMPTOMS?

- Prolonged crying that takes place at approximately the same time each day, usually in the evening
- Lack of response to comforting measures, such as holding or feeding
- Sometimes, drawing the legs up to the chest as if in pain
- The crying may be made worse if the baby is tired or in an unfamiliar environment

WHY MIGHT MY CHILD HAVE THIS?

PREDISPOSING FACTORS
- Living with smokers

TRIGGERS
- Food sensitivity
- Cow's milk

TREATMENT PLAN

PRIMARY TREATMENTS
- Soothe the baby (see *Helping Your Child, right*)
- Avoiding cow's milk

WORTH CONSIDERING
- Food elimination diet
- Stabilizing blood sugar levels
- Chiropractic and other forms of manipulation
- *Chamomilla* and other homeopathic medicines

For an explanation of how treatments are rated, see p.111.

WHY DOES IT OCCUR?

No one knows why colic occurs. It is not thought to be due to an illness, abdominal pain, or gas. In some instances, the baby may be sensitive to formula, cow's milk, or to a mother's milk that is less rich and filling in the evening. Colic often begins when a baby is a few weeks old and usually stops at about four to five months. Colicky babies typically eat and gain weight well and do not have more health problems than babies without colic.

HELPING YOUR CHILD

PRIMARY TREATMENT Simple measures to cope with colic include:
- Rock your baby, walk around with him, or go for a drive in your car.
- If you breast-feed, rest in the afternoon so your early evening milk is replenished.
- Burp your baby frequently.
- Give your baby plenty of back rubs.
- Gently massage your baby's abdomen.

TREATMENTS IN DETAIL

Conventional Medicine

The doctor will check that there is no underlying cause and that the baby is otherwise well. Over-the-counter remedies, such as simethicone, may provide relief, but are not backed up by medical evidence.

IMPORTANT

Consult your doctor for advice and support if you cannot cope with a colicky baby's prolonged crying. Consult your doctor if your baby develops symptoms that are not part of colic, such as a fever or vomiting.

Nutritional Therapy

PRIMARY TREATMENT **AVOID COW'S MILK** Babies may react to infant formulas based on cow's milk. Switching to a formula based on goat or cow's milk specially treated to break down the protein molecules within can be very effective. Breast-fed infants with colic often improve when cow's milk is eliminated from the mother's diet as well; rice milk, oat milk, and calcium-enriched soy milk make good alternatives.

FOOD ELIMINATION DIET Evidence suggests that eliminating cabbage, broccoli, cauliflower, onion, and chocolate from a breast-feeding mother's diet may help.

STABILIZE BLOOD-SUGAR LEVELS Feeding on demand may avoid a drop in blood-sugar levels and can dramatically reduce the incidence of colic. One study found that a teaspoon of sugar water improved symptoms more than plain water.

Bodywork Therapy

MANIPULATION Chiropractic can often speed up the resolution of colicky episodes. Cranial osteopathy or craniosacral therapy may also help, but as yet they are unsupported by research.

Homeopathy

CHAMOMILLA is the classical medicine for colic. Crush a pill of the 6C strength between two teaspoons and give a few granules on the tip of a spoon when the baby has colic. If the baby needs them more than four times a day, you probably need to increase the strength or use a different medicine, such as *Colocynthis* or *Magnesia phosphorica*. If you have any doubts, consult a qualified homeopath.

CHILDREN'S FEVERS

A fever, in which the body's temperature rises above 100.4° F (38° C), is not an illness in itself but is a symptom of one. Fever is one of the body's responses to infection and enhances its defense mechanisms. The body creates extra heat as the immune responses fight off viruses or bacteria. Less commonly, a child's fever may be a response to an inflammatory disease or other noninfectious diseases. The overall aim of treating a fever is to keep the child hydrated and to improve the immune response.

WHAT ARE THE SYMPTOMS?

- Body temperature rises above 100.4° F (38° C)
- Shivering
- Chills may result when the body temperature falls

WHY MIGHT MY CHILD HAVE THIS?

TRIGGERS

- Infection
- Inflammation
- Allergy

TREATMENT PLAN

PRIMARY TREATMENTS

- Fluids and other self-help measures (*see Helping Your Child, right*)

BACKUP TREATMENTS

- Vitamin C supplements
- Homeopathic medicines

For an explanation of how treatments are rated, see p.111.

WHY DO THEY OCCUR?

The body temperature is controlled by the hypothalamus, which is located in the brain. In a fever, the temperature is raised by moving blood from the skin to the interior, reducing the amount of heat radiating from the body. Shivering, which involves the muscles contracting, may also help increase heat production. When the hypothalamus resets the temperature to a lower level, the body throws off the extra heat by moving blood outward to the skin and sweating.

HELPING YOUR CHILD

PRIMARY TREATMENT If your child is uncomfortable, try the following measures:

- Keep your child cool and comfortable — give plenty of cool drinks (such as water with fresh lemon juice), loosen clothes, and cool the skin with a washcloth soaked in tepid water.
- Give liquid acetaminophen to children over three months.(do not give aspirin to children under 12 years of age due to the risk of Reye syndrome)

IMPORTANT

Call an ambulance or go straight to an Emergency Room if the child has possible meningitis symptoms (a fever plus severe headache, dislike of bright lights, neck pain on moving the head forwards, drowsiness or confusion, and a rash of flat spots that do not fade when pressed with a drinking glass).

If a baby under six months has a fever, consult a doctor without delay.

TREATMENTS IN DETAIL

Conventional Medicine

Children who develop a fever in response to an upper respiratory tract infection, such as a cold (*see p.200*), usually subside after 2–3 days without requiring any medical attention or treatment.

However, if your child runs a high temperature (over 102°F/39°C), consult your doctor. Also, if the temperature stays high for 48 hours, even if everything else seems normal, consult your doctor because a persistent fever may mean a bacterial infection that could be serious.

Nutritional Therapy

VITAMIN C SUPPLEMENTS Give a child 500–1,000mg of vitamin C a day, divided into three or four doses, to help resolve a fever associated with a minor infection.

Homeopathy

ACONITE AND BELLADONNA For the early stages of acute fevers, the two most commonly used medicines are *Aconite* and *Belladonna*. In both cases, the fever comes on quickly and the child's temperature may be quite high. These medicines should ideally be given in the 30C strength, in two pills or tablets every 1–2 hours until the fever settles. You can give 6C pills if the 30C strength is not available.

OTHER MEDICINES may be required after the initial stage of the fever and should be given in the 6C strength every two hours. These medicines include *Ferrum phosphoricum*, *Gelsemium*, and *Mercurius solubilis*.

TONSILLITIS AND ENLARGED ADENOIDS

The tonsils, located at the back of the throat, and the adenoids, at the back of the nasal cavity, form part of the body's defenses against infection. In tonsillitis, the tonsils are infected with bacteria or a virus, causing inflammation and a sore throat. The adenoids may become enlarged, often as a result of recurrent infections or an allergy. Mild cases may be helped with herbal and homeopathic remedies, antibiotics, or a food elimination diet. Severe, recurrent cases of tonsillitis may require surgery.

WHAT ARE THE SYMPTOMS?

Tonsillitis symptoms usually develop over 24–36 hours and may include:

- Sore throat and difficulty swallowing
- Fever
- Headache
- Enlarged lymph nodes in the neck

Symptoms of enlarged adenoids tend to appear gradually over time and may include:

- Breathing through the mouth and snoring during sleep
- Persistently blocked or runny nose

WHY MIGHT MY CHILD HAVE THIS?

TRIGGERS

- Food sensitivity
- Nutrient deficiency

TREATMENT PLAN

PRIMARY TREATMENTS

- Fluids and liquid acetaminophen (*see Helping Your Child, right*)
- Food elimination diet
- Herbal gargles

BACKUP TREATMENTS

- Surgery (for persistently enlarged tonsils or adenoids that are blocking airways)
- Antibiotics (in some cases)
- Vitamin and mineral supplements
- Homeopathy
- Herbal tinctures and teas
- Chinese herbal medicine
- Lymphatic pump techniques
- Massage and chiropractic

For an explanation of how treatments are rated, see p.111.

WHY DOES IT OCCUR?

Tonsillitis is common in childhood when the tonsils are exposed to many infections for the first time. The tonsils become smaller with age and tonsillitis occurs less frequently in adults. Symptoms tend to become milder as the child gets older and they have usually disappeared completely by adolescence.

Tonsillitis may be recurrent and eventually result in the enlargement of the tonsils. Enlargement of the tonsils and adenoids may block the upper airway. In some cases, it causes obstructive sleep apnea, in which breathing is interrupted for brief periods during sleep.

Enlarged adenoids may also predispose a child to recurrent middle ear infections and, in some cases, to otitis media with effusion (*see p.388*). Permanently enlarged tonsils and adenoids maay be caused by an allergy — commonly to dust mites or mold.

HELPING YOUR CHILD

PRIMARY TREATMENT You can relieve many symptoms of your child's tonsillitis with the following measures:

- Bring down your child's temperature by sponging with tepid water and giving liquid acetaminophen. (Do not give aspirin to children under 12 years because of the risk of Reye syndrome.)
- Relieve a sore throat in young children by giving them cold, nonacidic drinks such as milk.
- Older children can eat ice cream or suck ice cubes or throat lozenges.
- Give your child frequent drinks, such as water or diluted fruit juice, but in small quantities.
- Older children can gargle with warm, salty water, or with manuka honey, which is antibacterial and soothing to the throat.

TREATMENTS IN DETAIL

Conventional Medicine

Your doctor will diagnose tonsillitis from the symptoms and an examination. A throat swab may also be sent to a laboratory to look for a bacterial cause. Acetaminophen and similar drugs may help calm the fever and discomfort. In some cases, antibiotics are prescribed.

SURGERY Removal of the tonsils (tonsillectomy) is not commonly performed today. Although a doctor might recommend it if a child is repeatedly sick and missing school, in general, children tend to "grow out" of recurrent tonsillitis.

Tonsillectomy and adenoidectomy may be advised for severe, recurrent tonsillitis, in cases of persistent obstruction, or when obstructive sleep apnea is present.

Nutritional Therapy

PRIMARY TREATMENT **FOOD ELIMINATION DIET** Clinical experience suggests that recurrent tonsillitis is often related to food sensitivity, commonly to dairy products, such as milk, cheese, yogurt and ice cream. In practice, when these suspect foods are eliminated from the affected child's diet, the tonsillitis attacks generally become far less common or disappear altogether. (*For more details about food sensitivity, see p.39.*)

VITAMIN AND MINERAL SUPPLEMENTS
Children with recurrent tonsillitis infections may be helped if they take a multivitamin and mineral supplement each day to ensure proper nutrient levels. Studies indicate that the balance of many vitamins and minerals may be disturbed in individuals who have regular bouts of tonsillitis. A 2001 study found that patients who suffered with chronic tonsillitis had decreased levels of vitamins B$_1$, B$_2$, and C.

There is evidence that zinc levels can be especially low in individuals as a result of chronic tonsillitis. A 1998 study found that taking a vitamin E supplement was as effective as removal of the tonsils in treating chronic tonsillitis.

> **CAUTION**
>
> Consult your doctor before giving zinc or vitamin C with antibiotics (*see p.46*).

Homeopathy

In a 1994 clinical trial, homeopathic medicines, such as *Sulphur*, *Calcarea carbonica*, *Belladonna*, *Pulsatilla*, and *Silica*, were used to treat children (aged between 18 months and 10 years) who had repeated upper respiratory tract infections, such as tonsillitis, and ear infections. Not all the children had enlarged tonsils, but those who did required fewer tonsillectomies and adenoidectomies if they received homeopathy instead of placebo tablets. They also required fewer courses of antibiotics to recover from tonsillitis.

The following medicines can safely be used on a self (or family) treatment basis (*see p.77 for details of doses*). If you are in doubt or the response to treatment is poor, consult a qualified homeopath.

CALCAREA CARBONICA is one of the main medicines for children with chronically enlarged tonsils and adenoids. Those who respond to *Calcarea carbonica* are often big and chubby, and they sweat from their heads at night. They are often stubborn,

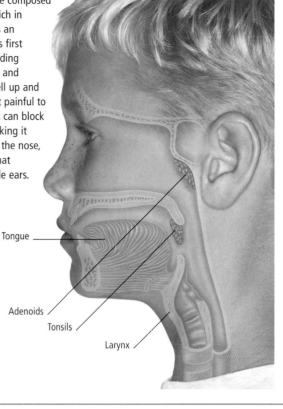

TONSILS AND ADENOIDS

The tonsils and adenoids are composed of lymphatic tissue that is rich in white blood cells and forms an important part of the body's first line of defense against invading organisms, such as bacteria and viruses. Infected tonsils swell up and become inflamed, making it painful to swallow. Enlarged adenoids can block both the nasal passage, making it difficult to breathe through the nose, and the eustachian tubes that allow air to reach the middle ears.

The location of the tonsils and adenoids

Tongue

Adenoids

Tonsils

Larynx

The tonsils are two almond-shaped glands of lymphatic tissue located at the back of the throat. The pair of adenoids are located above the throat at the back of the nasal cavity.

and may have various fears, waking at night crying and frightened. Many love eggs.

SILICA Children who respond to *Silica*, in contrast to those who respond to *Calcarea carbonica*, tend to be small and slim, with fine hair and delicate skin. Appearances may be deceptive because they can be quite determined and stubborn. But they often feel chilly and seem to "pick up every cold that is going around." They frequently have cold, clammy hands and feet, and may have weak or deformed nails.

BARYTA CARBONICA Children who respond to *Baryta carbonica* may have big tonsils and sometimes large, firm glands in the neck. They often have delayed development: they are slow to talk or read for no obvious reason, and they may be very shy. They may also have sweaty, smelly feet.

SULPHUR A number of other medicines may be required, including *Sulphur*. Children who respond to *Sulphur* are hot-blooded, throwing off their bedclothes

at night. They are generally strong-willed, determined, and messy. They often have skin trouble, particularly eczema.

PULSATILLA Children who respond to *Pulsatilla* tend to cry easily and become whiny, clinging to their mothers when ill. Their noses become blocked with excessive amounts of yellow or green mucus, which can trickle down into their throats, making them cough, particularly at night.

Western Herbal Medicine

Sore throats are much better treated when they first appear by herbal medicines than by antibiotics. This is a condition that is suitable for self-treatment, but consult a health-care professional if symptoms persist and do not respond to treatment.

PRIMARY TREATMENT **HERBAL GARGLES** are an effective way to alleviate sore throats. There are three main categories of herbs for gargles. One or two herbs from each category should be combined.

TANNIN HERBS In the first category are astringent herbs that contain tannin, which has the ability to coagulate the protein of infecting bacteria. These herbs include tormentil (*Potentilla tormentilla*), bayberry (*Myrica cerifera*) bark, agrimony (*Agrimonia eupatoria*), plantain (*Plantago major*), oak (*Quercus robur*) bark, and raspberry (*Rubus idaeus*) leaves.

HERBS WITH ESSENTIAL OILS In the second category are herbs with antibacterial essential oils. These herbs include sage (*Salvia officinalis*) leaf, hyssop (*Hyssopus officinalis*), thyme (*Thymus serpyllum*), chamomile (*Matricaria recutita*), marigold (*Calendula officinalis*) flowers, and myrrh (*Commiphora molmol*).

MUCILAGE HERBS In the third category are herbs with mucilage, which is a gum-like substance that can soothe an inflamed throat. These herbs include marshmallow (*Althea officinalis*) root or leaf, mullein (*Verbascum thapsus*), aloe vera (*Aloe vera*) juice, licorice (*Glycyrrhiza glabra*), slippery elm (*Ulmus fulva*), and Iceland moss (*Cetraria islandica*).

MAKING THE GARGLES Use two parts mucilage herbs, two parts tannin herbs, and one part of the herbs with essential oil. (If using myrrh, add 15 drops of tincture to a gargle.)

To make the gargles, boil the roots or barks first, then add the volatile oil-bearing and mucilage herbs in the last five minutes of the simmering period. Strain off the fluid and allow to cool. Gargle every 2–4 hours daily during the acute phase.

OTHER GARGLES
Sage Sore Throat Soother
Take a handful of fresh garden sage or half a handful of dried sage and simmer it for 20 minutes in 500ml of water with the lid on the pan. Strain and add a tablespoon of cider vinegar and a teaspoon of honey. Allow to cool, then gargle 3–4 times daily during the acute phase of the infection. Keep leftover fluid in the refrigerator.

Cider vinegar and honey gargle
Mix one tablespoon of cider vinegar in a glass of warm water and add 1–2 teaspoons of honey. Gargle the mixture 2–4 times daily during the acute phase.

INTERNAL TREATMENTS Take tinctures of one or more of the following herbs: echinacea (*Echinacea angustifolia*), wild indigo (*Baptisia tinctoria*), golden seal (*Hydrastis canadensis*), myrrh (*Commiphora molmol*), burdock (*Arctium lappa*) root, figwort (*Scrophularia nodosa*) herb and root, thyme (*Thymus serpyllum*), sage (*Salvia officinalis*), hyssop (*Hyssopus officinalis*), marshmallow (*Althea officinalis*), agrimony (*Agrimonia eupatoria*), and Andrographis (*Andrographis paniculata*).

All of these tinctures combat the bacteria that cause sore throats as well as ease soreness. Take 5ml of a tincture mixed with water 2–3 times a day. This dosage is for a 1:5 tincture. Tinctures vary in strength so if a particular tincture is stronger, reduce the dose.

Alternatively, teas made of thyme, sage, and hyssop will support the immune system's resistance and aid the mucous membranes in the throat.

> **CAUTION**
>
> See p.69 before giving a herbal remedy and, if your child is taking prescribed medication, consult an herbal medicine expert first.

Chinese Herbal Medicine

Chinese herbs for treating sore throat include burdock (*Arctium lappa*) seed, figwort (*Scrophularia ningpoensis*) root, puff ball (*Lasiosphaera fenzlii*), dyer's woad (*Isatis tinctoria*) root, pigeon pea (*Sophora subprostata*), honeysuckle (*Lonicera japonica*), forsythia (*Forsythia suspensa*), mint (*Mentha arvensis*), licorice (*Glycyrrhiza uralensis*), blackberry lily rhizome (*Belamcanda chinensis*), and balloonflower (*Platycodon grandiflorum*) root.

Sore throats are treated according to the pattern of symptoms they present. A "wind–heat" presentation is marked by aversion to cold, fever, headache, generalized aching, red tonsils, sore throat,

difficulty in swallowing, and a red tongue tip with a thin yellow coat. It is treated with Honeysuckle and Forsythia Powder (*Yin Qiao San*), which can be taken in pill form or as a decoction.

A more serious presentation is the development of "throat–fire toxin." The patient may have a high fever, thirst, restlessness, and swelling of the tonsils with an abscess or pus formation on the surface. The TCM doctor may use a variation of Coptis Decoction to Clear the Throat (*Huang Lian Qing Hou Yin*).

> **CAUTION**
>
> Do not treat a child with Chinese herbs without first consulting a Chinese herbalist for a correct diagnosis.

Bodywork Therapies

LYMPHATIC PUMP TECHNIQUES can be used, but only if a child happily tolerates bodywork. Evidence suggests that specific osteopathic methods, known collectively as "lymphatic pump technique," can increase the immune system's response to infection. They markedly increase the levels of defensive white blood cells for up to 24 hours.

MASSAGE AND CHIROPRACTIC Your child's immune system could also be boosted through a general, nonspecific massage by a qualified massage therapist or a spinal manipulation by a licensed chiropractor.

> **PREVENTION PLAN**
>
> The following may help prevent your child from developing tonsillitis:
> - Plenty of fresh fruit and vegetables
> - A regular multivitamin and mineral supplement

Tonsillitis in preschool children is usually caused by a virus

MUMPS

Mumps is a viral illness that was common in children before the MMR (measles, mumps, and rubella) vaccine was introduced. In most cases, the virus causes characteristic swelling and inflammation of the parotid salivary glands, located below and just in front of the ears. Swelling may be on both sides of the face or on one side only. Treatment depends on the severity of the symptoms and involves giving fluids, acetaminophen, vitamin C, and zinc. Homeopathic medicines may also help.

WHAT ARE THE SYMPTOMS?

Symptoms usually begin 2–3 weeks following infection with the virus and may include:

- Pain and swelling on one or both sides of the face, below and in front of the ear, lasting for about three days
- Pain when swallowing
- Sore throat
- Fever

TREATMENT PLAN

PRIMARY TREATMENTS

- Fluids and liquid acetaminophen (*see Helping Your Child, right*)

BACKUP TREATMENTS

- Vitamin C and zinc supplements
- *Mercurius solubilis* and other homeopathic medicines

For an explanation of how treatments are rated, see p.111.

WHY DOES IT OCCUR?

Mumps is caused by a paramyxovirus and is spread via coughs and sneezes or by direct contact with the saliva of an infected person. Symptoms are mild in most people and absent in a few. An individual with mumps is infectious from three days before swelling to seven days afterward.

HELPING YOUR CHILD

PRIMARY TREATMENT The following can make your child more comfortable.

- Plenty of cool fluids to help prevent dehydration.
- Give a nutritious diet.
- Liquid acetaminophen, if your child is over 3 months of age and has a fever.
- Do not give aspirin to children under 12 because of the risk of Reye syndrome.

TREATMENTS IN DETAIL

Conventional Medicine

Always consult your doctor if a child is very young or very ill and you suspect mumps. The diagnosis will be made from the swelling below and in front of the ears. The only therapy is treating the symptoms (*see above*). It is best to keep the child at home.

Adolescent boys may develop a severe inflammation of one or both testes, for which a strong analgesic is needed. If other sites of the body are affected, the relevant symptoms will be treated accordingly.

Nutritional Therapy

VITAMIN C AND ZINC SUPPLEMENTS Although no trials have been done, for children aged two and over it is safe to give

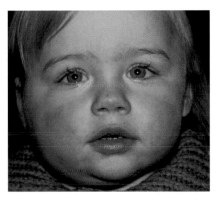

The characteristic swollen cheeks in mumps are the result of swollen parotid salivary glands, which are below and in front of the ears.

500–1,000mg of vitamin C divided into three or four doses during the day and 10–15mg of zinc once or twice a day for the period of the illness.

Homeopathy

The medicines *Mercurius solubilis*, *Pulsatilla*, and *Belladonna* may safely help a child with mumps and should be given as two pills in the 6C strength, 3 or 4 times a day. When in doubt, or the response to the treatment is poor, consult a qualified homeopath.

There is no evidence that homeopathic vaccination works. Your homeopath should not recommend them, since they will lull you into a false sense of security.

IMPORTANT

A boy or man who thinks he may have contracted the disease, or who has swollen testes and has been exposed to someone with mumps, should see his doctor immediately.

WHAT ARE THE SYMPTOMS?

Symptoms usually begin about 10 days following infection with the virus and may include:

- Fever, runny nose, and cough
- Red, watery eyes
- White spots on a red base on the inside of the cheeks (Koplik's spots)
- After 3–4 days, a red rash that starts on the face and behind the ears, before spreading down the body. The rash does not itch and lasts about a week

MEASLES

Measles is a viral illness that causes a fever and rash. It is a highly infectious disease that mainly affects young children. Measles is relatively rare in the developed world because of routine immunization, usually as part of the combined MMR (measles, mumps, and rubella) vaccine. However, the disease kills up to one million unimmunized children in the developing world each year. Treatment involves relieving the symptoms, boosting vitamin A levels, and increasing the immune system's response to infection.

WHY DOES IT OCCUR?

The measles virus is transmitted through minute airborne droplets of saliva that are scattered when an infected person coughs or sneezes. Measles is contagious from the onset of its coldlike symptoms until five days after the distinctive rash appears. The symptoms usually disappear after about a week, unless complications (*see below*) develop. One measles infection should confer lifelong immunity.

In children who are healthy and well nourished, measles is usually not serious although the child may feel very ill. However, complications, such as conjunctivitis, middle ear infections, and bacterial pneumonia, can occur, especially if the child is malnourished or if his or her immune system is depleted. In rare cases (about one in a thousand), the brain may be affected and inflamed with viral encephalitis, sometimes with permanent damage.

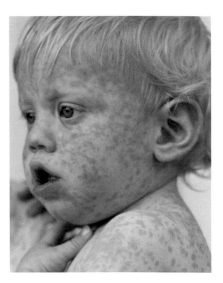

At first, the spots in a measles rash appear on the face and behind the ears, before spreading over the whole body. They are initially separate and then gradually merge together to form a blotchy, large-scale rash.

HELPING YOUR CHILD

PRIMARY TREATMENT Try the following measures to bring down your child's fever and to relieve discomfort:

- Let your child sleep as much as possible.
- Allow your child to rest in bed or be up but make sure he or she doesn't get too tired.

IMPORTANT

If your child vomits, develops an earache, has a severe headache, becomes drowsy, starts breathing abnormally, or experiences a febrile convulsion, call your doctor at once.

- Keep your child cool — give plenty of cool drinks, loosen his or her clothes, and moisten the skin with a washcloth soaked in tepid water.
- Give liquid acetaminophen to children over three months (aspirin should not be given to children under 12 years because of the risk of Reye syndrome).
- Encourage your child to drink plenty of cool fluids to prevent dehydration. Thirst is often absent and dehydration is a real danger, especially for babies. Offering lots of small sips is usually best, especially when nausea is a problem. A plastic medicine dropper that holds a few fluid ounces is useful.
- A child with a fever can go from cold to

TREATMENT PLAN

PRIMARY

- Fluids and liquid acetaminophen

BACKUP TREATMENTS

- Vitamin A supplements
- Vitamin C and zinc supplements (may protect or reduce the severity)
- Homeopathic medicines

For an explanation of how treatments are rated, see p.111.

hot very quickly; follow the cues and let him or her throw off the covers if desired.

- Don't force food on a child with a fever. Let him or her decide when and what to have, but avoid too much sugar which may slow immune responses down.
- Give liquid acetaminophen to children over three months (aspirin should not be given to children under 12 years because of the risk of Reye's syndrome).
- Rarely, if your child's temperature rises quickly, he or she may have febrile convulsions. Remove nearby objects and surround the child with pillows and cushions. The convulsions will soon subside. Consult a doctor promptly and prevent your child from getting cold afterward. (*See also Children's Fevers, p.391.*)

TREATMENTS IN DETAIL

Conventional Medicine

Doctors usually make the diagnosis from just the symptoms and an examination. However, blood tests may be used for confirmation. Keep your child at home and away from other people.

No treatment is usually needed, other than measures to relieve the symptoms (*see Helping Your Child, p.396*). Complications will need treatment, such as antibiotics for bacterial pneumonia.

IMMUNIZATION Babies in the US are immunized against measles with the MMR vaccine. An injection into the thigh or upper arm is given at 12–15 months, with a booster dose before going to school, usually between the ages of four and six years.

Fears that the MMR vaccine may contribute to the development of autism were shown to be unfounded by research published in 2004.

> **CAUTION**
>
> If you are concerned about letting your child be immunized with the MMR vaccine, consult your doctor.

Nutritional Therapy

Encourage your child to drink plenty of cool fluids, especially if he or she has a fever. This will help prevent dehydration and is likely to help speed the healing and recovery process. Sugar consumption can impair immune functions, so restricting refined sugar intake may help, despite the child's pleas for special treats while sick.

VITAMIN A SUPPLEMENTS have an important role in the treatment of measles. There is some thought that vitamin A deficiency makes measles, and its complications, more likely. A 1992 study undertaken in California found that 50 percent of supposedly well-nourished children with measles were relatively deficient in vitamin A.

In a 2002 review, vitamin A supplementation in young children with measles was described as one of the best-proven, safest, and most cost-effective interventions in international public health.

The World Health Organization recommends giving 200,000 IU per day for two days to children over the age of two (100,000 IU to infants) with measles when vitamin A deficiency may be present. At this dose there is evidence of a reduced risk of complications and mortality.

Half these doses can safely be given to children, even if they are not vitamin A deficient. Vitamin A can be given until the symptoms disappear.

VITAMIN C AND ZINC SUPPLEMENTS might help in the treatment of measles. Both have immune-stimulating and antiviral properties. Laboratory studies in 1983 revealed that vitamin C helped boost the activity of certain infection-fighting white blood cells that are often depressed during measles infection. Zinc supplementation may also help correct the loss of zinc through the diarrhea that can occur during and after measles infection.

For children two years old and over, it is safe to give 500–1,000mg of vitamin C in three or four doses a day and 10–15mg of zinc once or twice a day. If this loosens their bowels, reduce the dose until a normal bowel pattern returns. Stop giving the nutrients once the illness is over. Taking zinc supplements long-term can deplete the body of copper, so the child should take 1mg of copper for each 15mg of zinc.

> **CAUTION**
>
> Consult your doctor before giving vitamin C with antibiotics (*see p.46*).

Homeopathy

The following medicines should be given in a dose with pills of the 6C strength every 6 hours. If it seems to help but the effect does not last, increase the dosing schedule to every four hours.

PULSATILLA is the homeopathic medicine most commonly required for measles. As is often the case with homeopathy, *Pulsatilla* is prescribed on a "whole person" basis (*see Constitutional homeopathy, p.73*).

The child who is likely to benefit from *Pulsatilla* becomes whiny and weepy when he or she has measles, and becomes better with attention and affectionate cuddles. There is a thick, yellowish discharge from the nose and sometimes from the eyes, gumming them up.

There are several unusual paradoxical features that strongly suggest *Pulsatilla* would be helpful. For instance, the child has a dry, sticky mouth, but is not thirsty. Although the child is chilly and easily feeling the cold, she wants fresh air, her nose is less blocked, and she feels generally better from having the window open or a fan blowing on her.

OTHER MEDICINES that may be helpful include *Euphrasia* if the conjunctivitis (inflamed eyes), which is sometimes a feature of measles, is a problem and *Bryonia* for a dry, painful, hacking cough.

If the measles seems to drag on, then *Sulphur* may be helpful, again prescribed on "whole child" characteristics: the child feels hot and is lethargic. The rash is slow to clear up, turning purple, and may become itchy (the rash of measles is usually not itchy). The child may have an increased appetite, especially for sweets, and be thirsty for cold drinks.

> **PREVENTION PLAN**
>
> **The following measures may help to prevent measles:**
>
> - Arrange for your child to have the MMR vaccine
> - Give plenty of fruit and vegetables to ensure a plentiful supply of protective antioxidants

RUBELLA

Rubella, or German measles, is a virus that usually causes no more than a mild rash and fever, but if a pregnant woman contracts the disease, severe birth defects may result. Rubella is less common than it used to be due to routine immunization with the MMR vaccine. It usually settles by itself after a few weeks, and is treated by taking fluids, acetaminophen, and sometimes supplements. Homeopathy may also help.

Symptoms usually begin about 2–3 weeks following infection with the virus and may include:

- Fever that is usually mild in children but may be high in adolescents and adults
- Swollen lymph nodes, particularly those at the back of the neck and behind the ears
- After 2–3 days, a pink rash, which appears first on the face and then spreads down the body. The rash does not itch and usually clears up within three days

WHY DOES IT OCCUR?

The rubella virus is spread via coughs and sneezes. An individual with rubella is very contagious from roughly a week before the pink rash appears until a week after it goes. One infection confers lifelong immunity.

HELPING YOUR CHILD

PRIMARY TREATMENT The following can help your child feel more comfortable:

- As much sleep as possible.
- Give plenty of cool fluids, such as water with a little lemon juice, to help prevent dehydration.
- Make sure your child has a nutritious diet that includes plenty of fresh fruits and vegetables.
- Let your child sleep as much as possible.
- Allow your child to rest or to get up and play as he or she feels inclined.
- If your child is over three months and has a fever, give liquid acetaminophen (do not give aspirin to children under 12 years due to the risk of Reye syndrome).

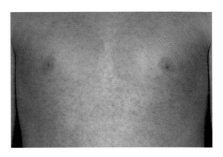

The pink rash of rubella first appears on the face. It gradually develops on the body and then on the arms and legs.

(diluted with the same amount of water) throughout the day may help a child recover.

However, supplemental vitamin C is likely to provide additional benefit. Give your child 500–1,000mg vitamin C each day, divided into three or four doses. If this loosens the bowels, reduce the dose until a normal bowel pattern resumes.

ZINC SUPPLEMENTS At the same time, give 10mg of zinc, once or twice a day for 1–2 weeks. This dose is safe for short-term use in children aged two or more.

TREATMENTS IN DETAIL

Conventional Medicine

Your doctor may arrange blood tests to confirm the diagnosis. There is no specific treatment except for dealing with the symptoms (*see above*). Keep your child at home, away from other people. Children should have the MMR vaccine, which is particularly important for girls.

Nutritional Therapy

VITAMIN C SUPPLEMENTS Orange juice may lessen the symptoms and accelerate the production of antibodies in the blood. Giving sips of freshly squeezed orange juice

Homeopathy

Rubella symptoms in children are often mild and do not require treatment. If symptoms are troublesome, consult a qualified homeopath or you can safely use medicines such as *Belladonna, Ferrum phosphoricum, Gelsemium, Pulsatilla,* and *Euphrasia.*

If you are pregnant, are not immune to rubella, and think you may have contracted the disease or been exposed to someone with it, see your doctor immediately.

TREATMENT PLAN

PRIMARY TREATMENTS

- Rest, fluids, and liquid acetaminophen (*see Helping your child*)

WORTH CONSIDERING

- Vitamin C supplements
- Zinc supplements
- *Belladonna* and other homeopathic remedies

For an explanation of how treatments are rated, see p.111.

PERTUSSIS

Pertussis, sometimes known as whooping cough, is a highly infectious bacterial illness that was common in children before immunization became routine. The infection causes characteristic attacks of severe coughing that end with a "whoop" as an affected child inhales. Pertussis is most serious in babies under the age of one year, when it can be life-threatening, and remains serious for children under the age of two. Integrated treatments include antibiotics and nutritional or other strategies to boost the immune system.

WHY DOES IT OCCUR?

Pertussis is caused by the bacterium *Bordetella pertussis*, which infects and inflames the mucous membranes of the windpipe and the airways of the lungs (the trachea, bronchi, and bronchioles). The bacterium are spread by coughs or sneezes. The initial stage of pertussis may last 1–2 weeks. During this time, the child is highly infectious. Symptoms then become worse before subsiding, usually within 4–10 weeks if there are no complications. However, a dry cough may persist for some time. An attack of pertussis does not give complete immunity, but a second attack is usually milder and may not be recognized as pertussis. There are possible complications including convulsions, pneumonia, and bronchiectasis (permanent widening of the airways). Babies may briefly stop breathing after coughing fits.

TREATMENTS IN DETAIL

Conventional Medicine

Your doctor will probably be able to diagnose this illness from the distinctive sound of the cough. The diagnosis can then be confirmed by testing swabs that are taken from the nose.

> **IMPORTANT**
>
> If your child is under a year old and seems to have whooping cough, contact your doctor immediately. Most children have the DTP immunisation at two, three and four months, as well as before they start school.

PRIMARY TREATMENT **ERYTHROMYCIN** If pertussis is diagnosed in the initial phase, the antibiotic erythromycin may stop the disease from progressing or decrease its severity. If an unimmunized child is exposed to the infection, erythromycin should be given as a preventive measure.

HOSPITAL TREATMENT Seriously ill children will be admitted to a hospital for monitoring and other measures, including intravenous fluids and oxygen if necessary.

Nutritional Therapy

MULTIVITAMIN/MINERAL SUPPLEMENTS Boost the child's immune system during an infection by restricting sugar intake and giving a children's multivitamin and mineral supplement. Some nutrients, especially vitamin C and zinc, may help maintain and stimulate immune function. If an ear infection accompanies pertussis, treat it in the same way as otitis media with effusion (*see p.388*).

Bodywork Therapy

LYMPHATIC PUMP TECHNIQUES can be used but only if the child will happily tolerate bodywork. Evidence suggests that specific osteopathic methods, known collectively as "lymphatic pump techniques," can increase the immune system's response to infection. This approach might be worth trying if coughing persists and causes muscular discomfort and tension.

A similar effect can be achieved either through a general, nonspecific massage by a qualified massage therapist or spinal manipulation by a licensed chiropractor.

CHICKENPOX

Chickenpox, also known as varicella, is a contagious viral illness that is common in children. It is caused by the varicella zoster virus and results in a characteristic rash of fluid-filled spots that are usually widespread over the body. Chickenpox is usually mild in children, but symptoms tend to be more severe in young babies, adolescents, and adults. The main aim of treatment is to fight the virus and enhance the function of the immune system.

WHAT ARE THE SYMPTOMS?

Symptoms usually begin 1–3 weeks following infection and may include:

- A mild fever, headache, or flulike symptoms
- Rash that appears as crops of small red spots. The spots become itchy and fluid-filled, then dry out and form scabs
- Discomfort in the mouth if spots develop there
- Possible complications include bacterial infections of the rash

WHY MIGHT MY CHILD HAVE THIS?

PREDISPOSING FACTORS

- Weakened immune system

TREATMENT PLAN

PRIMARY TREATMENTS

- Give fluids and acetaminophen (*see Helping Your Child, right*)
- Antiviral drugs (in some cases, e.g., where immunity is compromised by other illnesses or drugs)

BACKUP TREATMENTS

- Antibiotics (if a secondary infection occurs)
- Nutritional therapy
- Rhus *toxicondendron* and other homeopathic medicines

For an explanation of how treatments are rated, see p.111.

WHY DOES IT OCCUR?

The varicella zoster virus that causes chickenpox is transmitted through airborne droplets contained in the coughs and sneezes of infected people. It can also be transmitted by direct contact with the rash of spots and blisters.

Once the rash appears, the tiny red spots quickly turn into itchy, fluid-filled blisters. These dry out within 24 hours and form scabs. Several crops of spots can appear.

Someone with chickenpox is infectious from about two days before the rash appears until the last spots have formed scabs, usually 10–14 days after the onset of the rash.

COMPLICATIONS Bacterial infection of the blisters caused by scratching the itchy rash is the most common complication of chickenpox. Newborn babies and people with weakened immune systems (such as those who are undergoing chemotherapy) are likely to have more serious varicella infections and may also develop other complications, such as pneumonia.

THE RELATIONSHIP OF CHICKENPOX TO SHINGLES People who have had chickenpox are then immune to the disease and cannot catch it again. However, the virus remains dormant in nerve cells and may be reactivated later in life, causing shingles (*see p.165*). People who have not had chickenpox can catch it from someone with shingles, but only via direct contact with the shingles rash and not via coughs and sneezes. However, it is not possible to develop shingles without having first had chickenpox, even if it was only a very mild episode a long time ago.

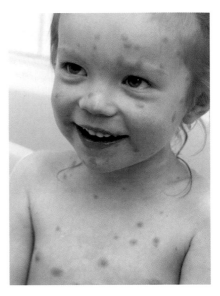

The chickenpox rash first affects the skin on the body, then spreads to the face and limbs. The spots become itchy, fluid-filled blisters that dry out and then form scabs.

HELPING YOUR CHILD

PRIMARY TREATMENT For a child with a mild infection who does not need to see a doctor, try the following measures:

- Let your child rest.
- Reduce the fever by dabbing the skin with a cool washcloth. Encourage your child to drink plenty of cool fluids to prevent dehydration. Thirst is often

IMPORTANT

Pregnant women who develop chickenpox, or who are exposed to the infection for the first time, should see their doctor.

absent and dehydration is a real danger, especially for babies. Offering a lot of small sips is usually best, especially when nausea is a problem. A plastic medicine dropper that holds a few fluid ounces is useful.

- To relieve discomfort, give acetaminophen to children over three months (do not give aspirin to children under the age of 12 years because of the risk of Reye syndrome).
- Give your child a warm-water bath that contains either a handful of bicarbonate of soda or two cups of powdered oatmeal to soothe itching.
- Use cotton to gently dab calamine lotion onto the spots to relieve itching. Alternatively, apply a gel of chickweed (*Stellaria media*) and/or a paste made from slippery elm (*Ulmus fulva*) powder, baking soda, and water to the spots.
- Keep your child's fingernails short and try to prevent him or her from scratching the spots and blisters to prevent skin infections. Babies may need to wear mittens to keep from scratching.

TREATMENTS IN DETAIL

Conventional Medicine

If your child is healthy, the infection is likely to be mild and will not need treatment. The child will normally recover fully between 10–14 days after the onset of the first crop of the chickenpox rash. Simply focus on relieving the itching and preventing your child from scratching the blisters (*see Helping Your Child, p.400*). Permanent scars may result from blisters that are scratched and become infected.

PRIMARY TREATMENT Babies or individuals with reduced immunity, such as those who are undergoing chemotherapy or who are HIV-positive, should see a doctor at once regarding possible treatment with antiviral drugs.

Chickenpox does not usually require any treatment, although antiviral drugs, such as acyclovir, may be considered for adults. Antiviral drugs may limit the effects of the varicella infection but they need to be administered in the early stages of the disease if they are to be of help.

Antibiotics are needed if a secondary bacterial infection of the rash occurs.

IMMUNIZATION Doctors in the US have introduced a program of chickenpox immunization as a routine measure for children between 12–18 months, with catch-up immunizations offered for children 13–18 years old who have not been previously vaccinated.

> **CAUTION**
>
> Antiviral drugs have potential side effects; ask your doctor to explain these to you.

Nutritional Therapy

PRIMARY TREATMENT **VITAMIN C AND ZINC SUPPLEMENTS** may help boost the immune system, which can encourage healing and speed recovery.

Give 500–1,000mg of vitamin C per day, divided into three or four doses, together

Chickenpox can be extremely dangerous in women who are pregnant

with 10mg of zinc, once or twice a day for 1-2 weeks. (This dosage of zinc is safe for children aged two years or more.) Taking zinc supplements over a long period can deplete the body of copper, so give your child 1mg of copper for each 15mg of zinc.

VITAMIN A SUPPLEMENTS Studies show that the chickenpox infection causes a lowering of vitamin A levels in children. Giving 3,000–5,000 IU of vitamin A every day for 10 days from the start of infection seems to help children with chickenpox. If given at the very start of the infection, vitamin A supplementation can help shorten the illness. Moreover, it may also help complications, such as pneumonia, conjunctivitis, and gasteroenteritis.

MULTIVITAMIN/MINERAL SUPPLEMENT In 2001, a study revealed that a daily multivitamin and mineral formulation made children much less likely to contract chickenpox when there was an outbreak at school. A multivitamin and mineral supplement are believed to help boost a child's immune defenses.

> **CAUTION**
>
> Consult your doctor before giving zinc or vitamin C with antibiotics (*see p.46*).

Homeopathy

Chickenpox is usually a mild disease in young children, settling without complications, but it can be a severe illness in people with a suppressed immune system (which occurs, for example, as a side effect of certain drugs).

RHUS TOXICODENDRON The classical homeopathic treatment for chickenpox is *Rhus toxicodendron*. This medicine is frequently helpful, particularly if the rash is very itchy, with small blisters. Give your child two pills of the 6C strength, 4 times a day until the rash heals (*see p.77*).

BELLADONNA AND ACONITE *Belladonna* and *Aconite* may help in the early stages of the infection, when there is fever and the child is generally unwell. *Aconite* is likely to help if the child feels both chilly and frightened. *Belladonna* is appropriate if the child feels hot and flushed.

PULSATILLA may help with children who are miserable, clingy, and tearful with the illness. They may have a fever, but are strangely not thirsty. *Antimonium tartaricum* has a reputation for helping when the skin rash is slow to subside.

> **PREVENTION PLAN**
>
> **The following may help prevent your children from catching chickenpox:**
>
> - Stay away from people infected with chickenpox or shingles
> - Give them a daily multivitamin and mineral supplement
> - Make sure they are immunized against varicella

ADHD

Attention deficit hyperactivity disorder (ADHD) is characterized by high levels of activity, impulsiveness, and inattention. In some cases, hyperactivity and impulsiveness predominate; in others, the child's main problem is difficulty concentrating on a given activity. ADHD is more common in boys than girls and seems to run in families. Treatment involves reducing and/or managing the symptoms through counseling, drugs, nutrition, manipulation, herbs, homeopathy, and psychological therapies.

WHAT ARE THE SYMPTOMS?

Symptoms of ADHD usually become apparent between the ages of 3 and 7 years and are often noticed after a child starts school. They may include:

- Almost constant physical activity
- Impulsiveness
- Short attention span and difficulty staying focused in a classroom situation
- Difficulty following instructions
- Inability to complete simple tasks
- Tendency to talk constantly and interrupt others
- Difficulty waiting and taking turns
- Startle response, in which a child is excessively jumpy from quite mild stimuli, such as sudden noises
- There may also be learning difficulties

WHY MIGHT MY CHILD HAVE THIS?

PREDISPOSING FACTORS
- Consumption of alcohol by mother during pregnancy
- Genetic factors
- Fetal hypoxia (inadequate oxygen reaching the brain) in the womb or during birth
- Family stress

TRIGGERS
- Food sensitivity
- Low levels of blood sugar
- Exposure to metals, such as lead, mercury, and manganese, in the environment

WHY DOES IT OCCUR?

ADHD belongs to a spectrum of behaviors that also includes attention deficit disorder (ADD) and hyperkinetic disorder (HKD). The causes of ADHD are not fully understood. It is not a result of poor parenting, as is sometimes believed, nor should it be confused with the normally boisterous activity of healthy children. Genetics, conditions in the uterus during pregnancy, and environmental factors, such as family stress and toxic metals, may play a part.

TREATMENT PLAN

PRIMARY TREATMENTS
- Behavior management
- Talking therapies
- Emotional support
- Methylphenidate or other drugs

BACKUP TREATMENTS
- Nutritonal therapy

WORTH CONSIDERING
- Massage
- Chiropractic
- Osteopathy
- Tai chi and yoga
- Individualized homeopathy
- Avoiding lead and other environmental hazards

For an explanation of how treatments are rated, see p.111.

Children can outgrow ADHD, although some may carry aspects of the disorder, such as attention problems and depression, into adulthood.

HELPING YOUR CHILD

The following techniques can help you manage your child's ADHD:
- Establish a routine that your child can understand and easily follow.
- Create simple rules and boundaries, and make sure that you stick to them.
- Reinforce acceptable behavior with rewards and discourage unacceptable behavior with sanctions.
- Organize activities that help increase your child's concentration.
- Keep distractions to a minimum.
- Arrange plenty of physical activities so that your child can let off steam.

TREATMENTS IN DETAIL

Conventional Medicine

The advice of various specialist professionals and consultants, such as a pediatrician and a child psychologist, may be needed to diagnose ADHD because there are many factors to consider and no single definitive test. ADHD may be diagnosed if a child consistently shows the distinctive symptoms of hyperactivity, impulsiveness, and attention difficulties over a period of six months or more and in more than one environment (for example, both at home and at school).

PRIMARY TREATMENT **COMBINED APPROACH** Treatment of ADHD requires a combined approach, which may include drugs in some cases. Therapy that aims to modify behavior may be recommended (see Psychological Therapies, p.405), while the parents may be given support and advice on managing the child, often through counseling and self-help groups.

PRIMARY TREATMENT **ORAL DRUGS** The drugs most commonly prescribed are stimulants, such as methylphenidate and dextroamphetamine, which may help reduce the symptoms of ADHD. These drugs are prescribed by specialists who will carefully monitor the child. Every year or so the drugs may be stopped for short periods of time to see whether they are still needed.

Tricyclic antidepressants, such as amitriptyline, may improve behavior in some cases.

> **CAUTION**
>
> Drugs for ADHD have a range of side effects; ask your doctor to explain these to you.

Nutritional Therapy

ELIMINATE FOOD SENSITIVITIES ADHD is very often amenable to a nutritional approach, because certain foods seem to be associated with an increased risk of mood and behavior disturbance. Eliminating caffeine, sugar, and food additives (artificial flavorings, colorings, and preservatives) from the child's diet often helps control his or her symptoms.

Studies show that ADHD is sometimes related to food sensitivity. Children suffering from food intolerance often have dark circles or bags under their eyes. During bouts of uncontrollable behavior or screaming their cheeks and/or ears may turn very red. While any food may give rise to these types of unwanted reaction, the most common problems are due to wheat, dairy products, chocolate, citrus fruits, and eggs. Children may often crave the foods to

which they are sensitive, so be especiaally suspicious of a child's favorite foods. (see The Elimination Diet, p.39).

STABILIZE BLOOD-SUGAR LEVELS Episodes of low blood sugar (hypoglycemia) appear to be a common feature in children with ADHD. Starving the brain tissue of its main fuel (sugar) can provoke significant problems with the child's mood. Low blood sugar levels also tend to cause the body to secrete the hormone epinephrine, which can make children anxious and/or aggressive.

Blood sugar problems are likely if a child either craves sweet foods or becomes very irritable if he or she does not eat regularly and on time. These children will often respond to a diet designed to stabilize blood-sugar levels (see p.42).

ESSENTIAL FATTY ACIDS Children with ADHD are often found to have nutrient deficiencies. They are especially likely to lack healthy fats known as essential fatty acids (EFAs). Common symptoms of EFA deficiency include dry, flaky skin; frequent urination; and excessive thirst.

EFAs (see p.34) are believed to play an important role in brain function. Possibly the most important in this respect are the omega-3 fatty acids eicosapentaenoic acid (EPA) and docosahexaenoic acid (DHA), which are found in oily fish, such as salmon, mackerel, and sardines, or in fish-oil supplements. In practice, about 1g of concentrated fish oils given two or three times a day may help improve behavior and learning in children.

NUTRITIONAL SUPPLEMENTS There is evidence that many children do not receive adequate amounts of key nutrients in their diets. Many vitamins and minerals, such as B vitamins, selenium, and magnesium, are important for brain function and are known to affect mood. Studies show that some children with ADHD have low levels of certain nutrients such as magnesium, zinc, and B vitamins.

Taking a daily multivitamin and mineral supplement may help ensure adequate nutrient intake and does seem to improve mood and behavior in some children.

Other evidence points to magnesium as being particularly helpful. Giving a child 100–200mg of magnesium per day is recommended in addition to a multivitamin and mineral supplement.

Homeopathy

Studies using homeopathic medicines, including *Stramonium, Hyoscyamus, Belladonna, Cina, Lycopodium, Calcarea carbonica, Sulphur,* and *Causticum,* indicate that homeopathy can help children with ADHD. Homeopathic treatment of ADHD is complex. Although these medicines can be safely used on a self-help basis it is best to consult a qualified practitioner.

STRAMONIUM is an important medicine when there has been a background of trauma, including abuse and desertion. Symptoms indicating that *Stramonium* may be appropriate include fear of the dark, water, or other things related to the original trauma. Children may also exhibit fits of destructive rage.

Other symptoms indicating *Stramonium* include "startle responses," night terrors, and intrusive thoughts or flashbacks to traumatic events.

HYOSCYAMUS Children who respond to *Hyoscyamus* are described as wild, manic, and difficult or impossible to control. They may talk very rapidly and display sexualized behavior.

BELLADONNA Children who respond to *Belladonna* are oversensitive to noise, light, and jarring, which make them "jump." They become very hot and flushed, and may be confused and delirious when they are excited.

CINA is useful for physically aggressive children who are constantly arguing and fighting, and who throw tantrums when disciplined or given orders.

CALCAREA CARBONICA Children who respond to *Calc. carb.* tend to be plump, with especially big heads. Characteristically, they sweat a lot from the head at night.

About 5 percent of children in the US have symptoms of ADHD

They are not typically hyperactive, but find it hard to concentrate, and they are often very stubborn. Their development may be delayed — for example, they may start talking late. They also have many fears, including fear of animals and death, or even a fear that their parents will die or desert them. As a result, they often experience nightmares.

> ## If one identical twin has ADHD, the other almost always has it as well

LYCOPODIUM is one of the most useful medicines for school phobia: the child screams and cries or complains of a stomachache when it is time to go to school. In fact, they often have a "tummy ache," particularly gas and bloating, and may have "bilious attacks," in which they vomit. They have difficulty concentrating, particularly in the afternoon. These children lack self-confidence and fear being alone. They are shy and awkward with strangers, but can be bossy and bad tempered with family and friends.

SULPHUR Children who respond to *Sulphur* are typically highly active, hot, and scruffy. They are "into everything" and seem to make a mess everywhere they go. No matter how carefully they are dressed in the morning, they soon get dirty. They like to be the center of attention and cause trouble if they are not. They are often irritable and self-centered; seeming to have no regard for the feelings of others, they may be bullies.

Children who respond to *Sulphur* are typically "hot-blooded," throwing off their pajamas at night and thirsty for cold drinks. They often have skin problems, especially eczema.

CAUSTICUM Children who respond to *Causticum* are sensitive and excitable. Unlike with *Sulphur*, they are very aware of, and intensely sympathetic to, the suffering of others. A *Causticum* child may burst into tears for the slightest reason, especially cruelty to animals, even in a story, and may have many fears, especially of the dark. Compulsive and perfectionistic behavior

may also occur. The *Causticum* teenager is both rebellious and highly idealistic.

Environmental Health

Hyperactivity is a disease in which various aspects of the modern environment appear to play a major role. For example, it may be triggered by exposure to organic toxins. At the same time, many people with attention and hyperactivity disorders are especially susceptible to distraction from electronic devices such as television.

A first step in dealing with hyperactivity should be to avoid or minimize exposure to heavy metals, such as lead, mercury, or manganese. This is especially important for pregnant women and for developing children whose bodies readily incorporate the toxic compounds.

LEAD can have a devastating effect on the development and function of nerves, especially those in the central nervous system. Evidence suggests that it is increasingly probable that a child exposed to lead will have problems with hyperactivity. Where possible, take the following steps to minimize your child's exposure to lead:

- Before using, run water for at least a minute through household pipes that may contain solder with lead.
- Make sure your child drinks cold, not hot, tap water (or filter your water with an approved portable filter, or reverse osmosis system).
- Do not let your child eat or drink from leaded crystal or improperly glazed ceramic dishes or containers.
- Check that remedies, including calcium supplements, are lead-free.
- Limit his or her exposure to paints containing lead, found in older homes.

Significant lead exposure can be detected in a child's blood or, in cases of long-term exposure, by measuring the amount of lead incorporated into the child's bones.

A technique called chelation (binding a metal and filtering it from the bloodstream

by chemical means) is one way of dealing with lead in the body, but there is no guarantee that this will work, even in acute high-dose lead poisoning.

Supplementing with calcium (*see p.37*) may work, since calcium takes preference over lead when the metals are absorbed and incorporated in the body.

MERCURY, like lead, is notorious for interfering with the normal development of nerves. The organic form is particularly dangerous. You can decrease your child's mercury exposure by limiting the fish, especially oily fish, that he or she eats.

Although many fish-oil supplements contain DHA (*see Essential Fatty Acids, p.403*), which has been shown to help with several behavioral issues, make sure the brand of fish oil you use has been conclusively determined not to contain heavy metals. If in doubt, look for a product that has been distilled.

MANGANESE has been associated with hyperactivity problems, according to a few studies. Since manganese is a recent addition to gasoline in the US and Canada, more evidence may emerge in the future about its role in ADHD.

ELECTRONIC STIMULATION There is ample research that demonstrates what common sense tells us: overstimulation by television, video games, or loud noises can exacerbate a child's problems with attention and hyperactivity. The rapid-firing bombardment of the senses and the neural circuitry by electronic entertainment devices could make anybody inattentive and "wired." If a child is prone to hyperactivity, this kind of stimulation can make the problem worse and should be discouraged.

PHYSICAL EXERCISE Another kind of stimulation, however, can ease the symptoms of hyperactivity problems: physical exercise can be highly therapeutic for people who are prone to hyperactivity and attention disorders. Encourage your child to play sports and get regular exercise.

Bodywork Therapies

MASSAGE is a very useful technique for helping children cope with ADHD. One 1998 study suggests that children who receive 15 minutes of massage after school each day for 10 days experience an improvement in their behavior and concentration, and a reduction in their hyperactivity. The massage consists of five minutes on the neck, five minutes across the base of neck and shoulders, and five minutes on the spinal region.

The researchers strongly urge the use of massage in helping children with ADHD, either in conjunction with a standard treatment or as a substitute, especially when medication is having undesirable side effects.

CHIROPRACTIC A number of research studies and case reports suggest that hyperactivity and associated behavioral conditions respond well to chiropractic care, often more effectively than when medication is used.

CRANIAL OSTEOPATHY and other craniosacral methods of manipulation have also demonstrated benefits in treating children with ADHD. Research strongly suggests that the problems being treated may be the result of obstetrically complicated deliveries.

Tai Chi and Yoga

Movement and bodywork can help calm children and adolescents with ADHD. For example, research at The Touch Research Institute at the University of Miami Medical School has shown that tai chi, as well as massage, can markedly reduce ADHD symptoms.

TAI CHI In a 2000 study, adolescents with developmental problems who had been diagnosed with ADHD engaged in tai chi exercise classes twice a week over the course of five weeks. Classes were in the early afternoon. During the 30-minute classes the adolescents improved their conduct and exhibited less anxiety, "day dreaming," displays of inappropriate emotions, and hyperactivity.

YOGA Research at the University of Sydney in 2003 suggested that yoga can help boys with ADHD manage their behavior while they are not taking any medication. Following 20 weeks of practicing yoga in weekly one-hour classes, the boys's restless

and/or impulsive behavior improved. However, their ADHD was still present.

Psychological Therapies

PRIMARY TREATMENT **BEHAVIOR MANAGEMENT** The main focus of various talking therapies is to help parents manage their child's behavior. All too often parents feel overwhelmed and powerless to help their children. This sometimes ends up in a spiral of "coercive parenting" in which parents try to force their children to do things or behave in certain ways — but the real result is that they bring out the worst

> ### Up to 30 percent of children with ADHD in the US may be clinically depressed

in each other. Most of the psychological research has been carried out using systems therapies (*see p.107*) because the focus of these is on family interactions.

Training both parents and children to manage their behavior simultaneously has been shown to reduce conflicts and noncompliance in children with ADHD. This form of training has also been evaluated for children with conduct and behavior problems, and has been shown to reduce problematic and oppositional behavior.

PRIMARY TREATMENT **INDIVIDUAL TALKING THERAPIES** for ADHD aim to help a child or young person regulate their behavior and become more reflective. There has been considerable interest in developing cognitive behavioral therapy (CBT) for these children, but the results have so far been disappointing, even when the children are also given medication.

There is some evidence to suggest that skills training with children alone has had some success in improving children's social skills. There is also some evidence that behavioral therapy, in which rewards are given for "acceptable" behavior, shows short-term improvement.

The use of a method known as anger-control training, in which children engage in role play to find ways of coping with situations, has shown initial promise in the treatment of ADHD.

The practice of some of the above skills in a school environment has also been attempted with some success. While some of the behavioral methods have only shown short-term improvement, their use in the classroom on a more regular basis has shown promise. This involves teaching behavioral techniques to teachers and instilling the techniques as part of the classroom culture.

MULTIMODAL TREATMENT is increasingly used for children and young people with ADHD. Here, a combination of medication and talking therapies becomes more effective than the sum of the treatments when they are used separately. One advantage of this multimodal approach appears to be that a lower dosage of medication can be used, thus reducing the occurrence of side effects.

Mind-Body Therapy

Biofeedback may benefit children with ADHD. A small controlled study of EEG (brainwave) biofeedback found that it was more effective than placebo treatment.

PREVENTION PLAN

The following may help prevent your child from developing ADHD:

- If you are a mother-to-be, avoid drinking alcohol during pregnancy

- Make sure your child's diet contains a minimum amount of caffeine, sugar, and additives

- Avoid excessive family stress caused by arguments, conflicts, etc.

- Avoid exposing your child to toxic levels of metals, such as lead, mercury, and manganese

- Limit the amount of time your child spends watching television or playing computer or video games

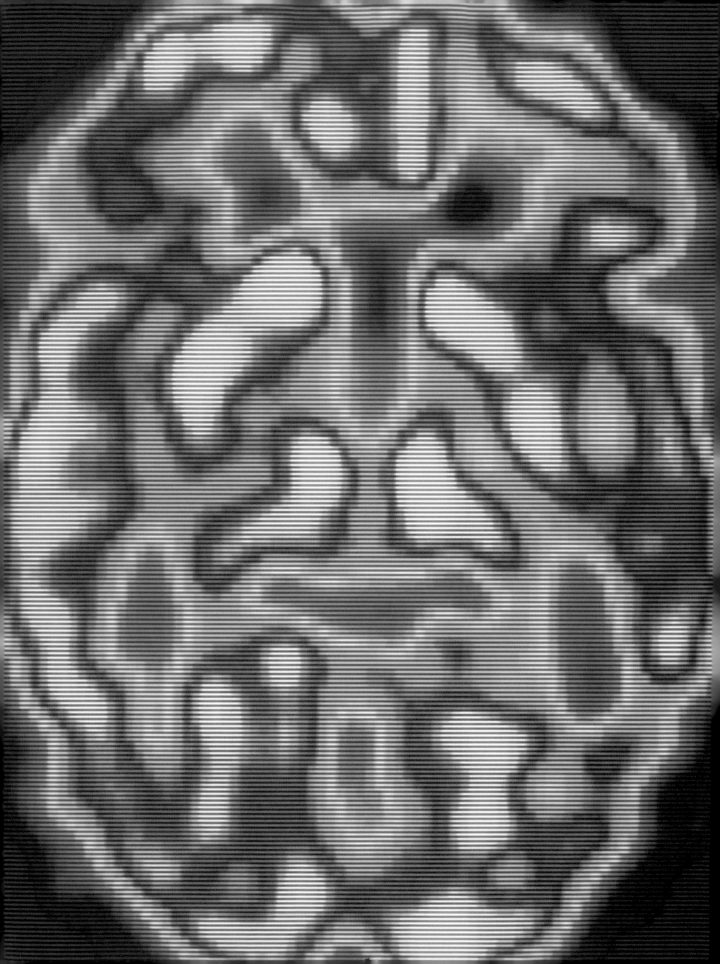

Mind & Emotions

Mental and emotional problems can disturb the roots of a person's existence, affecting his or her self-esteem and ability to cope with the pressures of the modern world. Advances in our understanding of the way the mind and body are interrelated have led to new ways of coping with these disorders, from touch and movement therapies to drugs, nutritional supplements, psychological therapies, and stress-management techniques.

EXCESS STRESS

A physical or mental challenge such as a car speeding toward us or a work deadline looming provokes the "fight or flight" stress response, which involves physical reactions, such as an increase in heart rate and sweating, and psychological reactions, such as intense concentration. Everyone faces a certain amount of stress and it only becomes a problem when it is too much for the individual to handle. There is a wide range of therapeutic measures that aim to reduce the symptoms and to help the person better manage stressful situations.

PHYSICAL SYMPTOMS OF STRESS INCLUDE:

- Fatigue
- Frequent headaches, caused by tension
- Muscle pains
- Increased symptoms of other diseases
- Inability to cope physically

PSYCHOLOGICAL SYMPTOMS OF STRESS INCLUDE:

- Anxiety
- Tearfulness
- Irritability
- Lack of concentration
- Difficulty making decisions
- Problems sleeping
- Loss of appetite
- Low energy levels and lack of motivation
- Inability to cope psychologically

WHY MIGHT I HAVE THIS?

PREDISPOSING FACTORS

- Anxious personality
- Poor general health
- Lack of social support

TRIGGERS

- A difficult event or situation
- Accumulation of many daily hassles

WHY DOES IT OCCUR?

In the "fight-or-flight" response, stress hormones, such as epinephrine, norepinephrine, and cortisol, pour into the body's systems. As digestion slows, the muscles tense up, the liver releases sugar and fats as energy for sudden action, and the heart rate rises. If this energy and tension are not discharged, the effects can accumulate and affect every major organ and body system, causing or worsening diseases or conditions such as gastrointestinal disorders, arthritis, diabetes, chronic back pain, angina, hypertension, sleep disorders, and cancer.

TREATMENT PLAN

PRIMARY TREATMENTS

- Self-help measures
- Counseling
- Psychotherapy
- Stress management programs

BACKUP TREATMENTS

- Nutritional therapy
- Breathing retraining
- Western herbal medicine
- Touch therapy
- Homeopathy
- Acupuncture
- Mind–body therapies

For an explanation of how treatments are rated, see p.111.

Stress is caused by events or situations, such as bereavement, divorce, giving a public presentation, or moving. It can result from boredom or many minor irritations, such as being stuck in a traffic jam or losing your keys. The extent to which people become stressed under such circumstances depends on their personality traits and how they cope with pressure. It only becomes a problem when it is too much for the indivdual and interferes with his or her ability to relax and cope with life.

People vary in their ability to cope with stress on both physical and emotional levels. Enhancing this ability in one area will improve the other as well, so getting more exercise to improve physical functioning will also increase the ability to cope with emotional stress.

SELF-HELP

PRIMARY TREATMENT The following measures may help you deal with stress:

- Aim for optimum health by eating a balanced diet and getting regular exercise (exercise is an excellent stress-reliever).
- Reduce your intake of caffeine and other stimulants, and cut down on other addictive substances, such as tobacco and alcohol.
- Make time to enjoy your hobbies — this will give your mind a break from the sources of stress.
- Keep in touch with your friends and family — this will make you feel supported and may help increase your self-confidence.
- Learn relaxation techniques (see p.99).
- Anticipate times of stress and consider how you will deal with them.
- List what you have to do and prioritize.

Conventional Medicine

PRIMARY TREATMENT **COUNSELING AND PSYCHO-THERAPY** If you are under stress and are having difficulty coping, or believe that stress is affecting your physical or emotional health, you may wish to speak to your doctor, who will discuss possible underlying causes with you and check your general health. Your doctor may recommend the preventive measures described (*see Self-Help, p.408*) and may advise you to have counseling or another form of psychotherapy.

Nutritional Therapy

MAGNESIUM Stress can lead to weakened adrenal glands and taking steps to strengthen adrenal function seems to help individuals cope better with the stress in their lives (*see p.44*).

Magnesium may help alleviate stress by improving the function of the adrenal glands and by counteracting the magnesium depletion in the body that can be induced by stress. One study with fighter pilots found that taking 400mg of magnesium supplements a day reduced the stress-induced rises in norepinephrine. You may find that taking 300–500mg of magnesium a day is helpful during times of stress.

CAUTION

Consult your doctor before taking magnesium with ciprofloxacin, warfarin, or spironolactone (*see p.46*).

PROBIOTICS Studies have shown that excessive stress can cause the depletion of beneficial bacteria, such as species of *lactobacillus* and *bifidobacteria*, in the intestinal tract. You may benefit from taking a probiotic in times of stress.

Homeopathy

It is difficult to generalize about treatments for stress, not only because of the individualized nature of homeopathy but also because of the wide variety of sources of stress and the different ways that people cope with stress.

HOW THE BODY RESPONDS TO STRESS

The brain and adrenal glands work together to control the stress responses. There are two types: the "fight-or-flight" stress response occurs when your brain detects an immediate threat. Epinephrine is released into the bloodstream to prepare your body for quick action. If stress is prolonged, for example as the result of a heavy workload, the hormone ACTH is released, which makes the adrenal glands secrete corticosteroid hormones. These can have a damaging effect on the body.

IMMEDIATE RESPONSE

Nerve impulses travel from the hypothalamus in the brain via the spinal cord to the adrenal glands, which then release epinephrine.

Effect of epinephrine Breathing and heart rate increase and blood pressure rises. Glucose is released for instant energy and the digestive system slows down.

KEY
- Nerve impulse
- ACTH

LONG-TERM RESPONSE

The hypothalamus triggers the pituitary gland to release ACTH (adrenocorticotropic hormone) into the bloodstream. In response, the adrenals release cortisol and other corticosteroid hormones.

Effect of corticosteroids The kidneys reabsorb water which raises blood pressure. Protein and fat metabolism increase, which can lead to plaque in the arteries. Memory and immune responses may be impaired.

Brain, Pituitary gland, Spinal cord, Adrenal gland, Epinephrine, Kidney, Adrenal gland, Corticosteroids, Kidney

NUX VOMICA is the classic homeopathic medicine for stress. The typical "picture" is of the efficient, hardworking business man who finds himself waking early in the morning, worrying about the problems of the day that lie ahead, and unable to get back to sleep. He may even feel physically ill in the morning and it takes several cups of coffee to get him going.

Very impatient and irritable, he is annoyed by what he perceives as inefficiency or stupidity. As the day wears on, he feels better, gradually relaxing, perhaps with the help of rich or spicy food, alcohol, nicotine, or other drugs. Yet the cycle starts again early the next morning.

There may be physical symptoms, such as a stuffy head cold, sore throat, indigestion, and bowel problems — in particular, a constant urge to pass stools, which may or may not be successful.

KALIUM PHOSPHORICUM In contrast to *Nux vomica*, this homeopathic medicine is useful for people who have a very different reaction to stress. Their main feature is fatigue, particularly mental exhaustion, combined with weak memory and trouble with concentration, headaches, disturbed sleep with bad dreams, and a tendency to pick up infections.

OTHER REMEDIES to consider for stress at work include *Calcarea carbonica* for the reliable worker who gets jaded with work, waking at night in a sweat worrying that he or she will be unable to cope. *Lycopodium* is for serious, conscientious people in responsible and intellectually demanding posts who get depressed and lose self-confidence. *Phosphoric acid* can be useful when intellectual and emotional stress combine — for instance, the stress of exams and relationship difficulties that teenagers experience. *Natrum muriaticum* is important for the consequences of bottled-up, long-term emotional stress, which the sufferer often does not like to discuss or reveal to other people, even medical professions.

Western Herbal Medicine

Adaptogenic herbs help the individual cope with stress often associated with fatigue, debility, anxiety, and depression. Overall, they improve vitality, staying power, memory, and concentration. They include ginseng (*Panax ginseng*), Siberian ginseng (*Eleutherococcus senticosus),* astragalus (*Astragalus membranaceus*), and withania (*Withania somnifera*).

The so-called nervine herbs support an overtaxed nervous system. They include skullcap (*Scutellaria laterifolia*), wild oat (*Avena sativa*), vervain (*Verbena officinalis*), and damiana (*Turnera diffusa*).

Stress with anxiety and depression can be treated with valerian (*Valeriana officinalis*), lemon balm (*Melissa officinalis*), and St. John's wort (*Hypericum perforatum*).

Passionflower (*Passiflora officinalis*), hops (*Humulus lupulus*), valerian, chamomile (*Matricaria recutita*), and lemon balm can all help improve the quality and duration of sleep, which, in turn, will ease stress and nervous tension.

Cramp bark (*Viburnum opulus*) relaxes the tense muscles that are often associated with stress. Soaking in a lavender oil bath (add 10–15 drops of the essential oil to a hot bath) can help relieve the stresses of a busy day.

CAUTION

Do not take any type of ginseng for more than six weeks without a break. See p.69 before taking an herbal remedy, in particular before taking St. John's wort. If you are already taking prescribed medication, consult an herbal medicine expert first.

Breathing Retraining

If you are affected by stressful feelings and events, then learn deep breathing techniques *(see p.62)*. Certain breathing patterns can have an "antiarousal" effect that reduces the sympathetic (alarm) response of the body when faced with stressful events or stimuli.

Touch Therapies

EFFECTS OF TOUCH Research into the calming, antistress effects of touch therapies, such as massage and reflexology, has consistently shown that they commonly lead to a reduction in production of cortisol and other stress hormones. Touch therapy has helped people with asthma, anorexia, breast cancer, burns, depression, chronic fatigue, diabetes, and HIV. It is also useful for preterm infants and during labor, as well as in people suffering posttraumatic stress disorder.

When individuals who are stressed are taught to give massage — for example, parents massaging their hyperactive children or grandparents massaging their grandchildren — both the givers and the receivers of the massage show reduced stress levels.

Massage and/or acupressure may also reduce stress in the workplace, delivering benefits such as an improved ability to concentrate, a greater sense of well-being, increased job satisfaction, fewer work-related injuries or absences, and improved productivity.

REFLEXOLOGY has been shown to produce a calming effect in people with a variety of stressful problems, including hospitalized patients, parents of babies in intensive care units, and a range of health conditions, such as migraine, and bowel, and sleep disturbances. When reflexology is compared with general foot massage, the benefits seem very similar.

Acupuncture

There is some evidence that acupuncture helps relieve depression, anxiety, and sleep disorders, all of which are common symptoms of stress. It would therefore be logical to consider acupuncture in situations of great stress, although there are no clinical trials specifically highlighting the benefits. Acupuncture can be given to help balance an individual's energy and possibly avoid stress, and this may be part of regular maintenance acupuncture. In situations of acute anxiety and concern, acupuncture may be given daily or every other day but in general, weekly treatments are the preferred option, and benefit should be apparent in six to eight sessions. If no benefit is seen within that time, the therapy should be stopped.

Mind–Body Therapies

While some patients visit their doctors actually complaining of stress, more often they complain of various physical symptoms, such as gastrointestinal disturbances, pain, insomnia, and fatigue. The mainstay of treatment is based on appropriate counseling, lifestyle advice, reassurance, addressing specific issues, and other non-pharmaceutical treatments.

PRIMARY TREATMENT **STRESS-MANAGEMENT PROGRAMS** using behavioral and mind–body approaches are widely employed to reduce stress. Among the mind–body skills and therapies that have been found to be effective are regular physical exercise, clinical biofeedback, muscle relaxation, and psychotherapy.

Guided imagery *(for a sequence, see p.99),* which combines deep relaxation with positive suggestion, is a powerful technique for managing stress. Eight studies found that, relative to control groups, guided imagery sessions were effective at reducing the physical and emotional signs of stress in groups of smokers, surgical patients, cardiac, and cancer patients, as well as in otherwise healthy people who said they had high stress levels. Moreover, the effects were stronger when patients could practice the skills on their own.

Relaxation, whether it is practiced with or without guided imagery, is highly recommended, because it can improve the ability to cope with the inevitable stresses of everyday life.

PREVENTION PLAN

The following may help to prevent the development of excess stress:

- Eat a nutritious diet
- Get regular exercise
- Practice relaxation regularly

PHOBIAS

A phobia is a persistent, irrational fear of an object, situation, or activity that compels a person to avoid it obsessively. A fear of something, such as dogs or high places, that causes occasional unease but does not disrupt everyday life is not a phobia. People with genuine phobias can be severely restricted, with their lives affected in many different ways. Their phobias usually develop in late childhood or early adulthood. Phobias are principally treated with exposure therapy but breathing retraining may also be helpful.

WHAT ARE THE SYMPTOMS?

Exposure to the object of the phobia, or sometimes even thinking about it or imagining it, may cause the following symptoms:

- Dizziness and feeling faint
- Palpitations (awareness of an abnormally rapid heartbeat)
- Sweating, trembling, and nausea
- Shortness of breath

WHY MIGHT I HAVE THESE?

PREDISPOSING FACTORS

- Traumatic childhood experience
- Lack of self-esteem
- Anxious personality

TREATMENT PLAN

PRIMARY TREATMENTS

- Exposure therapy, sometimes in combination with certain antidepressants
- Breathing retraining

WORTH CONSIDERING

- Nutritional therapies
- Homeopathy
- Other psychological therapies

For an explanation of how treatments are rated, see p.111.

WHY DO THEY OCCUR?

SIMPLE OR COMPLEX PHOBIAS Phobias are often classed as being either simple or complex. Simple phobias are specific to a single object, situation, or activity, such as a fear of flying, fear of spiders or fear of enclosed spaces. Complex phobias involve several component fears.

A fear of open or public spaces (agoraphobia) is a complex phobia that may involve, for example, fear of being alone in a public place and of being trapped in a public place with no exit. Social phobias, in which people are afraid of embarrassing themselves or being humiliated, are also considered complex phobias.

CAUSES Phobias often have no identifiable cause. Sometimes, however, a simple phobia can be traced back to a traumatic experience in childhood. Simple phobias appear to run in families, but this is thought to be because children learn the fear from a family member. The causes of complex phobias are less clear, but they seem to develop from a general tendency to anxiety. People who lack self-esteem are more likely to develop social phobias or agoraphobia.

AVOIDANCE A phobic person is aware that his fear is irrational but is still compelled to avoid the object or situation that he fears. Exposure to the object of the phobia causes a physical reaction ("fight-or-flight"), often with sweating and a rapid heartbeat. A factor that is common to all phobias is avoidance of the object of the phobia and this may severely limit a person's activities. Anxiety and panic attacks (*see p.414*) sometimes develop in relation to the phobia.

TREATMENTS IN DETAIL

Conventional Medicine

PRIMARY TREATMENT Your doctor will suggest psychological therapies, which are the mainstay of treatment for phobias (*see Psychological Therapies, p.412*). When there are symptoms of depression (*see p.436*), certain antidepressants may be helpful when they are prescribed in combination with psychological therapy. Most commonly, these medications are tricyclic antidepressants, such as clomipramine; however, selective serotonin uptake inhibitors (SSRIs) are used in some cases.

Nutritional Therapy

The nutritional measures described for anxiety (*see p.415*) are also relevant for people with phobias. These include balancing blood-sugar levels, avoiding caffeine, and taking supplements such as magnesium, selenium, or a multivitamin.

Homeopathy

Homeopathy is helpful for treating the phobic "terrain," i.e., the background of anxiety. Some homeopathic medicines may help with specific fears, among them *Argentum nitricum*, *Phosphorus*, *Stramomium*, *Lycopodium*, *Calcarea carbonica*, and *Silicea*.

ARGENTUM NITRICUM Probably the most useful medicine is *Argentum nitricum* It is suitable particularly for claustrophobia and fear of heights, especially if associated with a distressing impulse to jump. People who respond to this medicine are hot, twitchy, and impulsive. They seem to have a problem managing their time, always seeming to be in a hurry and getting into a terrible state before any important event. The anxiety associated with the phobia may express itself in physical manifestations, including diarrhea, burping, vertigo, and tremor.

PHOSPHORUS may be appropriate for people who have a fear of the dark. People who respond to *Phosphorus* are excessively sensitive, both to their physical and their human environment. They may be hypersensitive and sense that they can "feel vibes," though not always accurately. They are greatly affected by thunderstorms: they may fear them or develop a headache before a storm breaks.

STRAMONIUM may also be appropriate for people who fear the dark. *Stramonium* may help when someone is praying and trembling and really beside themselves with fear. Apart from the dark, they may also fear animals, ghosts, or water.

LYCOPODIUM Various fears make up parts of the "picture" of other homeopathic medicines. For instance, *Lycopodium* is frequently a valuable medicine for children with a phobia about school and for adults whose stage fright makes them anxious before appearing in public.

CALCAREA CARBONICA People whose constitution fits the *Calcarea carbonica* "picture" tend to have many fears, especially of disease and death.

SILICEA People who respond to *Silicea* (also called *Silica*) fear needles and pins, and may feel faint at the suggestion of a blood test. But in all cases, the person's overall "picture" must fit the remedy if the treatment is to be of help. It is therefore essential to consult an experienced homeopath (*see p.73*).

Breathing Retraining

PRIMARY TREATMENT A great deal of evidence confirms that a combination of breathing retraining and manual therapy (to assist in freeing the muscles of the chest and other respiratory structures) can reduce the anxiety and help people cope with phobic reactions. This will often com-

pletely eliminate phobic behavior. When a phobia has deep-rooted emotional or psychological causes, breathing retraining might have to be used alongside psychotherapy or cognitive behavioral therapy.

In one major study, more than 1,000 phobic patients (mainly people suffering from agoraphobia — the fear of open/public places) were treated using techniques such as breathing retraining, physical therapy, and relaxation. One the whole, their symptoms took one to six months to disappear, with some younger patients requiring only a few weeks. A year after the treatment, 75 percent of former patients were free of all their symptoms; a further 20 percent had only mild symptoms. Only about one patient in 20 failed to respond to the treatment.

HYPERVENTILATION It has been estimated that approximately 60 percent of people with phobic behavior have hyperventilation as part of their symptom picture. The main characteristic of hyperventilation is a habitual tendency to breathe shallowly with just the upper chest, rather than the deeper breathing that uses the diaphragm. This leads to excessive exhalation of carbon dioxide, so that the person gets used (habituated) to having low levels of this important regulatory gas in their bloodstream.

TESTING CARBON DIOXIDE TOLERANCE A low tolerance to carbon dioxide can help identify people who hyperventilate. A simple test can be used in which a person is asked to exhale and wait until there is a an urgent "need to breathe." During the holding time, carbon dioxide levels will be rising, and the "need to breathe" represents that moment when the level of carbon dioxide triggers a message to the respiratory center in the brain, requesting that breathing start again.

This test is a reasonably accurate way of assessing a person's current tolerance to carbon dioxide. "Normal" is thought to be between 25 to 30 seconds. Under 15 seconds is thought to represent a low tolerance of carbon dioxide.

Another test for carbon dioxide tolerance is to ask a person to breathe air that contains increased levels of carbon dioxide and then to assess the reaction by finding out when feelings of panic and phobia

start. Using this approach, researchers have reported that, childhood anxiety disorders are all associated with carbon dioxide hypersensitivity.

YOGA AND THE BUTEYKO METHOD A major part of breathing retraining involves using techniques, such as slow exhalation as in yoga-type exercises and periodic holding of the breath, that help the person slowly, over a period of months, to become accustomed to increasingly higher levels of carbon dioxide in the blood. The breath-holding method forms a part of the Russian Buteyko breathing retraining method (*see also Asthma, p.205*).

When breathing retraining is used regularly, the benefits include reduced feelings of anxiety, fewer panic attacks, and, most importantly, a lessening or vanishing of the phobia. (*For a breathing sequence, see p.62.*)

Psychological Therapies

Phobias can be severely restricting, creating a powerfully negative impact on a person's life in many ways. They are divided into two main categories: simple or specific phobias and complex or social phobias.

Therapies from the cognitive behavioral model (*see p.106*) have been shown to be particularly effective for both categories. Exposure therapy is probably the most commonly used for simple or specific phobias, which include animal phobias and fear of flying. Eye movement desensitization and reprocessing (EMDR) may also be effective (*see p.413*).

The more complex social phobias, such as the fear of open spaces (agoraphobia), are more difficult to disentangle and need more psychological reprogramming of a person's thinking and perception.

You can try to tackle your phobia if you think it is mild enough by following the three steps of the phobia desensitization sequence (*see box, p.413*).

PRIMARY TREATMENT **EXPOSURE THERAPY** is most commonly used as a treatment for simple phobias. As the name suggests, exposure therapy (or graded exposure) consists of gently introducing patients to the very thing, situation, or event that makes them anxious. For example, people with spider phobias will initially be asked to imagine a spider, then

PHOBIA DESENSITIZATION

The aim of this phobia desensitization sequence is to reduce your fear response and replace it with a relaxation response. Take it slowly: do not attempt all the steps in a single day. Spread them over several days or more if you prefer. You need to feel completely comfortable with each step before moving on to the next. As you feel ready, you can use photos or video clips of the object or situation that triggers your phobia before attempting to encounter it in real life. This self-desensitization sequence is only suitable if you have a mild phobia. Do not hesitate to seek professional help if you need it.

DESCRIBE YOUR PHOBIA

Anxious situations

- List all the situations that could trigger your phobia. For claustrophobia, these might include being trapped in an elevator or taking the subway during rush hour.

Feelings and thoughts

- Think about these situations and list sensations — e.g. rapid heartbeat — and concerns, for example "If I were trapped in an elevator, I might die of dehydration."

Response to the fear

- Make a list of how you might respond if faced with the object or situation you fear. For example, "I might scream."

ORDER YOUR FEARS

- Write down the situation that would make you most anxious.
- Then list the others according to how much they scare you. For people who are phobic about spiders, the number one fear might be a large spider running across their face, whereas seeing an illustration of a spider's web might be fairly low down on the list.

ADDRESS YOUR PHOBIA

- Choose the least fearful thought on your list.
- Relax deeply and concentrate on your breathing.
- Start to think about your fearful thought. Try to control your responses using relaxation techniques.
- Deepen your relaxation.
- When you can approach this thought without any discomfort, move up your list to the next thought and repeat the process.

---

to view a drawing of a small spider until they stop feeling anxious. Next, they are asked to look at a more detailed drawing while their anxiety reduces to a manageable level and they become desensitized. The patient progresses at their own pace and eventually may be presented with a real spider. The therapist may hold the spider until the patient's anxiety subsides sufficiently (a technique known as modelling) and may invite the patient to touch or hold it (a technique known as *in vivo*).

Video and virtual reality technology have been used to expose patients to their fears and a review found that 70–80 percent of patients showed significant clinical improvement. The *in vivo* method seems to be particularly effective.

Video and virtual reality technology have been used to expose patients to their fears, and a review found that 70–80 percent of patients showed significant clinical improvement. The *in vivo* method seems to be particularly effective.

One advantage of exposure therapy is that it can be brief. For instance, dental phobia can be treated using just two or four sessions. People with animal phobias have been treated in a two-hour session and in one study using exposure and modeling, 90 percent of the individuals were free of their phobias a year later.

EYE MOVEMENT DESENSITIZATION AND REPROCESSING (EMDR) is based on exposure therapy (*see p.412*) and has shown promising results. The mode in which the exposure therapy is delivered — whether it is carried out in an individual, couple, or family, or in a group setting — has also been examined and the use of group treatment has been shown to be effective. (*For more details of EMDR, see Post-Traumatic Stress Disorder, p.422.*)

COGNITIVE THERAPY Although the use of cognitive therapy (which is CBT without a behavioral component such as exposure

therapy) has not been shown to make a significant difference with simple phobias, it appears to help people who are affected by the more complex social phobias. Cognitive therapy focuses on how the patient perceives and thinks about an event. Facilitating the patient to review his or her thoughts and change them has been shown to help as an adjunct to exposure therapy in social phobias.

According to one review, cognitive behavior therapy (CBT) is an effective method of treating social phobias. It appears that a combination of cognitive and exposure methods, rather than either one or the other alone, is the most effective form of treatment. Training in social skills in order to promote more productive and positive interaction with other people may also have an effect on social phobias.

HYPNOSIS There have been many studies of the effectiveness of hypnosis as a treatment for phobias.

ANXIETY AND PANIC DISORDER

Feeling worried or anxious occasionally and with reason is appropriate and normal. When anxiety becomes the usual response to ordinary situations and interferes with everyday life, it is considered a disorder. Panic disorder is a common, recurrent, and unpredictable type of anxiety. Anxiety disorders may be present without panic attacks. Treatment involves psychological therapies, the occasional use of drugs, control of blood-sugar levels, supplements, massage, breathing exercises, homeopathy, herbs, and mind–body therapies.

WHAT ARE THE SYMPTOMS?

Symptoms of anxiety disorder include:

- Headaches
- Abdominal cramps, sometimes with diarrhea and vomiting
- Frequent urination
- Sweating, flushing, and tremor
- Constricted feeling in the throat
- Being on edge, with a sense of foreboding
- Inability to concentrate
- Repetitive worrying thoughts
- Disturbed sleep patterns, sometimes with nightmares

Symptoms of a panic attack include:

- Intense anxiety
- Shortness of breath
- Sweating, trembling, and nausea
- Rapid heartbeat
- Dizziness and fainting
- Constricted feeling in the throat
- Feeling of unreality and fears about loss of sanity

WHY MIGHT I HAVE THIS?

PREDISPOSING FACTORS

- Genetic factors
- Stress overload
- Trait anxiety

TRIGGERS

- Caffeine
- Blood-sugar imbalance
- Stressful event, such as a death in the family

WHY DOES IT OCCUR?

The term "anxiety disorders" covers a group of psychological conditions that are related to excessive concerns and fears. These conditions include generalized anxiety disorder, panic disorder, acute stress disorder, post-traumatic stress disorder (*see p.422*), phobias (*see p.411*), and obsessive-compulsive disorder (*see p.419*).

TREATMENT PLAN

PRIMARY TREATMENTS

- Self-help measures (*see Self-Help, p.415*)
- Cognitive behavioral therapy
- Drugs, such as benzodiazepines
- Breathing retraining

BACKUP TREATMENTS

- Drugs, such as beta-blockers and antidepressants (short term only)
- Nutritional therapy
- Exercise and massage
- Acupuncture
- Western herbal medicine

WORTH CONSIDERING

- Homeopathy
- Environmental health measures

For an explanation of how treatments are rated, see p.111.

All of these conditions are marked by feelings of apprehension, uneasiness, or tension, which range from being mild to being incapacitating. Physical symptoms can include muscle tension, shaking or trembling, shortness of breath, palpitations (*see p.258*), and sweating.

Anxiety disorders usually start in middle age and are more common in women than in men. Sometimes, an anxiety disorder develops after a stressful event, such as a death in the family. However, often the anxiety has no identifiable cause. In some cases, it is associated with a depressive illness.

Poor bonding between parents and children or an abrupt separation of a child from a parent may also play a part in some anxiety disorders.

TRAIT ANXIETY Anxiety disorders appear to be caused by a complex interaction of psychological, physical, and genetic influences. Some people are more prone to anxiety than others. For example, the likelihood of developing an anxiety disorder is increased if you have close relatives with anxiety disorders or phobias (*see p.411*) or if you experienced a traumatic event during your childhood.

Those with high "trait anxiety" (a long-standing tendency rather than simply being temporarily anxious) are more likely than most to perceive a stressful situation or sensation as dangerous or threatening. Their response is to feel apprehensive, upset, or distressed. Also called neuroticism, this trait often runs in families and involves a rapid and excessive "fight-or-flight" arousal response.

GENERALIZED ANXIETY DISORDER (GAD)

Some anxiety is normal. Persistent, exaggerated worry is not. Everyone feels some anxiety, even on a daily basis. But people with generalized anxiety disorder (GAD) have a constant anxiety, often without any obvious cause, yet enough to interfere with normal life. Typical symptoms of GAD are:

- Persistent worry and anxiousness about events that are unlikely to occur.
- Inability to shut off these constant anxious thoughts.
- Muscular tension, aches, and soreness.
- Restlessness, an inability to relax, and a lack of energy.
- Feelings of dread.
- Sweating, hot flashes, or a dry mouth.
- Dizziness and lightheadedness.
- Insomnia (having trouble falling or staying asleep).
- Shakiness or trembling.
- Concentration problems.
- Irritability or can be startled easily.
- Stomach problems (nausea, diarrhea).

SELF-HELP

PRIMARY TREATMENT The following measures may help if you have panic attacks:
- Practice relaxation exercises (*see p.99*).
- Try "rebreathing" into a paper bag.
- Slow your breathing to 10 breaths or less per minute.
- Try one of the homeopathic medicines discussed below.

TREATMENTS IN DETAIL

Conventional Medicine

A doctor may recommend relaxation exercises together with counseling to help with stress management or other psychological therapies, such as cognitive behavioral therapy (*see Mind–body Therapies, p.418*), to help control anxiety and panic attacks.

PRIMARY TREATMENT **BENZODIAZEPINES** In rare cases, when an individual is undergoing an extremely stressful period,

benzodiazepines, such as diazepam, may be prescribed, but only on a short-term basis since they are associated with high risks of dependence. If dependence occurs, increasing doses are needed to achieve the same effect and withdrawal symptoms such as restlessness and severe anxiety may occur.

BUSPIRONE Studies have shown that the drug buspirone helps relieve anxiety; it takes about two weeks to have an effect and is used for short periods only.

BETA-BLOCKERS are prescribed in some cases to help control the physical symptoms of anxiety, but they have no effect on the psychological features of the condition.

ANTIDEPRESSANTS When anxiety is part of a depressive illness, antidepressants may be prescribed. Some, such as paroxetine, venlafaxine, and other selective serotonin uptake inhibitors (SSRIs), have been found to help relieve the symptoms of anxiety and panic disorders.

Some antidepressants, for example the tricyclic antidepressants group, have been shown to help improve the symptoms of panic disorders in some people.

> **CAUTION**
> Drugs to relieve anxiety and panic attacks may have side effects; ask your doctor to explain these to you.

Nutritional Therapy

BALANCE BLOOD-SUGAR LEVELS An imbalance in the levels of blood sugar is a common factor associated with anxiety. The body generally attempts to correct a fall in blood sugar by secreting epinephrine, which stimulates the release of sugar from the liver. Epinephrine is certainly one hormone in the body that is well known to provoke feelings of anxiety and even panic.

Several studies show that one of the symptoms of hypoglycemia (low levels of

sugar in the blood) in diabetes is anxiety, and clinical experience suggests that even nondiabetics can be prone to anxiety at times when blood-sugar levels are lower than ideal. (*For a diet to steady blood-sugar levels, see p.42.*)

In practice, individuals prone to anxiety will tend to put more strain on their adrenal glands. This seems to be especially true for individuals who feel weak or anxious if a meal is skipped. (*For more on adrenal function, see p.44.*)

AVOID CAFFEINE A very important dietary factor that often features in anxiety is caffeine. It is a stimulant and can provoke symptoms of anxiety and nervousness. A 2002 study found that it may exaggerate responses to the stressful events of normal daily life. In the study, caffeine (equivalent to that found in four small cups of coffee) raised blood pressure and elevated the production of epinephrine.

> ### COPING WITH ANXIETY
>
> Anxiety is a normal response to a worrying event or threatening situation. However, it is not the situation or event itself but the accompanying thoughts that generate anxiety. Here are four steps to help you reduce a panic attack.
>
> - Is the problem actually yours? Sometimes, people get needlessly upset over distressing events that do not actually threaten their well-being.
> - Write down the essence of the problem and the worst-case scenario.
> - Then list ways to solve the problem. For example, if you are worried about intruders, could you install window locks or a burglar alarm? Choose the solution that seems most practical and break it down into steps.
> - To gain a sense of perspective, talk through your anxieties with a sensible friend.
> - Stress-management measures, such as getting plenty of exercise and relaxing regularly, can also help restore your calm and well-being.

Anxiety disorders and related illnesses affect 5 percent of the population

Individuals suffering from anxiety and panic attacks seem to be sensitive to the amount of caffeine found in just one cup of coffee. If you are prone to anxiety and panic attacks, it is probably advisable to avoid caffeine altogether.

MAGNESIUM SUPPLEMENTS Studies show that magnesium deficiency can enhance stress reactions and that emotional stress, such as anxiety, can increase the need for magnesium. Supplementating the diet with magnesium may be valuable for sufferers of anxiety. Taking about 200mg of magnesium supplements twice daily may help reduce symptoms. Too much magnesium can cause diarrhea.

MULTIVITAMIN/MINERAL SUPPLEMENT A good nutritional status may be helpful to those who suffer from anxiety and panic attacks. A 2000 study showed that a multivitamin and mineral supplement taken for 28 days was associated with a consistent and significant reduction in anxiety and perceived stress.

SELENIUM SUPPLEMENTS The trace mineral selenium seems to have a particular role to play in regulating mood. A 1991 study found that taking 100mcg a day of selenium lead to a general improvement in mood and a reduction in feelings of anxiety, especially in those individuals with low levels of selenium in their diet. Supplementation may be particularly beneficial for those whose diet is low in this mineral.

> **CAUTION**
>
> Consult your doctor before taking magnesium with ciprofloxacin and warfarin, or with iron and warfarin, or with spironolactone (*see p.46*).

Homeopathy

COMPLEX HOMEOPATHY In a clinical trial, a complex homeopathic medicine called Anti-Anxiety, which contains *Ignatia, Asa foetida,* and *Valeriana officinialis,* was found to be effective in treating anxiety.

IGNATIA Many homeopathic medicines may be helpful in anxiety, depending on the type of anxiety and the person who has it. Perhaps the most frequently appropriate medicine for acute anxiety triggered by an emotional shock is *Ignatia (for dosages, see p.77).* Typically, the anxiety this medicine relieves is characterized by hypersensitivity of all the senses: noises seem too loud, lights too bright, and so on. There is also great emotional hypersensitivity and changeability, as well as various kinds of spasms, including nervous coughs and tics. The "keynote" is said to be paradoxicality — for instance, there is a sensation of a lump in the throat, but liquids are more difficult to swallow than solids.

ACONITE is another homeopathic medicine that is useful in acute situations, often triggered by a physical shock or acute physical illness. Typically, the patient is very anxious, feels very chilly, and thinks she or he is about to die.

CONSTITUTIONAL TREATMENT If anxiety is long-term, you may need to visit a homeopath for constitutional treatment (*see p.72*). Perhaps the most common medicines are *Argentum nitricum, Calcarea carbonica,* and *Arsenicum album.*

ARGENTUM NITRICUM patients often have many fears, particularly claustrophobia and fear of heights, associated with a distressing impulse to jump from high places. They typically suffer from severe anticipation, getting into a terrible state in advance of important events, with physical symptoms often emanating from the intestines, including bloating, belching, and diarrhea. They also tend to feel too hot.

CALCAREA CARBONICA presents a very different picture. The anxiety may be less obvious on the surface but is deep seated. These people are often solid, conscientious types but have many fears, particularly about being seriously or incurably ill. They tend to "niggle" — they turn small things over and over in their minds. On the physical side they tend to be chilly but sweat easily, especially on the head and neck.

ARSENICUM ALBUM patients are different again. They tend to be perfectionists who get very upset if everything is not neat and organized. They get very anxious if they have even minor illnesses; where there is nothing to worry about, they will find something. On the physical side, they are usually very chilly and may have skin problems, including eczema, psoriasis, or just dry, flaky skin.

> **CAUTION**
>
> Some homeopathic medicines, including *Ignatia,* are antidoted by coffee. This means that the medicine is rendered ineffective.

Western Herbal Medicine

RELIEVING SYMPTOMS It is unrealistic to expect a herbal medicine to "cure" an anxiety that is disrupting someone's life. Herbal medicines can help relieve the symptoms of anxiety, such as muscle tension, headaches, palpitations, and sleep disturbance, and to reduce the intensity with which anxiety can grip the person's mind.

SHORT-TERM RELIEF to enable the person to implement changes that will lower anxiety levels is an aim of the herbal approach. For example, better quality and duration of sleep usually lead to improved self-confidence and vitality, increasing the person's chances of exercising more, improving his or her diet, getting through a relationship breakdown, and so forth.

In the longer term, the aim would be to prescribe herbs that will strengthen the function of the neuroendocrine system (nerves and hormones), while helping the person develop life patterns in order to become less dependent on an "epinephrine economy" — in other words, overactivity of the sympathetic nervous system.

Typically, herbal remedies are selected to match the specific anxiety exhibited by the individual patient. Lindenflowers (*Tilia*

> **People with panic disorder may become so afraid of an attack that they develop a phobia**

ANTIANXIETY BREATHING

One of the effects of experiencing anxiety and panic disorders is to change your pattern of breathing, forcing you to breathe more quickly and more shallowly from the upper chest. This has an effect on your body chemistry, leading to a cycle of tension and stress. If you feel that you are about to become anxious or are on the verge of a panic attack, try to practice the two steps of the antianxiety breathing technique shown here. You can stand, sit, or lie down on your back — whatever is most appropriate and comfortable for you at the time.

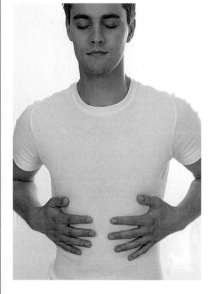

Place your hands, with the fingers spread out, below your ribcage and either side of your torso. Concentrate on your diaphragm and breathe deeply for several breaths.

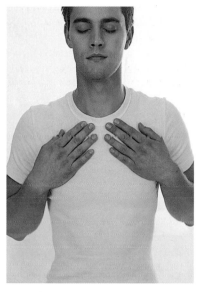

Then, with your eyes closed, place your hands on your upper chest and concentrate on sending several breaths down through your lungs to the diaphragm.

---

europea) or lemon balm (*Melissa officinalis*) relieve anxiety (anxiolytic). Both can also treat nervous palpitations, strengthening parasympathetic nervous activity on the heart, dampening the nervous irritability producing heart irregularity.

OVER-THE-COUNTER REMEDIES A range of herbal medicines can be used to relieve anxiety. Most of them are suitable for self-medication as well as for practitioner use, but if you have any doubt, consult an herbal medicine expert. Among the herbs that can be used are kava, chamomile, sage, lavender, California poppy, vervain, lemon balm, as well as those profiled below.

VALERIAN (*Valeriana officinalis*) is a relaxant and mild sedative, taken for nervous overactivity, insomnia, and muscle tension. Clinical trials have shown valerian extracts improve sleep quality and duration, with few side effects. A 1995 clinical study found valerian combined with St. John's wort (*Hypericum perforatum*), was as effective as amitryptyline in treating depressive anxiety, yet with far fewer side effects.

PASSION FLOWER (*Passiflora incarnata*) is a sedative herb that is used principally for combating sleep disturbance, but it is equally useful in relieving anxiety.

WITHANIA (*Withania somnifera*) is a relaxant and restorative herb. It is particularly useful in treating the exhaustion and enervation that accompany long-term anxiety.

> **CAUTION**
>
> Before taking a herbal remedy, see p.69 and, if you are taking prescribed medication, consult an herbal medicine expert first.

Environmental Health

TOXIC EXPOSURES Anxiety, weakness, fatigue, and difficulty concentrating are common symptoms in people after they have been exposed to toxic compounds. The symptoms result either from toxic injury to the nervous system, or to emotional or psychological responses to the exposure, or to both.

According to some research, an acute exposure that requires medical care is more likely to result in psychological symptoms, such as anxiety, than chronic low levels of toxic exposure. In fact, there is still doubt about whether or not chronic exposures could lead to an anxiety disorder. Anxiety responses to toxic exposures show some similarity to post-traumatic stress disorder (*see p.422*).

Anxiety problems may develop in people with a history of past serious exposures to environmental toxicants, or who live in close proximity to known environmentally dangerous sites.

There are many factors that affect whether or not someone will develop anxiety or other psychological problems from living or working close to a hazardous site. For example, symptoms may be more likely if the exposure was accidental or involuntary, or if there was a feeling of a lack of community control over the safety regulations in place. In addition, anxiety and concern that develop near such sites may depend on whether or not the person has a history of acute exposure to the relevant compounds or if the compounds from the site have a perceptible odor. Some people may continue to have psychological symptoms, such as anxiety, after toxic exposures; these symptoms are more likely if the person was stressed before the event happened, or if he or she had a severe enough exposure to warrant a visit to a hospital emergency room.

CHEMICALS Panic attacks may be brought on by certain chemicals, such as the cyanoacrylate and organic solvents in Superglue®. Research into other compounds, such as ammonia from a diazo printer, ozone from a photocopier, or chlorine from a pulp mill factory, support this finding. The panic reactions were often unpredictable and the particular compounds irritated skin and mucous membranes.

If you have panic attacks, it is not necessary to avoid all possible chemical triggers because people react to them in an unpredictable fashion. There is no evidence that avoidance helps prevent panic attacks from developing or improves the symptoms of panic attacks.

However, some people have a learned or conditioned response to a particular chemical so that when they smell, inhale, or contact the chemical again at a later date, they experience a panic attack.

Just as a particular chemical can elicit a panic attack, classical (Pavlovian) conditioning can be used to allay anxiety. For example, if a distinct essential oil is used during a series of relaxing massages, then

Anxiety and panic disorders can be greatly eased with professional help

the scent of the oil will come to be associated with relaxation. A small bottle of the oil can then be carried around and smelled at the first sign of anxiety to help induce a state of relaxation.

Exercise and Massage

People who are anxious or prone to panic attacks are urged to do regular aerobic exercise and to receive a regular massage. Both practices have been shown to be effective ways of reducing feelings of anxiety and apprehension, on their own and in combination with each other, or in combination with medication.

For example, research at the Touch Research Institute in Miami has shown in numerous studies that massage reduces feelings of anxiety, as well as the presence of elevated levels of "stress" hormones, such as cortisol. In a 2003 study, the effects of massage and movement therapy (50-minute sessions, twice weekly, for three weeks) were compared with the effects of relaxation on anxiety experienced by people with chronic pain. The results showed that the greatest reduction in anxiety (and pain) levels was achieved by those receiving massage and movement therapy.

A 2002 study showed that over 50 percent of a group of middle-aged men and

women with a background of depression and anxiety were much better after a four-month program of aerobic exercise combined with appropriate medication.

Breathing Retraining

PRIMARY TREATMENT Breathing retraining is a valuable tool for easing anxiety states. If your breathing is too shallow, it disrupts your body's biochemistry, which can contribute to feelings of anxiety (*for breathing exercises, see pp.57 and 62*).

In 1999, a Dutch study involved a combination of breathing retraining (learning to slow down the rate and to improve abdominal breathing) together with physi-

cal therapy designed to release tense muscles that were hampering the breathing process. The researchers found that there was a clear link between the rate of breathing and the development of symptoms of anxiety, and that slowing this rate was the key to the successful treatment.

In 1993, research looked at the effects of breathing retraining on anxiety experienced by people with chronic fatigue, compared with nonfatigued anxious individuals. The results were varied and the researchers concluded that breathing retraining benefited these people, not only in restoring more normal patterns of breathing but also in reducing anxiety, particularly in those who were not suffering from chronic fatigue.

Acupuncture

Clinical experience suggests that acupuncture is often useful to help people cope with anxiety and panic attacks. In addition, there are good scientific theories explaining how acupuncture could alter the balance of chemical messengers in the brain in a way that would be likely to benefit people with these conditions.

Often, several acupuncture treatments are required, given on a weekly basis — unless the particular anxiety disorder is

very acute, in which case treatment can be given two or three times a week. In general, you would usually expect some benefit to emerge over six to eight treatment sessions, with the possibility that long-term maintenance may be required.

Mind–Body Therapies

PRIMARY TREATMENT **COGNITIVE BEHAVIORAL THERAPY** The most effective nondrug approaches involve cognitive behavioral therapy (CBT). Many research studies confirm the effectiveness of CBT for treating anxiety disorders. In some circumstances, it may even replace medication in treating the symptoms of anxiety related ailments such as obsessive-compulsive disorder and post-traumatic stress disorder.

OTHER APPROACHES Studies confirm the efficacy of mind–body treatments, such as guided imagery, relaxation, hypnosis, meditation, and clinical biofeedback, in all types of anxiety and across all age ranges. They work well combined with CBT and medication — the latter is sometimes required if the anxiety is disabling. Patients report feeling more in control of their symptoms; positive benefits have been sustained in follow-ups as long as six years. Self-help audiotapes and/or multimedia self-help programs have also been effective.

Meditation can relieve and prevent anxiety and panic attacks. Some forms may be more effective than others, but it is important to adopt a technique that you feel comfortable doing on a regular basis.

PREVENTION PLAN

The following may help you prevent an anxiety or panic disorder:

- Do plenty of regular exercise to relax muscle tension
- If you feel a panic attack is imminent, practice slow, diaphragmatic breathing
- Reassure yourself that the feelings you are having in your body are not dangerous and will soon disappear
- Avoid caffeine and other stimulants
- Eat a nutritious diet to help you maintain steady blood-sugar levels

OBSESSIVE–COMPULSIVE DISORDER

In obsessive–compulsive disorder (OCD), unwanted thoughts repeatedly enter the mind. People may experience anxieties about safety, hygiene, or security of possessions. The unwanted thoughts are often accompanied by anxiety and irresistible urges to carry out compulsive actions over and over again. Treatment may involve psychotherapy techniques and adopting ways of relieving anxiety, including breathing retraining and controlling blood-sugar levels.

WHAT ARE THE SYMPTOMS?

The most common symptoms of obsessive–compulsive disorder are:

- Intrusive and irrational mental images
- Repeated attempts to resist irrational or unwanted thoughts
- Repetitive behavior that cannot be resisted

WHY MIGHT I HAVE THIS?

PREDISPOSING FACTORS

- Genetics
- A personality that is perfectionistic or inflexible
- Stress
- Blood-sugar imbalance
- Impaired adrenal function

TREATMENT PLAN

PRIMARY TREATMENTS

- Exposure, ritual prevention, and other cognitive behavioral techniques

BACKUP TREATMENTS

- Antidepressants (in some cases)
- Exercise
- Breathing retraining
- Keeping a diary

WORTH CONSIDERING

- Homeopathy
- Nutritional therapy

For an explanation of how treatments are rated, see p.111.

WHY DOES IT OCCUR?

People with OCD are obsessed with something in their lives. The obsession returns like repetitive bouts of mental hiccups while a thought, urge, or fear keeps them in its grasp. Their attempts to banish an obsession turn into ritual compulsions.

The likelihood of developing obsessive–compulsive disorder sometimes runs in families. The disorder is often associated with depressive illness although it is possible to have an obsessive–compulsive personality, which is characterized by inflexibility and continually striving for perfection. People with this type of personality are at an increased risk of developing the disorder.

Examples of common compulsive actions are hand washing, checking that windows and doors are locked, making sure that keys are safely in their place, and arranging items on a desk in a precise manner. The same action is performed over and over again — sometimes hundreds of times a day — because each time it brings only a temporary sense of relief from anxiety. The disorder can interfere with normal life, which may cause a great deal of distress.

IMPORTANT

OCD is not a condition that is suitable for self-diagnosis and self-treatment. Consult your doctor if you think you have the symptoms of OCD. As with all personality and mental health problems, expert advice and supervision is essential in treating OCD.

TREATMENTS IN DETAIL

Conventional Medicine

Your doctor should be able to diagnose OCD from a description of your symptoms. He or she will recommend psychological treatments, such as "ritual prevention," in which the individual must resist performing a compulsive action (*see Psychological Therapies, p.421*).

PRIMARY TREATMENT **ANTIDEPRESSANTS** Although psychological therapy is the main treatment for OCD, certain types of antidepressant drugs may help some people. Drugs include clomipramine and selective serotonin reuptake inhibitors (SSRIs), including fluoxetine.

CAUTION

Antidepressant drugs may cause side effects; ask your doctor to explain these to you.

Nutritional Therapy

Nutritional strategies have not been shown to help OCD, but since the condition usually involves an underlying anxiety, they are worth considering as part of an overall self-help program.

RELIEVING ANXIETY Anxiety (*see p.414*) is a prominent feature in some individuals with OCD and one nutritional factor that commonly occurs in conjunction with anxiety is blood sugar imbalance. When blood sugar levels fall, the body generally attempts to correct this by secreting the hormone epinephrine, which stimulates the release of sugar from the liver. Epinephrine is one hormone in the body that is well known to provoke feelings of anxiety and panic. Clinical experience suggests that even nondiabetics can be prone to anxiety at times when blood sugar levels are lower than ideal. (*For more on blood sugar balance, see p.42.*)

IMPAIRED ADRENAL FUNCTION In practice, individuals who are prone to OCD or anxiety may have weakened adrenal glands. This seems to be especially true for individuals who feel weak or anxious if a meal is skipped. (*For more on impaired adrenal function, see p.44.*)

AVOID CAFFEINE Caffeine is a stimulant, and can provoke symptoms of anxiety and nervousness. People suffering from anxiety seem to be sensitive to the amount of caffeine found in just one cup of coffee. Individuals prone to OCD or anxiety should avoid caffeine.

MAGNESIUM SUPPLEMENTS Studies show that magnesium deficiency can enhance the way some people react to stress and that emotional stress, such as anxiety, can increase the need for magnesium. Magnesium supplementation may be valuable for people prone to anxiety. Taking 200mg of magnesium supplements twice daily may help people with OCD reduce their anxiety.

> **CAUTION**
>
> Consult your doctor before taking magnesium with ciproflaxin, warfarin or spironolactone (*see p.46*).

EICOSAPENTAENOIC ACID (EPA) has also been shown to help, as demonstrated in a placebo-controlled crossover trial.

Homeopathy

Although there is no research on the homeopathic treatment of OCD, some practitioners report that homeopathy has helped their patients. Treatment requires a trained and experienced practitioner (*see p.73*). Among the medicines that may help are *Thuja occidentalis, Aurum metallicum, Anacardium,* and *Silicea.*

OBSESSIONS AND COMPULSIONS

People with OCD become obsessed with something that takes over their lives. They attempt to deal with these obsessions by endlessly repeating a ritual action known as a compulsion. The table below lists some of the more common obsessions and some of the particular compulsive actions that may be expressed in OCD.

ANXIETY	ACTIONS
Germs and cleanliness	• Repeatedly washing and scrubbing hands, sometimes until the skin is raw and bleeding
Security and safety	• Repeatedly checking that doors and windows are locked • Repeatedly checking that keys are put in the "safe place" • Repeatedly checking that the oven/iron has been turned off
Preoccupation with exactness, or perfect order	• Rearranging objects, e.g. lining shoes up, straightening pictures • Counting or sorting objects
Religious anxieties	• Overly time-consuming mental rituals and prayers • Repeating "good" thoughts in order to counteract "bad" thoughts
Concerns about harm to self or others	• Repeatedly checking that self or others are all right
Running out of things	• Buying more than necessary, shopping in a ritualistic pattern
Concerns about diseases, e.g. cancer	• Repeated self-examinations, e.g. blood pressure

THUJA OCCIDENTALIS is perhaps the most commonly indicated homeopathic medicine for both obsessive and intrusive thoughts. The patients who respond to it may be fixated by diseases, such as cancer, and feel the need to follow rituals in order to avoid them. They may have strange feelings about their body — for instance, that there is an animal moving around inside their abdomen, or that they are very fragile. The skin on their face may be greasy and they may have multiple warts and other skin blemishes. The problems sometimes seem to have been triggered by immunizations or other long-term medical treatment.

AURUM METALLICUM is often the medicine of choice when the patient is very depressed and obsessed with thoughts of death or suicide. Frequently, the problem is worse in winter and at night. The patient may become very angry over minor things. The compulsive behavior may be associated with sinusitis or palpitations.

SILICEA People who respond to *Silicea* (also called *Silica*) may be obsessed with counting or sorting small objects. These patients tend to be shy and experience fatigue. They may feel the cold, but they have cold, clammy hands and feet, as well as weak nails and hair.

ANACARDIUM Patients who respond to *Anacardium* have a curious sensation that their mind and body are separated, or that they are being controlled by an external force. They may also suffer from bouts of violent anger, gaps in their memory, and sometimes skin problems, especially hives.

Exercise

Both physical exercise and breathing exercises (*see Breathing Retraining, right*) can be very useful in managing OCD, but they should be incorporated into a general program of treatment; cognitive behavior modification (*see Psychological Therapies, right*) as well as medication must not be overlooked as treatment options when dealing with OCD.

Canadian researchers report that regular exercise may help many people who suffer from psychiatric disorders, including pho bias (*see p.411*) and OCD. A review of all major studies of anxiety disorders and exercise, dating back to 1981, reported that strength training, running, walking, and other forms of aerobic exercise can help alleviate mild to moderate depression (*see p.436*), and may also help relieve other mental disorders, including anxiety, OCD, and substance abuse.

Some experts are concerned that a devotion to regular exercise may itself represent a form of obsessive–compulsive behavior. However, several research studies refute this belief. One evaluated the personalities of more than 200 men and women, recruited from health and fitness clubs. Results of the study showed that, contrary to expectations, excessive exercisers were not more likely to have low self-esteem or obsessive-compulsive tendencies than their moderately exercising counterparts. Accordingly, regular exercise is not an indication of having OCD.

To support this, a different Canadian study that involved 55 aerobics class regulars concluded that people who regularly attend aerobic classes are not more likely to have OCD.

Breathing Retraining

Since OCD is classified as an anxiety disorder, and since evidence for the anxiety-relieving influence of breathing retraining is overwhelming, breathing exercises (*see p.62*) are a useful strategy and should be part of the treatment program for OCD.

Psychological Therapies

One of the most important steps in helping people with OCD is to have them recognize that there are effective ways to treat their condition. This is when family members can be most useful — they need to learn as much as possible about the causes and treatment of OCD and keep informed of developments.

When people with OCD continue to deny that they have a problem or persistently refuse treatment, there is little that can be done for them. However, once the person accepts that he or she has OCD, there is a good chance that the disorder can be brought under control and managed effectively.

Family members can also join therapy sessions to help them understand the ritual behaviors and to introduce them to step-by-step ways of gradually (not abruptly) disentangling normal family life from the OCD rituals.

It is important to avoid making negative comments. In order to bring about positive outcomes with treatment, calm support and encouragement are needed. Joining a support group provides an opportunity for family members to share experiences and concerns, to learn new ways of coping, and to help them lead their own lives.

PRIMARY TREATMENT **COGNITIVE BEHAVIORAL THERAPY (CBT)** By far the most common form of treatment for OCD comes from cognitive behavior therapy (CBT) techniques, which combine behavioral therapy, such as exposure and ritual prevention, with cognitive therapy.

Exposure often helps the patient cope with the anxiety and the obsession, while ritual prevention works on reducing the compulsive behaviors.

Exposure and ritual (or response) prevention consists of gradually exposing the patient to the thing or the event that they find distressing, and asking the patient to avoid responding with the ritual that they normally use to alleviate the anxiety.

For example, some people who have obsessive–compulsive disorder may respond to anxious thoughts about having germs on their skin by washing their hands over and over again. In this case, the patient would be asked to think deliberately about the germs and then to refrain from hand washing. While this is likely to be distressing in the beginning, the distress usually subsides and eventually the patient is able to have the thought without feeling a compulsive need to wash their hands.

KEEPING A DIARY is another important aspect of treating OCD, especially if combined with CBT. Patients may be asked to keep a diary between therapy sessions, recording their thoughts and how they were triggered. They may also be asked to note how they responded to the thoughts as a way of alleviating the anxiety. This diary would then be used in the following therapy session to plan the next stage of the treatment.

A typical diary entry might have the following headings: time; thought; trigger (what initiated the thought?); response (what were your actions?); duration (how long did your response last?); and feelings.

For example, someone who is obsessed with cleanliness might have the following diary entry:

- Time: 8:30 A.M.
- Thought: The table is dirty.
- Trigger: Crumbs on the breakfast table.
- Response: Repeatedly scrubbed the table.
- Duration: How long did the response last? 20 mins
- Feelings: Initially relief, then anxiety and anger because I was late for work.

Regular entries in a diary may help you recognize patterns of behavior and identify the ways in which you can make changes. For example, if each bout of compulsive behavior lasts an average of 30 minutes, you could aim to gradually reduce this time until the behavior is under control.

> ## Up to one half of adults with OCD say that their disorder began during childhood

POST-TRAUMATIC STRESS DISORDER

Post-traumatic stress disorder (PTSD) occurs as a persistent reaction to a traumatic and highly stressful experience. Sometimes, the reaction is delayed. The kinds of event that cause PTSD include natural disasters, serious accidents, and physical assault. Treatment may involve counseling, psychological therapy, homeopathy, and measures such as breathing retraining and massage which help relieve anxiety.

WHY DOES IT OCCUR?

Witnessing or being involved in a stressful event, such as a traffic accident, mugging, or an earthquake, can trigger intense emotions. Sometimes, symptoms last for years. Children and elderly people are at higher risk of developing PTSD, as are people with anxiety disorders (*see p.414*) and those who lack support.

People with PTSD may feel emotionally numb, detached from life, and distanced from family and friends. However, they may also experience great anxiety in response to reminders of the traumatic experience and they may become depressed. Sometimes, the disorder can lead to drug or alcohol abuse. People who have had PTSD once are more likely to experience it again if faced with another traumatic event.

TREATMENTS IN DETAIL

Conventional Medicine

PRIMARY TREATMENT Through discussion, a doctor can diagnose PTSD and determine the severity of symptoms. The main part of treatment is likely to be psychological (*see Psychological therapies, p.423*).

> **IMPORTANT**
>
> PTSD is not a condition that is suitable for self-diagnosis and self-treatment. Consult your doctor as soon as you suspect you have the symptoms of PTSD. If the symptoms are disabling, don't hesitate to seek urgent medical advice.

Certain antidepressants, such as selective serotonin reuptake inhibitors (SSRIs), may be recommended in some cases.

> **CAUTION**
>
> Drugs for PTSD have side effects; ask your doctor to explain these to you.

Nutritional Therapy

Nutritional treatment of PTSD is similar to treatment for other ailments where anxiety is a significant factor. See also anxiety (*p.414*), depression (*p.436*), phobias (*p.411*), and coping with stress (*p.408*). (*For more on adrenal imbalance, see p.44.*) PTSD may also be associated with reductions in immune function and can be treated accordingly (*see p.45*).

AVOID CAFFEINE Caffeine is a stimulant that can provoke symptoms of anxiety and nervousness. If you are suffering from PTSD, you should stay away from caffeinated substances such as tea, coffee, certain carbonated drinks such as colas, and chocolate.

SUPPLEMENTS Studies show that magnesium deficiency can exacerbate stress reactions and that emotional stress can increase the need for magnesium. In practice, magnesium supplementation seems to be valuable for individuals who are persistently anxious. Taking 200mg of magnesium twice daily can help.

A healthy nutritional status is important for those who suffer from anxiety and stress. If you have PTSD, take a multivitamin and mineral supplement each day; in one study, doing this for 28 days was associated with a consistent and significant reduction in anxiety and perceived stress.

> **CAUTION**
>
> Consult your doctor before taking magnesium with ciprofloxacin, warfarin, or with spironolactone (*see p.46*).

Homeopathy

There are a number of reports that homeopathic medicines help people with PTSD, particularly children in foster care who have suffered physical or sexual abuse and adult survivors of childhood sexual abuse. Medicines used include *Stramonium*, *Platina*, *Ignatia*, *Staphysagria*, *Causticum*, and *Opium*. You should consult an experienced homeopath who can make a constitutional diagnosis (*see p.73*).

STRAMONIUM is an important medicine for some of the most distressing symptoms of PTSD, such as night terrors, startle responses, and intrusive thoughts or flashbacks to traumatic events. The person may have fears of the dark, water, or other things related to the original trauma, as well as fits of destructive rage.

IGNATIA People who respond to *Ignatia* may appear hysterical. They are hypersensitive, both emotionally and physically. It is said to be a medicine of paradoxes — for instance, there is often a sensation of a lump in the throat, making swallowing difficult, yet liquids can be harder to swallow than solids.

STAPHYSAGRIA The "keynote" of *Staphysagria* is "suppressed indignation." It is suitable for people who may have suffered a sexual assault or abusive relationship as an adult and are tremendously angry about what has been done to them. This may be bottled up and expressed through physical symptoms, particularly recurrent sterile cystitis or urethral syndrome. Sometimes, the anger is expressed, making these people prickly and difficult to deal with.

CAUSTICUM complements *Staphysagria* because it is often appropriate for use after *Staphysagria*. A typical feature of people who respond to *Causticum* is their strong sense of justice and feelings of empathy with those who have been unjustly treated.

OPIUM When physical injury is involved — for instance, PTSD triggered by a traffic accident or war experience — homeopathic *Opium* may be indicated as a medicine. A typical feature of people who respond to *Opium* is that they may feel "spaced out" or withdrawn, becoming either very timid or else reckless by losing their sense of danger. They may also abuse alcohol or other drugs.

> **CAUTION**
>
> Some homeopathic medicines, including *Ignatia*, are antidoted (rendered ineffective) by coffee.

Breathing Retraining

PTSD involves a great deal of anxiety, which responds favorably to strategies for breathing retraining (*see p.62*).

Many experts believe that the quality of an individual's sleep is extremely important in the PTSD process, and that sleep disruption, whatever its cause, has important influences on the trauma recovery process for many people.

Disturbed sleep is often associated with sleep-disordered breathing (SDB), which may involve sleep apnea (brief periods when breathing stops), snoring, and a tendency to have nightmares. Feeling sleepy during the day is a consequence and exaggerates PTSD symptoms.

Treating the breathing component of SDB might help sleep quality and thereby the PTSD symptoms. To find out if this is true, one research study evaluated the benefits of using a CPAP (continuous positive airway pressure) breathing mask that delivers oxygen and helps maintain normal airflow during sleep. The results were remarkable, not just in terms of better sleep, daytime well-being, and reduced nightmares, but also in relation to all the PTSD symptoms.

Other research has found similar benefits — when a person's breathing improves, his or her sleep improves and so, usually, do the PTSD symptoms.

Massage Therapy

Researchers evaluated the benefits of massage therapy for children affected by a major hurricane who had severe symptoms of PTSD, such as anxiety, depression, and behavioral outbursts. A group of 60 children were divided into two groups, one of which received massage (30 minutes of back massage administered twice weekly for a month). The other group spent the same amount of time watching nonstimulating video cartoons — the children sat quietly with psychology graduate students, who maintained physical contact either by placing the child in his or her lap or holding an arm around the child.

After one month of treatment, children who had received massage showed significant differences compared to the other group. Their anxiety and depression had improved, their stress hormone (cortisol) levels were lower, and they were better able to relax. The researchers in the study noted that parents, if trained, could continue the massage therapy.

Psychological Therapies

PRIMARY TREATMENT The talking therapies used to treat PTSD include cognitive behavioral therapy (CBT) techniques, such as systematic desensitization, exposure therapy, anxiety management, and stress inoculation. Eye movement desensitization and reprocessing (EMDR) as well as psychodynamic approaches are used.

EXPOSURE TECHNIQUES In a review of treatments for PTSD, three studies of exposure therapy showed mixed results.

> Survivors of a trauma who blame themselves may be more at risk of severe or long-term PTSD

STRESS INOCULATION TRAINING

People with PTSD can benefit from stress inoculation training. It not only helps them cope with the aftermath of their particular trauma but also inoculates them against future stressors. The technique follows three stages: understanding the stress that is affecting them; learning and practicing the skills needed to cope with the particular stressful event; and applying the coping skills to future situations. SIT can take up to 12 months to be effective and may need booster sessions or numerous follow-ups.

PHASE 1	PHASE 2	PHASE 3
Understanding your stress Discussions with a therapist will cover: • The nature and impact of the stress • Education about stress • How you may be exacerbating the stress • How to view perceived threats as problems to be solved	**Learning and rehearsing coping skills** The therapist will show you skills such as: • Relaxation techniques • Role play • Mental rehearsal of stressful situations and positive ways of dealing with them • Learning how to stop negative thoughts • Problem solving	**Application and follow-through** The therapist will set short, intermediate and long-term goals that will involve: • Applying the coping skills in a series of increasingly stressful situations • Relapse prevention procedures (identifying high-risk situations, the warning signs, and learning ways to cope with lapses)

Another study found that, after having exposure therapy, patients reported a significant reduction in the frequency of PTSD symptoms they experienced. *(For a description of the techniques used, see Phobias, p.411).*

STRESS INOCULATION TRAINING (SIT) consists of helping patients respond in different ways to traumatic and stressful situations (*see box, above*). SIT combines role play, relaxation techniques, modeling (when the therapist literally shows the patient different ways of responding), and some techniques used in changing thought patterns. SIT therapy has been effective in reducing PTSD symptoms, such as anxiety and intrusive thoughts, in rape victims. Compared to exposure therapy, SIT appears to be the most promising technique.

ANXIETY MANAGEMENT uses techniques, such as relaxation training (*see p.99*), biofeedback, and stress management, which provide significant benefit to people with PTSD.

SYSTEMATIC DESENSITIZATION (SD) is a cognitive technique that uses relaxation to help patients gradually and systematically desensitize their trauma under controlled conditions. The use of SD as a treatment for SD has been studied by a number of researchers and there is some evidence that it is effective.

Other studies showed that SD may be used in the treatment of victims of rape. Although the research is promising, there are a number of problems with the design of these studies and the results are therefore far from conclusive.

PRIMARY TREATMENT **EYE MOVEMENT DENSENSITIZATION AND REPROCESSING** is a relatively new therapy that was designed specifically for the treatment of PTSD. It is beginning to accrue an evidence base suggesting it may be a rapidly effective treatment for people with PTSD.

According to the theory, rapid eye movements (which are known to occur when dreaming) take place when the brain moves information in short-term memory to long-term memory. The former type of memory tends to be emotional, whereas the latter is not.

In EMDR, the person treated thinks about the trauma's most important features while the therapist moves his fingers in front of the person's eyes, producing rapid eye movements. This reawakens the memory and it may cause a minor reaction, which the experienced practitioner must carefully control.

According to the theory, however, EDMR helps move the traumatic memories into long-term storage, defusing their emotional charge. Emerging research suggests that patients who receive a few sessions of EDMR are able to recall their trauma without the feelings of terror experienced previously.

PSYCHODYNAMIC METHODS are widely used for the treatment of PTSD. One of the problems of treating this condition is that it is sometimes unclear how much the traumatic incident itself has created the problems and how much symptoms are due to earlier difficulties which the traumatic incident has exacerbated. It seems likely that the people most likely to develop PTSD are those who have been previously traumatized or who have an anxious personality.

Psychodynamic methods help people distinguish between the two. The therapist listens to the person's account of his or her experiences and explores the connections between what the person is thinking, doing, and feeling in his or her present life compared with past experiences.

Evidence is promising but limited and the research has had some criticisms. However, psychodynamic methods have been found to be just as effective as hypnotherapy and systematic desensitization.

SCHIZOPHRENIA

Schizophrenia is a severe mental illness that impairs the person's sense of reality, leading to irrational behavior and disturbed emotional reactions. Contrary to popular belief, it does not mean that people have split personalities. People with schizophrenia may hear voices, which contributes to their bizarre behavior. They often have problems maintaining relationships with other people and holding down jobs. Treatment with antipsychotic drugs aims to control symptoms. Supplements, exercise, and massage may also be used.

WHAT ARE THE SYMPTOMS?

- Hearing voices that do not exist
- Having irrational thoughts or beliefs, usually of being controlled by other people
- Belief that trivial events are of great significance
- Expressing inappropriate emotions, such as laughing at bad news
- Rambling speech
- Difficulty concentrating
- Agitation and restlessness
- In some cases, the condition develops gradually, with apathy, poor motivation, and withdrawal as predominant features

WHY MIGHT I HAVE THIS?

PREDISPOSING FACTORS

- Genetic factors
- Substance abuse
- Omega-3 fatty acid deficiency
- Folic acid deficiency
- Abnormal levels of histamine

TRIGGERS

- Stressful life event

IMPORTANT

Because of their irrational thoughts and delusions, schizophrenics may behave in ways that are dangerous to themselves or others. In this situation, they should be seen urgently by a psychiatrist or other appropriately trained professional.

WHY DOES IT OCCUR?

Schizophrenia is a brain disorder that is often mistakenly described as a split personality. It can develop at any age, but most commonly develops in the late teens and early twenties. The onset in women may be later than in men. At first, there may be signs of confused, shocking, or irrational behavior, involving a loss of sense of reality and an inability to function socially, either at work or in relationships with family and friends. This sense of social isolation may occur with a number of other symptoms (*see left*), involving disturbed emotional reactions, hallucinations, delusions, and unusual speech patterns.

No single cause of schizophrenia has been identified, but genetic factors are implicated (*see chart, p.426*) and certain neurotransmitters in the brain, such as dopamine and serotonin, may also be involved. A stressful life event, such as a bereavement or serious illness, can trigger the disorder in a person who is susceptible. Substance abuse may also be a factor in the development of schizophrenia.

The condition affects approximately one in 100 people worldwide and may begin gradually or come on suddenly. Some people have episodes of illness with periods of complete recovery in between, while in others the disorder is continuous. Left to themselves without treatment, people with schizophrenia are prone to self-neglect or even self-harm, and about 10 percent commit suicide. Rarely, there may be violence toward others.

BRAIN ABNORMALITIES Advances in brain imaging techniques have revealed that schizophrenia may, in part, be a result of the development of the brain. Some of those with schizophrenia have enlarged ventricles (fluid-filled cavities) deep within the brain — but this feature is not exclusive to the disease. Research also suggests that inappropriate nerve connections in the brain, made while the fetus was developing, could cause abnormalities during puberty and adolescence.

In 2004, researchers reported that there were distinct abnormalities in the auditory cortex (the area of the brain that decodes impulses from the inner ears and thereby governs hearing) in those with schizophrenia. These anatomical findings may lead to an accurate diagnostic test that will help pinpoint the condition.

TREATMENT PLAN

PRIMARY TREATMENTS

- Emotional and practical support
- Antipsychotic and other drugs
- Cognitive behavioral therapy in some cases and psychosocial treatment

BACKUP TREATMENTS

- Nutritional therapy

WORTH CONSIDERING

- Homeopathy
- Exercise
- Massage
- Mind-body therapies

For an explanation of how treatments are rated, see p.111.

RISKS OF DEVELOPING SCHIZOPHRENIA

Schizophrenia is a disease with a strong family link as the chart below shows. If you have an identical twin with schizophrenia, you stand an almost 50 percent chance of developing the disease yourself. This risk drops as the degree of relationship decreases. A person's susceptibility to schizophrenia is closely linked with a range of genes, so susceptibility can be passed through family lines. However, family dynamics can also strongly influence the development of psychological problems.

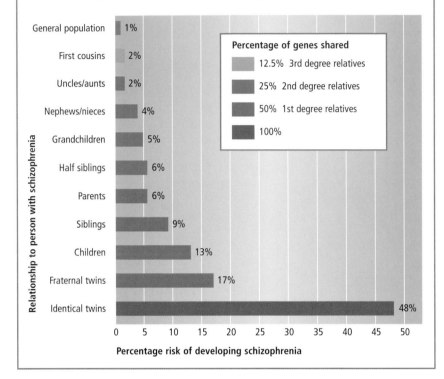

Percentage of genes shared
- 12.5% 3rd degree relatives
- 25% 2nd degree relatives
- 50% 1st degree relatives
- 100%

Relationship to person with schizophrenia:
- General population — 1%
- First cousins — 2%
- Uncles/aunts — 2%
- Nephews/nieces — 4%
- Grandchildren — 5%
- Half siblings — 6%
- Parents — 6%
- Siblings — 9%
- Children — 13%
- Fraternal twins — 17%
- Identical twins — 48%

Percentage risk of developing schizophrenia (0 5 10 15 20 25 30 35 40 45 50)

If you have schizophrenia, the following may prove useful once you have discovered the particular treatment that suits you:
- Discuss your condition with your family, friends, employer, and colleagues. Try to establish a good balance of support — you don't want to feel smothered by their attention, but if people are too remote, you may feel isolated.
- Don't put yourself under too much pressure or stress by trying to do too many things. On the other hand, avoid boring and meaningless activities — try to do things that suit you and your temperament.
- Identify situations that make you feel stressed and ask your friends and family to help you establish ways of dealing with them.
- Join a self-help group that can provide you and your family with support.

Conventional Medicine

The doctor will be able to make a full assessment by talking to the patient as well as to a close relative or friend, if possible. Hospital admission is usually a necessary precaution when drug treatments are initially prescribed.

PRIMARY TREATMENT **EMOTIONAL AND PRACTICAL SUPPORT** play an important role in long-term care for a person who has schizophrenia. There is a range of services available, from helplines, self-help groups, and residential care, as well as organizations that can offer practical help with both employment issues and financial benefits (*see p.486*). Such services also assist the families of people with the disease, who often find they require amounts of support and help.

PRIMARY TREATMENT **ANTIPSYCHOTICS** are the main drugs used to treat schizophrenia. They block the action of the neurotransmitter dopamine. Control of symptoms may take up to three months.

Antipsychotic drugs include phenothiazines, such as chlorpromazine; butyrophenones, such as haloperidol; and thioxanthines, such as thiothixene. If individuals have problems remembering to take their medication, they can receive haloperidol or fluphenazine in the form of intramuscular injections every 1–5 weeks. In some cases, drugs are combined with cognitive behavioral therapy (*see Psychological Therapies, p.427*), which may help with delusions.

> **CAUTION**
>
> Antipsychotic drugs for treating schizophrenia have a range of side effects; ask your doctor to explain these to you.

Nutritional Therapy

OMEGA-3 FATTY ACIDS, known as eicosapentaenoic acid (EPA) and docosahexaenoic acid (DHA), have been shown to be deficient in schizophrenic patients. These omega 3-fatty acids (*see p.34*) can be found in oily fish, such as mackerel, salmon, and sardines.

One study showed that the lower the levels of these fatty acids are in the body, the more severe the symptoms of schizophrenia tend to be. Studies suggest that people with schizophrenia who take EPA supplements alone or in combination with normal medication show improvement in their symptoms. Taking 1 or 2g of EPA supplements per day may be useful (in combination with normal medication) in the treatment of schizophrenia.

FOLIC ACID (FOLATE) Studies suggest that folic acid deficiency is also common in those with the disease. Good sources of folic acid are leafy green vegetables, organ meats, whole grains, fortified bread, and nuts. One study showed that giving supplements to folate-deficient schizophrenics (in addition to standard treatment) brought significant improvements in their condition and their ability to function normally. Moreover, the folic acid supplement appeared to increase the effectiveness of standard pharmaceutical drugs given for schizophrenia. Taking 400–800mcg of folic acid per day is recommended.

VITAMIN C Studies have shown that many people with schizophrenia excrete vitamin C more quickly than others. As a result, those with the disease may benefit from taking 1g of vitamin C per day.

HISTAMINE Evidence suggests that a relationship exists between histamine and schizophrenia, so asking a nutritionist for a blood test to assess "histamine type" and then appropriate supplementation is of value. About half of patients have low levels of histamine in their blood. They are often helped with supplements containing vitamin B_3, folic acid, vitamin B_{12}, zinc, and manganese, that can help increase histamine levels.

Paradoxically, about 20 percent of people with schizophrenia seem to have high levels of histamine in their bodies. Nutrients that may help decrease histamine levels include vitamin C, calcium, and the amino acid methionine.

> **CAUTION**
>
> Consult your doctor before taking vitamin C with antibiotics or warfarin, or omega-3 fatty acids/fish oils with warfarin, or folic acid with anticonvulsants or methotrexate (see p.46).

Homeopathy

Schizophrenia is a serious condition, so support from trained professionals, such as psychiatrists, nurses, and psychiatric social workers, is required. There is no published research on the homeopathic treatment of schizophrenia, and certainly homeopathic medicines should not be used alone. But some homeopaths report being able to help people with long-term problems related to schizophrenia.

Exercise

Studies have shown that people with schizophrenia have increased rates of gastrointestinal, respiratory, and cardiovascular disease. This is likely to be due to high rates of smoking and obesity, accompanied by a poor diet, lack of exercise, and the side effects of medication.

If it is possible to achieve higher levels of physical activity, along with a better diet and improved lifestyle habits, general health should improve as well. Since increased exercise alone has been shown to be helpful in a variety of mental illnesses, such as depression (see p.436), it is possible that people with schizophrenia will also benefit.

Treatment allows about one in five people with schizophrenia to make a full recovery

Massage

A German study has found that massage may be useful in the treatment of chronic schizophrenia. Ten people with chronic schizophrenia were given massage to their feet, back, and neck, in an attempt to increase awareness of their own body limits. Some people with schizophrenia lose the awareness of where their body begins and ends — so that being touched not only helps them reconnect with their body but is also calming.

Massage therapy was clearly relaxing, as recorded by physiological measurements of skin conductance (the skin's capacity to conduct an electric current) and slower heart rate. The patients reported they felt more relaxed, too. Although the number of patients who participated in the study was too small to draw any firm conclusions, the results do indicate that massage and other forms of body therapy should be considered as a method for helping schizophrenic patients.

This German study supports Swiss ideas that have been put forward for a more holistic approach to treating schizophrenia. The approach incorporates different forms of bodywork and movement therapies as part of the overall care of the individual.

Mind-Body Therapies

Mind-body therapies, such as yoga, relaxation, and guided imagery (see p.99), may have a role in reducing the stress associated with schizophrenia. Expressive therapies, such as art, music, dance, and drama, have been widely used in psychiatric settings. They can help release suppressed emotions and stimulate the flow of endorphins, improving mood.

Psychological Therapies

PRIMARY TREATMENT **COGNITIVE BEHAVIORAL THERAPY (CBT)** Although talking therapies are not recommended as the main treatment for complex mental health problems such as schizophrenia, cognitive behavioral therapy, which helps people change their patterns of belief and behavior, may be useful in reducing delusions.

PRIMARY TREATMENT **PSYCHOSOCIAL TREATMENTS** Once antipsychotic drugs (see Conventional Medicine, p.426) have reduced or relieved their psychotic symptoms, people with schizophrenia will need help fitting in with the world at large. They need to develop their communication skills, build self-confidence, discover internal motivations, and establish relationships with other people. In addition, because their illness has probably developed during the crucial years of their education and training, they may have been prevented from following a particular career path.

Various forms of psychosocial therapy can help improve social functioning. Such treatments may take place at home, in the workplace, in the community, or at a medical facility. They include rehabilitation (which helps with everyday skills, such as money management), as well as vocational training and psychotherapy, which involves regular appointments with a mental health professional. He or she can help people with schizophrenia learn about themselves and how best to deal with day-to-day problems as they arise.

OTHER PSYCHOLOGICAL THERAPIES are available both for people with schizophrenia and for their caregivers. These include counseling, family intervention, and group therapy. Doctors can advise on the suitability of each depending on individual needs.

SUBSTANCE DEPENDENCY

Addiction is the excessive and compulsive use of a substance, such as alcohol or heroin, which may take priority over all other things in a person's life. Addiction is distinguished from abuse by a craving for the substance and withdrawal symptoms when the substance is unavailable. Dependence on alcohol and drugs is more common in men. Treatment varies according to the substance involved, but in each case the addict needs support, counseling, and, commonly, the short-term use of medication to help with withdrawal.

WHAT ARE THE SYMPTOMS?

Alcohol dependence

- A compulsion to drink; lack of control over amount consumed; drinking in the morning; blackouts
- Increased tolerance to the effects of alcohol; larger amounts needed to achieve desired effects

As dependence increases:

- Night sweats; vomiting in the morning
- Withdrawal symptoms, including tremors, nausea, and sweating, sometimes only a few hours after the last drink
- A severe withdrawal state, delirium tremens, can develop up to three days after the last drink. Addict has severe tremors, agitation, sweating, and hallucinations. Requires urgent hospital treatment.

Recreational drug dependence

- Mood changes
- Changes in energy levels
- Changes in ability to concentrate
- Faster or slower speech
- Increased or decreased appetite
- Withdrawal symptoms may include: anxiety and restlessness; sweating that alternates with chills; confusion; muscle aches and abdominal cramps; vomiting; diarrhea; seizures

Nicotine dependence

- Cravings
- Irritability, mood swings, anxiety

WHY MIGHT I HAVE THESE?

PREDISPOSING FACTORS

- Genetic predisposition
- Culture of drinking or drug taking
- Psychological problems

TRIGGERS

- Blood-sugar imbalance
- Nutrient deficiencies
- Prostaglandin (PGE$_1$) deficiency

WHY DO THEY OCCUR?

The causes of addiction are complex and depend on the substance involved. For example, alcohol addiction may run in families, as a result of genetics and/or cultural influences. It can also develop in response to anxiety (see p.414), low self-esteem, or depression (see p.436). Social drinking and stress (see p.408) may increase the risk of dependence.

Similar factors cause addition to drugs, whether the drug is taken for recreational or medical reasons. Sleeping pills to cure insomnia (see p.448) and addictive antide-pressants can affect brain chemistry. Prolonged use will influence behavior, making it difficult to choose not to take the drug. As with alcohol addiction, drug abuse is often chronic, with periods of abstinence followed by periods of relapse.

ALCOHOL DEPENDENCE Alcohol has a direct effect on the body and may cause a number of diseases when used in excess. The symptoms begin with a compulsion and can gradually worsen through to del-rium tremens (see Symptoms, left) when alcohol is withdrawn. Long-term dependence on alcohol is the most common cause of severe liver disease and may also damage the digestive system, causing peptic ulcers.

People who drink heavily tend to have poor diets and may be deficient in vitamins, in particular vitamin B$_1$. Deficiency of this vitamin can cause neuropathy (see p.127) and dementia (see p.133). Several psychiatric disorders are also related to alcohol addiction, including anxiety (see p.414), depression (see p.436), and suicidal behavior. Alcohol dependence is likely to lead to social problems, including relationship and work difficulties.

NICOTINE DEPENDENCE Smoking can be highly addictive because it releases nicotine into the bloodstream. Once in the body, nicotine affects the transmission of nervous impulses and sets up a pattern of dependency that is hard to break.

Toxic substances in tobacco smoke damage the mucous membranes that line the lungs, preventing the tiny hairs (cilia) from clearing mucus from the alveoli, bronchioles, and bronchi. Smokers commonly develop a distinctive cough and shortness

TREATMENT PLAN

PRIMARY TREATMENTS

- Advice and emotional support
- Drugs when appropriate
- Psychological therapies

BACKUP TREATMENTS

- Nutritional supplements

WORTH CONSIDERING

- Diet to balance blood sugar
- Homeopathy
- Acupuncture
- Breathing retraining and yoga
- Mind–body therapies
- Massage

For an explanation of how treatments are rated, see p.111.

of breath. Carcinogens in the smoke are likely to cause lung cancer in heavy smokers, while pipe and cigar smokers are prone to developing mouth cancer and cancer of the larynx.

Smoking can cause permanent damage to the heart and blood vessels, probably through the actions of nicotine and carbon monoxide. Smokers are at risk of developing atherosclerosis (narrowing of the arteries), coronary artery disease (*see p.252*), and stroke (*see p.148*).

Smoking may be implicated in a number of other problems, such as peptic ulcers and reduced fertility in both men and women, while pregnant women who smoke put their unborn babies at risk.

DRUG DEPENDENCE Many drugs can cause dependency in people who take them, and this is true of some prescription drugs as well as illegal and recreational drugs. For example, benzodiazepines (anti-anxiety and sleeping drugs) have strong addictive qualities; analgesics (painkillers) can also cause addiction.

The risk of dependence depends on the drug being used. For example, heroin may cause addiction after only a few doses. Once in the brain, it binds to the opioid receptors on certain nerves. At first, this process may cause a pleasurable sensation. However, increasingly large quantities of this addictive drug are often needed to produce the desired effect, and physical withdrawal symptoms may develop if the drug is stopped. In contrast, LSD does not create a physical addiction, but prolonged use may cause a psychological dependancy

The use of certain drugs, such as cocaine, amphetamines, and LSD, can induce a state of psychosis in which the person who takes them experiences hallucinations, feelings of persecution, and extreme excitement or lack of emotion.

In addition to mental problems, misuse of certain drugs may cause physical damage; for example, repeated snorting of cocaine can result in destruction of the nasal septum that separates the nostrils, and the use of ecstasy may cause kidney and liver failure. The sharing of needles by intravenous drug abusers carries a risk of hepatitis B and HIV infection (*see p.470*). Repeated needle injections can damage veins in the arm, often visible as bluish needle tracks.

IMMEDIATE RELIEF

When you have cravings, try:
- Massaging your ear or hands to stop the craving if you are a smoker.
- The homeopathic medicine *Nux vomica* to help reduce withdrawal symptoms, such as nausea and retching.
- Distracting yourself with exercise, chewing gum, reading, watching TV, etc.
- Calling a friend or a helpline (*see p.486*).

TREATMENTS IN DETAIL

Conventional Medicine

PRIMARY TREATMENT **ALCOHOL DEPENDENCE** Attempting to overcome alcohol addiction requires recognition of the problem, a great deal of support and understanding, and motivation to follow the program through. In addition to psychotherapy on an individual basis, support groups, such as Alcoholics Anonymous

(AA for address, see p.486), play an important role in treatment for many people. At AA, recovered alcoholics guide uncontrolled drinkers through a 12-step program in a bid to give up alcohol (*see Mind-Body Therapies, p.431*)

Your doctor may prescribe benzodiazepine drugs, such as diazepam, on a reducing schedule to help you cope with the symptoms of alcohol withdrawal. However, these drugs must be used only for a short period because they rapidly cause addiction.

Certain drugs are prescribed to prevent a return to drinking. These include acamprosate, which, when used in combination with counseling, may help maintain abstinence. The drug disulfiram may also be prescribed. It causes unpleasant symptoms, including vomiting, flushing of the face, palpitations, and severe headaches when combined with even a small amount of alcohol. The effects of drinking larger amounts of alcohol with the drug are serious and may include abnormal heart

rhythms and collapse. Therefore, it is important not to drink for some time before and after taking disufiram.

PRIMARY TREATMENT **DRUG DEPENDENCE** The treatment depends to an extent on the drug involved, but in all cases emotional support and advice on withdrawal will be beneficial. Specific treatment may be required for some individuals; for example, the drug methadone may be prescribed in a schedule of reducing doses to help those withdrawing from heroin.

CAUTION

Drugs aimed at preventing dependency may have side effects; ask your doctor to explain these to you.

PRIMARY TREATMENT **NICOTINE DEPENDENCE** Although it is very hard to stop smoking, it is never too late to quit. If you need help consult your doctor, who

About 20 percent of alcohol is absorbed by the stomach and 80 percent by the small intestine

may recommend one of the various aids that help prevent nicotine cravings. These include special nicotine-containing chewing gum or patches. You may also benefit from joining a support group or contacting a telephone helpline that is staffed by ex-smokers (*see p.486 for contact details*).

Nutritional Therapy

BALANCING BLOOD SUGAR Alcohol cravings can be associated with fluctuations in the level of sugar in the bloodstream. When blood-sugar levels drop, the body tends to crave foods that replenish sugar quickly, such as sweet foods or alcohol. Clinical experience and scientific research suggests that many individuals can successfully reduce their alcohol consumption by eating a wholesome diet, which balances their blood sugar (*see p.42*).

INCREASING NUTRIENT INTAKES Research demonstrates that alcoholics frequently lack key nutrients, especially the

B vitamins, zinc, and magnesium. Studies of alcoholics show that adding supplements to their diet leads to reduced alcohol consumption.

Increasing nutrient intake through eating a balanced diet is also associated with reduced alcohol craving and increased abstinence from alcohol. Individuals who want to reduce their alcohol consumption should try a balanced multivitamin and mineral, combined with a B-complex supplement which provides 25–50mg of vitamins B_1, B_2, B_3, B_5, and B_6 each day.

ESSENTIAL FATTY ACIDS Alcoholics may also be deficient in essential fatty acids (EFAs). One of the final breakdown products of EFAs is a hormonelike molecule, known as prostaglandin E_1 (PGE_1). This is thought to have mood-enhancing and antidepressant actions in the brain. Alcoholics are often deficient in both PGE_1 and gamma-linolenic acid (GLA), the molecule from which it is made.

Studies suggest that supplementing the diet with EFAs can help reduce alcohol intake and prevent symptoms of withdrawal. Taking 1g of evening primrose oil, which is rich in GLA, three times a day might help control alcohol consumption in the long term.

> **CAUTION**
>
> Consult your doctor before taking omega-3 fatty acids/fish oils with warfarin (see p.46).

GLUTAMINE The amino acid glutamine appears to help reduce alcohol cravings. In a 1957 study, nine out of ten alcoholics thought that glutamine, taken at a dose of 1g per day, reduced their desire for alcohol.

Homeopathy

Case series reports show that individualized homeopathic treatment may be helpful for alcoholism, reducing cravings and the frequency of relapses. If you are trying to overcome an addiction of any kind, visiting a homeopath for advice may help (see p.73).

NUX VOMICA In the treatment of hangover and alcohol withdrawal symptoms, the most commonly used medicine is *Nux vomica*. It is helpful for symptoms includ-

---

ACUPRESSURE FOR SMOKING CESSATION

Researchers from the Touch Research Institute at the University of Miami in the US have demonstrated that massaging particular areas of the hand can help relieve the stress and anxiety in smokers who crave the nicotine in tobacco. Benefits include reductions in both the intensity and the frequency of the nicotine craving. Regular practice of the sequence shown here has a soothing effect and may help smokers who are trying to quit. Try the sequence at the first sign of a craving.

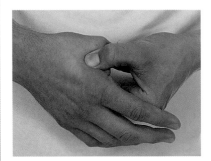

Place one thumb and forefinger at the junction of the other thumb and forefinger. Squeeze thumb and forefinger together for 30 seconds. Change hands and repeat.

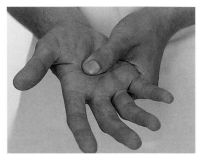

Hold one hand in the other hand, with the thumb on top. Press down with the thumb and rotate it around the palm for 30 seconds. Change hands and repeat.

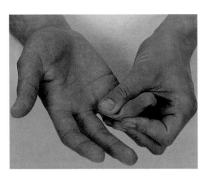

Use the thumb and fingers of one hand to massage, from base to tip, each of the fingers of the other hand (above). Massage each joint thoroughly. Change hands and repeat.

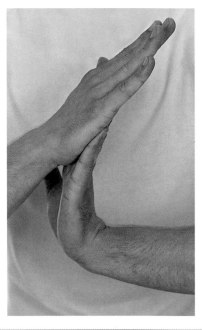

With the palm of one hand gently massage the fingers of the other hand by pushing them up and stretching them back. Do this five times. Change hands and repeat.

---

ing nausea, retching, headaches, muscular twitching, and cramps. Symptoms are usually associated with irritability, poor sleep, and early waking.

SULPHUR is usually prescribed on a constitutional basis (see p.73). It is said that *Sulphur* may decrease addictive tendencies. Indviduals who respond to this treatment are warm and do not feel the cold. They are untidy (sometimes to the point of being smelly), argumentative, and thirsty. They often have skin problems that may be very itchy.

STAPHYSAGRIA is another useful medicine. The main feature of patients who respond to this medicine is that they are angry and indignant about what they see as injustices done to them in the past.

PREVENTION Constitutional treatment, particularly with *Sulphur*, may decrease addictive tendencies.

Massage

Massage induces calm, eases anxiety, and generally reduces feelings of stress. There are many reports of how massage and other "antiarousal" methods help people break their addictions. However, research evidence is limited.

Stopping smoking can involve marked withdrawal symptoms, including intense cravings, anxiety, and depressed mood. Anecdotally, massage has been shown to reduce anxiety and to improve mood.

A simple self-massage of the hand (*see illustration, p.430*) during the period of cravings may reduce anxiety and withdrawal symptoms and may result in smoking fewer cigarettes per day.

Breathing Retraining and Yoga

Learning to breathe slowly (10 breaths per minute) and rhythmically can ease the feelings of anxiety related to addictions, such as alcohol dependency. Antianxiety exercises involving yoga-type breathing induce calm and reduce feelings of apprehension, anxiety, and panic (*see p.62*). A 2002 survey done by The Yoga Biomedical Trust showed that yoga therapy can benefit both people who are addicted to tobacco and those addicted to alcohol.

Acupuncture

Acupuncture can help people seeking to break their addiction to a drug, alcohol, or to smoking cigarettes. Many studies suggest ear acupuncture is useful, although a review of the current research concluded it is too early to make definitive recommendations as to its effectiveness.

Curiously, it does not seem to matter whether the acupuncturist uses specifically selected acupoints or "sham acupuncture" (the needles are placed in points not believed to cause any relief) — the benefits appear to be the same.

Acupuncture, whether real or sham, has often been shown, particularly in smoking trials, to help roughly the same percentage of people as other approaches, such as hypnosis and chewing nicotine-containing gum. At least one study indicates that a traditional Chinese acupuncture approach appears to work very well in controlling the relapses of people who are alcoholics.

Treatment may need to be provided very frequently — for instance, one study on alcohol abuse provided treatment every other day for two months. However, this can be expensive and time-consuming so consider carefully before commiting to trying acupuncture.

Mind–Body Therapies

STRESS People may develop addictions to a wide array of substances, ranging from tobacco and smoking to cocaine and alcohol. When an individual is already vulnerable to addiction, or recovering from a previous addiction, stress is likely to cause a relapse or new pattern of substance abuse. (*see also Excess stress, p.408*).

Most major theories of addiction agree that stress has an important role in increasing drug use and relapse. Many animal studies and some human laboratory studies (where people enter a structured setting) have clinically demonstrated the detrimental effects of stress.

Research that has attempted to explore the relationship between stress and addiction in humans outside of a structured enviornment is largely correlational (not causal), often anecdotal, and sometimes contradictory. However, these studies may soon provide more conclusive evidence supporting the belief that stress influences addictive behavior. The exact psychological and/or biochemical mechanisms underlying this association remain unclear.

TREATMENTS Mind–body therapies that can reduce stress are evidently useful in treating addictions. A few important research studies indicate that mind–body techniques and self-care practices, such as transcendental meditation (TM) and clinical biofeedback, are useful complementary additions to the Alcoholics Anonymous (AA) treatment for addictions.

Sufferers of addictions sould try meditation techniques (*see p.98 for a sequence*) or taking up yoga. When practiced regularly, these mind–body therapies may be able to help with detoxification, treatment, and relapse prevention.

Psychological Therapies

PRIMARY TREATMENT Talking therapies account for much of the treament for substance abuse. The therapy adopted depends on whether the practitioner interprets the substance abuse using the disease model or the learned behavior model.

DISEASE MODEL This is probably the most commonly used model. Substance abuse is viewed as a disease that, once developed, cannot be "cured" (i.e. "once an alcoholic or addict, always an alcoholic or addict"). The focus is on how to cope with the disease and how to manage life while "in recovery." The goal is total abstinence. The main proponent of this view is known as the 12-step, or Minnesota, model and is practiced by the collective "anonymous" groups, such as Alcoholics Anonymous.

Much of the research on treatments using the Minnesota model has been criticized for poor methods. However, several more robust studies support it, with about a third of clients maintaining abstinence after one year. More research is needed.

LEARNED BEHAVIOR MODEL The learned behavior model has gained popularity since its creation but it has also been the subject of controversy. It views substance abuse as a learned behavior that can be unlearned. While it recognizes that the substance can have addictive properties, the main focus is on practicing different ways of behaving and thinking, i.e. cognitive behavioral therapy (CBT) and a return to "controlled use" is considered a relevant goal alongside abstinence. The main theory — the Cycle of Change — focuses on the cyclical nature of dependence (be it on a substance, such as alcohol, or a behavior, such as eating, gambling, or sex). At first, people are unaware of the potential problems of their behavior (Precontemplative), followed by a period of thinking about the dependency (Contemplation); then they may decide to act to change (Action). They may maintain this change, but more often they return to their original pattern (Relapse) and start the cycle again.

The cycle may be repeated several times before the person is addiction free. At each stage of the cycle, different interventions may be used, including motivational interviewing, CBT, and relapse prevention.

SEASONAL AFFECTIVE DISORDER

In seasonal affective disorder (SAD), episodes of depression occur in the fall and winter months. This is thought to be because of reduced daylight. While many people experience SAD as a mild "blue" feeling, others have disabling symptoms. The aim of treatment is to lift the mood and to relieve depression. Light therapy is the main treatment for SAD and has good results, but exercise, vitamin D, homeopathy, and psychological therapies can also help bring relief.

WHAT ARE THE SYMPTOMS?

- Feelings of sadness and apathy
- Fatigue and lethargy
- Sleep problems, often oversleeping but also disturbed sleep and early waking
- Overeating, with a craving for sweet foods and carbohydrates, leading to weight gain
- Loss of self-esteem
- Tension and irritability
- Decreased sex drive

WHY MIGHT I HAVE THIS?

TRIGGERS
- Lack of sunlight

TREATMENT PLAN

PRIMARY TREATMENTS
- Bright light therapy
- Antidepressants

BACKUP TREATMENTS
- Vitamin D and other nutritional measures

WORTH CONSIDERING
- Homeopathy
- Exercise
- Psychological therapies

For an explanation of how treatments are rated, see p.111.

WHY DOES IT OCCUR?

Many functions of the body, such as temperature and the secretion of hormones into the bloodstream, follow an approximately 24-hour cycle, known as a circadian rhythm. The organs, tissues, and cells of the body seem to respond to the slow environmental cycle of day and night. This response is coordinated by a biological clock in a part of the brain called the hypothalamus, which links the nervous system and the endocrine system of hormones. Like the conductor of an orchestra, the hypothalamus, together with the pituitary gland to which it is connected, synchronizes the physiology and biochemistry of the body.

There are two general categories of SAD: one that starts in the winter and another that starts in the summer. The second is much rarer than the first but both have similar symptoms.

MELATONIN is thought to be a key hormone in the development of SAD because of its importance in the regulation of sleep (*see p.448*). The pineal gland in the brain produces melatonin mostly at night when there is no daylight and the body is asleep. The blood level of melatonin reaches its peak in the middle of the night but is almost undetectable during the day.

When melatonin sleep cycles are out of sync, an imbalance in the hypothalamus may result and the depression associated with SAD may develop. This asynchrony and imbalance is thought to be due to fewer hours of daylight and a lack of sunlight in the fall and winter months. When longer days return in spring, some people with SAD experience a short-lived period of high levels of physical activity. For others, the symptoms of SAD disappear gradually with the spring.

SELF-HELP

The following may help you cope with the symptoms of SAD:

- Buy a light box for use at home. Make sure you follow the manufacturer's instructions and work with your doctor to derive the most benefit.
- Try to establish whether you are more of a "lark" (more active in the morning) or an "owl" (more active in the evening). Owl types begin to produce melatonin later then lark types — synchronizing the time when you use the light box with the timing of your melatonin cycle can be beneficial.
- Get regular exercise, preferably outside in natural daylight.

TREATMENTS IN DETAIL

Conventional Medicine

Your doctor will ask you about the history of your symptoms to exclude any other psychological causes or an underlying physical cause. Various tests may also help the doctor make a diagnosis.

PRIMARY TREATMENT **BRIGHT LIGHT THERAPY** SAD may be treated successfully with a course of bright light therapy (phototherapy), which is given on a daily basis, usually early in the morning. The

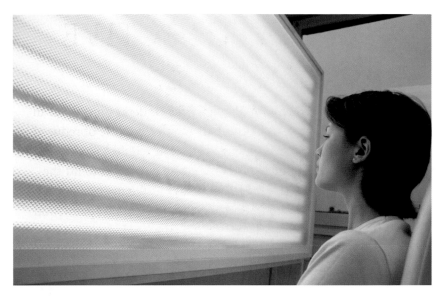

People with seasonal affective disorder can be treated by exposure to a bright light. Each day, they sit in front of a bright screen for a period of time to compensate for lack of sunlight.

individual is exposed to fluorescent light from a light box with a spectrum similar to that of daylight. It is thought that the light needs to be at least 2,500 lux (a measurement of light intensity). Each treatment usually lasts from 30 minutes to an hour. Light therapy may be helpful in treating both mild and severe SAD.

PRIMARY TREATMENT **ANTIDEPRESSANTS** Selective serotonin reuptake inhibitors (SSRIs), such as fluoxetine, may also help relieve depressive symptoms. Several drugs may need to be tried before finding the one that works best for you.

> **CAUTION**
>
> SSRIs may have side effects; ask your doctor to explain these to you.

Nutritional Therapy

Depression is the primary symptom of SAD, and its effects can be alleviated using various approaches (*see Depression, p.436*). Some people with SAD may have low thyroid function, and taking steps to maintain thyroid health may be helpful (*see p.319*). Overeating, craving sweet foods, and weight gain are also characteristic of SAD. Regulating blood-sugar levels may help control these (*see p.42*).

VITAMIN D supplements may be useful for improving mood in people with SAD. It has been suggested that the seasonal symptoms of SAD are due to changing levels of vitamin D_3, a nutrient made by the action of sunlight on the skin, and that this can improve mood through the brain chemical serotonin. In one study, subjects were given 400 IU, 800 IU, or no vitamin D_3 for five days during late winter. Results showed that the vitamin significantly enhanced positive mood. In another study, 30 days of treatment with vitamin D completely resolved depression in a group of people with SAD, whereas light treatment did not. If you have SAD, a daily dose of 400–800 IU vitamin D_3 may help.

> **CAUTION**
>
> Consult your doctor before taking vitamin D with verapamil (*see p.46*).

Homeopathy

AURUM METALLICUM Although there is no published research, some homeopaths report good results in the treatment of SAD. The medicine most often recommended is *Aurum metallicum*. People who respond to this medicine may be seriously depressed, even to the extent of brooding about death or suicide. Although depressed,

they may fly into a rage because of a minor annoyance or from being contradicted. In addition to SAD, they may have palpitations and/or sinusitis.

Exercise

Exercise can usually improve mild to moderate depressive symptoms (*see Depression, p.436*), so a study was performed to evaluate the relative benefits of exercise and bright light on the mood of people affected by seasonal changes in light availability. Ninety-eight people completed an eight-week study in which it was found that both exercise and bright light effectively relieved depressive symptoms. However, bright light seemed to be more effective, suggesting that SAD is not quite the same as mild clinical depression and that tailored treatment is needed.

Psychological Therapies

While the main methods of treating SAD use light (or phototherapy) and medication, promising research suggests that including talking therapies in the treatment plan can be beneficial. For example, interpersonal therapy has helped patients cope with the interpersonal implications of SAD, such as feelings of isolation or alienation. Cognitive therapy has also been used with promising results.

There are also potentially promising results for a combination of talking therapies and medication for people who do not respond to light therapy.

Having a family member who is depressed can have a profound effect on the rest of the family and systemic therapy as a means of support is recommended. In this form of psychological therapy, a practitioner helps the group cope better with the depressed person.

> **PREVENTION PLAN**
>
> **The following may help prevent SAD:**
>
> - Use a light box at home, with advice from your doctor
>
> - Get plenty of exercise, preferably in natural daylight and when the sun is shining

- Shock
- Feeling numb and detached
- Anxiety symptoms, such as inability to sleep and loss of appetite
- Sadness, anger, guilt, or fear

COPING WITH BEREAVEMENT

Adjusting to a loss or bereavement takes time. The grieving process usually has several stages, the length of which varies depending on the individual. Throughout the grieving process, people may vacillate between focusing on their loss and distracting themselves with work or making plans for the future. Strong emotions may abruptly emerge, including sadness, confusion, or even apathy. Help is available in the form of support, counseling, breathing retraining, and homeopathy.

WHY DOES IT OCCUR?

Loss and bereavement can occur in many forms. A person may suddenly lose his or her job, children may leave home to go to college, or a loved one may pass away. The initial reaction to a bereavement is usually one of shock and of feeling numb and detached. Some people may even pretend that nothing has happened. This is normal and provides a shield from the immediate impact of the loss. Stages of grief (*see p.435*) are common at this stage, including inability to sleep and loss of appetite.

INTENSE EMOTIONS Following the initial shock, a person may be overcome by intense emotions. The most common feeling is sadness but anger, guilt, and fear are also frequently experienced. Thinking constantly about the loss is normal as your mind challenges the fact that the event occured. As the mind adjusts to the idea of loss and accepts the reality of it, a bereaved person may feel bleak, apathetic, confused, and have no hope for the future. In extreme cases a bereaved person may become suicidal.

ACCEPTANCE As time passes, the bereaved person comes to accept the loss and achieves a new normality. He or she may hope to be happy again without forgetting the departed loved one. In the end, people often feel stronger after coping with a loss.

If you know that you may suffer a loss, for example the death of a loved one who has a terminal illness, it may be wise to familarize yourself with the grieving process in advance. This can help you cope with the event when it actually occurs.

All these feelings are part of the normal grieving process. However, if very intense emotions last for a very long time; if a person does not stop grieving, even after several years; or if a person cannot grieve at all, this process has been interrupted. These may be signs of depression and advice from a health-care professional is needed.

IMPACT ON HEALTH The sense of loss a person experiences in bereavement can provoke strong physical and emotional reactions, which may have serious effects on health. Bereaved persons may also feel run down and become susceptible to minor illnesses. Spouses who are bereaved, especially widowers, are at increased risk of dying from disease or suicide in the year following the loss. Bereavement also increases a person's risk of developing depression (*see p.436*).

SELF-HELP

PRIMARY TREATMENT Everyone grieves differently — there is no "normal" way — but the following may help:

- Talk to family and friends — even if it is painful — don't bottle up feelings.
- Keep up regular routines and avoid making sudden changes in your life.

IMPORTANT

You should consult your doctor if you feel you need help or advice coming to terms with a bereavement, and particularly if you develop overwhelming feelings of helplessness or depression or if you feel suicidal.

TREATMENT PLAN

PRIMARY TREATMENTS

- Self-help measures (*see right*)
- Support and counseling

WORTH CONSIDERING

- Breathing retraining
- Homeopathy

For an explanation of how treatments are rated, see p.111.

- Try to get plenty of sleep and exercise.
- Accept that ugly emotions, such as feeling angry and bitter, are normal and will pass in time.
- However tempting, don't drown your sorrow in alcohol or drugs.
- Keep a diary or write poetry — some people find pouring out their grief on paper helpful. Others prefer to put together a photo album of the person who they miss.
- Give yourself plenty of time: it can take months or years to fully accept the death of someone close.
- For some, the homeopathic medicine *Ignatia* may relieve symptoms.
- Join a self-help group (*see p.486 for details*).
- Read about other people's experiences of grief and bereavement, and join in discussions on the internet if you like. (*See p.486 for useful websites.*)

TREATMENTS IN DETAIL

Conventional Medicine

People often see their doctor after the death of a loved one. Doctors may have long-standing relationships with the family and can provide important emotional support and time talking with family members. The doctor may also recommend bereavement counseling to help individuals come to terms with their loss. Emotional support and understanding are also available through organizations for those who have been bereaved. It is possible to attend a group session or have counseling on a one-to-one basis.

Homeopathy

IGNATIA is the most frequently indicated homeopathic medicine for immediate reactions to bereavement. People who respond to *Ignatia* may feel numb and unreal, emotionally hypersensitive, with occasional paradoxical reactions, such as inappropriate or hysterical laughter. They may experience a sensation of a lump in their throat, and muscular twitching.

NATRUM MURIATICUM is the classical medicine for long-standing unresolved grief. Typically, those people who benefit from *Natrum muriaticum* could not express grief at the time — for instance,

STAGES OF GRIEF

Not everyone will pass through each grief stage, and not necessarily in the order below. A grieving person may cycle between stages, appearing to progress, then move back to an earlier stage. Some psychologists see grieving as a series of tasks that must be accomplished before the bereaved can reach acceptance and recovery.

STAGE	BEHAVIOR	POSSIBLE DURATION
Shock	Usually the first response. May include numbness, pain, or apathy.	Usually lasts no more than 2 weeks
Denial	Refusal to acknowledge the death ("It can't be true").	Usually an early feature. Duration varies
Disorganization	Inability to do the simplest thing. May feel restless, aimless, helpless, and lonely.	
Anger/Guilt	Includes self-blame, irritability, or anger toward God, fate, doctors, or the deceased.	Begins almost at once. Peaks after 2–4 weeks
Bargaining	Acknowledges the loss, but tries to bargain ("If only I could…" or "If only I had…").	
Mourning/Depression	As denial breaks down, grief, mourning, and depression set in. A painful and lonely stage.	Can recur at any time, but becomes less frequent and intense
Anxiety	Worry about control of feelings or of going crazy. Apprehension about the future.	
Restitution	Attending rituals, such as the funeral, and accepting the reality of the loss.	
Resolution	Gradual acceptance of the death and that life goes on.	
Reintegration	Forging new relationships and goals. The deceased has a special place in one's memory.	Can take many months or years

they may not have cried at the funeral. They may have found themselves considered a source of strength for family and friends. They may put on a brave face, coping and caring for others, but privately feel desperately depressed.

CAUSTICUM is another medicine that may be useful. It is often appropriate for caregivers who looked after a relative or friend with great dedication for a long period before the bereavement. Anger, particularly about injustice, may be a strong feature in people who respond to *Causticum*.

CAUTION

Some homeopathic medicines, including *Ignatia*, are made ineffective by coffee.

Psychological Therapy

PRIMARY TREATMENT **COUNSELING** is available (*see p.104*). Talking to someone outside the immediate family can help the bereaved to express their feelings, cope with the reactions of others, and adjust to life without the person who has died.

DEPRESSION

Depression is a state of mind in which persistent feelings of sadness are accompanied by a loss of interest in life and a lack of energy. Repetitive, worrying thoughts and a constant sense of foreboding may also be present. It affects about one in five people in the US and is one of the most common mental health disorders. Women are twice as likely as men to develop depression. A range of treatments may be called upon to tackle depression — from counseling, medication, and supplements to aerobic exercise, homeopathy, herbs, and psychological therapies.

WHAT ARE THE SYMPTOMS?

In depression, feelings of sadness are often worse in the morning and persist to some degree for the rest of the day. Other symptoms include:

- Loss of interest and enjoyment in work or leisure activities
- Difficulty concentrating
- Low self-esteem
- Feeling guilty
- Tearfulness
- Difficulty making decisions
- Early waking or excessive sleeping
- Decreased sex drive
- Low energy levels, decreased appetite, and constipation
- Symptoms of anxiety and panic attacks are common

WHY MIGHT I HAVE THIS?

PREDISPOSING FACTORS

- Genetics
- Stress or violence at home or work
- Isolation

TRIGGERS

- Stressful life events
- Loss of a family member or friend
- Recent childbirth
- Seasonal affective disorder
- Food sensitivity
- Blood-sugar imbalance

IMPORTANT

You should consult your doctor if you develop overwhelming feelings of helplessness or depression or if you feel suicidal.

WHY DOES IT OCCUR?

Depression may occur in response to a particularly stressful event or situation. The trigger for depression is often a loss of some kind, whether through the breakup of an important relationship or a bereavement (*see p.434*). Other factors include genetic predisposition, stress, chronic pain, or having a disability. However, often there is no apparent cause.

TREATMENT PLAN

PRIMARY TREATMENTS

- Lifestyle measures (*see Self-Help, right*)
- Support
- Antidepressant drugs
- St. John's wort

BACKUP TREATMENTS

- Nutritional therapy
- Exercise
- Acupuncture
- Homeopathy
- Western herbal medicine
- Mind–body therapies
- Psychological therapies

WORTH CONSIDERING

- Environmental health measures
- Massage

For an explanation of how treatments are rated, see p.111.

Some factors may cause an increased susceptibility to depression. These include a family history of depression or a traumatic experience in childhood, such as the death of a parent. Hormonal changes in women that occur after childbirth (*see p.362*) may also increase the chances of developing depression.

How depression develops is not yet fully understood, but low levels of neurotransmitters (chemicals released from nerve endings that transmit impulses to other nerves) in the brain, such as serotonin and norepinephrine, and hormones are thought to play a role.

SELF-HELP

PRIMARY TREATMENT If you are recovering from depression, the following measures may help you:

- Make a list of the tasks you have to do each day. Put the most important things at the top of the list.
- Complete these tasks one at a time and think about what you have achieved.
- Practice relaxation every day (*see p.99*).
- Exercise regularly to relieve stress.
- Eat a nutritious diet (*see p.44*).
- Get involved in an activity (sport, pastime, hobby, etc.).
- Join a support group to share your thoughts and experiences.

TREATMENTS IN DETAIL

Conventional Medicine

Your doctor may arrange for blood tests to rule out physical illnesses that can affect your mood and energy levels. He or she will also suggest one or a combination of

SELECTIVE SEROTONIN RE-UPTAKE INHIBITION

Depression is thought to be associated with low levels of the chemical serotonin in parts of the brain. Serotonin is normally produced by the brain and helps to control mood. When serotonin is reabsorbed, in a process known as reuptake, too quickly by the nerve endings that produce it, the level of stimulation falls. Specific drugs that selectively inhibit this reuptake can help to reduce the likelihood of depression.

How SSRIs work

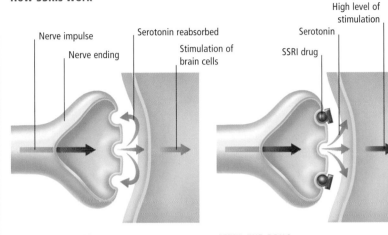

BEFORE THE DRUG

When a nerve impulse reaches the nerve ending, serotonin is released. It crosses the synaptic space, stimulates the next nerve cell and is then reabsorbed.

AFTER THE DRUG

An SSRI drug can block the reuptake of serotonin by occupying the exact places on the nerve ending where the molecules of serotonin would be reabsorbed.

---

treatments. A reduction in alcohol intake may be advised, since alcohol can aggravate depression. Exercise may also be recommended as an effective treatment.

PRIMARY TREATMENT | **SUPPORT** Psychotherapy may be suggested; for example, cognitive therapy (see Mind–Body Therapies, p.440) has been shown to be beneficial. Emotional support from family and friends is very important; support groups may also help. Other services are available to help with specific problems, such as unemployment and financial problems. Although depression often causes feelings of worthlessness and makes it difficult to seek help, it is extremely important that you do not suffer alone.

PRIMARY TREATMENT | **ORAL DRUGS** may be prescribed: the exact drug selected depends on symptoms and possible side effects. Symptoms may start to improve after about two weeks. In some cases, the drug may need to be changed if it is not effective (sometimes, more than one drug needs to be tried), or if it causes undesirable side effects.

Your doctor may prescribe a drug from one of several groups of antidepressants:
- Selective serotonin reuptake inhibitors (SSRIs), such as fluoxetine and paroxetine, affect serotonin (see box, above).
- Tricyclic antidepressants, such as amitriptyline and nortriptyline, are also commonly prescribed. They interfere with the reabsorption of serotonin and norepinephrine, maintaining high levels of these neurotransmitters in the body.
- Monoamine oxidase inhibitors (MAOI), such as phenelzine, can be used when other drugs fail to work. They block the action of an enzyme that makes serotonin and norepinephrine inactive.

There are various newer drugs, including venlafaxine, which may help when energy levels are low, and mirtazapine, which can be used to help sleep.

ELECTROCONVULSIVE THERAPY (ECT) is occasionally recommended for very severe depression when other treatments fail. A course of ECT is carried out under a general anesthetic and involves passing an electrical current briefly between two electrodes applied to either side of the head. This brief period of electrical stimulation produces a generalized seizure. The beneficial results of ECT are often quicker to take affect than other forms of treatment, such as antidepressants. Another technique, transcranial magnetic stimulation, is an alternative to ECT.

> **CAUTION**
>
> ECT and drugs used to treat depression can cause side-effects: ask your doctor to explain these to you. Conventional antidepressants should not be taken at the same time as herbal ones, such as St John's wort.

Nutritional Therapy

While depression is generally considered a predominantly psychological problem, it can also have physiological and/or biochemical triggers. Common problems encountered in clinical practice include low thyroid function (see p.319), anemia and/or iron deficiency, SAD (see p.432), food sensitivity (see p.39), and blood sugar imbalance (see p.42). Apart from these disorders there may be a vitamin deficiency or even too much of an essential nutrient.

FOOD ELIMINATION DIET Certain food intakes, such as sugar, caffeine, alcohol, and artificial sweeteners, may upset brain chemistry. Removing these from the diet can lead to a significant improvement in mood (see p.39).

OMEGA-3 FATTY ACIDS Evidence is accumulating to link depression with abnormalities in fatty acid metabolism and deficiencies in dietary fatty acid intake. The omega-3 essential fatty acids, such as EPA and DHA (see p.34), found in oily fish like salmon and mackerel, seem to be most important in this respect.

Countries where people eat plenty of oily fish, such as Japan and China, have substantially lower rates of depression, and, in general, people who eat fish regularly are less likely to report feeling depressed. In addition, the blood of depressed individuals commonly has low

Consult your doctor before taking omega-3 fatty acids or fish oils with warfarin, or folate (folic acid) with anticonvulsant drugs or methotrexate (see p.46).

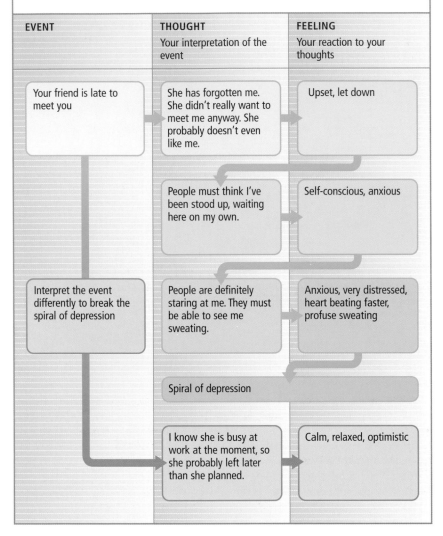

SPIRAL OF DEPRESSION

One of the features of depression is the spiral of negative thoughts and feelings that is triggered by a seemingly innocuous event. Thoughts and feelings feed off each other until the spiral goes out of control. One way of preventing this is to interpret the event differently as soon as possible and to think positively about it.

EVENT	THOUGHT Your interpretation of the event	FEELING Your reaction to your thoughts
Your friend is late to meet you	She has forgotten me. She didn't really want to meet me anyway. She probably doesn't even like me.	Upset, let down
	People must think I've been stood up, waiting here on my own.	Self-conscious, anxious
Interpret the event differently to break the spiral of depression	People are definitely staring at me. They must be able to see me sweating.	Anxious, very distressed, heart beating faster, profuse sweating
	Spiral of depression	
	I know she is busy at work at the moment, so she probably left later than she planned.	Calm, relaxed, optimistic

levels of omega-3 fatty acids. Supplementing the diet with omega-3 fatty acids, especially EPA, is often useful in treating depression. A daily dose of 1g of EPA (found in about 3g of concentrated fish oil) may be helpful.

THIAMINE (VITAMIN B₁) Studies have shown mood improvement with thiamine supplementation (varying from 2mg to 50mg a day), even in people who were not previously deficient in this nutrient. Taking a daily dose of 25mg of thiamine would be safe in the long term.

FOLATE (FOLIC ACID) is another vitamin that seems to be involved in depression. Studies reveal that a large percentage of depressed individuals have low folate levels. Supplementing the diet with 500mcg per day of folate may be of benefit in the relief of depression.

SELENIUM A deficiency of selenium is associated with a significantly greater incidence of depression and other negative mood states. Although selenium deficiency is rare in the US, selenium supplements may have a beneficial impact on mood in

people who are only slightly deficient in the mineral. Eating plenty of foods rich in selenium, such as shellfish, eggs, and mushrooms, or taking selenium supplements appears to improve mood. If you have depression, try taking 100mcg of selenium per day.

Homeopathy

Case series suggest that depression responds to homeopathic treatment. However, depression has many variations and different homeopathic medicines are potentially appropriate depending upon the symptoms to be treated. Unless you have extensive knowledge of homeopathy, you will need to consult a practitioner before beginning treatment.

Among the more commonly suggested homeopathic medicines are *Natrum muriaticum, Sepia, Aurum metallicum, Lachesis,* and *Pulsatilla.*

NATRUM MURIATICUM is often the medicine for "copers" — people who seem in control, kind and caring to others, yet hiding the dark mood they feel inside. Their concerns are often triggered by relationship problems. Sometimes, they have the unfortunate habit of falling in love with unsuitable people for the wrong reasons, such as misplaced pity. They are good listeners but have difficulty expressing their own feelings and may get annoyed if others pry or try to help.

SEPIA People who respond to *Sepia* also resent fuss and sympathy. But in other respects, patients who benefit from *Sepia* are different. For instance, *Natrum muriaticum* people empathize (perhaps too much) with others, but *Sepia* people are emotionally flat — they cannot be bothered with others, even their close family.

A very important feature of *Sepia* is the temporary improvement brought on by vigorous activity: working out or dancing lifts the mood. In women, there is a loss of sex drive; in men, there may be sexual promiscuity. In women, the depression may have been triggered by having a baby.

LACHESIS If depression is associated with menopause, a woman may respond to *Lachesis*. There are often severe hot flashes and depression may be accompanied by jealousy or excessive suspiciousness. People who respond to this medicine are often talkative, and for some reason hate tight clothes, especially collars.

PULSATILLA Depression that responds to *Pulsatilla* is often characterized by great weepiness, dithering, and indecision. People who are helped by the medicine may feel temporarily much better around company and after talking about their problems (unlike patients who respond to *Natrum muriacum* and *Sepia*).

AURUM METALLICUM may be useful for people with serious depression who have suicidal thoughts. In people whom it helps, depression is often seasonal, worse in winter and at night. It may be accompanied by painful sinusitis.

Western Herbal Medicine

PRIMARY TREATMENT **ST. JOHN'S WORT** (*Hypericum perforatum*) Many studies have shown the benefit of St. John's wort in treating mild to moderate depression. If your depression is recent and not severe, St. John's wort is worth a try. The usual dose is an extract standardized with 0.3% hypericin or 3–5% hyperforin. Take 300mg three times daily. Although it has been found effective for treating mild depression, a recent US trial found that neither St. John's wort nor sertraline were as effective as placebo when used to treat longstanding severe depression.

Used for depressive states since the time of the ancient Greeks, herbal practitioners also consider St. John's wort an herb of choice in conditions where the nervous system is under stress, such as shingles (*see p.165*), sciatica (*see p.272*), and nervous exhaustion. It combines well with valerian (*Valeriana officinalis*) in depression to promote sleep and relaxation and with black cohosh (*Cimicifuga racemosa*) in depression linked to menopause. While St. John's wort may increase the effect of a few drugs, it is also known to decrease the effects of

several, such as digoxin, cyclosprorine, and some antidepressants. Consult a healthcare professional before taking it

> **CAUTION**
>
> See p.69 before taking an herbal remedy and, if you are already taking prescribed medication, consult an herbal medicine expert first. Do not take St. John's wort with antidepressants, warfarin, antibiotics, birth control pills, or any medication that is taken daily.

OTHER HERBAL MEDICINES that have proven valuable in treating depression include: lemon balm (*Melissa officinalis*), which is a gentle sedative with a positive uplifting effect; licorice (*Glycyrrhiza glabra*), which is a tonic and restorative that supports liver and adrenal gland function; and ginkgo (*Ginkgo biloba*), which stimulates the circulation, protects the nerves, and has some antidepressant activity. Schisandra (*Schisandra chinensis*) is another medicine that may help. It works as a nerve tonic that improves memory and mental performance.

Herbal practitioners will combine these with other herbs that strengthen liver function and elimination, support circulation, particularly to the central nervous system, and stimulate adrenal gland activity.

Environmental Health

STRESS The majority of research demonstrates higher rates of depression in individuals who are unable to cope with stressful situations or who have lower than average levels of self-esteem.

Research also suggests that individuals who lived near the Chernobyl power plant in Ukraine, a site of a major nuclear disaster in 1986, experienced depression from chronic stress. It is important to note that during holidays, emotional and physical stress and loneliness can trigger a recurrence of depressive symptoms.

SEASONAL PATTERNS, such as changes in weather, temperature, and light, affect the body and mind in numerous ways and may lead to symptoms of depression. They may result in physiological changes that sometimes lead to reduced mental stability and increases in symptoms of depression. Case studies indicate that lack of natural light may cause increased anxiety and depression (*see also SAD, p.432*). Evidence also suggests that walking outside in the sunlight can help alleviate depression.

WAR Nonmilitary personnel may experience symptoms of depression during times of war. Some researchers claim that the many symptoms, including depression and memory loss, that have appeared in the Gulf War syndrome may represent injury to the nervous system. Among the possible causes for this injury are exposure to chemical warfare agents, pesticides, extremes of heat and cold, blowing dust,

> Depression and suicide are increasing faster among young people than any other age group

and smoke from oil well fires. Studies showing that these substances may have caused damage to soldiers' nervous systems support other studies showing a possible connection between exposures to certain solvents in the workplace and symptoms of depression.

ENVIRONMENT People who are poor and/or live in low-income housing have demonstrated a higher prevalence of depressive symptoms. Higher rates of depression can also be found in areas of high crime or community violence. Relocating will not necessarily resolve depressive symptoms, but re-evaluating your surroundings is an important step to improving the symptoms you may be experiencing.

Another daily factor that may influence depression is the amount that families watch television. For example, as children spend more time watching TV, they are less likely to participate in enriching activities with their parents, strengthening the parent-child bond. This can commonly lead to depression in parents.

Massage and Exercise

MASSAGE has been shown in numerous research studies to be a useful treatment for depression. It has helped relieve depression in child and adolescent patients, adolescent mothers, people with chronic fatigue and immune dysfunction, cancer patients, people with chronic pain, and people who are depressed due to work-related stress.

AEROBIC EXERCISE has been shown to be important in alleviating even major depression. It increases self-esteem, improves mood, reduces anxiety, enhances the ability to handle stress, and encourages better sleep patterns, in both adults and children. If you suffer from depression, try walking, running, or other aerobic exercise, for 20 minutes three times a week.

People who are depressed dream up to 3 times more often than people without depression

Other forms of exercise, including martial arts, also have the potential to offer similar benefits.

Acupuncture

There is evidence that acupuncture has fundamental effects on the brain's chemical messages, making it a reasonable treatment for depression. In fact, there are at least three clinical trials indicating that acupuncture is as effective in relieving the symptoms of depression as some conventionally used antidepressants. Usually, prolonged treatment is needed.

Acupuncture treatment should be given on a weekly basis for eight to ten weeks. If it proves to be valuable, then maintenance treatments may be required, depending on how the symptoms respond to the treatment.

Mind–Body Therapies

RELAXATION AND GUIDED IMAGERY (see p.100) have improved mood and decreased depressive symptoms in women who have recently had a baby, those with cancer or who have just had surgery, people with multiple sclerosis, healthy adults, and college students. The antidepressant effects of guided imagery and relaxation may result from reduced anxiety and an increased sense of control.

A very low cost program, which is based on mind–body skills, such as relaxation and/or guided imagery, can provide people with powerful self-help tools for overcoming depression. People who are able to practice these techniques at home on a regular basis are likely to require fewer medical resources and have increased quality of life, better overall health, and longer life spans.

Psychological Therapies

PSYCHOTHERAPEUTIC APPROACHES include cognitive behavioral therapy, behavioral therapy (especially mind–body stress management programs), psychodynamic approaches, and solution-oriented brief therapy. Many experts believe that combining psychotherapy or behavioral therapy with selective serotonin reuptake inhibitors (SSRIs) is more beneficial for treating depression than either treatment alone — at least in women.

AVOIDING ISOLATION Some individuals may become depressed if they lead an isolated life with minimal social interaction. Doctors recommend that those prone to depression try to participate in community events with stable group dynamics that will provide both excitement and release for the tension in their lives.

TALKING THERAPIES Four of the five talking therapy approaches (see p.106) are of value in depression: psychodynamic, cognitive behavioral therapy (CBT), interpersonal therapy (IPT), and humanistic therapy. A great deal of research has been done to examine the use of talking therapies for the treatment of depression. Overall, reviews suggest that therapies from the CBT group tend to be more effective in creating long-term results than other talking approaches.

THE PSYCHODYNAMIC APPROACH recognizes that depressed people have developed a very negative self-image, which usually begins in childhood. They are often highly critical of themselves, engaging in self-punishment that is expressed as a kind of internal battle. They may "invite" other people to join in criticizing them in order to confirm their negative self-image.

This process is largely unconscious and the goal of therapy is to make the process more conscious: the therapist "declines the invitation" and gains an understanding of the internal conflict via the therapeutic relationship. As a result, new opportunities for emotional assimilation and insight open up for the client. Evidence suggests that this form of therapy is effective in both an individual and a group setting.

THE COGNITIVE BEHAVIORAL THERAPY APPROACH is similar to the psychodynamic approach and is used to address a person's negative thinking patterns. The therapist's goal is to help clients identify their negative thoughts, often by using a "thought diary," and thinking about alternatives. Other people's behavior patterns, which often confirm the negative thoughts, are also identified — alternative behavior is generated and tried out by the client in "homework tasks." Problem-solving techniques help clients manage their lives so that they feel less overwhelmed. A wealth of evidence supports the use of CBT in the treatment of depression, both with individuals and in groups.

THE HUMANISTIC APPROACH aims to provide a supportive and nonjudgmental environment in which clients can explore their difficulties and provide a solution for themselves. Research suggests that a humanistic therapy, such as client centered therapy, helps people who are depressed and that no significant advantage is gained by combining it with medication.

INTERPERSONAL THERAPY tends to focus more on the client's present relationships and how these contribute to the feeling of depression. The goal of therapy is to review these relationships and explore new ways of relating to other people. IPT has been proven particularly effective with adolescents, although people of any age may benefit from its effects.

EATING DISORDERS

People with eating disorders use overeating, purging, or rigidly restricting their food intake to help cope with their problems. Those with anorexia deliberately lose weight until they are unhealthily thin, while people with bulimia repeatedly binge on food, after which they may force themselves to vomit or take laxatives. Some people have anorexia and bulimia at the same time. The multidisciplinary approach to treatment, which involves support, psychotherapy, medication, and supplements, aims to help them cope better with underlying feelings.

WHAT ARE THE SYMPTOMS?

Anorexia nervosa:

- Refusal to eat, especially foods that are high in calories
- Obsession with food and food-related activities, such as cooking
- Preoccupation with body weight and shape
- Weight loss — which may be concealed with baggy clothing
- Distorted view of body shape
- Use of appetite suppressants and laxatives
- Rigid routine of excessive exercise

If anorexia continues for some time:

- Extreme weight loss
- Wasting of the muscles
- Swollen ankles
- Fine body hair on limbs and trunk
- Irregular periods or lack of menstruation

Bulimia:

- Frequent weight fluctuations
- Eating alone and in secret
- Guilt/self-disgust after binge-eating
- Vomiting
- Use of laxatives

If binge-eating and purging become established:

- Abdominal pain and swelling following a binge
- Physical weakness
- Eroded teeth
- Abrasions on fingers from using them to induce vomiting
- Bleeding from esophagus lining
- Disturbed heart rhythm and impaired kidney function

WHY MIGHT I HAVE THESE?

PREDISPOSING FACTORS

- Low self-esteem
- Perfectionistic, high-achieving personality

WHY DO THEY OCCUR?

ANOREXIA NERVOSA usually develops in adolescence and is more common in girls and women. The condition can cause changes in hormone levels that may affect growth and development during adolescence and may interfere with normal menstruation. In severe cases, the weight loss caused by anorexia is life threatening. Anorexia occurs almost solely in developed countries and is more prevalent in the middle and upper classes.

Anorexia often develops after weight loss dieting. The importance placed on having a perfect, slim body in many countries can lead people of normal size to diet without reason, especially if they have low self-esteem. Anorexia often occurs in young people, especially girls, who are under pressure to succeed in a family where success is overemphasized. The condition is also common in professions where being slim is important, such as dance, gymnastics, and modeling. Sufferers of anorexia may enjoy preparing food for others but refrain from eating the meal themselves.

BULIMIA usually develops in early adulthood and is more common in women. People with bulimia are often of normal weight with low self-esteem and often feel a great need to control their surroundings and their emotions. Bouts of bulimia are sometimes triggered by stress. The pattern of binge-eating and purging may become habitual and the cycle may be difficult to break. Unlike anorexia, bulimia does not usually lead to severe weight loss. However, repeated vomiting can cause dehydration and chemical imbalances in the blood, as well as cause teeth erosion.

COMPULSIVE OVEREATING People who overeat as a means of coping with the stress of their feelings end up in a cycle of secret binge-eating and depression. The overeating eases stress but a short time later feelings of guilt take over, culminating in depression. The cycle is complicated by worries about weight.

TREATMENT PLAN

PRIMARY TREATMENTS

- Emotional support
- Psychotherapy and counseling
- Antidepressants (in some cases)
- Hospital therapy (for severe anorexia)
- Blood-sugar stabilizing diet (bulimia)

BACKUP TREATMENTS

- Nutritional therapy

WORTH CONSIDERING

- Massage and exercise
- Homeopathy

For an explanation of how treatments are rated, see p.111.

IMPORTANT

As soon as you suspect you have an eating disorder, consult your doctor. If you don't feel able to do this, talk to a sympathetic friend or relative first.

TREATMENTS IN DETAIL

Conventional Medicine

PRIMARY TREATMENT **ANOREXIA NERVOSA** is often difficult to treat. Studies suggest that only about 40 percent of those treated make a full recovery. In some cases the disease can be fatal.

Psychotherapy (*see Psychological Therapies, p.443*) may be recommended to address the emotional problems behind the disorder — for example, to examine the underlying reasons for a distorted body image. Another aim of treatment is to encourage the person to eat a balanced diet and return to an acceptable weight.

Hospital admission may be needed if weight loss is very severe and there are physical symptoms, such as dizziness and extreme weakness. There may also be chemical imbalances and vitamin deficiencies that must be treated.

Antidepressant drugs may be prescribed if there are symptoms of depression.

PRIMARY TREATMENT **BULIMIA** Cognitive behavioral therapy and other forms of psychotherapy are likely to be recommended (*see Psychological Therapies, p.443*). Certain antidepressants, such as monoamine oxidase inhibitors (MAOI) and fluoxetine, may also be helpful. The prognosis for bulimia tends to be better than for anorexia.

Nutritional Therapy

ANOREXIA NERVOSA Individuals with anorexia often have multiple nutrient deficiencies, a factor that may have a major impact on both psychological and physical health. Taking a high potency multivitamin and mineral supplement each day may help prevent or reverse these effects.

One nutrient that appears to be particularly beneficial for people with anorexia is zinc, which has many important functions in the body, such as the normalization of brain function and perception. In a 1990 study, a daily dose of 45–90mg of zinc led to weight gain in 17 out of 20 anorexic people after periods ranging between eight months and five years. In a 1994 double-blind study, 14mg of zinc per day doubled the speed of weight increase in a group of women with anorexia.

A 2002 review concluded that zinc therapy should be included in the treatment of anorexia because during recovery it increases weight gain and reduces levels of anxiety and depression.

Anorexic individuals may benefit from taking 45–90mg of zinc per day. Because zinc can induce copper deficiency, about 3–6mg of copper should be taken with this dose of zinc. Once improvement is seen, the dose of zinc may be reduced, and the anorexic individuals should try to eat a nutritious, varied diet.

BULIMIA Blood-sugar imbalance seems to play an important role in treating sufferers of bulimia. In a 1984 study, a group of bulimic women were put on a diet designed to maintain stable blood sugar levels. It excluded all alcohol, caffeine, refined sugar, white flour products, monosodium glutamate, and flavor enhancers. All women in the study stopped binge-eating while they were on this regimen, and were still binge-free two and a half years later. (*For more information on blood-sugar instability, see p.42.*)

Another factor that may play a part in bulimia is low levels of the brain chemical serotonin. This chemical, which generally induces feel-good emotions, is made in the brain from an amino acid called tryptophan, found in foods such as meat, tofu, almonds, peanuts, pumpkin seeds, sesame seeds, and tahini (a paste made from seasme seeds). Tryptophan is absorbed into the brain most efficiently when there are carbohydrates present, which might explain why certain individuals gravitate toward sweet or starchy foods when upset or stressed.

In a 1989 study, bulimic women were given either 3g of tryptophan or a placebo each day for about a month. Those taking tryptophan were also given 45mg of vitamin B_6 per day, because this nutrient is thought to aid the conversion of tryptophan into serotonin. Those who took tryptophan and vitamin B_6 found that their mood, eating behavior, and feelings about eating improved as compared to the bulimic women taking the placebo.

Tryptophan is not available over the counter in many countries, including the US and the UK. However, 5-hydroxytryptophan (5-HTP), which is the substance tryptophan is converted into before it is made into serotonin, is a good alternative. The recommended dose is 50mg of 5-HTP, taken two or three times a day.

> **CAUTION**
>
> Consult your doctor before taking 5-HTP with zolpidem, venlafaxine, fluvoxamine, fluoxetine, sumatriptan or paroxetine, and before taking zinc with antibiotics (*see p.46*).

ANOREXIA CYCLE

A person with anorexia is trapped in a cycle where mistaken views of being overweight become reinforced by changes in the physique. These changes are due to malnutrition and, possibly, diet drugs and laxatives. Once this cycle of dieting, fluid retention, and muscle deterioration is established, it is very difficult to break.

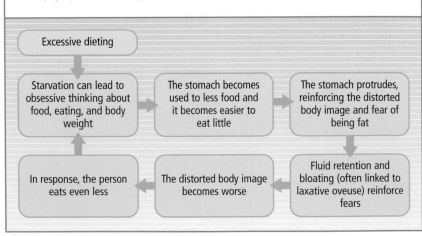

Homeopathy

Individualized homeopathy may be helpful in conjunction with other methods. Generally, treatment of eating disorders requires skilled treatment from a qualified homeopath. Among the most frequently indicated medicines are *Ignatia, Arsenicum album, Tarentula, Pulsatilla,* and *Phosphorus.* These are prescribed according to the individual's constitution and characteristics (*see p.73*).

IGNATIA Conditions that respond to *Ignatia* are often triggered by an emotional shock, such as bereavement (*see p.434*) or a relationship breakup. The person is emotionally and physically oversensitive. This is a medicine of paradoxes: for instance, there is often a sensation of a lump in the throat, making swallowing difficult, but liquids are more difficult to swallow than solids.

ARSENICUM ALBUM People who respond to *Arsenicum album* are often perfectionists, making impossible demands on themselves. They tend to be very tidy and organized — great planners who get upset if their plans go awry. They feel the cold excessively and often have dry, flaky skin.

TARENTULA is made from a tincture of the living spider of the same name. People who respond to it are restless even to the point of being twitchy and making involuntary movements. They love music and dancing, and feel much better after engaging in these activities.

PULSATILLA is appropriate for people whose symptoms and moods change easily. People who respond to it may be extremely finicky eaters and particularly dislike fatty and rich food. Despite having a dry mouth, they are not thirsty. They are weepy, but quickly cheer up after a sympathetic chat.

Women who respond to this medicine often have disturbed menstrual cycles, particularly very irregular or variable periods. They frequently feel worse right before their menstrual period.

PHOSPHORUS may be helpful for bulimics, particularly those whose favorite binge food is ice cream. People who respond to this medicine tend to feel better in the morning and following a short nap. They often have irrational fears and phobias, particularly of being alone in the dark and of storms. They may be oversensitive.

> **CAUTION**
>
> Some homeopathic medicines, including *Ignatia*, are antidoted by coffee. This means that the medicine is rendered ineffective.

Massage and Exercise

Regular massage is recommended for people with eating disorders. In various studies, massage has been shown to reduce dissatisfaction with body image in people with both anorexia and bulimia. It also reduces associated levels of anxiety and depression.

Research also shows that exercise therapy significantly improves the anxiety associated with bulimic behavior, although it did not produce any change in the bulimic behavior itself. The exercise recommendations for people with eating disorders are the same as for anyone else: aerobic exercise of some form for 20 minutes at least three times a week.

Psychological Therapies

PRIMARY TREATMENT **ANOREXIA** People with anorexia often have a distorted view of their body shape — what to most people would be considered thin, they may view as excessively fat. They may respond to various approaches, particularly to systemic and psychodynamic therapies (*see p.106*). Approaches vary: someone with anorexia can have therapy with her family, on a one-to-one basis, or in a group with others who have the disease.

Anorexia is a very serious condition and can be life threatening, so sufferers may require hospital admittance to bring their weight under control. Hospitalization may last for months and require repeated admittance. Once weight loss is no longer a danger, outpatient treatment may begin. Initially, treatment consists of medical care and programs designed to increase weight, while talking therapies aim to address long-term problems.

A 1991 review examined a variety of treatments for patients with severe anorexia. One group received inpatient treatment with an outpatient follow-up and another group received solely outpatient treatment, consisting of psychodynamic individual, family, or group therapy. All forms of treatment were effective, although members of the solely outpatient group (who were probably less severely anorexic) remained well for a longer time.

A 2000 review of treatments for younger patients (aged 12 to 30) with anorexia concluded that the most effective method of treatment was a family therapy that used a mixture of systemic interventions and education about the risks of anorexia. There has been remarkably little research on the

About half of all those with anorexia are able to recover and maintain a healthy body weight

effectiveness of cognitive behavioral therapy (CBT) for anorexia, although this is now being addressed.

PRIMARY TREATMENT **BULIMIA** For people with bulimia, fear of gaining weight is alleviated by self-induced purging, which consists of vomiting and/or taking laxatives. The purging normally follows a period of binge eating.

Many studies support the use of CBT when treating bulimia, either given to individuals or to people in groups. It is effective when combined with psychoeducation, which is usually carried out in a group setting and attempts to explain psychological theory in a user-friendly, often experiential, way. For example, participants are invited to have an anxiety-provoking thought and to notice what happens in their body.

Interpersonal therapy (*see p.107*) also shows promising results and compared favorably when researched against CBT. Psychodynamic therapy is also an effective treatment for bulimia.

OBESITY

Obesity is an accumulation of excess body fat with a body mass index (BMI) of over 30 (*see p.445*). Carrying excess weight puts a strain on the body's organs and joints, and increases the risk of potentially fatal disorders. A surfeit of appetizing and widely available fatty and sugary foods combined with sedentary lifestyles are making obesity increasingly common in the developed world. Treatment involves changing to a healthy diet and getting regular exercise. Drugs, acupuncture, stress-reduction techniques, and surgery may also be used.

WHAT ARE THE FEATURES?

- BMI of over 30 (*see box, p.445*)
- Accumulation of excessive body fat
- Higher than average metabolic rate

WHY MIGHT I HAVE THIS?

PREDISPOSING FACTORS

- Overeating
- Sedentary lifestyle
- Diet rich in partially hydrogenated fat
- Diet rich in sugary foods (high-glycemic index carbohydrates)
- Genetic factors
- Stress and other psychological factors
- Dietary imbalances
- Low thyroid function (rarely)

TREATMENT PLAN

PRIMARY TREATMENTS

- Lifestyle measures (*see Self-Help*)
- Weight-reducing diet (on rare occasions in combination with drugs or surgery)
- Exercise and increased lifestyle activity

BACKUP TREATMENTS

- Nutritional therapy
- Mind–body therapies

WORTH CONSIDERING

- Acupuncture
- Homeopathy

For an explanation of how treatments are rated, see p.111.

WHY DOES IT OCCUR?

Obesity is defined as having a BMI of 30 or more, but a BMI between 25 and 30 can also have detrimental effects on health (*see right*). The risks are greater if fat collects around the abdomen, which may be increase the likelihood of developing high blood pressure.

Obesity occurs when food intake (in calories) provides more energy than the body needs. It is usually brought about by overeating and lack of exercise. Lifestyle and psychological factors, such as stress, depression, and anxiety, which often lead to "emotional eating," may also play a role.

Obesity is only rarely the result of a medical disorder, such as an underactive thyroid gland (*see p.319*). Some drugs, such as oral corticosteroids, can cause an increase in weight. Obesity appears to run in families; bad eating habits learned in childhood and genetics are both likely to play a role.

FAT CELLS (adipocytes) in white adipose tissue, which protects joints and organs, store the body's excess energy. Babies are born with around five billion fat cells, which contain an oily globule composed mostly of triglycerides (*see p.254*). Throughout childhood, the number of fat cells increases so that an average adult has between 25–30 billion.

Normally, the body establishes an energy equilibrium and a steady body mass index (*see right*). However, when calorie intake consistently exceeds energy needs, the adipose tissue multiplies, in number or size of fat cells, or both. Fat cells, once formed, are not lost but stay in the body for life. As a result, someone who is obese may have as many as 200 billion fat cells.

FETAL PROGRAMING Babies who do not receive enough nutrients during their first six months in the womb are more likely to become obese later in life. It seems that this shortage of nutrients causes their organs (brain, heart, kidneys, liver, and pancreas) to be programmed differently, as if their development and function were primed for a life of scarcity. If they then face a life where food is plentiful, their appetite malfunctions and they find it hard not to overeat. As a result, mothers who are obese, diabetic, or malnourished may be passing obesity on to future generations.

OBESITY EPIDEMIC According to the World Health Organization, obesity threatens to overwhelm both developed and developing countries. It predicts there will be approximately 300 million cases by 2005. The country most affected by this epidemic is the US. The Centers for Disease Control and Prevention (CDC) estimate that 64 percent of all Americans and 15 percent of American children are overweight. In addition, more than 30 percent of people in the US are considered obese. These numbers have risen steadily since the 1980s and in the year 2000 caused an estimated 400,000 deaths. Childhood obesity is also on the increase and in the past two decades the percentage of overweight children in the US has almost doubled.

DETRIMENTAL EFFECTS ON HEALTH Increasingly, governments need to make healthy eating choices easier. Obesity (along with smoking) is one of the major public health problems of this century. Obesity contributes to conditions such as osteoarthritis (*see p.289*) because it increases strain on the knees and hips. It also increases the risk of developing serious health problems, including coronary artery disease, strokes, and high blood pressure.

Obesity is also a factor for type 2 diabetes (*see p.314*) and some cancers, including cancer of the colon. Of particular concern is the increasing incidence of type 2 diabetes among children.

SELF-HELP

PRIMARY TREATMENT For sustained, permanent weight loss, focus on making long-term changes to your eating habits.

- Don't try a crash/fad/starvation/liquid diet. They don't work and could damage your health in the long term.
- Aim to lose about 5–7 lb a month.
- Eat a nutritious diet based on whole grains, low-fat dairy products, lean meat, and plenty of fruit and vegetables. Concentrate on quality rather than quantity.
- Cut out foods that only deliver calories without nutritional value, such as soft drinks, potato chips, sweets, and alcohol.
- Keep on hand a stock of nuts, fruit, granola bars, and other healthy snacks.
- Eat some protein with every meal and limit your intake of high-glycemic index foods such as bagels and pasta.
- Put away the skillet and grill, bake or steam food instead.
- Increase the amount of regular exercise you get. Try using a pedometer to get feedback on the amount of physical activity you have performed each day. You can set targets, such as 10,000 steps a day, and use it to as motivation.
- Diet with a friend or join a weight loss program for morale-boosting support.

TREATMENTS IN DETAIL

Conventional Medicine

Your doctor will measure your height and weight to calculate your BMI (*see above*) and will discuss your diet with you and the amount of exercise you get Your blood may be tested for the level of sugar, cholesterol, and, rarely, hormones.

PRIMARY TREATMENT **DIET** The mainstay of treatment is a reduction in calorie intake, while ensuring a balanced intake of nutrients, and a permanent change in eat-

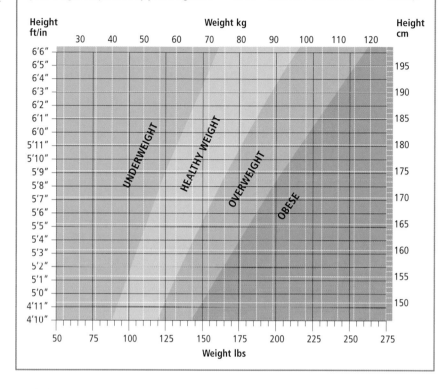

BODY MASS INDEX (BMI)

Examine the chart below to see if your weight is healthy. A BMI of 20 to 25 is healthy, 25 to 30 is overweight, and over 30 indicates obesity. To figure out yours, divide your weight (in pounds) by your height (in inches) squared. Then multiply by 703. For example, a woman who is 5 feet 3 inches tall (63 inches) and weighs 143lbs has a BMI of 25 (63 x 63 = 3969. 143 divided by 3969 = 0.03603. 0.03603 x 703 = 25.33).

ing habits to maintain weight loss. Your doctor can advise you about healthy eating habits and how to lose weight slowly and steadily. He or she may give you a diet sheet or refer you to a dietician. A balanced diet should be combined with an exercise program. Psychotherapy may also play a role in modifying attitudes to food and eating patterns. Losing a great deal of weight is a long-term venture and a great deal of support is needed from doctors, dietitians, relatives, or by joining a weight loss program.

DRUGS are occasionally considered for obesity, but they must be combined with a strict diet. Some have been banned in the US due to their potential effects on the heart and circulatory system. Two that are available in the US are sibutramine, which acts on the brain to suppress appetite, and orlistat, which reduces the absorption of fat in the gut. However, weight tends to be regained after the drugs are stopped.

SURGERY may be used for very severe obesity. There are various options. The jaws may be wired together, but weight is often regained afterward. In gastroplasty, the stomach is stapled to limit the amount of food that can be eaten at one time — eating small but very frequent meals may put the weight back on. Liposuction is relatively common, but weight is often regained.

CAUTION

Drugs and surgical procedures for obesity have potential side effects and risks; ask your doctor to explain these to you.

Nutritional Therapy

Obesity is caused by consuming more calories than are burned in the body. The main conventional approaches to treat this are centered around restricting calorie intake and/or increasing exercise. However, experience suggests that specific imbalances can be very common in cases of overweight and obesity, and correcting them can aid long-term weight loss. They may include low thyroid function, food sensitivity, or imbalance of blood sugar or gut flora.

FAT, CARBOHYDRATES, AND OBESITY Many weight-loss diets restrict the intake of fat because it contains nine kilocalories per gram, whereas carbohydrates contain four. However, in 2002, a comprehensive review concluded that dietary fat was not a major factor in weight gain, and that restricting fat alone is unlikely to bring long-term weight reduction.

HEALTHY FATS The fats to use in a healthy diet designed for weight loss are the essential fatty acids found in extra-virgin olive oil, nuts, seeds, avocadoes, and in oily fish, such as salmon, trout, mackerel, herring, and sardines. Saturated fats, such as those in red meat and dairy products, appear not to be as harmful as is often said, and may be included in moderation.

UNHEALTHY FATS Probably the most harmful fats (and the ones most important to avoid) are the trans-fatty acids of partially hydrogenated fats. These can be found in most margarines and in fast and processed foods. (*For more on types of fat and their effects on health, see p.34.*)

EXCESS CARBOHYDRATES Growing evidence suggests that the burgeoning rate of obesity in industrialized nations is fueled by excessive consumption of carbohydrates (starches and sugars). High-glycemic-index foods (*see chart, p.43*), which release sugar quickly into the blood, seem to be the most problematic. They cause the body to secrete large amounts of insulin, which encourages the conversion of sugar into fat. Studies show that high insulin secretion is associated with weight gain.

High blood-sugar levels also tend to indicate that the body is using carbohydrates (sugar) as its energy source instead of fat. Long-term studies in animals have shown that diets based on high-glycemic index starches are more likely to promote weight gain. In general, diets based on low-glycemic index foods may promote weight loss. Low-glycemic index starches contain more fiber and help control the

---

BURNING THE CALORIES

Choosing simple everyday activities rather than the labor-saving alternatives can make a big difference to your calorie balance (the difference between the number of calories you take in and burn off). The table below provides some everyday examples that compare the sedentary option with the more active, calorie-burning alternative. Try examining your lifestyle for possible changes.

SEDENTARY	KCAL	ACTIVE	KCAL
Driving to work (20 mins)	50	Biking to work (30 mins)	140
Taking the elevator up one floor	0.1	Walking up a flight of stairs	5
Using a car wash	10	Washing and waxing car by hand	300
Employing a gardener	0	Yardwork and mowing the lawn (30 minutes)	150
Employing a cleaner	0	Heavy housework, e.g. scrubbing floors (1 hour)	225
Sitting and waiting 30 minutes for pizza delivery	30	Cooking for 30 minutes	100
Letting the dog run around the yard (30 mins)	30	Taking dog for brisk 30-minute walk	125
Shopping online (1 hour)	90	Shopping in supermarket (1 hour)	200
Taking the bus (20 mins)	30	Walking, carrying shopping (30 mins)	120
Using remote control to change TV channel	0.1	Walking across room to change channel	3
Total calories expended:	**240.2**		**1368**

---

appetite, so that fewer daily calories are consumed. (*For more information about blood-sugar balance, see p.42.*)

SNACKING AND WEIGHT GAIN Most weight-loss regimens advise against eating between meals on the basis that this puts additional calories into the body. However, healthy snacking may help control your appetite and prevent overeating at meals, and may also help stabilize the body's levels of sugar and insulin. A 1964 study found that people eating six small meals instead of three normal-sized ones lost weight and had more stable levels of blood sugar.

Snacking may also reduce the appetite and the overall quantity of food eaten in a day. In a 1999 study, overweight men ate a large breakfast and then nothing for five hours. Another group ate the same food but it was divided into five hourly meals. At an "all you can eat" lunch, the men who had eaten regular hourly snacks ate a quarter less than the men who just had one large breakfast. The "snackers" also had more favorable insulin and blood sugar levels. A 1996 review on this subject concluded that healthy snacking has distinct benefits for weight loss.

OVERWEIGHT CHILDREN face major health problems. Research has shown that by addressing the problems of obesity and low fitness levels early in a child's life, a significant step can be taken toward reversing the negative trends of this potentially dangerous condition. It is not easy to help children change their eating habits. The extra few grams of fat deposited every day become the pounds that cause disability in the long term.

Homeopathy

There is little scientific evidence indicating that homeopathy helps in obesity, and it is no substitute for diet and lifestyle changes. However, some practitioners feel they can help, usually by prescribing the medicines *Calcarea carbonica* and *Graphites* (*see p.73*).

Exercise

PRIMARY TREATMENT There is some disagreement regarding the precise role of exercise. Some studies suggest that it helps reduce weight, while others say its chief benefit is to maintain (rather than to assist) weight loss. However, there is no doubt that regular exercise is important. If you are obese, exercise should not be extreme or prolonged, but brisk walking for half an hour a day will make a substantial difference to your well-being and should assist weight loss and maintenance. In a 2003 study, a combination of increased general exercise and an appropriate diet were shown to offer major health benefits. Weight loss, improved cardiorespiratory fitness, and reduced cholesterol levels were all maintained after the program for a period of six months.

PRIMARY TREATMENT **LIFESTYLE ACTIVITY** Studies indicate that incorporating more activity into your daily life could be even more beneficial than formal exercise sessions. A 1999 study examined the short- and long-term benefits produced by a low-fat diet of about 1,200 calories per day when it was combined with either structured aerobic exercising or moderate intensity lifestyle activities (for example, walking to stores instead of driving, performing more work outdoors, and using stairs instead of the elevator when possible). Changes in body weight, body composition, cardiovascular risk profiles, and physical fitness were assessed at 16 weeks and again at one year. Overall, those doing more lifestyle activity lost significantly more weight and managed to keep it off for longer compared to those doing

aerobic exercise. Cholesterol levels reduced significantly in both groups.

It is crucial to encourage overweight children to exercise regularly. Try to incorporate enjoyable activities and exercise, such as playing games or going swimming together, into the family routine.

OSTEOARTHRITIS Joints carrying excess weight are at an increased risk of developing osteoarthritis (*see p.289*). Research in 2000 showed that even relatively minor weight loss, combined with appropriate exercise, can decrease this risk, as well as the symptoms and progression of OA in people who already have the condition.

Acupuncture

Acupuncture over the stomach meridian point in the ear has been used to help suppress appetite. The treatment involves wearing a tiny "ear stud" that is left in place. Pressing it whenever you feel hungry can help control appetite. However, the four clinical trials that evaluated this approach indicated only marginal benefit. It is worthwhile persisting with acupuncture, for four to six weeks, but discontinue treatment if there is no apparent effect.

Mind–Body Therapies

BEHAVIOR MODIFICATION has traditionally been used for weight management, along with diet, exercise, nutritional education, and other techniques. Individual and/or group psychological treatment is often recommended, especially for people who are significantly obese.

Diet, exercise, and other strategies will often achieve some short-term weight loss but long-term weight management is not usually possible without tackling the factors that cause overeating in the first place. Most people struggle through the "yo-yo process" of repeatedly losing and gaining weight, becoming more frustrated each time. Weight-management treatments are often unsuccessful in the long run because they focus on reducing excessive and unhealthy eating instead of on understanding the forces that produce such behavior.

STRESS (*see p.408*) is one of the major forces that can negatively influence weight.

Stress and unsuccessful efforts to manage it have a "double whammy" effect. First, stress affects the body directly through hormonal changes that can have profound and negative effects on the body's metabolic systems, even influencing how and where fat is stored. Second, psychological stress and distress can affect weight indirectly by encouraging people to comfort eat and to avoid getting exercise.

Mind–body practices, such as autogenic training and visualization, can engage the full power of the mind to help you better manage your weight. Practicing yoga, relaxation breathing, or guided imagery (*for details, see p.100*) is recommended as part of an overall weight-loss plan. This is not to suggest that effective weight management is simply a case of "mind over matter," or that you can somehow magically lose weight by thinking or visualizing your fat cells melting away. However, when it comes to managing weight, there is a growing body of scientific research showing that the mind does matter.

STRESS EATING Studies have shown that continual high levels of stress may contribute to the tendency to accumulate fat, particularly in the abdominal region. Stress hormones, such as cortisol, are released, which alter the metabolic processes responsible for the proper utilization of fat. Research in 2000 also suggests that leptin, a neurotransmitter produced in fat cells and involved in regulating appetite, is also released. With plenty of cortisol and leptin circulating in the body, food intake is increased, a phenomenon scientists term "stress eating." Frequently, when individuals are under stress, they will eat to excess or consume high-calorie foods, triggering weight gain. Mind–body practices, used both at home and as part of a supervised weight-loss program, can reduce stress and enhance the ability to lose weight and maintain a lifelong desirable weight.

PREVENTION PLAN

The following may help prevent you from becoming obese:

- Eat a nutritious diet
- Get plenty of exercise

SLEEP DISORDERS

Adequate sleep is important for maintaining good health. If you sleep well, you wake up feeling refreshed and ready to deal with the day ahead; if you sleep badly on a regular basis, your ability to cope with life can suffer. Common sleep problems include difficulty falling asleep, waking up during the night or too early in the morning, and feeling tired during the day. Sometimes sleep disorders can be treated with simple lifestyle measures such as exercise and dietary changes. There is a range of therapies that may also help.

WHAT ARE THE SYMPTOMS?

Symptoms of insomnia include:
- Regular inability to fall asleep or to stay asleep
- Excessive fatigue

Symptoms of sleep apnea include:
- Breathing during sleep is interrupted for 10 seconds or more at least five times an hour
- Sleep is restless and not refreshing
- Loud snoring
- Sleepiness during the day
- Morning headaches

WHY MIGHT I HAVE THESE?

PREDISPOSING FACTORS

Insomnia:
- Stress
- Illness, such as asthma, that causes problems at night
- High intake of caffeine or alcohol
- Food sensitivity
- Blood-sugar instability

Sleep apnea:
- Being male, especially between 40 and 60 years of age
- Being overweight
- Drinking alcohol
- Smoking

TRIGGERS
- Depression and anxiety
- Emotional upset

IMPORTANT

If you think your sleeping problems may be associated with depression, see your doctor.

WHY DOES IT OCCUR?

Most people experience changes in their sleep patterns at some point in their lives. These may be due to, or made worse by, behavior associated with stress, such as drinking too much alcohol or working late into the night. Sleep disorders are caused by, and may contribute to, other problems, such as depression (see p.436), anxiety (see p.414), SAD (see p.432), and fibromyalgia (see p.298). In some cases, a sleep disorder is caused by an underlying medical disorder, such as an overactive thyroid gland (see p.319).

Sleepiness during the day may simply be a reflection of difficulty getting to sleep or difficulty staying asleep at night. In a few cases, it is caused by sleep apnea, a condition mainly affecting middle-aged men in which breathing is repeatedly interrupted during sleep. This is often due to the soft tissues of the throat relaxing and blocking the flow of air.

THE RIGHT AMOUNT OF SLEEP Adults generally should sleep for seven or eight hours each night. Teenagers need an hour or so more, whereas babies need as much as 16 hours a day. Pregnant women in their first trimester usually sleep for a few more hours a day than normal. Older people usually sleep less than younger adults. If you feel sleepy during the day, or fall asleep the moment your head hits the pillow, it is likely that you need more sleep.

TREATMENT PLAN

PRIMARY TREATMENTS
- Simple lifestyle measures (see Self-Help, right)
- Treatment of underlying disorders
- Caffeine withdrawal
- Blood-sugar stabilizing diet
- Valerian
- Behavioral therapy (for chronic insomnia)

BACKUP TREATMENTS
- Sleeping tablets
- Massage and exercise
- Bodywork and movement therapies
- Homeopathy
- Acupuncture
- Mind–body therapies
- Western herbal medicine

For an explanation of how treatments are rated, see p.111.

SELF-HELP

PRIMARY TREATMENT — If sleep eludes you, the following measures might help:
- Avoid drinking large amounts of tea, coffee, and cola after lunchtime.
- Give up smoking; nicotine is a stimulant that can keep you awake.
- Do not eat large meals late in the evening — you won't have time to digest them.
- Get plenty of regular exercise, preferably in the late afternoon so there is time to relax afterward.
- Go to bed at the same time each night and wind down first by listening to music or soaking in a warm bath.

- Add five drops of lavender oil to your evening bathwater or burn it in an aromatherapy vaporizer to scent the room.
- Avoid drinking alcohol.
- Keep your bedroom for sleeping rather than eating, watching TV, reading, etc.
- If you are unable to fall asleep, get up and do something rather than lie in bed awake and frustrated.
- Invest in heavy curtains if early morning light bothers you.
- Practice yoga eye exercises (*see p.451*).

TREATMENTS IN DETAIL

Conventional Medicine

Tackling problems that are worrying you may help you sleep better, as may following preventive advice (*see Self-Help, p.448*). Counseling may be appropriate to help resolve issues that are troubling you.

PRIMARY TREATMENT **TREATING AN UNDERLYING DISORDER** If sleeping problems are persistent, it may be worth seeing your doctor, who will discuss your symptoms with you to look for evidence of an underlying physical or psychological cause. Investigations may be arranged if necessary. For example, if sleep apnea is suspected, sleep studies may be performed, in which breathing, heart rate, and blood oxygen levels are monitored during sleep. Underlying conditions are then treated when possible.

SLEEPING TABLETS do not treat the cause of the sleep disorder but may be prescribed occasionally to help restore a normal sleep pattern. Benzodiazepines may be prescribed, but only on a short-term basis because they are associated with a high risk of dependence. When dependence occurs, patients find that increasing doses are needed to achieve the same effect while refraining from taking the drug causes withdrawal symptoms such as restlessness and severe anxiety.

Your doctor may prescribe other sleeping tablets, such as zopiclone and zolpidem. However, these drugs may also cause dependence when taken for too long and prolonged use is not recommended.

In elderly patients, sleep medications can cause accidental falls or respiratory depression. They can interact with other medications or alcohol, and can disrupt natural circadian rhythms. The next-day aftereffects of sleep medications can be similar to the effects of sleep deprivation itself. For these reasons, sleeping tablets are not recommended for the elderly.

OTHER DRUGS Over-the-counter drugs containing antihistamines are also available. When poor sleep is associated with depression (*see p.436*), antidepressants may help.

CAUTION

Sleeping pills (including ones bought over the counter) can affect the ability to drive and operate machinery. These effects can last until the next day and are made worse by drinking alcohol. Sleeping pills may cause other side effects; ask your doctor to explain these to you.

Nutritional Therapy

CAFFEINE Dietary factors can play an important part in determining the ability to fall asleep. A common cause of sleeplessness is caffeine, which has stimulant effects on the body. Studies have shown that coffee and tea drinkers are more likely to suffer from sleep disruption, an effect that is related to caffeine's ability to enhance arousal. The effects of caffeine can linger for up to 20 hours, so cutting it out or at least avoiding it after breakfast may be necessary to regularize sleep patterns.

FOOD SENSITIVITY/ALLERGY may also be an underlying problem in sleep disorders. Foods causing allergic reactions are known to increase the heart rate, which can cause or aggravate insomnia. Children and infants suffering from persistent sleeplessness may be intolerant to cow's milk. Studies show that exclusion of cow's milk from the diet may normalize sleep in some children. (*For more information on food sensitivity, see p.39.*)

STABILIZE BLOOD-SUGAR LEVELS Some people find that getting to sleep is not a problem but that they tend to wake up in the middle of the night. They often feel alert at this time and have difficulty getting back to sleep. In practice, this problem is related to a drop in blood-sugar level during the night. If the level falls, the body secretes certain hormones, notably epinephrine (which increases arousal), to correct this.

The secret to ensuring a good night's sleep for many people is to maintain a stable blood-sugar level throughout the night. An evening meal based on protein (meat, fish, eggs), vegetables, and a limited amount of starch should help. A snack of some fruit and/or nuts eaten an hour before bedtime seems to help maintain blood-sugar levels through the night, and therefore may help sleep. (*For more information about how to stabilize blood-sugar levels, see p.42.*)

TRYPTOPHAN SUPPLEMENTS Sleep is induced by the production of certain brain chemicals, including a substance called serotonin. In the body, serotonin is made from the amino acid tryptophan. Low levels of tryptophan in the body can lead to insomnia. Supplementing with 5-hydroxytryptophan (5HT), an intermediary in the production of serotonin from tryptophan, may help induce sleep and enable sleeping through the night. The normal recommended dose is 50mg of 5HT, taken an hour before bedtime. Malted milk products are high in tryptophan and may promote sleep.

CAUTION

Consult your doctor before taking 5-HTP with zolpidem, fluoxetine, paroxetine, venlafaxine, fluvoxamine or sumatriptan (*see p.46*).

Homeopathy

There are a number of homeopathic remedies available for sleep disorders. For the medicines described below, take two 6C pills twice a day. In addition, there are proprietary remedies available in the US. Avena sativa compound, made by Viable Herbal Solutions, has a similar composition, and comes in a capsule form. The usual dose is 5–10 drops in a little warm water. Take this solution about one hour before bed.

NUX VOMICA For insomnia, one of the most commonly suitable remedies is *Nux vomica*. The type of person this medicine helps typically wakes at 5 or 6 A.M. They may feel grouchy and "out of sorts," perhaps with a headache or indigestion.

COFFEA helps when the problem is difficulty falling sleep — often, there has been too much mental stimulation during the day and the person lies awake, too excited to sleep and with many thoughts spinning around their head.

KALIUM PHOSPHORICUM may help when the person is exhausted, "too tired to sleep," and woken by bad dreams.

CALCAREA CARBONICA is a medicine for bad dreams. Typically, the person it helps wakes up in a cold sweat from vivid, anxious dreams. There are often other constitutional features suggesting this medicine (*see Constitutional Medicines and Polychrests, p.73*).

KALIUM BROMATUM is another useful medicine for vivid, disturbing dreams that are often of a sexual nature. In addition to having sleep problems, the people whom *Kalium bromatum* helps often have acne and difficulty concentrating.

RHUS TOXICODENDRON AND LACHESIS Medicines for unrefreshing sleep include *Rhus tox.* and *Lachesis.* The former is suitable when the problem is restlessness — the person feels he or she has "tossed and turned all night." *Lachesis* patients may complain of "waking up feeling more tired than when they went to bed," or waking up feeling wretched, often with a headache on the left side of their head. These patients sometimes awake with a jerk, just as they are dropping off to sleep. There may also be constitutional features (*see p.73*).

NUX MOSCHATA is a useful medicine for attacks of overpowering drowsiness during the day. An unusual feature of the people who respond to this medicine is an extreme dryness of the mouth.

Western Herbal Medicine

Herbal medicines are used worldwide for sleep disorders and can be a safe, effective, and nonaddictive solution to the problem. An herbal approach is likely to work well in relieving or at least ameliorating temporary sleep disorders — the occasional disturbed night's sleep or short-term insomnia resulting from an emotional upset. They are less likely to help with entrenched sleep disorders but should still be tried for long-term problems.

Most sleep disorders involve difficulty getting to sleep, waking for variable lengths of time during the night, or early waking and an inability to return to sleep. Preparing for sleep by relaxing and unwinding beforehand is important.

> People who have sleep apnea may briefly wake hundreds of times every night

Most commonly available herbal remedies that aid sleep (*see below*) can be safely used at home. If self-medication proves ineffective, seek professional advice. An herbal practitioner will consider factors not directly linked to sleep, such as the state of the circulation, digestive, liver, and nervous systems, and prescribe appropriate remedies to treat the symptoms.

PRIMARY TREATMENT **VALERIAN** (*Valeriana officinalis*) has a long history of use for sleep disorders, proving especially useful when nervous overactivity and anxiety are factors. It has been fairly well researched and is extremely safe. Clinical studies indicate that extracts improve sleep quality and increase the time spent in deeper sleep. Drowsiness upon waking is not common but can occur, since people have different levels of sensitivity to the herb.

In one double-blind clinical trial, 44 percent of those taking valerian reported excellent sleep, while 89 percent reported improved sleep. Valerian combines well with St. John's wort (*Hypericum perforatum*) for sleep disturbance that is linked with depression (*see p.436*), which typically results in poor-quality sleep and early morning waking.

OTHER HERBAL REMEDIES that are commonly used to improve sleep include passionflower (*Passiflora incarnata*), Californian poppy (*Eschscholzia california*), scullcap (*Scutellaria lateriifolia*), and hops (*Humulus lupulus*). These and other sedative remedies are often combined in proprietary blends and are available in tablet and capsule form. For the best results, make sure you purchase quality herbs from reputable manufacturers.

Alternatively, you can make an infusion of one of the following and drink a cup before retiring. Chamomile (*Matricaria recutita*) is a gentle, relaxing, and antispasmodic herb, which is helpful when tension is a factor. It is a traditional remedy for nightmares and is valuable for children with disturbed sleep. Lemon verbena (*Lippia citriodora*) is pleasant tasting and mildly sedative. Linden flower (*Tilea cordata*) is a mild sedative that helps when anxiety is a factor. If required, these herbs may also be taken during the night, since they are mild-acting and the exact dosage is not critical.

CAUTION

See p. 69 before taking an herbal remedy and, if you are already taking prescribed medication, consult an herbal medical expert first. Do not take St. John's wort with antidepressants, digoxin, cyclosporine, warfarin, antibiotics, birth control pills, or any medication that is taken daily (*see p.46*).

Bodywork and Movement Therapies

MASSAGE may help restore normal sleep patterns. Studies have shown a benefit of massage therapy in improving disturbed sleep patterns in those who have chronic migraines (*see p.119*) and those with fibromyalgia (*see p.298*).

When sleep is disturbed as part of a serious illness, acupressure in combination with massage has been shown to be helpful — for example, in one study it helped people with kidney disease who were receiving regular dialysis.

MODERATE EXERCISE or physical activity may be useful for those with sleep disorders. Regular exercise is important.

EYE EXERCISES

These yoga eye exercises will keep your eye muscles strong and active and will also help you sleep. In each case, do not move your head, only your eyes. Close and relax your eyes for about 30 seconds before moving on to the next exercise.

Exercising your eye muscles

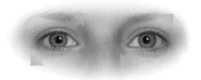

3. Move the eyes diagonally 10–15 times one way, then the other.

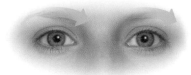

4. Move the eyes in a 180-degree arc looking upward 10–15 times.

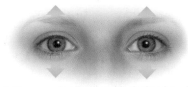

1. Keep your head still and look ahead. Look up and then down 10–15 times.

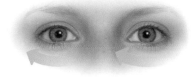

5. Finally move the eyes in a 180-degree arc looking downward 10–15 times.

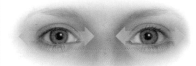

2. Look left and right as far as possible. Repeat 10–15 times.

YOGA EYE EXERCISES Traditional Hatha yoga eye movement exercises can effectively induce a sense of relaxation to help you fall asleep. The eye exercises consist of "drawing" a vertical line, with the head held still, for 10 or 15 repetitions, by moving the eyes up and down as far as they will go (*see illustration, above*).

The procedure is repeated making a horizontal line (side to side), and then two diagonal lines, relaxing the eyes in their normal posture in between exercises. After the linear exercises, make two 180 degree arcs, upper and lower, making a clockwise and then a counterclockwise circle. In studies, 90 percent of individuals report sleep to be rapidly approaching by the time the latter part of the exercise is performed.

YOGA MEDITATION Practicing yoga meditation may help insomnia. A study in 2000 showed that people who regularly practiced yoga meditation experienced an increase in melatonin levels. Melatonin assists in normalizing sleep patterns.

CHIROPRACTIC AND OSTEOPATHY Some reports suggest that chiropractic and osteopathy may treat sleep disorders, if the cause lies in disturbed mechanics of the spine having an adverse effect on the nervous system. For example, a case report discussed the effectiveness of spinal adjustment in the relief of poor sleeping patterns (and disturbed behavior) of a 12-month-old toddler.

Acupuncture

Acupuncture has been widely used in the treatment of insomnia and other sleep disorders, although there are only a small number of clinical trials for these specific conditions. First, it is necessary to visit a traditional Chinese doctor for a diagnosis (*see p.81*), and then therapy and treatment may be needed over a prolonged period. Acupuncture can give immediate relief from sleep disorders and may have a long-term beneficial effect, making it a useful means of prevention.

Treatment should initially be given on a weekly basis, and some improvement should be observed after six to eight sessions of acupuncture. If this is effective, then long-term maintenance treatments may be required to prevent the insomnia from returning.

Mind–Body Therapies

There are three types of clinical sleep disturbance. In the first, there is a "sleep latency period" of greater than 30 minutes, i.e., it takes 30 minutes to fall asleep. In the second, the person wakes up after 30 or more minutes of sleep. The third involves waking earlier than desired over a period of 30 or more days. This is accompanied by feelings of fatigue and drowsiness during the day.

Although certain medical conditions need to be ruled out, long-term insomnia is most commonly behavioral or psychophysiological. Temporary sleeplessness during stressful life events is usually the result of anxiety (*see p.414*) and must be treated accordingly.

Insomniacs tend to have higher than normal levels of anxiety and depression, low self-efficacy (when a person feels unable to influence or control their behavior or the course of daily events), and high performance anxiety — all of which can be either a cause or an effect of sleeplessness. Hormonal changes and drug use, including prescription drugs, cigarettes, and alcohol, can also cause insomnia.

PRIMARY TREATMENT **BEHAVIORAL THERAPY** is reputably the most effective long-term approach to chronic insomnia, in both general and specific groups. The main categories of behavior therapy for insomnia are stimulus control (using a bed only for sleeping), a sleep hygiene program (advice to help you sleep), keeping a sleep log, cognitive control (turning off the "racing" mind), and progressive relaxation. These methods are often combined.

RELAXATION has been found to reduce sleep-onset insomnia (not being able to fall asleep), with or without stimulus control measures. Effects are better when the two are combined. Guided imagery programs combine progressive relaxation with pleasant suggestions for cognitive control, turning off the "racing mind" that characterizes much chronic insomnia.

Practicing relaxation skills can help individuals of all ages cope with chronic insomnia, although effects will be stronger if lifestyle changes are also followed (*for a detailed relaxation and guided imagery sequence, see p.100*).

STUTTERING

Stuttering is a disorder that interferes with the continuous flow of speech. It is a common problem — about one percent of the adult population is affected. Stuttering usually emerges at a young age, when a child is first developing language. It varies between individuals, but is often characterized by the repetition of sounds, pausing, and lengthening of words that are different from normal fluid speech. Speech and language therapy aims to build self-confidence, nurture social skills, improve communication, and develop fluency control.

WHY DOES IT OCCUR?

There is no single reason why a person stutters, but given that speech is a complex process involving 37 muscles and thousands of nerves, it is not surprising that sometimes there is a problem.

Each stutterer is different and the disorder seems to be caused by a combination of many factors. Having a close relative with a speech disorder increases the risk of a person developing a stutter and the condition is much more prevalent in men and boys. Emotional stress in childhood may be a factor in some people. Stuttering is often made worse by stress, fatigue, or particular situations.

DEVELOPING A STUTTER The disorder usually starts in early childhood (between two and six years of age), when it may not cause much concern to the child. In fact, it can be difficult to spot because as they learn to speak, all young children naturally pause and repeat sounds or words.

Between eight and twelve years, stuttering may start to cause concern. In adolescence and adulthood, the speech disorder and lack of fluency can cause considerable frustration and embarrassment, and usually affects self-confidence.

THE PROCESS OF SPEAKING seems to involve a "planning" and an "articulation" stage, which need to be synchronized to be effective. If a significant gap develops between these two stages, or the timing of the synchrony is disrupted, stuttering may result. One theory suggests that too much self-monitoring is a factor. Stutterers may find themselves caught in a vicious circle — they feel self-conscious and worried about making mistakes which in turn causes stuttering.

IMAGING THE BRAIN Research with techniques such as transcranial magnetic stimulation (TMS) reveal there may be a "neurologic switch" in the brain that affects how we monitor speech. The fact that the presence of people activates some mechanism that makes stutterers stumble over words seems to support this. PET (positron emission tomography) scans reveal that people who stutter may be using the wrong side of their brains when they try to speak. It seems as though the right hemisphere is interfering with the left hemisphere, which is usually more active in the production of speech. During times when stutterers are fluent, their PET scans appear to show similarities with those of people who do not stutter.

TREATMENT PLAN

PRIMARY TREATMENT

- Self-help measures (see *Helping your Child, p.453*)
- Speech and language therapy

BACKUP TREATMENTS

- Psychological therapies

WORTH CONSIDERING

- Homeopathy
- Relaxation and breathing

For an explanation of how treatments are rated, see p.111.

PRIMARY TREATMENT Speech therapists recommend the following:

- Encourage everyone in the family to take turns talking. If a young child is constantly interrupted by older siblings, he or she may not be getting enough practice speaking.
- Give your child your full attention: make eye contact and speak slowly.
- Play with your child and make plenty of time to talk together.
- Listen carefully and respond positively to what your child says instead of criticizing how he or she says it.
- Give your child the opportunity to speak voluntarily instead of repeatedly asking him or her questions.
- Develop a daily routine and make family life at home as calm as possible. Try to avoid making your child feel rushed and under pressure.
- Praise your child for things he or she does well in order to build up his or her self-confidence.

Conventional Medicine

If a child is stuttering that is causing distress or concern to the child or to the parents, a doctor can refer them to a speech and language therapist. Older children and adults who stutter should also consult speech and language therapists.

PRIMARY TREATMENT **SPEECH AND LANGUAGE THERAPY** Therapists talk and play with a child in order to assess his or her speech. They also watch to see how parents and other caregivers interact with the child. They will offer advice and support to parents on the types of measures that help prevent stuttering.

When treating an older child or an adult, therapists take a more holistic approach, looking not only at the speech itself, but also at how the stuttering is affecting the individual's life. The subsequent treatment focuses on building up self-confidence and developing social skills as well as finding ways of coping with the stutter. Treatment may be given on an individual basis or in groups and there are various techniques that are taught to the stutterer, such as slowing down the rate of speech and paying particular attention to breathing patterns.

Speech and language therapy has a high success rate if provided when someone who stutters is young. In teenagers and adults, the problem is more complex to treat because the stuttering is now likely to be inextricably linked with the feelings it has caused, such as a lack of self-confidence. However, in many cases progress can still be made.

Homeopathy

Some homeopathic medicines, such as *Stramonium*, *Hyoscyamus*, *Agaricus muscarius*, and *Zincum metallicum*, are said to help with stuttering. You may need to consult an experienced homeopath before beginning treatment.

STRAMONIUM is suitable for excitable children who flail their limbs when they try to get words out, and may have night terrors.

HYOSCYAMUS may be used for excitable children who try to talk too fast and "trip over their words."

AGARICUS MUSCARIUS AND ZINCUM METALLICUM are both suitable for people whose stuttering is associated with twitchiness. People who respond to *Agaricus muscarius* may have facial twitching or twitches in other parts of their body, and suffer from itchy chilblains. People who respond to *Zincum metallicum* may have fidgety, restless legs.

CAUSTICUM, LYCOPODIUM, AND SULPHUR may help adults and children when prescribed on a constitutional basis (*see p.73*).

Relaxation and Breathing

Breathing patterns are inextricably linked with speech. Speech and language therapists teach deep breathing techniques as part of their treatment, but in addition individuals striving for long-term speech fluency may benefit from relaxation and diaphragmatic breathing. Both of these methods may help reduce anxiety when practiced correctly (*see pp.62, 98, and 99*).

Psychological Therapies

Speaking problems can have significant social and psychosocial consequences. As a result, talking therapies need to treat the effect of stuttering on self-image and self-esteem as well as the process of stuttering itself. Therapists may use one or a combination of the following therapies.

HUMANISTIC THERAPIES emphasize the importance of the therapeutic relationship rather than technical expertise of the therapist (*see p.107*). The client-centered approach focuses on giving the patient who stutters the space to provide their own solutions to their difficulties.

Gestalt therapy (*see p.102*) may be combined with a 12-step approach similar to that used in recovery from substance use (*see p.428*). The emphasis is on achieving three essential stages of recovery — awareness of the process of stuttering, acceptance of the problem, and change.

HYPNOSIS has had some positive results and is used to help the person who stutters relax and increase his or her self-esteem, as well as attempt to address the stuttering directly. Hypnosis has also been used successfully in conjunction with other therapies, such as rational emotive behavior therapy (*see p.103*).

COGNITIVE BEHAVIORAL THERAPY is probably the most widely used and most researched form of psychological therapy for stuttering. CBT focuses on stutterers' beliefs about themselves, their ability to speak fluently, and other people's reactions to their stuttering. It also aims to help patients reassess their perception of themselves as potential fluent speakers, and to overcome any critical and judgmental notions that can inhibit change.

> **Two-thirds of children grow out of stuttering by the time they reach adulthood**

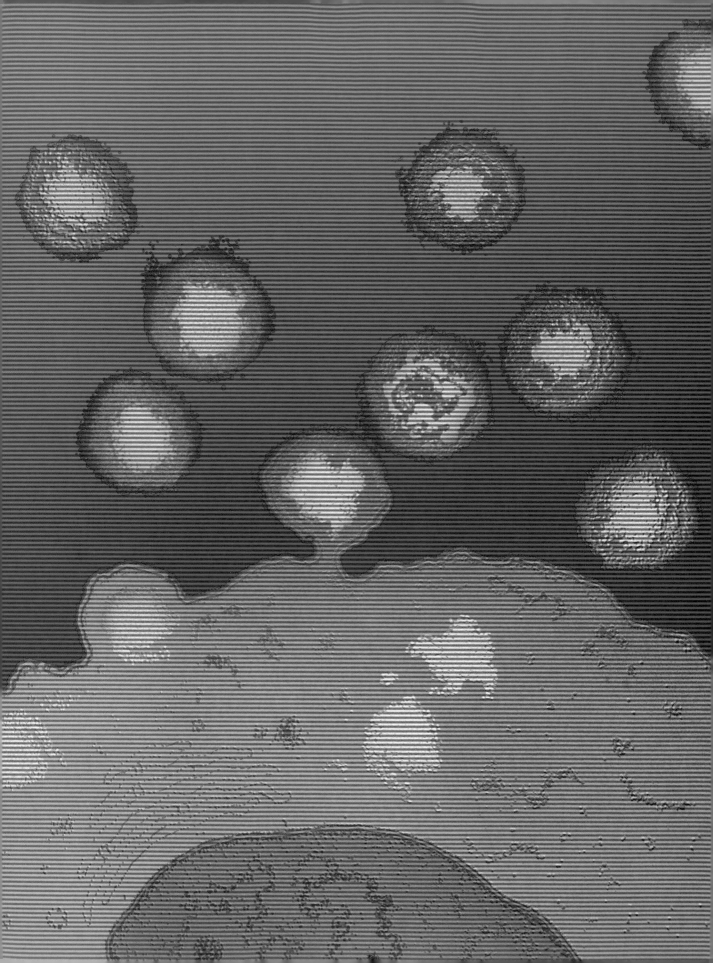

Allergies & Systemic Disorders

The holistic nature of integrated medicine is
particularly appropriate for conditions that affect
the whole body. Allergies can often be controlled
through diet, and for chronic illnesses, the
alternative treatments such as acupuncture,
homeopathy, herbs, and talking therapies can
ease symptoms and offer enhanced emotional
stability, support, and a sense of control.

WHAT ARE THE SYMPTOMS OF FOOD ALLERGIES?

Symptoms occur almost immediately

- Iching and swelling of the lips, mouth, and throat
- Itchy red rash (*see Urticaria, p.176*)
- Shortness of breath and wheezing

WHAT ARE THE SYMPTOMS OF FOOD INTOLERANCES?

Symptoms usually occur a few hours after eating the food

Lactose intolerance

- Stomach cramps
- Bloating and gas
- Diarrhea

Amine intolerance

- Irritation of the skin, mouth, stomach, and intestinal tract
- Hives
- Mouth ulcers
- Nausea and stomach cramps
- Diarrhea
- Headaches

WHY MIGHT I HAVE THIS?

PREDISPOSING FACTORS

- For food allergies, having other atopic conditions, such as asthma (*see p.205*)
- Temporary lactose intolerance may follow gastroenteritis
- Genetic predisposition

FOOD ALLERGIES AND INTOLERANCES

True food allergy can be very dangerous. When it occurs, the immune system reacts instantly to the food, forming immunoglobulin E (IgE) antibodies that may cause the skin and the mucous membranes to swell. In a severe reaction, blood pressure may suddenly drop, causing anaphylactic shock. Food intolerances are more common and are not true allergies; intolerances do not involve an immune response. Symptoms occur after eating certain foods, but these are never acute or severe. In both cases, identifying and avoiding problem foods is essential.

WHY DOES IT OCCUR?

FOOD ALLERGIES The symptoms of food allergies are caused by an abnormal or exaggerated immunological response to one or more proteins in a particular food. Food allergies generally develop in infancy rather than later in life and various theories have been put forward to explain why this happens. It has been suggested that babies have a less mature immune system and that their stomachs produce fewer acidic juices, allowing more proteins to reach the small intestine and trigger allergic responses. Most food allergies tend to disappear in early childhood, but some, such as peanut allergy, may be lifelong.

Food allergies are more common in children who are affected by other allergy-related conditions, such as asthma (*see p.205*) and eczema (*see p.167*). Relatively few foods are responsible for the majority of allergic reactions. Common allergenic foods include cow's milk, eggs, peanuts, nuts, fish, and shellfish.

FOOD INTOLERANCES may have a variety of causes, including a lack of certain chemicals in the body. One example of this is lactose intolerance. It is caused by insufficient amounts of the enzyme lactase, which is needed to break down the milk sugar lactose. Lactose intolerance is common in people of African, Caribbean, Asian, and Mediterranean descent. Also, as people grow older they produce less lactase and, as a result, they may be more likely to develop lactose intolerance. Diarrhea can also cause temporary lactose intolerance.

Amines (found in bananas, tomatoes, oranges, avocados, mushrooms, wine, and Parmesan cheese) can cause intolerances, as can the chemical MSG, an additive in canned soups, frozen meals, and Chinese

TREATMENT PLAN

PRIMARY TREATMENTS

- Avoiding allergenic or sensitive foods
- Drugs

BACKUP TREATMENTS

- Osteopathy and chiropractic
- Massage and reflexology

WORTH CONSIDERING

- Homeopathy
- Acupuncture

For an explanation of how treatments are rated, see p.111.

IMPORTANT

If someone with a known food allergy develops swelling in the lips or face, or difficulty breathing, administer adrenaline using an Epipen in the thigh and call for an ambulance. If no Epipen is available, call for an ambulance immediately.

HOW FOOD SENSITIVITY MIGHT ARISE

One theory concerning the development of food sensitivity concentrates on the permeability of the intestinal lining. Some researchers believe that if the intestinal lining is more permeable than normal, it allows incompletely digested food proteins to be absorbed into the bloodstream, where the immune system reacts to them and becomes sensitized to them. According to the "leaky gut" theory, this then gives rise to an allergic reaction whenever the food concerned is eaten. The theory has yet to be widely accepted.

Absorption of food in the intestine

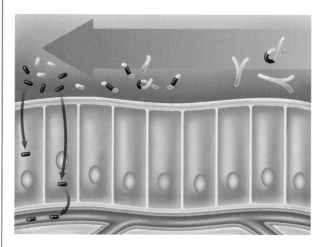
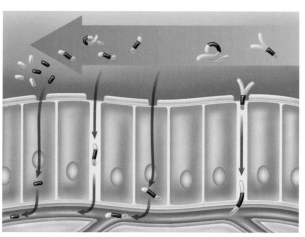

Food particles, represented here by colored shapes, are broken down as digestion progresses (*arrow*). When they are small enough, they pass through the intestinal wall and into the bloodstream.

The "leaky gut" theory states that if the intestinal wall becomes more permeable than normal, it allows incompletely digested food proteins to enter the bloodstream, provoking an immune response.

---

food. Intolerance of gluten, which is found in wheat products, is known as celiac disease and is another form of severe food intolerance.

TREATMENTS IN DETAIL

Conventional Medicine

DIAGNOSING FOOD ALLERGY To investigate the possibility of food allergy, the doctor will first take a careful history to determine what the offending food might be and whether the time between eating the food and the onset of symptoms suggests an allergic response. Possible investigations include skin-prick tests, in which diluted solutions are made from foods. A drop of a each solution is put on the skin, which is pricked with a needle; the skin is then monitored for a reaction. These tests are not always reliable because a significant number of people who test positive to a certain food will not have allergic symptoms when they eat that food. However, negative results are more reliable and virtually rule out the possibility of an allergy to the food tested.

In some cases of suspected food allergy, blood samples are taken and antibody levels to certain proteins measured. Known as RAST tests, these investigations are less reliable than skin tests. If a skin test or a RAST test for a particular food is positive and the diagnosis is backed up by the symptoms described, the food should be tested using a double-blind food challenge. In this test, responses to the food and to a placebo are monitored. These are presented so that neither the patient nor the investigator knows which is which.

DIAGNOSING FOOD INTOLERANCE There is no specific group of tests to investigate food intolerance apart from testing for gluten and lactose intolerance. Often, the diagnosis is made from a description of symptoms. In certain cases, such as lactose intolerance, testing may be appropriate.

PRIMARY TREATMENT | **TREATMENT FOR FOOD INTOLERANCE AND ALLERGY** The aim of treatment for both food allergies and food intolerances is to avoid the offending food. Difficulty breathing, or swelling of the mouth, face, or whole body, is an emergency situation that must be treated immediately with injected epinephrine (adrenaline). Self-injecting devices called Epipens should be carried all the time by anyone with severe allergies; this treatment can be lifesaving.

Nutritional Therapy

Food intolerances are more likely to occur when the mucous membrane lining the intestines becomes excessively permeable, allowing large food-derived molecules and breakdown products to pass from the intestines into the bloodstream and trigger intolerance responses. This is known as the "leaky gut" hypothesis.

Many food intolerance reactions of this nature are thought to be mediated by the immune system, although not through the production of IgE antibodies (as occurs in true allergic reactions). Certain nonimmune mechanisms may also be involved.

PRIMARY TREATMENT | **ELIMINATION DIET** There are many tests that can be used to identify sensitive foods (*see p.39*). However, the elimination diet is regarded by many practitioners of nutritional medicine as the most accurate way of testing for food intolerance. In this approach, all likely problem foods are removed from the diet for several weeks. Symptoms may initially worsen, but an improvement is usually seen and foods are added back into the diet, one at a time. A note is made of which foods cause a recurrence of the symptoms. (*See p.39 for further details of elimination diets.*)

Improving digestive capacity can help reduce food intolerance because more complete digestion of food ensures that it is not absorbed in a partially digested form. (*See p.39 for ways to improve digestion.*)

LACTOSE INTOLERANCE Lactase pills are available for those who are lactose intolerant, to be taken with lactose-containing food. People who are lactose-intolerant may be able to tolerate yogurt and some cheeses, in which the lactose has been broken down. Lactase-treated liquid milk is also available.

Homeopathy

Homeopathy is often helpful for children who are intolerant of cow's milk protein (this is not the same as lactose intolerance, in which the body cannot digest the milk sugar lactose). The most commonly appropriate medicines are *Silica, Calcarea carbonica, Magnesia carbonica*, and *Natrum*

SILICA AND CALCAREA CARBONICA In children who respond to *Silica* and *Calcarea carbonica*, milk often causes vomiting. Children who respond to *Silica* tend to be small and wiry, with fine hair and delicate skin. Appearances may be deceptive because they can be quite determined and stubborn.

By contrast, children who respond to *Calcarea carbonica* are often big and chubby, and they may sweat from their heads at night. They are often stubborn, and may have various fears that cause them to wake at night, crying and frightened. Another key feature of these children is that they love eggs.

NATRUM CARBONICUM AND MAGNESIA CARBONICA In children who respond to *Natrum carbonicum* and *Magnesia carbonica*, the problem is more likely to be diarrhea. Features that suggest *Natrum carbonicum* include nasal congestion and symptoms such as headaches brought on by the sun. Symptoms that suggest *Magnesia carbonica* include abdominal swelling and diarrhea that resembles frog spawn. An affected baby may also have a sour smell.

Bodywork Therapies

MASSAGE AND REFLEXOLOGY If you think that emotional factors may play a part in your food intolerance, regular massage or reflexology sessions may help.

aggravated by a number of structural factors, including spinal restrictions, which cause the nerves supplying the digestive organs to become "irritable."

Clinical experience suggests that another structural factor that can contribute to digestive dysfunction is the presence of trigger points (particularly sensitive areas) in the muscles of the abdominal wall. Bodywork practitioners believe that these can influence the underlying digestive organs, such as the stomach and pancreas, and reduce their secretion of digestive juices. This in turn has an impact on how well the body is able to digest food.

Osteopathic, chiropractic, and soft-tissue manipulation methods can help treat both spinal restrictions and trigger points. If you have long-standing food intolerances, visiting a practitioner may be worthwhile.

Acupuncture

Acupuncture does not cure food intolerance, but it can help relieve many of the symptoms caused by it.

Food intolerance is usually associated with a specific traditional Chinese diagnosis called "damp heat" that involves the lung, large intestine, spleen, and stomach, as well as the liver and gallbladder meridians. Treating these organs with repeated acupuncture, based on a traditional Chinese diagnosis, can help relieve many symptoms caused by food intolerance.

Acupuncture may sometimes strengthen an individual's constitution, and as such should be given on a weekly basis for eight or ten weeks, before deciding whether it is effective or not.

> Food intolerance may cause discomfort but it is never life-threatening, unlike a food allergy

carbonicum. In order to get a correct diagnosis it is best to take your child to a homeopath. If sensitive children continue to drink milk, other problems may develop, including runny nose, asthma, and skin rashes.

Homeopathic pills usually include lactose, which theoretically might cause problems if you are lactose intolerant. However, the amount of lactose is very small and is unlikely to cause trouble. If there is a problem, homeopathic medicines made from sucrose pills or in liquid form can be obtained.

Sustained negative emotions, such as anxiety, anger, and fear, influence the intestinal tract and lead to the increased likelihood of intestinal permeability and intolerance reactions. Numerous studies have shown that massage and reflexology can reduce stress levels and thereby improve the function of the digestive tract.

OSTEOPATHY AND CHIROPRACTIC Food intolerances may be related to incomplete breakdown of food, which can result from inadequate production of digestive enzymes and acids. This can be caused or

PREVENTION PLAN

The following measures may help prevent your child from developing food sensitivities:

- Breast-feed your baby exclusively for the first six months. If possible, avoid giving formula or introducing solid food before six months

- When introducing solids, begin with only rice-based foods. Do not give milk (as a drink) until after the first year, or nut products until three years

ALLERGIC RHINITIS

In allergic rhinitis, the membrane lining the nose becomes irritated and inflamed due to an allergic reaction when certain airborne substances are inhaled. Some people are affected only at a particular time of year (this is seasonal allergic rhinitis or hay fever), while others have it throughout the year (perennial allergic rhinitis). The first line of defense against allergic rhinitis is identifying and avoiding allergens. Once this has been done, other measures including drugs, herbs, dietary changes, and homeopathy may help relieve symptoms.

WHAT ARE THE SYMPTOMS?

- Itching sensation in the nose
- Frequent sneezing
- Blocked, runny nose
- Itchy, red, watery eyes
- Headaches
- Nosebleeds, if nasal lining becomes very inflamed

WHY MIGHT I HAVE THIS?

PREDISPOSING FACTORS

- Genetic tendency
- Food sensitivities (*see p.456*)

TRIGGERS

- Exposure to allergens, such as dust mites or pollen

TREATMENT PLAN

PRIMARY TREATMENTS

- Lifestyle changes
- Drugs
- Dietary changes

BACKUP TREATMENTS

- Nutritional supplements
- Western herbal medicine

WORTH CONSIDERING

- Hydrotherapy
- Massage
- Cranial manipulation
- Breathing retraining
- Acupuncture
- Homeopathy

For an explanation of how treatments are rated, see p.111.

WHY DOES IT OCCUR?

When a trigger substance is inhaled, specialized immune cells, called mast cells, release histamine, a chemical that triggers inflammation and the other symptoms of allergic rhinitis.

Seasonal allergic rhinitis, commonly called hay fever, is usually due to pollen from grass, trees, flowers, or weeds. In contrast, perennial allergic rhinitis may be caused by dust mites, animal dander, feathers, and mold spores.

It is important to confirm with your doctor that your symptoms are truly due to an allergy. Often, people with non-allergic rhinitis are misdiagnosed, since they experience the same runny nose, nasal congestion, sneezing, and watery eyes that someone with allergic rhinitis experiences. In these cases rhinitis may be due to a viral infection instead of an allergy.

Several factors may influence allergic rhinitis. For instance, food sensitivity seems to be a common component of allergies in people who also have hay fever.

Some practitioners believe that shallow breathing using just the upper chest may also be a factor, because it causes the blood to become too alkaline and makes histamine levels in the body rise. This makes allergic responses such as rhinitis more likely. Other practitioners believe that trigger-point activity in the muscles of the face may make rhinitis symptoms worse by altering mucous secretion from mucous membranes in the nose and sinuses.

Both seasonal and perennial allergic rhinitis are more common in people who have other conditions with an allergic component, such as asthma. Both types of allergic rhinitis may run in families, suggesting that genetic factors may play a role in their onset, which commonly occurs in a person's mid-twenties.

SELF-HELP

PRIMARY TREATMENT Once you have identified the triggers for your allergic rhinitis, you can take appropriate steps to avoid them. For perennial allergic rhinitis try the following:
- Avoid furry animals if you are allergic.
- Only use pillows containing synthetic stuffing and cover pillows and mattresses with nonallergenic fabric.
- Have bare wood floors instead of carpet, particularly in the bedroom, and wash the floor often.

For seasonal allergic rhinitis:
- In summer, avoid going outside before 10am (when the pollen count is at its highest).
- Keep doors and windows closed at night when possible.
- Wear dark glasses outside to help prevent eye irritation.

(*See also Environmental Health, p.462*)

TREATMENTS IN DETAIL

Conventional Medicine

PRIMARY TREATMENT Your doctor will take a careful history to identify possible allergens. Skin-prick tests may be arranged to help identify allergens. In these tests, small amounts of allergens are applied to the skin to see if there is a reaction.

Specific allergens should be avoided as much as possible, but clearly it is not always practical to avoid some triggers, for example, pollen.

HOW ALLERGIC REACTIONS OCCUR

In an allergic reaction, the immune system responds inappropriately to a substance that normally would cause no reaction at all. After the first exposure to the substance, the immune system becomes sensitized and produces antibodies against it. Further exposure to the substance then causes an allergic reaction, in which the antibodies bind to specialized immune cells known as mast cells. The allergens link the antibodies and destroy the mast cells, which release a substance called histamine. Histamine causes an inflammatory response in the body and is responsible for the symptoms associated with allergy, such as sneezing, a runny nose, and itchy, watery eyes. Antihistamine drugs work by blocking histamine receptor sites on tissue cells, preventing histamine from attaching to them.

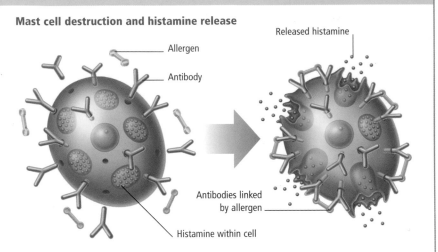

Mast cell destruction and histamine release

Released histamine

Allergen

Antibody

Antibodies linked by allergen

Histamine within cell

Repeated exposure to an allergen causes antibodies that were previously produced in response to it to bind to the surface of mast cells, which contain histamine.

The allergens bind to and link the antibodies, which causes the cell to burst and release the histamine that it contains. Histamine causes inflammation in the body.

PRIMARY TREATMENT **DRUGS** Various treatments help relieve the symptoms of allergic rhinitis. Oral and topical antihistamines (applied locally) can be bought over the counter. You should bear in mind that topical treatments may irritate the lining of the nose.

Your doctor may prescribe anti-inflammatory drugs, decongestants, or corticosteroids. Sodium chromoglycate is one example of an anti-inflammatory drug that is available to treat allergies. Decongestants, such as xylometazoline, are available as drops to relieve nasal blockage. However, don't use decongestants for more than a week, or symptoms may worsen when the drug is stopped — what is known as the rebound effect. Low-dose corticosteroids can be applied to the lining of the nose as a spray or drops. Small amounts of corticosteroid may be absorbed into the bloodstream but are unlikely to cause side effects unless use is excessive or prolonged. If symptoms persist, a short course of oral corticosteroids may be prescribed.

CAUTION

Drugs for allergic rhinitis can cause a range of possible side effects; ask your doctor to explain these to you.

Nutritional Therapy

PRIMARY TREATMENT **FOOD ELIMINATION DIET** A diet that excludes common problem foods has been shown to help some people with allergic rhinitis. While the effect of such a diet on allergic rhinitis symptoms has not been studied specifically, identification and elimination of problem foods often seems to help control symptoms. Dairy products are renowned for their ability to stimulate mucous formation and experience shows that eliminating them from the diet is often beneficial. *(For more information about food sensitivities, see p.456).*

VITAMIN C The chemical histamine triggers the body's allergic response. Vitamin C has a mild antihistamine effect and has been used to control hay fever symptoms and symptoms of perennial allergic rhinitis. If you have allergic rhinitis, take 1g of vitamin C two to three times a day while symptoms persist.

QUERCETIN Another useful natural agent for the treatment of hay fever and allergic rhinitis is quercetin. Quercetin seems to have the ability to reduce the release of histamine from mast cells and has been used for alleviating symptoms of both seasonal allergic rhinitis and perennial allergic rhinitis. If you have allergic rhinitis, try taking 400mg of quercitin two or three times a day.

Homeopathy

There is strong evidence that several homeopathic approaches to hay fever are successful. These include isopathy, in which hay fever is treated with homeopathic dilutions of pollen, and the homeopathic medicine *Galphimia glauca.* There are also studies indicating that homeopathic complexes are effective.

ISOPATHY In clinical trials conducted by Dr. David Reilly of the Glasgow Homeopathic Hospital, *Mixed Grass Pollen* 30C had a beneficial effect on the symptoms of allergic rhinitis.

COMPLEX HOMEOPATHY involves taking a combination of homeopathic medicines that are likely to be beneficial. It is often the most practical form of homeopathy for simple self-treatment. Many homeopathic treatment sources offer an allergy-relief pill containing *Allium,* *Euphrasia,* and *Sabadilla* in combination with other medicines. These pills can bring fast relief when nasal congestion is due to allergy. However, chronic or recurrent allergies may necessitate visiting an expert for individualized treatment with medicines such as *Arsenicum album*, *Arsenicum iodatum*, or *Sulphur*.

Western Herbal Medicine

Allergic rhinitis often responds well to herbal treatment. Appropriate herbs can reduce the severity of symptoms even in those who have had allergic rhinitis for a long time. An herbal medicine expert will assess the state of the mucous membranes, digestive system, and immune function. You may be advised to avoid sugar and dairy products, which can exacerbate symptoms. The practitioner will consider emotional factors, including anxiety and depression, which can exacerbate allergic conditions and may need to be treated with herbs or other therapies. A practitioner will combine herbs according to your specific needs.

EYEBRIGHT (*Euphrasia officinalis*) **AND PLANTAIN** (*Plantago major*) are often prescribed to strengthen mucous membranes and relieve irritability and inflammation. Eyebright is an astringent, tonic herb which helps dry up excessive watery secretions. Plantain, which is rich in a soothing substance called mucilage, can soothe sore, dry mucous membranes. Both can also help relieve sneezing. Pharmacological research into these herbs suggests that they have significant anti-inflammatory, antioxidant, and immune-modulating effects.

ELDERFLOWER (*Sambucus nigra*) **AND ECHINACEA** (*Echinacea* spp.) are both thought to have a direct antiviral action. Elderflower is given to treat chronic upper respiratory infection and echinacea is given to restore normal immune function.

NETTLE, GINKGO (*Ginkgo biloba*), **AND GERMAN CHAMOMILE** (*Matricaria recutita*) help reduce the allergic tendency. They have antiallergenic, antihistamine, and anti-inflammatory actions. A 1990 placebo-controlled clinical trial involving 69 patients investigated nettle as a treatment for allergic rhinitis. It was found to be "moderately effective" by 58 percent of those taking it, compared to 37 percent in the placebo group. The anti-inflammatory effects of both ginkgo and chamomile have been established in numerous studies.

MILK THISTLE (*Silybum maritum*) **AND DANDELION** (*Taxacum officale*) may also be recommended by herbalists.

> **CAUTION**
>
> See p.69 before taking a herbal remedy and, if you are taking prescribed medication, consult a herbal medicine expert first.

Bodywork Therapies

TRIGGER-POINT DEACTIVATION AND MASSAGE Trigger points (sensitive areas) in certain muscles of the face can increase secretions from the mucous membranes lining the nose and sinuses. Trigger points can be deactivated by acupuncture, as well as by manual pressure and stretching techniques such as those used by osteopaths, massage therapists (particularly those with neuromuscular therapy training), and some physical therapists and chiropractors. Additionally, therapeutic massage can assist the drainage of lymphatic fluid, and may help decongest the area that is massaged.

Breathing Retraining

Rapid, deep breathing (hyperventilation) can cause respiratory alkalosis, in which the blood becomes too alkaline. This causes histamine levels in the body to rise, heightening allergic responses. Learning yoga-type diaphragmatic breathing exercises can be beneficial. They reduce respiratory alkalosis by improving the mechanics and efficiency of breathing.

To do this, breathe in through the nose after fully exhaling through pursed lips ("kiss" position). Take as long as is comfortable to exhale fully, and when you sense that it is time to breathe in, close the mouth and pause for a count of one, then inhale through the nose.

TRIGGER POINTS

The symptoms of allergic rhinitis may be made worse by trigger points, which are sensitive areas in muscles that can affect nearby tissues and cause pain. Trigger points in facial and neck muscles may be responsible for causing pain in various areas of the head. They may also cause an increase in secretions from the mucous membranes in the nose. Osteopaths, acupuncturists, and other practitioners can deactivate trigger points using a variety of different methods.

Areas affected by trigger points

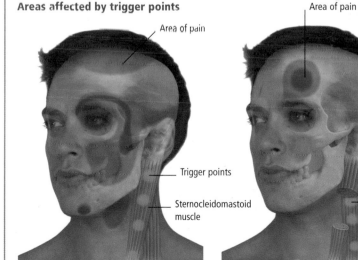

Trigger points in the sternocleidomastoid muscle in the neck may be responsible for pain that is felt in the area of the sinuses and on the back and top of the head.

Trigger points in other muscles in the neck may be responsible for pain that is felt in the forehead above the left eye, behind the ear, and at the back of the head.

Hydrotherapy

A traditional yoga technique involving nasal saline inhalation, in which a warm saltwater solution is poured through the nose, usually offers rapid relief from allergic rhinitis. A special ceramic pot, known as a "neti lota" pot, makes this procedure easy to perform. Fill the pot with warm water and add salt until the solution tastes like tears. Stand over a sink, tilt your head far to one side so your ear is parallel to the floor, and pour the solution into the upper nostril, allowing it to drain through the lower nostril. Repeat on the other side. This procedure may be safely performed two or three times a day.

> **CAUTION**
>
> Nasal saline inhalation should not be done by children under the age of 12.

Acupuncture

Acupuncture has been used for both chronic sinusitis and perennial and seasonal allergic rhinitis (hay fever). Although no reliable clinical trials have assessed this technique, acupuncture may be worth trying in treating this acute condition.

A traditional Chinese diagnosis is usually required, and treatment will need to be repeated on several occasions. If you

Environmental Health

The severity of allergic rhinitis is greatly affected by the environment. Consequently, avoidance of environmental triggers that you have the ability to control is the most effective strategy.

POLLEN If your allergic rhinitis is seasonal (hay fever), avoid being outside when local pollen counts are highest; concentrations of airborne pollen usually peak between 5 and 10 A.M. Throughout the allergy season it is best to be in an air-conditioned environment and keep the windows shut. A high-efficiency particle air (HEPA) filter may be helpful.

You should get someone else to mow the lawn if you have outdoor seasonal allergies. If you must do outdoor work when the pollen count is high, a respirator-type mask may be useful, but remember that allergens can enter the body and trigger symptoms via the eyes as well as the nose and mouth. Allergic conjunctivitis, which causes teary and itchy eyes, often accompanies allergic rhinitis. The use of sealing goggles may look strange but they can help you avoid an attack of allergic rhinitis and conjunctivitis.

Keep in mind that many people unknowingly bring outdoor allergens into the home. For example, people with tree allergies may attribute their increase in symptoms at Christmastime to dust mites

perennial allergic rhinitis. If you are sensitive to dust mites, consider removing the carpet and installing wood floors. If this is not possible, have someone else vacuum regularly while you are out of the house. Do not return for two or three hours to allow any airborne particles to settle (or use a HEPA filter). If you need to vacuum yourself, wear a mask while doing so, then leave the house for a few hours afterward. Use double-thickness vacuum bags or special allergy bags to limit the spread of airborne allergens.

It helps to keep the humidity in your home below 40 or 50 percent, because this limits dust mite reproduction. You can control humidity levels with a dehumidifier and by using air conditioning in the summer. Wash your bedding weekly in water that is at least 130°F (60°C) hot, and remove any stuffed animals or decorative pillows from the bed. The use of mite-impermeable mattress covers and pillowcases alone is not helpful, but is probably beneficial when used along with other measures.

PETS If you have tested positive for allergy to pets (usually cats), it would be best not to have a pet. However, some breeds of cats and dogs cause a midler reaction than others. Barring this, the bedroom at least should become a pet-free haven. Special preparations containing tannic acid may help reduce allergens on pet fur. A weekly bath for your pet also seems important.

INDOOR MOLDS (fungi) are another indoor allergen worth noting, although they typically cause asthma more than rhinitis symptoms. There are numerous species of fungi that can be found in the home, either from spore entry through windows or through growth indoors. Mold can often be seen around leaky pipes, on basement carpets, and in bathrooms lacking adequate ventilation. Wipe away any obvious mold using a solution of diluted bleach (make sure the room is adequately ventilated), and eliminate damp conditions that favor its growth by using a dehumidifier. Maintain heating, ventilation, and air-conditioning systems with regular inspections. When cleaning mold, be sure to wear a particle mask to limit exposure to this allergen.

> Allergic rhinitis is the sixth most common chronic illness in the US, affecting 20 to 40 million Americans.

have seasonal allergic rhinitis and want to use acupuncture as a preventive treatment, you should have two or three sessions before the hay fever season in preparation, and two or three sessions during the season itself. If acupuncture works during a particular hay fever season, then try a similar regimen each summer, just prior to when you are expecting the hay fever to occur. If treatment works for three or four years, it might be worthwhile to try a hay fever season without acupuncture. Sometimes acupuncture can have a long-term effect.

or other indoor allergens, when actually the Christmas tree is the culprit. Fresh flowers may have the same effect.

OUTDOOR MOLDS, such as *Alternaria*, can also cause problems. If they trigger your symptoms, stay clear of places where mold may be found, such as old sheds, barns, and storage areas.

DUST MITES In the home, dust mites (microscopic organisms that live in bedding, upholstered furniture, and carpeting) and pets are leading causes of

MONONUCLEOSIS

Caused by infection with the Epstein-Barr virus (EBV), mononucleosis is characterized by a sore throat, swollen lymph glands, and fatigue, which in some cases can persist for weeks. It is most common in adolescents and young adults; one attack provides lifelong protection against getting the infection again. The integrated approach involves treating the symptoms, eating a nutritious diet to help the immune system fight the virus, taking homeopathic remedies, and having osteopathic treatment or massage therapy.

WHAT ARE THE SYMPTOMS?

Symptoms usually begin 4–6 weeks following infection with the virus. They may come on gradually or suddenly, and include:

- Fever and sweating
- Sore throat that may cause difficulty swallowing
- Enlarged and tender lymph glands in the neck
- Headache
- Fatigue
- Poor appetite
- Complications are uncommon but include bacterial throat infections

WHY MIGHT I HAVE THIS?

TRIGGER

- Contact with someone who has the Epstein-Barr virus

TREATMENT PLAN

PRIMARY TREATMENTS

- Analgesics
- Fluids
- Rest
- Antibiotics (for a throat infection)

BACKUP TREATMENTS

- Dietary changes
- Multivitamin and mineral supplements

WORTH CONSIDERING

- Lymphatic pump techniques
- Homeopathy

For an explanation of how treatments are rated, see p.111.

WHY DOES IT OCCUR?

Infection with EBV is very common — about 90 percent of the population is infected by the age of 50. However, many people with EBV infection do not develop symptoms and therefore do not know that they have the infection. Mononucleosis, which may result from infection with EBV, has been associated with chronic fatigue syndrome (*see p.474*).

The virus is transmitted in saliva, which is why it is called the "kissing disease." It enters the body through the nose or throat, and causes B lymphocytes to multiply rapidly and produce IgM antibodies to fight the virus. As a result of the huge number of lymphocytes in the body, the lymph nodes in the neck, throat, and nose swell and the throat feels sore. The spleen is also enlarged. In some people, the symptoms clear up within two weeks; in others, there is persistent lethargy that lasts for weeks or months.

TREATMENTS IN DETAIL

Conventional Medicine

A diagnosis may be made from the symptoms alone. Your doctor may also arrange for blood tests to confirm the diagnosis.

PRIMARY TREATMENT **SYMPTOM RELIEF** Measures to relieve symptoms include analgesics for headaches, drinking plenty of fluids, and prolonged rest. Vigorous exercise should be avoided while the spleen is enlarged and for a few weeks afterward. Any complications should be treated; for example, antibiotics may be given for a bacterial throat infection.

Nutritional Therapy

DIETARY CHANGES Support the immune system by eating a nutritious diet, based on whole, unrefined foods, and restrict sugar, which can impair immune function.

Support for the immune system can be supplied by taking a high-potency multivitamin and mineral preparation every day. Alternatively, take a daily dose of 500–1,000mg of vitamin C and 10–25mg of zinc (balanced with 1mg of copper for every 15mg of zinc) while symptoms last.

Homeopathy

MERCURIUS SOLUBILIS Of the several medicines that may be helpful, *Mercurius solubilis* is probably the most frequently used. People who respond to it have a sore throat with swollen glands and excessive saliva that is painful to swallow. *Merc. sol.* is best taken in the 30C dilution, two pills four times a day. If the 30C dilution is not available, use the 6C dilution instead.

OTHER REMEDIES People who respond to *Ailanthus* may have a blotchy red rash, headache, and muscular pain, with throat ulcers that make swallowing difficult. *Baryta carbonicum* is useful for persistent mononucleosis.

Bodywork Therapies

Evidence suggests that osteopathic methods known as lymphatic pump techniques can increase immune response. They markedly increase blood levels of B and T lymphocytes for up to 24 hours. Nonspecific massage by a trained practitioner may have a similar effect.

CANCER SUPPORT

In cancer, cells grow out of control because their normal regulatory mechanism has been damaged. Most types of cancer form solid tumors in a specific area of the body. The options for treating cancer are increasing and research continues into new types of treatment. Some people with cancer can now be cured and in others, the disease can largely be controlled. Dietary changes, acupuncture, bodywork therapies, and talking therapies can play important roles in supporting conventional cancer treatment.

WHAT ARE THE SYMPTOMS?

The symptoms of cancer depend mainly on when it arises and what type of cancer it is. However, the following symptoms may be associated with cancer:

- A lump, which is often firm and painless, e.g. in the breast
- Changes in the appearance of a mole, as well as itchiness or bleeding
- A wound that does not heal
- Blood in the urine
- Blood in sputum
- Unexplained changes in bowel habits
- Blood-stained discharge or bleeding from the vagina or anus
- Persistent hoarseness or changes in the voice
- Difficulty swallowing
- Unusual or very severe headaches

There may also be more general symptoms, including:

- Weight loss
- Fatigue
- Nausea and loss of appetite

WHY MIGHT I HAVE THIS?

PREDISPOSING FACTORS

These depend on the type of cancer.

- Genetic predisposition for some types of cancer
- Smoking for lung cancer
- Being over 65 for prostate and many other cancers
- Exposure to strong sunlight for skin cancer
- Various poorly understood dietary and environmental factors

WHY DOES IT OCCUR?

There are many factors that contribute to the development of cancer. In some cases, a susceptibility to develop cancer may be genetic; the genes that play a role in the development of breast cancer, ovarian cancer, bowel cancer, and prostate cancer, have been identified. Sometimes an environmental cause can be found. For example, smoking has been shown to be the main cause of lung cancer in as many as 70 percent of cases, and exposure to the ultraviolet rays in strong sunlight causes most cases of malignant melanoma (the most serious type of skin cancer). In many instances, avoiding the cancer-causing agents can significantly reduce the chances of developing a specific type of cancer.

Cancer develops more often in older people because their cells have had more time to accumulate genetic damage and the immune system, which repairs damaged cells, becomes less efficient with age. As life expectancy has increased in the developed world, the incidence of cancer has increased.

Common sites for cancer include the skin, breast, lung, bowel, and prostate gland. It may also affect the lymph nodes (leukemia) or blood-forming cells in bone marrow (lymphoma). Once established in a concentrated location, cancer cells may spread through the blood and lymphatic systems, causing secondary cancers, which are known as metastases. These often occur in the liver, lungs, bone, and brain.

TREATMENT PLAN

PRIMARY TREATMENTS

- Surgery
- Chemotherapy
- Radiation therapy
- Hormonal and biological therapies
- Drugs for pain relief and other symptoms
- Talking therapies

BACK-UP TREATMENTS

- Nutritional therapy
- Exercise

WORTH CONSIDERING

- Western and Chinese herbal medicine
- Homeopathy
- Lymphatic drainage and massage
- Acupuncture and acupressure

For an explanation of how treatments are rated, see p.111.

TREATMENTS IN DETAIL

Conventional Medicine

Cancer may be identified during routine screening, for example during a mammogram. The aim of screening is to identify cancer or precancerous changes that may later lead to cancer (in the case of cervical smears) before symptoms develop. However, in many cases, the disease is diagnosed when symptoms are investigated.

A number of options are available for cancer treatment. Which is most appropriate depends on several factors, including the type of cancer and whether it has spread. The goals of treatment are to cure the cancer, slow its growth, or relieve symptoms.

The support of medical and nursing staff, friends and family, support workers, and self-help groups is often key to helping a person come to terms with a diagnosis of cancer and cope with treatment. Friends and family may also need support. (*For details of support organizations, see p.486.*)

INVESTIGATIONS for cancer vary depending on the symptoms. Blood tests are commonly performed to check for anemia and assess the function of various organs, including the liver and kidneys. Imaging tests, such as X-rays, ultrasound, or CT scanning, may be used to look at an area of the body in more detail.

In some cases, viewing instruments are passed into a part of the body (such as the airways, the bladder, or the digestive tract) and samples of tissue (biopsies) are taken to look for cancer cells. If cancer is found, the type of cancer cell will be identified, which will help when recommending the most appropriate treatment option. Further tests may be needed to look for evidence of cancer spread to nearby lymph nodes or to other parts of the body.

PRIMARY TREATMENT **SURGICAL TREATMENT** Solid tumors diagnosed at an early stage are often removed surgically. Some of the surrounding tissue may be taken to improve the chances of removing all the cancer cells. Nearby lymph nodes may also be removed, to see if the cancer has spread through the lymphatic system.

In some cases, surgery is performed to relieve symptoms. Other treatments, such as chemotherapy and radiation therapy (*see below*), may be given in addition to surgery; these additional therapies are known as adjuvant therapies.

PRIMARY TREATMENT **CHEMOTHERAPY** is done to destroy cancer cells by damaging the genetic material they contain. A combination of cytotoxic (cell-destroying) drugs is often given through an I.V. into the bloodstream. In addition to destroying cancer cells, these drugs can damage other rapidly dividing cells in the body, such as those in the hair follicles and those that line the mouth. The side effects caused by chemotherapy depend on the drug or drugs that are used but fertility may be affected.

Cytotoxic drugs may affect the production of blood cells close to bone marrow, causing anemia and predisposing to infections. Nausea is often a side effect of these drugs but can usually be relieved successfully by the antinausea drugs now available. Hair loss may occur as well, but this is only temporary.

PRIMARY TREATMENT **RADIATION THERAPY** Like chemotherapy, radiation therapy is done to destroy cancer cells by damaging their genetic material. During radiation therapy, high-intensity radiation is delivered to the site of the cancer by a machine as a series of treatments. Alternatively, some cancers are treated with sources of radiation placed inside the body in or very near the affected area. The specialist carefully calculates the necessary dose to keep the radiation delivered to nearby healthy tissues to the minimum possible.

PRIMARY TREATMENT **HORMONE THERAPY** can be used to treat certain cancers. In some cases of breast cancer, growth of the tumor is influenced by the female hormone estrogen. Drugs, such as tamoxifen, can be given to suppress the action of estrogen. Hormone therapy may also be used to treat prostate cancer.

PRIMARY TREATMENT **BIOLOGICAL THERAPY** is a term that covers a variety of treatments. Some of these can help the body's immune system react against and destroy cancer cells. The use of these drugs is limited to specific cancers.

The protein erythropoietin may be given as a biological therapy. Erythropoietin occurs naturally in the body and causes bone marrow to produce red blood cells. It can therefore be helpful when anemia develops as a side effect of cytotoxic drugs.

PRIMARY TREATMENT **OTHER TREATMENTS** may be given to relieve symptoms caused by cancer; for example, analgesics such as morphine relieve pain caused by the spread of cancer to the bone.

HOW CANCER DEVELOPS

Our cells divide to produce new cells. Cancer arises when cells divide faster than is necessary to replace lost cells. In the example of skin cancer shown below, the cells that form skin are dividing uncontrollably. As the number of rapidly dividing cells increases, a tumor forms.

Skin cancer

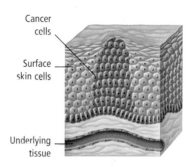

Cancer cells

Surface skin cells

Underlying tissue

Cancerous cells in the skin are dividing too fast.

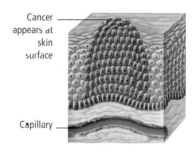

Cancer appears at skin surface

Capillary

The cancerous cells accumulate and eventually form a mass, which is known as a tumor.

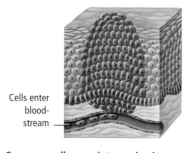

Cells enter bloodstream

Cancerous cells grow into nearby tissues. If they reach the bloodstream and lymph system, they may spread.

COMPLEMENTARY THERAPIES FOR SIDE EFFECTS

Chemotherapy and radiation therapy are powerful anticancer treatments but they have a range of side effects. Try the following therapies and self-help measures to relieve these.

SIDE-EFFECTS	HELPFUL TREATMENTS
Chemotherapy	
Nausea and vomiting	• Acupuncture • THC (the active ingredient in marijuana) • Ginger • Fennel • Slippery elm • *Ipecac* 6x • Acupressure to wrist (*see p.154*)
Loss of appetite	• THC (the active ingredient in marijuana)
Diarrhea	• Slippery elm • Acidophilus capsules to balance gut flora
Decreased immune function	• Echinacea • Astragalus • Pau d'arco • Andrographis • Cat's claw
Sore mouth	• Tincture of myrrh and golden seal as mouthwash
Sensitivity to sun	• High-factor sun block
Hair loss	• Scalp cooling during chemotherapy treatment
Fatigue	• Relaxation and gentle exercise • Nourishing diet with plenty of B vitamins • Siberian ginseng
Pain (chemotherapy can sometimes damage nerves, which can produce a burning sensation or a tingling or shooting pain; and peripheral neuropathy (*see p.127*)	• Acupuncture • Imagery, visualization, and other mind–body techniques (*see p.100*) • Hypnotherapy and meditation (*see p.98*) • Psychological support, e.g. counseling • Relaxing herbal remedies, e.g. valerian
Lymphedema (swelling of arms, legs or other body parts due to buildup of lymph fluid)	• Exercises • Massage • Lymphatic drainage
Damage to fertility	• Cryopreservation of sperm or ovarian tissue
Depression, anxiety	• Talking to supportive friends, family and clergy • Counseling, prayer, healing • Herbal remedies, e.g. St. John's wort
Radiation therapy	
Skin problems (red, blotchy, itchy, and irritated, like sunburn)	• Aloe vera gel • Comfrey or pine ointment
Internal burning sensation	• Sage extract • *Belladonna* 6x • Liquorice

Nutritional Therapy

For cancer to grow and spread in the body it must penetrate a mesh of tissue fibers known as the extra-cellular matrix. Cancer cells have the ability to secrete certain enzymes that allow them to spread. Several nutrients have the potential to block the action of these enzymes, which can help inhibit the growth and spread of cancerous tumors. Foods that may help include citrus fruits and soy-containing foods such as soy milk, tofu, and miso.

Cancer cells also need a blood supply to survive. Certain compounds known as angiostats can help prevent the formation of new blood vessels thereby "starving" existing tumors. Soy foods contain a substance called genistein, which has angiostatic properties.

Certain nutrients also seem to have the capacity to inhibit the growth of cancer cells. Some of these nutrients also seem to help convert abnormal cancerous cells into normal cells (a process known as re-differentiation). Some of the most important nutrients are carotenoid nutrients such as beta-carotene, alpha-carotene, and lycopene. Foods rich in carotenoid nutrients include yellow, pink, orange, and red fruits and vegetables such as tomatoes, carrots, apricots, red peppers, and squash.

ANTIOXIDANTS AND CANCER Evidence suggests that the development of cancer can be related to destructive molecules called free radicals. Certain nutrients, including beta-carotene, vitamins A, C, and E and the minerals zinc and selenium have the ability to quell free radicals through antioxidant action. In theory, higher levels of antioxidants can help combat cancer. In practice, a group taking high doses of nutrients including vitamins A, C, E, and zinc had half the risk of bladder cancer recurrence compared with a group not taking these nutrients. In another study, 200mcg of selenium, compared with a placebo, halved the risk of dying from cancer in patients with a history of skin cancer.

Homeopathy

Homeopathy is one of the most investigated therapies for breast cancer. It has been researched for hot flashes due to tamoxifen, a drug used to treat breast cancer; as a therapy for improving cancer patients' quality of life; and for its ability to reduce the adverse effects of radiation therapy. You should see a homeopath for treatment.

Hot flashes are common for women taking tamoxifen. Cancer patients commonly experience depression, anxiety, and fatigue. *Amyl nitrosum, Lachesis, Calcarea carbonica, Natrum muriaticum, Sepia, Pulsatilla,* and *Sulphur* are often prescribed for hot flashes and maintaining quality of life.

AMYL NITROSUM AND LACHESIS *Amyl nitrosum* is specifically prescribed for hot flashes. Women who respond to it have a sensation of blood surging to their head, sometimes with a throbbing headache, followed by profuse sweating and chilliness. Women who respond to *Lachesis* usually have hot flashes too, but they also have migraines, particularly left-sided ones. In fact, in women who respond to *Lachesis* all symptoms tend to be worse on their left side, and they are also intolerant of tight clothes. They may bruise easily.

CALCAREA CARBONICA Women who respond to *Calcarea carbonica* may also have hot flashes, but even without them, these women sweat, particularly from their head and neck at night. They are anxious and tend to obsess about little things. They may be woken regularly by bad dreams.

NATRUM MURIATICUM Women who respond to *Natrum muriaticum* are usually depressed, although this may be well hidden. These women have a "stiff upper lip" and do not like to talk about their problems. They often have vaginal dryness. Other possible symptoms include recurrent cold sores on the lips (*see p.162*).
SEPIA Women who respond to *Sepia* may have the same features, including depression and vaginal dryness. However, while women who respond to *Natrum muriaticum* are generally caring and sympathetic to those around them, women who respond to *Sepia* may be bad-tempered and less affectionate to their families.

PULSATILLA AND SULPHUR Women who respond to *Pulsatilla* may vascillate widely, both in mood and symptoms. These women are typically soft-spoken and easily moved to tears. Patients who respond to *Sulphur* may become lethargic and depressed but are usually strong-willed and hot (both in temperature and temperament). Their feet are especially hot and may be smelly, and they kick off their shoes at every opportunity and may stick their feet out of bed at night. They get burning pains at various sites and may have smelly discharges. They often have skin trouble, and rashes are often very itchy.

BELLADONNA A clinical trial done in Italy showed that a combination of *Belladonna* and a homeopathic medicine made from water irradiated with X-rays reduced the side effects of radiation therapy to the breast, including swelling, heat, and discoloration.

Western and Chinese Herbal Medicine

There is no evidence that herbal medicines can cure cancer. However, herbalists use three strategies to help people with cancer: support the immune system, inhibit cancer cell growth, and detoxify the body.

POLYSACCHARIDES AND SAPONINS Polysaccharides in medicinal mushrooms such as ganoderma (*Ganoderma lucidum*), also known as reishi or ling zhi, and shiitake (*Lentinus edodes*), as well as semipurified polysaccharide extract (PSK and PSP) obtained from *Coriolus versicolor*, have immunostimulating properties.

Maitake (*Grifola frondosa*), an edible mushroom, has anticancer, antiviral, and immune-enhancing properties, and may also reduce blood pressure and blood sugar. Shiitake (*Lentinula edodes*), widely available fresh or dried in grocery stores and Asian markets, has immune-modulating, antiviral, and cholesterol-reducing properties. Certain extracts are used in Japan as adjunctive therapy to strengthen immunity of cancer patients during chemotherapy and radiation. Agaricus (*Agaricus blazei*) is a medicinal mushroom with antitumor and antiviral activity widely used by cancer patients in Japan and Brazil. Reishi (*Ganoderma lucidum*) is too woody and bitter to eat as food, but are available in tea bags, capsules, and liquid extracts. Animal studies have shown that it improves immune function, inhibits the growth of some malignant tumors, and is a natural anti-inflammatory.

Polysaccharides are an active constituent of Siberian ginseng (*Eleutherococcus senticosus*) and astragalus (*Astragalus membranaceus*), both of which have immune-supporting potential. In addition, ginseng has a nonspecific tonic effect.

PHENOLS AND FLAVONOIDS A number of other Chinese herbs said to have anticancer activity are rich in phenolic compounds including flavonoids. *Scutellaria barbata*, a traditional Chinese herb, may have some anticancer activity, as might rhubarb root (*Rheum palmatum*).

Green tea and its polyphenolic components have demonstrated antimutagenic activity and can inhibit tumor growth in the laboratory. They may increase the effectiveness of chemotherapy drugs. Green tea consumption has been found to enhance the survival of women with ovarian cancer.

Western herbalists believe that herbs rich in phenols and flavonoids, such as garlic and onions, can reduce the risk of cancer. Milk thistle (*Silybum marianum*) is used to detoxify the liver. (*See also Nutritional Therapy, p.466.*)

PROANTHOCYANIDINS AND PHYTOESTROGENS Opinion is divided as to whether taking herbal antioxidants rich in proanthocyanidins, such as grapeseed extract, interferes with chemotherapy and radiation therapy. There is recent evidence of beneficial interactions between the herbal and drug treatments.

TYPES OF CANCER

There are several hundred types of cancer. Doctors classify and name them according to the body tissue where they form. A few of the most common types are explained below.

TYPE AND LOCATION	NAME OF CANCER
Carcinomas Cancers of the epithelial cells. A thin layer of these cells covers the body; they also form skin. Epithelial cells line the gut, inside of the chest, and other body cavities.	• Squamous cell carcinoma (Squamous cells are block-shaped cells that form skin, as well as mouth, gut, and lung linings.) • Adenocarcinoma (Adenomatous cells are glandular cells that are found in stomach, breast, and other organs that produce secretions.) • Transitional cell carcinoma (Transitional cells are layers of stretchy cells that line the bladder and urinary tract.) • Basal cell carcinoma (Basal cells form the lowest of the skin layers.)
Sarcomas Grow in supporting tissue, which include bones, ligaments, cartilage, tendons, fibrous (connective) tissues, and fat.	• Fibrosarcoma (Fibrocytes make up fibrous tissue.) • Liposarcoma (Lipocytes are fat cells.) • Rhabdomyosarcoma (Mycocytes are muscle cells.) • Osteosarcoma (Osteocytes are bone cells.) • Chondrosarcoma (Chondroblasts are cartilage cells.)
Leukemias Cancers of the white blood cells (leukocytes).	• Lymphocytic leukemia (There are two groups of leukocytes: lymphocytes and granulocytes.) • Myeloid leukemia (Granulocytes develop from blood-forming cells called myeloblasts.) • Lymphoblastic leukemia (Blast cells, or blasts, are immature white blood cells.)
Lymphomas Arise in the lymphatic system. They may affect lymph tissues, lymph nodes, the spleen, bone marrow, and the thymus gland.	• Hodgkin's disease (Affect lymphocytes, which are infection-fighting white blood cells found in lymph glands.) • Non-Hodgkin's lymphoma

The possibility that phytoestrogens found in medicinal plants such as black cohosh (*Cimicifuga racemosa*) and red clover (*Trifolium pratense*) may be contraindicated in women with pre-existing breast tumors is also contentious. It now appears that some phytoestrogens may help protect against breast cancer.

Acupuncture

Acupuncture has a number of important uses in alleviating some of the symptoms associated with cancer, but it cannot treat or cure the disease. Some hospices offer acupuncture as part of their program of palliative care (treatment to relieve symptoms). It is often difficult to judge how much acupuncture speeds up the resolution of acute symptoms and how effective it is as a constitutional "pick-me-up" in terminal illness.

RELIEF FROM NAUSEA There is evidence to suggest that activating a specific acupuncture point just above the wrist on the inside of the arm (P6) will alleviate the nausea and vomiting frequently produced by anticancer drugs. A medical device that electrically stimulates this point is also available. Clinical trials have suggested that acupuncture is as effective as some of the modern and expensive antinausea drugs.

PAIN RELIEF Acupuncture has been used extensively to ameliorate pain associated with cancer. Acupuncture for cancer pain needs to be repeated frequently, but it can provide a safe and effective form of treatment with few side effects.

Sometimes the use of anticancer drugs or radiation therapy may cause pain that can be relieved by acupuncture. Distressing symptoms, such as the suffocating breathlessness experienced by many patients dying from lung cancer, also may be helped by acupuncture.

If acupuncture is being used to treat acute pain, or postchemotherapy nausea, then daily, or even twice daily, treatment is best. If it is used as a general treatment, a weekly session is perfectly acceptable.

Bodywork Therapies

LYMPHATIC DRAINAGE After surgery or radiation therapy, for example following partial or total mastectomy, the lymph glands under the arm may be damaged or removed. This can mean that normal lymph drainage from the region becomes impeded, leading to fluid accumulation and swelling (edema) of the limb. If you have had such surgery, talk to a cancer care nurse about having manual lymphatic drainage. The methods used, involving very carefully targeted and light massage techniques, are capable of rapidly improving such conditions.

MASSAGE Living with cancer is often a stressful experience and, if massage appeals to you, it is to be recommended. Massage therapy, sometimes coupled with the use of various essential oils, has been shown in a number of research studies to be beneficial to cancer patients. It eases pain, reduces anxiety and depression, and helps create a sense of well-being. However, a tumor or metastasis site should never be massaged.

A study undertaken in 2000 looked at children with leukemia who received massage from their parents (who were taught basic techniques). Both the children and the parents had lower anxiety levels and fewer signs of stress. Parents felt less helpless by having an opportunity for contribute to their child's recovery.

In another study, women in the early stages of breast cancer were given three massages weekly for five weeks. They reported much reduced anxiety levels and were found to have increased numbers of immune cells. The researchers believe that a decrease in cortisol stress hormones, which may destroy immune cells, was responsible for the greater number of immune cells. Massage was shown to improve quality of life and may in turn prolong survival.

ACUPRESSURE The nausea often resulting from chemotherapy or anesthetics may be reduced by applying firm thumb pressure for several minutes to the acupressure point P6 on the front of each forearm (*see p.154*).

Yoga

Gentle yoga exercise can help calm the mind and the body, and may help promote a sense of well-being.

Psychological Therapies

| PRIMARY TREATMENT | The use of talking therapies in the treatment of patients with cancer is aimed mainly at addressing the pain and subsequent depression associated with cancer. It has not been shown that psychological therapies can influence the progression of the disease itself.

However, a growing body of evidence supports the view that therapies can improve quality of life by improving the patient's ability to cope with the illness. This in turn may have an effect on length of survival. In a study into breast cancer survival rates, women who had group therapy and learned pain management

Many cancers can now be cured, and others can be successfully controlled for many years

Exercise

A large study found that exercise improves physical functioning and well-being for many breast cancer patients. Researchers in Canada found that women undergoing treatment for early stage breast cancer who maintained a regular exercise program had a significant improvement in cardiac conditioning and overall functioning. The program consisted of hour-long walking sessions three to five times per week for six months

Rest is apparently not the best medicine for the fatigue caused by treatment such as chemotherapy. The researchers found that inactivity contributed to the weakening of those patients who followed the traditional medical advice to do little or no exercise during cancer treatment. However, the researchers warn that this does not mean that more is better. Anyone with cancer beginning an exercise program should first consult a doctor, along with someone, such as an exercise physiologist, who can evaluate his or her level of fitness.

techniques lived on average two years longer than those in the control group.

GROUP THERAPY In a research study, 50 women with metastatic breast cancer who participated in professionally led support groups survived twice as long (36.6 months) as those who did not participate. The researchers provided "supportive-expressive group therapy" to allow time for the women to express their deepest fears and emotions. Patients in the support group also reported experiencing 50 per cent less pain than those not participating.

COGNITIVE BEHAVIORAL THERAPY Psychoeducation, which is a type of cognitive behavioral therapy, teaches patients to become more aware of how they may develop anxiety or depression by how they think and behave. Meta-analysis of studies examining the use of psychoeducation in cancer patients concluded that it was beneficial for patients with cancer and helped with anxiety, depression, mood swings, nausea, vomiting, and pain.

RELAXATION THERAPY There are few well-designed studies into the use of relaxation along with conventional medication for pain control. However, one study found that patients who received either relaxation or were trained in cognitive behavioral skills reported less pain than people in a control group who did not have training in these skills.

If you have cancer, it may be worthwhile practicing daily relaxation (*see p.99 for details of a relaxation sequence*). You could also learn cognitive behavioral techniques.

Mind–Body Therapies

VISUALIZATION Although much has been written and researched about the use of imagery to boost the body's power to destroy cancer tissue, its effects are not well established, scientifically speaking.

Nonetheless, when it is incorporated into a relaxation and group support program, use of imagery may be an effective way of improving immune function or calming a tense and nervous body and mind. For some people with cancer, using imagery for relaxation and to help with focus can be a very important adjunct to some form of psychological treatment (*see left*).

The important point is that for many people, cancer becomes a turning point in their lives when they actively seek ways of working more effectively with their minds and bodies. Visualization can be a significant component of rediscovering the link between the body and the mind.

PREVENTION PLAN

The following measures may help reduce the likelihood of developing cancer:

- Eat a healthy, balanced diet, including at least five portions of fruit and vegetables each day (*for further nutritional advice, see p.44*)

- Avoid known environmental hazards, such as excessive sun exposure and tobacco smoke

- Attend any screening appointments you are offered (such as pap smears and mammograms for women)

HIV AND AIDS

Infection with the human immunodeficiency virus (HIV) usually leads to the development of acquired immune deficiency syndrome (AIDS), in which the immune system is severely weakened. This allows serious infections to develop, often from organisms that do not usually pose a danger to health. At present, antiretroviral drugs can limit HIV infection for many years, but there is no cure for the disease or vaccine against it. Drug treatment may be supported by a variety of complementary approaches, aimed at boosting well-being and general health.

WHAT ARE THE SYMPTOMS?

Initial symptoms may include:

- Swollen lymph glands
- Fever
- Fatigue
- Rash
- Muscle aches
- Sore throat

Symptoms that may develop as the disease progresses include:

- Persistent swollen lymph glands
- Mouth ulcers and mouth infections, such as oral yeast (see p.383)
- Gum disease (gingivitis)
- Bouts of herpes simplex infections (see p.162), such as cold sores or genital herpes
- Extensive genital warts
- Itchy, dry skin
- Weight loss and diarrhea
- Recurring vaginal yeast infections

Illnesses occurring with AIDS include:

- *Pneumocystis carinii* pneumonia
- Candidiasis that affects the respiratory tract or esophagus
- Tuberculosis
- Herpes simplex infection of the lungs or esophagus
- Infection of the brain with the *Toxoplasma gondii*
- Kaposi's sarcoma (a cancer that usually causes purplish lesions on the skin)
- Lymphoma (cancer of the lymph nodes)
- Cervical cancer

WHY MIGHT I HAVE THIS?

PREDISPOSING FACTORS

- Unprotected sexual intercourse (anal or vaginal)
- Sharing needles for injectable drugs
- Blood transfusions

WHY DOES IT OCCUR?

TRANSMISSION The HIV virus is transmitted through bodily fluids, including blood, semen, vaginal secretions, and breast milk. It is most commonly transmitted through sexual intercourse (vaginal and anal), but can also be passed on through the sharing of contaminated needles by intravenous drug users. A woman infected with HIV can pass the infection on to her baby during pregnancy or, more often, at birth. It may also be transmitted through breast-feeding.

HIV infection is not caught from everyday contact, such as touching an infected person, or from coughs and sneezes from an infected person or by working or living with someone who has HIV or AIDS.

TREATMENT PLAN

PRIMARY TREATMENTS

- Antiretroviral drugs and treatment of specific symptoms
- Emotional and practical support

BACKUP TREATMENTS

- Dietary changes and supplements
- Mind–body therapies

WORTH CONSIDERING

- Homeopathy
- Acupuncture

For an explanation of how treatments are rated, see p.111.

CD4 LYMPHOCYTES HIV enters the bloodstream and infects cells that have the CD4 receptor on their surfaces. The cells include a type of white blood cell called a CD4 lymphocyte, which fights infection in the body. HIV reproduces in these cells and destroys them. At first, the immune system can still function normally despite the infection, and symptoms may not arise for years. However, eventually the number of CD4 lymphocytes in the body begins to fall, especially if the infection remains untreated. This increases susceptibility to other infections and to some types of cancer. A person with HIV infection is said to have developed AIDS if the CD4 lymphocyte count falls below a certain level or if he or she develops an AIDS-defining illness (see left).

DISEASE DEVELOPMENT The first symptoms of HIV may appear within four weeks of infection and may include vague, flulike symptoms (see left), such as muscle aches and swollen glands.; in many cases there are no symptoms at this stage. They usually clear up in a few weeks. Many people feel perfectly healthy, often for years, but other symptoms may develop (see left), such as persistent swollen glands and weight loss.

The time between initial infection with HIV and the development of AIDS varies from person to person and can last only a few years or develop over the course of 15

IMPORTANT

If you suspect you have HIV, see your doctor or attend a clinic as soon as possible. Prompt diagnosis and early treatment are both essential.

to 20 years. Some people are unaware that they are infected until they develop a serious infection or cancer (*see p.470*). Once AIDS develops, nerve damage may result in tingling, pain, and numbness in the legs, feet, and hands. Dementia (*see p.133*) may also develop; symptoms vary from mild memory problems to personality changes and diminished intellectual ability in more severe cases.

SELF-HELP

If you are diagnosed with HIV, the following measures can help you stay healthy.
- Even if you feel well, don't miss regular health checkups.
- Get regular exercise, such as swimming or walking, three times a week.
- Eat nutritious, well-balanced meals and snacks (*see p.44*), even if you find that your appetite is poor.
- Keep the strain on your immune system to a minimum: avoid other infections as much as possible.
- Stay positive and if anxiety or depression become a factor, seek support (*see p.486 for organizations offering help*). Stress management or meditation can also help you deal with your feelings.

TREATMENTS IN DETAIL

Conventional Medicine

HIV infection is usually diagnosed by looking for the antibody to the virus in the bloodstream. If it is found, regular blood tests will be done to monitor the CD4 lymphocyte count.

Powerful antiretroviral drugs are now available that keep the virus under control so that the development of AIDS is delayed, sometimes indefinitely.

If the CD4 count becomes low or is decreasing rapidly, drug therapy is likely to be recommended. It may also be considered during early infection when the first symptoms appear. Pregnant women who are HIV positive may take antiretroviral drugs that reduce the risk of transmitting HIV to the fetus. Cesarean section and refraining from breast-feeding are other precautionary measures.

A course of antiretroviral treatment is recommended for anyone who suspects that he or she has been exposed to the HIV virus.

HOW ANTIRETROVIRAL DRUGS WORK

Antiretroviral drugs block enzymes that the virus needs to reproduce. Different types of these drugs work at different stages of the virus "production line." The process begins when the HIV virus attaches to a CD4 cell, then empties its genetic material (RNA) into the cell. This RNA is converted into DNA by an enzyme called reverse transcriptase. Reverse transcriptase inhibitor drugs stop this enzyme from working.

However, once the virus's RNA has been converted into DNA it can enter the cell's nucleus, where it combines with the cellular DNA. The virus then turns the cell into an "HIV factory," making billions of viral RNA particles. As these leave the cell, they are coated with protein. The drugs called protease inhibitors block the protease enzyme, thereby keeping the protein coat from forming.

Preventing viral replication

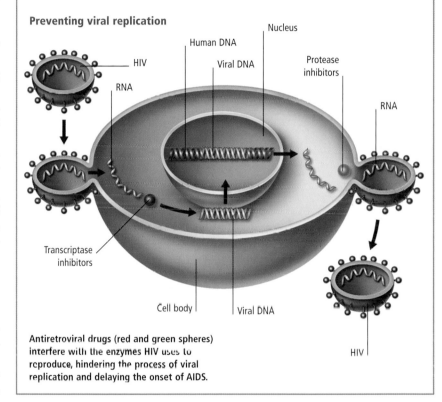

Antiretroviral drugs (red and green spheres) interfere with the enzymes HIV uses to reproduce, hindering the process of viral replication and delaying the onset of AIDS.

Drugs cannot eradicate the virus but they can keep it under control by interfering with its replication (*see box, above*). Various drugs for HIV infection have been shown to be particularly beneficial when used in combination. Side effects can be a problem, and regular monitoring with blood tests will be necessary. The drugs will need to be changed if side effects are unacceptable or if there is not an adequate response, which may be due to resistance of the virus to one or more of the drugs.

PRIMARY TREATMENT **ANTIRETROVIRAL DRUGS** There are two main groups of antiretroviral drugs used, both of which aim to disrupt viral replication.

Reverse transcriptase inhibitors, such as zidovudine and lamivudine, alter the genetic material both within the infected cell, which is needed by the virus to replicate, and within the virus itself.

Protease inhibitors, such as indinavir and ritonavir, prevent production of the viral proteins necessary for it to replicate.

PRIMARY TREATMENT **OTHER TREATMENT** Treatments will be needed for specific problems and may include topical corticosteroids for mouth ulcers and antibiotic or antiviral drugs for infections. Kaposi's sarcoma or lymphoma may be treated with radiation therapy or in some cases chemotherapy.

PRIMARY
TREATMENT **EMOTIONAL SUPPORT** is crucial, not only to help the affected individual come to terms with the disease but also for the individual's family, friends, and caregivers. The many HIV and AIDS organizations and support groups can give invaluable help and understanding.

> **CAUTION**
>
> Drugs for HIV and AIDS can cause a range of possible side effects; ask your doctor to explain these to you.

Nutritional Therapy

NUTRITIONAL SUPPLEMENTS Emaciation and weight loss are common and important complications of HIV infection and AIDS, and they seem to have a bearing on survival. Emaciation is believed to worsen immune function and increase the risk of further infection. However, it is possible for HIV and AIDS patients to regain weight, and when accomplished it seems to help improve immune function. One study found that a protein-based liquid nutritional formula containing omega-3 fatty acids, taken as a 236ml dose three times per day, increased weight and CD4 count in HIV-infected patients. However, another study of supplements containing a large amount of omega-3 fatty acids and arginine found no improvement in immune function.

In developed countries where appropriate care is available, HIV can be seen as a chronic illness

DIETARY CHANGES AIDS-related weight loss is thought to be partly due to reduced intake of food. However, there is some evidence that it is also linked to abnormal fat and protein metabolism in the body. People with HIV and AIDS can benefit from eating a nutritious diet based on whole, unprocessed foods. (*For more details, see p.44*).

OMEGA-3 FATTY ACIDS (found in oily fish such as mackerel, salmon, and sardines) can influence immunological and inflammatory processes. Studies have shown that levels of omega-3 fatty acids are generally very low in AIDS patients. Eating extra omega-3 fatty acids may help those with AIDS and HIV. Either have at least three portions of oily fish a week or take 5–10g per day of fish oil.

VITAMINS AND MINERALS People with HIV or AIDS often have multiple nutritional deficiencies. One study found that developing a vitamin A and B_{12} deficiency was associated with a reduced CD4 count, and restoring levels of vitamin A, B_{12}, and zinc to normal was associated with an increased CD4 count. The authors of this study concluded that nutrient deficiencies are associated with the progression of HIV.

Other research has found that low levels of vitamin B_{12}, vitamin A, niacin (vitamin B_3), and zinc are associated with faster HIV disease progression. A broad-spectrum multivitamin and mineral supplement may help prevent and/or reverse nutrient deficiencies and might also help slow the progression of the disease. However, a study of vitamin A found no effect on CD4 count or viral load; another study of vitamin E and vitamin C found no difference in viral load between treatment and a placebo.

GLUTAMINE The amino acid glutamine appears to be important for optimal functioning of the immune system, especially in the critically ill. Taking glutamine-enriched supplements may maintain and improve immune function in AIDS patients. They may also reduce weight loss from muscle and increase body weight and body cell mass in AIDS-related weight loss. One of the studies showed benefit from supplementation with 14g L-glutamine twice daily for eight weeks. If you have HIV or AIDS, taking 4–6g of L-glutamine each day may help maintain your weight and well-being.

N-ACETYL CYSTEINE The amino acid N-acetyl cysteine (NAC) may also be beneficial for people infected with HIV. NAC can inhibit the replication of the HIV virus in the test tube and studies show that supplementation may help people with HIV. NAC may work better in combination with glutamine, since these two amino acids promote the synthesis of glutathione, a naturally occurring antioxidant that may be protective in individuals with HIV. HIV-positive individuals may benefit from taking 600mg of NAC three times per day.

> **CAUTION**
>
> Consult your doctor before taking fish oil supplements with blood-thinning drugs, such as warfarin (*see p.46*).

Homeopathy

A clinical trial done in India suggests that homeopathy may have a favorable effect on CD4 count when used early in the development of AIDS. The most commonly used medicines were *Phosphorus*, *Pulsatilla*, *Sulphur*, and *Lycopodium*.

COTRIMOXAZOLE AND HOMEOPATHIC MEDICINES Cotrimoxazole is an antibiotic often required to treat or prevent the severe infections that people with AIDS develop, and it is a serious problem if someone with AIDS is allergic to this drug. There is evidence that homeopathic treatment can help control this allergy, enabling AIDS patients who are allergic to cotrimoxazole to take it.

KALIUM CARBONICUM AND MERCURIUS SOLUBILIS In industrialized countries, homeopathy is often used in a supportive role to treat HIV infection and AIDS. Among medicines that have been found helpful are *Kalium carbonicum*. Typically the patient is run down and tired, with a persistent wheezy cough, and often wakes up coughing at 3 or 4 A.M.

Mercurius solubilis may be given for infections, particularly for sore throats and tonsillitis, especially if the lymph glands in the neck are swollen. Excessive saliva in the mouth is a very characteristic feature in people who respond to *Mercurius solubilis*. In these people, the tongue feels sore and swollen and imprints of the teeth may be visible around its edge. Bad breath may also be a problem. These patients are said to be "human thermometers" because they are always too hot or cold and sweat very freely as soon as they get hot.

PHYTOLACCA AND THUJA OCCIDENTALIS may also be helpful for sore throats and other infections with a lot of rheumatic pain. *Thuja occidentalis* may be useful for recurrent infections and particularly for persistent urethritis in men or vaginal discharge in women. In people for whom it is suitable there is often widespread swelling of the lymph glands, numerous warts and polyps, and stubborn nasal stuffiness. These are sometimes accompanied by strange fixed ideas and obsessions.

PHOSPHORUS is sometimes helpful to aid general well-being and reduce the frequency of infections. People who respond to *Phosphorus* are tired and weak, although a bit better after rest and hence feel better in the morning. There may be hepatitis or a history of hepatitis, or diarrhea, often with blood. They often bleed easily and may get bruises for no apparent reason. They may have a loss of appetite, although they are often thirsty, especially for cold, refreshing drinks. People who respond to *Phosphorus* are very sensitive, both to the physical and human environment. They are often emotionally volatile, as well as sympathetic and vivacious.

Chinese Herbal Medicine

There are a number of trials and ongoing research indicating the possible efficacy of Chinese herbs as part of a total treatment protocol for HIV. One recent pilot study focused on an herbal formulation, SH Instant, which combines three medicinal herbs from China and two from Thailand. In a phase III study of 60 patients, the 40 people who took the drug fared better in fighting the virus than the 20 who did not and it reduced the participants' viral load by 43%. However, researchers noted that it does not eliminate the need for standard antiretroviral drugs.

Acupuncture

Acupuncture cannot cure HIV infection and AIDS, but it is sometimes used to alleviate many of the associated symptoms.

The traditional Chinese approach is to "balance the meridians" and hence provide immune balance, helping the immune system perform to its maximum ability within the constraints of the illness.

There are specific complaints that may be associated with HIV infection or AIDS, such as fatigue, chest infections, and irritable bowel syndrome, which acupuncture may help to alleviate and/or manage.

There are no specific randomized controlled trials in this area, but a number of studies have looked at whole treatment packages for HIV and AIDS, which include nutritional and herbal remedies and may involve acupuncture. In general, these natural approaches to managing HIV and AIDS have been claimed to be of substantial benefit by proponents, but compared to sham acupuncture, true acupuncture was no more effective for treating peripheral neuropathy (see p.127) related to HIV.

Probably the best way of using acupuncture is as part of a program designed to maintain a healthy lifestyle. If acupuncture is for long-term health maintenance, a monthly session is best.

HIV and AIDS can be passed on by contaminated needles, so you should ensure that the therapist uses only disposable needles.

Mind–Body Therapies

Mind–body therapies such as biofeedback and relaxation appear to be able to enhance the immune response by calming anxiety and stress.

Given the devastating psychological and biological impact of HIV and AIDS and the demonstrated effectiveness of mind–body therapies (see below) in helping people cope with these conditions, it is recommended that affected individuals practice regular relaxation (see p.99 for a relaxation sequence), yoga, or meditation.

STRESS MANAGEMENT One of the earliest studies indicating that mind–body therapies might be useful for people who are HIV positive and/or have AIDS was conducted in 1995.

This study evaluated the effects of a stress-management program on anxiety, mood, self-esteem, and T-cell count in a group of HIV-positive men who had no symptoms except for T-cell counts below 400. This early, innovative program consisted of 20 twice-weekly sessions of progressive muscle relaxation and electromyograph biofeedback-assisted relaxation training, meditation, and hypnosis. The treatment group showed significant improvement when compared to a group that did not receive any mind–body treatment. All of the positive changes were maintained after a month.

Later studies suggested that mind–body practices, such as relaxation exercises done at home, reduce stress levels and have a positive effect on immune response. Since stress is known to compromise the immune system, these results suggest that stress management to reduce arousal of the nervous system and anxiety is an important part of a treatment regimen for HIV infection.

Infection with herpes simplex virus type 2 (HSV2) is common in people with HIV and has negative implications for their health. A study examined the effect of a ten-week course of mind–body therapies on a group of men with mild HIV symptoms. Overall, those who practiced the most relaxation had the greatest reduction in symptoms from herpes simplex.

In 2001 a study looked at the effects of a seven-week self-management and coping skills training program in people with HIV or AIDS. The study aimed to discover whether a self-management program would have any impact on the mood and attitude of participants. Those who completed the program showed significant positive changes in terms of their mood, the way they coped with the disease, and their attitudes. Treatment significantly improved participants' coping strategies and they became noticeably less pessimistic and anxious.

PREVENTION PLAN

The following may help:

- Do not have sex, especially unprotected sex, with multiple partners

- Always use condoms during sex

- Couples who wish to have unprotected sex should have an HIV test first. Remember, it can take three months after infection for the antibodies that are usually measured to be detectable

- Never share needles if you use injectable drugs

CHRONIC FATIGUE SYNDROME

People with chronic fatigue syndrome (CFS) have severe fatigue that has caused substantial disability for at least six months. The term CFS is now preferred to myalgic encephalomyelitis (ME), because in most cases of CFS no underlying disease of the muscles or nervous system can be found. The condition affects more women than men. There is no single treatment for CFS. Instead, improvement in symptoms often comes from a combination of approaches, including cognitive behavioral therapy, dietary changes, supplements, and exercise.

WHAT ARE THE SYMPTOMS?

- Fatigue that is severe enough to interfere with work or home life and lasts at least six months
- Muscle aches and pains
- Irritability and mood changes
- Sleep disturbances
- Headaches
- Poor concentration
- Poor short-term memory
- Depression

WHY MIGHT I HAVE THIS?

PREDISPOSING FACTORS

- Low adrenal gland function
- Food sensitivity (see p.456) see p.000
- Candidiasis
- Magnesium deficiency
- Essential fatty acid deficiency
- Vitamin B deficiency

TREATMENT PLAN

PRIMARY TREATMENTS

- Self-help measures (see right)
- Graduated exercise
- Psychological therapy
- Nutritional therapy

BACKUP TREATMENTS

- Drugs and other treatment for symptoms

WORTH CONSIDERING

- Homeopathy
- Western herbal medicine
- Breathing retraining
- Environmental health measures
- Massage
- Acupuncture

For an explanation of how treatments are rated, see p.111.

WHY DOES IT OCCUR?

One in five people consult their doctor about fatigue but only a small proportion will have CFS, which is profound fatigue that makes any physical and mental activity very difficult and is not improved by bed rest. There does not appear to be a single cause of the disease; instead, it seems to be the result of a combination of physical and psychological factors. It can follow a viral illness, such as infectious mononucleosis (see p.463), in which case it may be known as post-viral fatigue syndrome. CFS usually begins suddenly, although the onset can sometimes be gradual.

SELF-HELP

PRIMARY TREATMENT Try the following measures to improve the condition:

- Find a sympathetic doctor. Try contacting the CFS organizations (see p.486), some of whom keep databases of doctors with an interest in CFS.
- Join a CFS support group.
- Pace yourself: be prepared for good days and bad days.
- Get regular relaxation and follow a graded exercise program to reduce stress.
- Practice cognitive behavioral techniques, which can help reduce fears and pessimism.
- Compile a list of the things you want to achieve and break it down into phased, achievable goals. Keep goals manageable so that you do not become discouraged.
- Talk to your employer about a phased return to work.

TREATMENTS IN DETAIL

Conventional Medicine

The diagnosis of CFS is made by ruling out other causes of persistent fatigue, such as an underactive thyroid. (This is diagnosed by a blood test.) A program aimed at gradually increasing physical activity is likely to be recommended to try to reduce fatigue and improve quality of life (see Exercise, p.477). The doctor may also make a referral for psychotherapy, in particular cognitive behavioral therapy (see Psychological Therapies, p.477). Drugs may be prescribed to treat specific problems, such as depression.

Nutritional Therapy

Some of the most common underlying problems associated with CFS that nutritional therapists see include low adrenal gland function, food sensitivity (see p.456), low thyroid function (see p.319), and gut flora problems (see p.40). Identifying and correcting any underlying problem is often effective in restoring energy and combating fatigue.

PRIMARY TREATMENT **MAGNESIUM** There is some evidence that many CFS patients have low levels of magnesium. Studies also show that giving magnesium injections into muscle can improve symptoms in most people with CFS. In one study, 80 percent of those receiving magnesium reported increased energy, better mood, and a reduction in pain. Taking supplements can also improve symptoms. If you have CFS, you may benefit from taking 500–750mg of magnesium each day.

ESSENTIAL FATTY ACIDS Supplementation with essential fatty acids (EFAs) might also benefit people with CFS. Low levels of essential fatty acids, specifically the omega-3 type, may be found in people with CFS. One study found that taking high doses of omega-3 fatty acids over a three-month period brought about an improvement in 85 percent of CFS patients. A diet rich in foods high in omega-3 fatty acids, such as oily fish (e.g. salmon, trout, mackerel, herring, and sardines), seeds, and walnuts may help reverse CFS symptoms in time. In addition, it may help to take essential fatty acid supplements. Taking 1g of concentrated fish oil once or twice a day might help in the long term.

PRIMARY TREATMENT **VITAMIN B** People who have CFS tend to be deficient in B vitamins. In practice, supplementation with a high-potency B-complex supplement that contains at least 25–50mg of vitamins B_1, B_2, B_5, and B_6 appears to be beneficial in improving symptoms of CFS, possibly because B vitamins are involved in many metabolic pathways that generate energy in the body.

CARNITINE Carnitine, an amino acid, is required for energy production in the mitochondria of body cells (the parts of the cell concerned with generating energy). Deficiency of carnitine has been found in some people with CFS. Taking 1g of carnitine three times daily has been found to improve CFS symptoms in one study, although improvement generally takes 4–8 weeks to become apparent. Try taking 1,000mg once or twice a day.

CAUTION

Consult your doctor before taking fish oil and magnesium supplements with blood-thinning drugs, such as warfarin. (See p.46.)

Homeopathy

Evidence from clinical trials and case reports suggest that homeopathy can be helpful in treating CFS. However, CFS is a

CFS AND ADRENAL GLAND FUNCTION

The pituitary and adrenal glands work together to determine how much energy the body uses and also how it responds to stress. Some experts link CFS to lowered adrenal gland function, but the evidence is far from clear. The adrenal glands produce several hormones that control energy levels, including cortisol and epinephrine. Cortisol is increased when the body is under stress.

Epinephrine alerts the nervous system and mobilizes sugars and fats. However, in the long term, adrenal overload may deplete the body's energy reserves. Cortisol also reduces the normal immune system responses. It is possible that CFS patients develop a lowered "stress threshold," leading to overworked adrenal glands and eventual "adrenal exhaustion."

Hormonal feedback and the adrenal glands

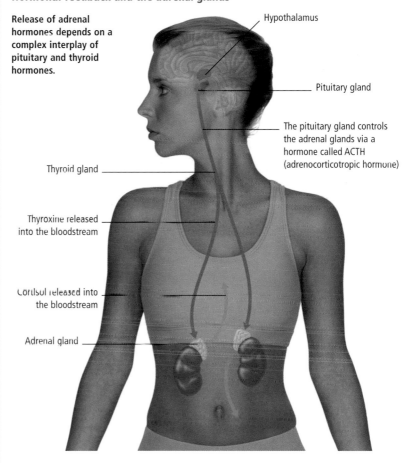

Release of adrenal hormones depends on a complex interplay of pituitary and thyroid hormones.

Hypothalamus

Pituitary gland

The pituitary gland controls the adrenal glands via a hormone called ACTH (adrenocorticotropic hormone)

Thyroid gland

Thyroxine released into the bloodstream

Cortisol released into the bloodstream

Adrenal gland

complex problem and often responds best to a combined approach including dietary changes, graded exercise programs, lifestyle management, homeopathy, and certain other therapies.

It is necessary to visit a homeopath for constitutional homeopathic treatment if you have CFS. Many medicines may be appropriate for treating this condition, including *Phosphorus* medicines, such as *Phosphoric acid*, *Kalium phosphoricum*, and *Calcarea phosphorica*.

KALIUM PHOSPHORICUM is one of the most frequently given basic medicines for CFS. It is suitable when there is general weakness and weariness, possibly with blurring of vision and humming or buzzing noises in the ears, a tendency to be startled by sudden noises, and a curious symptom of very yellow urine.

CALCAREA PHOSPHORICA may be appropriate when the person has a lot of aches and pains; it is useful for young people who seem to have developed CFS after a growth spurt. People who respond to *Calcarea phosphorica* may crave smoked or salted food, such as salami and anchovies.

PHOSPHORIC ACID AND PICRIC ACID In people who respond to *Phosphoric acid*, the initial problem is mental exhaustion, evidenced by weak memory and poor concentration. There is often diarrhea or looseness of the bowels, which may be diagnosed as irritable bowel syndrome.

In people who respond to *Phosphoric acid*, CFS is often triggered by an emotional upset, such as divorce or an unhappy relationship, and in men there is often impotence. If impotence is a prominent feature, *Picric acid* may be another possible treatment.

CFS can affect people of all ages, but women are more frequently affected than men

SILICEA A number of other medicines may be prescribed for CFS, including *Silicea*. People who respond to *Silicea* are pale and weak, with fine hair. They are usually chilly and feel cold even in a warm room. Their hands and feet are cold and clammy. They tend to catch infections easily; their immune systems are weak and their coughs and colds are very slow to clear up. If they get a boil or pimple, it is very slow to resolve and usually does not burst. Although they may be very tired, they are determined and will push themselves hard.

ZINCUM METALLICUM is another possible medicine for CFS. A particularly characteristic feature of these people is that they have fidgety, twitchy feet.

Western Herbal Medicine

Herbal practitioners view CFS as a disease resulting from neuroendocrine exhaustion — the body, mind, and spirit lack the resources needed to restore normal immune and nervous function. There has been little formal research specifically into the use of herbal medicine for CFS, but herbalists traditionally use cayenne (*Capsicum frutescens*), echinacea (*Echinacea*

spp.), ginkgo (*Ginkgo biloba*), and schisandra (*Schizandra chinensis*) in conditions such as this that are characterized by neurological and immune dysfunction.

Many people with CFS are highly sensitive to treatment, and it often needs to be started at a low dose, using well-tolerated remedies. Your precise treatment will depend on your symptoms but it is likely to include the following herbs.

IMMUNE-STIMULATING HERBS To stimulate immune resistance and detoxification, you may be given astragalus (*Astralagus membranaceus*), burdock (*Arctium lappa*), and echinacea. If a viral cause is suspected, antiviral remedies such as St. John's wort (*Hypericum perforatum*) and thuja (*Thuja occidentalis*) may be appropriate.

CIRCULATORY STIMULANTS Cayenne pepper, ginkgo, and prickly ash (*Zanthoxylum* spp.) increase blood flow (and thus nutrient supply) to the peripheral parts of the body, especially to the head. They also have helpful antioxidant actions. Relatively large doses may be prescribed.

The use of ginkgo in CFS, due to its circulatory stimulant and neuroprotective actions within the brain, is especially important. Cayenne — and in particular capsaicin, which is one of its key active constituents — has potent antioxidant and anti-inflammatory actions.

GLANDULAR TONICS Dandelion (*Taraxacum officinale*) root, kelp (*Luminaria* spp.) and licorice (*Glycyrrhiza glabra*) support and strengthen the liver and endocrine glands, in particular the thyroid and adrenal glands.

ADAPTOGENS American ginseng (*Eleutherococcus senticosus*), Siberian ginseng (*Panax quinquefolius*), and schisandra (*Schizandra chinensis*) are important for people with CFS because they help the body respond effectively (adapt) to things that cause stress such as cold, chemical toxins, and anxiety.

> **CAUTION**
>
> See p.69 before taking a herbal remedy and, if you are taking prescribed medication, consult an herbal medicine expert first.

Environmental Medicine

There are many possible environmental triggers for chronic fatigue syndrome that are still being investigated and are the subject of some controversy. It is possible that individuals with sensitivities to certain environmental chemicals and/or a genetic predisposition to CFS may have an adverse reaction to paints and other chemicals at a level that would not normally be considered toxic.

Treatment for CFS involves identifying the likely cause and avoiding it. You may need the support of an expert who can take an environmental and occupational history looking for relevant environmental exposures (*see p.86*).

SICK BUILDING SYNDROME This causes a set of general symptoms, similar to those of CFS, as a result of exposure to compounds from building materials. Your symptoms may improve with the use of low-emitting building materials, continuous ventilation, using nontoxic office supplies, and careful storage of chemicals.

MERCURY People may be exposed to mercury by consuming fish; the US Food and Drug Administration recommends that pregnant women and other vulnerable groups do not consume suspect fish (*for details, see p.86*).

People who work in mining, ore smelting, and in dental offices are at risk of mercury poisoning. If you work with dental amalgam, it is important to take precautions to prevent releasing mercury into the environment. You should ensure your workplace is adequately ventilated.

However, it is probably not necessary to remove dental amalgam fillings. Although leaching of mercury from them is often mentioned as the cause of a variety of health problems, this claim is doubted by many researchers.

It can be difficult to know if mercury is contributing to your CFS because some forms of mercury level testing, such as hair analysis and some urine tests, are unreliable. Some researchers also doubt the effectiveness of chelation therapy in removing mercury from the body.

DETOXIFICATION To improve the symptoms of chronic fatigue syndrome it is important to remove possible environmental toxins from the body (or "detoxify"). This can be done through changes in the diet (for example, following one of the many possible low-allergenic diets). It is also a good idea to take liver-tonic herbs such as milk thistle and supplements, such as vitamin C, vitamin E, selenium, green tea, and mixed carotenes. (*For help with detoxification, consult a qualified herbalist or nutritionist.*)

LIGHT THERAPY When over 100 people with CFS were studied, it was found that major symptoms in about a third of the participants were strongly influenced by season. It appears that a subgroup of patients with CFS show seasonal variation in symptoms resembling those of seasonal affective disorder (*see p.432*), in which symptoms are worse in the winter. Light therapy has been found to provide some people with CFS with an effective alternative or additional treatment to antidepressant drugs.

Acupuncture

CFS has many associated symptoms, in particular irritable bowel and muscle pain. While there are no rigorous clinical trials of acupuncture and the treatment of CFS, many individuals who experience this condition use acupuncture and report considerable benefit. There is no doubt that there is evidence for the treatment of individual symptoms, such as muscle pain, with acupuncture. There is also a clear case for the use of acupuncture within the context of a traditional Chinese approach to CFS, in that "rebalancing the body's energy" is likely to be of benefit. However, acupuncture alone will not prove effective and needs to be used in association with other approaches.

Acupuncture in general should be given weekly for six to eight weeks as the only new treatment, to enable both the patient and the therapist to judge whether it is having any real benefit.

Massage

Massage therapy, which is noted for its ability to improve well-being, has been found to be very helpful in the overall treatment of CFS. In one study, there was an immediate improvement in feelings of depression and anxiety after a single massage was given to participants. After ten days of daily massage, researchers noted that fatigue-related symptoms, particularly emotional stress, were reduced, as were depression, pain, and difficulty sleeping.

Breathing Retraining

Researchers have found that hyperventilation (shallow, fast breathing) is common in CFS patients. Such patterns of breathing can create or contribute to a variety of CFS symptoms, including anxiety, fatigue, poor stamina, and muscle pain. Breathing retraining of one sort or another, often yoga-based, can be very helpful in easing these symptoms (*see p.62*).

Exercise

PRIMARY TREATMENT People with long-term CFS withdraw from all activity and lose fitness and muscle strength. A program aimed at gradually increasing physical activity is likely to be recommended; research shows this helps reduce fatigue and improves quality of life.

However, exercise needs to be carefully controlled for people with CFS. People with CFS respond poorly to anything more than exercise within current tolerance and can feel even more exhausted unless the process is carefully monitored.

In one study, the response to exercise of a group of 15 people with CFS was compared to that of a group of 15 healthy people of the same age and gender. The CFS patients had weaker heart function and respiratory responses during and after exercise compared to the control group.

On the positive side, in three trials involving 350 adults, patients with CFS had weekly exercise sessions for 3–4 months. They also had advice on coping with the condition and pacing themselves. The results suggest that graded exercise programs reduce fatigue and improve quality of life, and may be as helpful for CFS as cognitive behavioral therapy.

Psychological Therapies

PRIMARY TREATMENT Psychological therapies are useful in treating CFS. The most successful treatment strategies for CFS involve cognitive behavioral therapy.

The goal of treatment is to overcome illness-perpetuating behaviors. The most important starting point is usually to promote a regular pattern of nonstressful activity, rest, and sleep, with a gradual return to normal activity. At the same time, it is important to reduce anxiety and depression.

COGNITIVE BEHAVIORAL THERAPY helps people recognize their habitual reactions to the illness and then change negative patterns of thinking. It does not work for everyone: there is no satisfactory evidence for the effectiveness of CBT in patients with milder CFS or in patients who are so disabled by the condition that they are unable to come to treatment as outpatients. There is also no satisfactory evidence for the effectiveness of group cognitive behavioral therapy in treating CFS.

For some people, however, CBT can be very effective. A 1991 study showed that it led to substantial improvements in overall physical and psychiatric symptoms. These improvements depended on the strength of the participants' belief that their symptoms were due exclusively to physical causes and were not influenced by the length of illness. The study also suggested that advice to avoid physical and mental activity in CFS is not appropriate.

A later study reviewed the psychological treatments for treating CFS. The results showed CBT significantly improved physical functioning in people with CFS compared to conventional medical management or just relaxation therapy alone.

A recent study also showed that CBT was significantly more effective than guided support groups in relieving fatigue and functional impairment.

If you have CBT, you will probably attend weekly sessions, which last about 50 minutes each. How long initial treatment continues depends on the individual. It is generally necessary to continue with less frequent treatment for about six months after the end of the initial treatment. It is important to keep practicing the technique daily after regular treatment ends.

JET LAG

The condition known as jet lag occurs as a result of long-distance air travel in which time zones are crossed. Many people find that jet lag is worse when they fly from the west to the east, or when they take an overnight flight. Some symptoms that are often associated with jet lag, such as a dry nose and throat or muscle aches, are probably due to being in the dry and often cramped atmosphere of the jet itself and not to crossing time zones. Many simple measures, such as lifestyle adjustments and exercise, can help make jet lag symptoms less severe.

WHAT ARE THE SYMPTOMS?

- Insomnia
- Fatigue
- Headaches
- Irritability
- Problems concentrating

WHY MIGHT I HAVE THIS?

TRIGGERS

- Long-distance air travel in which time zones are crossed

TREATMENT PLAN

PRIMARY TREATMENTS

- Self-help measures (see right)

BACKUP TREATMENTS

- Melatonin
- Light therapy

WORTH CONSIDERING

- Exercise
- Chiropractic
- Acupressure
- Acupuncture

For an explanation of how treatments are rated, see p.111.

WHY DOES IT OCCUR?

The body's sleep-wake cycle is controlled by the suprachiasmatic nucleus (SCN), a tiny structure located in the hypothalamus of the brain. In the morning when light is detected by the retina at the back of the eye, signals are transmitted to the SCN via the optic nerve. Messages are then relayed to the pineal gland to switch off production of melatonin, a hormone that induces drowsiness. When darkness falls, levels of melatonin start to rise again.

Jet lag arises because normal patterns of eating, sleeping, and waking are not yet synchronized with the local time, giving rise to a range of symptoms that may include difficulty sleeping, fatigue, and headaches. It can take up to five days before the sleep–wake cycle is reset to the new time. It is not the length of the flight that determines whether jet lag occurs, but how many time zones one passes through.

In addition, general health, age, and lifestyle play a part in susceptibility to jet lag. Overeating, smoking, and drinking alcohol tend to make it worse.

SELF-HELP

PRIMARY TREATMENT The following tips may help keep jet lag to a minimum.

- Get plenty of sleep before you travel and take it easy when you arrive.
- When you board the flight, try to adjust your eating and sleeping patterns to the local time at the destination.
- Drink two glasses of water before the flight and plenty of fluids during it. Avoid alcohol and caffeinated drinks.
- Get up and walk around at regular intervals during the flight. This also helps you avoid the dangers of deep vein thrombosis.
- Make sure you get some exercise outside in daylight after you arrive at your destination and try to resist having a nap during the day.

TREATMENTS IN DETAIL

Conventional Medicine

ADVICE Your doctor may give you advice on how to minimize the effects of jet lag (see Self-Help, left) and how you can cope if you have to take medication at regular intervals.

MELATONIN, the hormone that is largely responsible for regulating sleep, has been found to be useful for jet lag. It is available without a prescription in the US but is not regulated by the Food and Drug Administration and may have adverse side effects. Research suggests that it may be helpful for people flying across five or more time zones, especially if they are flying east. Jet lag symptoms associated with crossing time zones have been found to be reduced with quick recovery of preflight energy and alertness levels.

Homeopathy

The homeopathic medicine most often recommended for jet lag is *Nux vomica*. This medicine is appropriate for sleep disturbance (especially when this involves waking too early), digestive disturbances, and a dry, stuffy nose.

Other medicines that may help are *Kalium phosphoricum*, which is suitable when the person is exhausted and too tired to sleep, or may have disturbing dreams. *Arnica* is indicated when there are bruise-like aches and pains, which may be so severe that even the bed feels too hard.

Exercise

A study looked at the effect of exercising for a few hours on the day after a plane trip from Tokyo to Los Angeles (which is an eight-hour time difference). The researchers concluded that outdoor exercise hastens the resetting of the body's internal "clock," helping people become synchronized to a new time zone.

In general, it is important to get as much exercise as you can during a flight. Walking up and down the aisle, standing for a while from time to time, and doing small twisting and stretching exercises in your seat can all help reduce discomfort, especially swelling of legs and feet, and prevent blood clots. Get off the plane if possible at stopovers and do some exercises or take a walk. It is also helpful to get some exercise outside when you land.

Light Therapy

A most effective treatment for the general malaise of jet lag seems to be exposure to natural light, or exposure to the light from a natural full spectrum light box or bulb. Stimulus from natural light is needed for the pineal gland to reduce secretion of melatonin, and a lack of light is a recognized cause of jet lag. Prolonged exposure to bright artificial daylight has proved effective in easing jet lag symptoms.

Acupuncture

While there are no clinical trials supporting the use of acupuncture in jet lag, acupuncturists believe that it is effective and there are good reasons for believing this is the case. For example, acupuncture can be used to balance minor energetic dysfunctions. It has also been used extensively in the treatment of insomnia and anxiety, symptoms that are frequently associated with jet lag. Acupuncture also has fundamental effects on neurotransmitters, the chemical messengers within the brain, and appears to balance and normalize the release and uptake of these chemicals within the brain.

MELATONIN LEVELS AND JET LAG

Melatonin is a hormone produced in the pineal gland that is largely responsible for regulating the sleep–wake cycle. Melatonin is normally produced at night and seems to act as a signal to the body that it is dark. Levels of melatonin therefore tend to rise and fall with the hours of darkness and daylight. When people travel by plane across many time zones, their melatonin levels will initially be out of step with their new local time zone, making it difficult for them to sleep and wake at the right times.

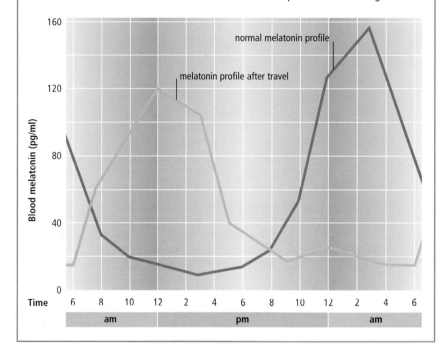

Ideally, acupuncture should be given to balance the body a day or two before a flight across several time zones, and then daily for three or four days after the flight. This may be part of a generalized acupuncture course to strengthen the whole body.

Bodywork Therapies

ACUPRESSURE Traditional Chinese Medicine (TCM) has identified what it calls a horary cycle. In this cycle, energy circulates through the main acupuncture meridians, or energy pathways, in a very specific order. Acupressure on particular "horary (time-related) points" is used to treat or to prevent jet lag. An informal study was conducted by a group of acupuncturists who were traveling from the US to China. They divided themselves into two groups, with one group acting as a control. The other group used acupressure treatments on their horary points while traveling.

After arrival, the control group experienced jet lag symptoms lasting from three days to two weeks. The group who treated themselves with acupressure experienced no jet lag symptoms. On the return trip, the groups switched and the results were similar, with those who used acupressure experiencing no jet lag symptoms.

CHIROPRACTIC It may be helpful to have a chiropractic session before and/or after you fly: one study evaluated the benefits of chiropractic treatment in relation to jet lag in athletes. One group of athletes received chiropractic treatment before flying, compared to two other groups, one of which received placebo (false) treatment and the other no treatment at all.

The results showed that the chiropractic care group had fewer jet lag symptoms and felt better overall than those in either of the other two groups. Those athletes who received chiropractic treatment also slept an average of one hour longer per night and experienced fewer disruptions in sleep patterns than athletes in either the placebo group or the control group.

GLOSSARY OF TERMS

A

Acupoint Term used in Traditional Chinese Medicine for a specific point on a meridian where the flow of *Qi* is accessible. Acupoints are stimulated by acupressure and acupuncture.

Acupressure Ancient Chinese massage that uses the thumbs and fingertips on acupoints to restore a healthy balance to an individual's energy.

Acupuncture Cornerstone therapy of Traditional Chinese Medicine in which ailments and disorders are treated by using needles to stimulate acupoints.

Acute A symptom or disorder that comes on suddenly.

Adaptogenic Restores balance within the body.

Adipose Relating to fat tissue, which is composed of cells called adipocytes.

Agglutination Term meaning sticking together — for example, sperm or red blood cells.

Aggravation A homeopathic term that means a worsening of symptoms.

Alexander technique Method of correcting imbalances in posture, with the aim of restoring health to both body and mind.

Alkaloids Organic compounds, such as nicotine and caffeine, that can be toxic yet are medicinally useful.

Allergen An environmental or dietary irritant that can trigger an allergic reaction in sensitive people.

Allergenic Sensitive to an environmental or dietary irritant.

Alpha blockers Drugs that interfere with nerve signals to the muscles. Used in the relief of urine retention, they work by relaxing the sphincter muscle of the bladder.

Alterative Term used in herbal medicine meaning restorative.

Amitriptyline Tricyclic antidepressant that is used to improve mood and activity levels, and encourage sleep in long-term depression.

Analgesics Drugs that relieve pain.

Androgen Male sex hormone.

Anemia Blood disease in which hemoglobin is deficient or abnormal.

Angiotensin-converting enzyme (ACE) inhibitors Powerful vasodilators that block an enzyme involved in blood-vessel constriction.

Antacids Mildly alkaline compounds that neutralize excess stomach acid.

Antibiotics Drugs that kill bacteria.

Antibody Protein in the blood that destroys an invading substance or pathogen that the body considers harmful.

Anticonvulsants Drugs that inhibit excessive activity in the brain and are used to prevent and stop epileptic seizures.

Antidepressants Drugs for treating moderate to severe depression.

Antifungals Drugs for killing fungi or inhibiting their growth.

Antigen Protein located on the surface of an invading micro-organism that stimulates the white blood cells to produce antibodies.

Antihistamines Drugs that counter the effects of histamine, a chemical released in the body during an allergic reaction.

Antihypertensives Drugs that reduce high blood pressure.

Anti-inflammatories Drugs, such as NSAIDs and corticosteroids, that relieve inflammation.

Antioxidants Chemicals that neutralize free radicals and are thought to prevent cancer.

Aphthous ulcers Ulcers in the lining of the mouth; they may occur in oral yeast.

Aqueous Relating to water.

Arachidonic acid Derivative of an essential fatty acid that produces substances causing inflammation.

Arginine Amino acid essential for sperm formation.

Arrhythmia Disrupted heart rhythm.

Arterial plaque Deposit of fat on the inner wall of an artery.

Arteriosclerosis Hardening of the arteries.

Asana Physical posture in yoga.

Astringent Substance that contracts tissue and reduces a discharge or secretion.

ATP Adenosine triphosphate, a high-energy molecule in cells.

Atria The two upper chambers of the heart.

Autogenic training Relaxation therapy. Six mental exercises relieve stress and promote self-healing.

Autoimmune Term applied to disorders in which the body's immune system produces antibodies that attack its own tissues.

Autonomic nervous system Part of the nervous system that controls body functions that are not under conscious control; for example, breathing and heart rate.

Anxiolytic Term used to describe a chemical that relieves anxiety.

B

Balneotherapy Traditional spa therapy in which bathing improves well-being and helps heal disorders of the skin, muscles, and joints.

Benign Of no danger to health i.e. cell growth that is under control and noncancerous.

Benzodiazepines Antianxiety drugs that reduce excessive activity in the part of the brain that controls emotion.

Beta blockers Drugs that reduce heart rate and prevent dilation of blood vessels by blocking the action of the neurotransmitter norepinephrine in the sympathetic nervous system.

Beta-endorphin Pain-relieving chemical found in the brain.

Biofeedback Interactive relaxation therapy in which feedback machines enable individuals to control their own body functions, such as muscle tension, brainwave patterns, and electrical skin resistance.

Bioflavonoid Chemical that aids the absorption of vitamin C by the body.

Bisphosphonates Drugs used to treat bone disorders, such as osteoporosis.

Bodywork Term used to describe manipulative therapies or techniques, such as massage.

Bone mineral density (BMD) Measure of bone mass, often tested in osteoporosis.

Breathing retraining Learning to control the rate of abdominal breathing.

Bronchiectasis Permanent widening of the airways associated with a persistent productive cough and eventually shortness of breath.

C

Calcium-channel blockers Drugs that block the entry of calcium into muscle cells, allowing blood vessels to dilate.

Candida albicans A yeastlike microorganism that occurs naturally in the mouth, gut, and vagina, and on the skin. It is normally controlled by "friendly" bacteria.

Cardiorespiratory Relating to the heart and respiration.

Cardiovascular Relating to the heart and circulation.

Carminative A herb or drug that calms cramps or induces gas expulsion from the stomach or the intestines.

Cauda equina Array of nerves at the bottom of the spinal cord.

Chelation Binding of a metal and filtering it from the bloodstream by chemical means.

Chemonucleolysis Chemical breakdown of the nucleus of a vertebral disk.

Chiropractic Manipulation therapy that diagnoses and treats disorders of the spine and other joints of the body.

Cholesterol One of the major fats found in the blood and most tissues.

Chronic Symptoms and conditions that are long-lasting and slow to change.

Chronic venous insufficiency Persistent lack of blood in the veins.

Clinical trial A scientific study to assess the safety and effectiveness of a medical treatment.

Clot Semisolid mass of blood, also called a thrombus.

Coenzyme Q$_{10}$ An antioxidant nutrient, also known as ubiquinone, that the body makes to help it release energy from food. Also available as a supplement.

Cognitive behavioral therapy (CBT) Form of psychotherapy pioneered in the 1960s and based on a belief in the ability of the mind to change negative patterns of thinking and behavior.

Collagen Tough protein found in bone and cartilage.

Compress Pad of fabric (usually cold) for relieving pain or inflammation

Coronary Relating to the arteries that supply the muscles of the heart.

Coronary thrombosis Blood clot that lodges in a coronary artery.

Corticosteroids (or steroids) Anti-inflammatory drugs that suppress allergic responses and the immune system, and help in the treatment of conditions caused by deficiency of adrenal gland hormones.

Cranial osteopathy Otheopathy that focuses on correcting distortions in the bones of the skull (cranium) and face.

Craniosacral therapy Form of cranial osteopathy that adjusts the pressure on the membranes and fluids surrounding the brain and spinal cord.

Crossover trial A form of clinical trial in which patients receive both treatments in sequence, half taking one treatment first, and the other half the other treatment first.

CT (Computer Tomography) scans Diagnostic technique that uses X-rays and computers to produce a cross-sectional image of a tissue under examination. Also called CAT (Computer Axial Tomography) scans.

Cyst Small, benign tumor filled with fluid or soft tissue.

Cytokine Drug that stimulates the immune system to attack the cells of certain cancers.

Cytotoxic test Diagnostic technique in which damage to white blood cells when mixed with extracts of a possible allergen is said to suggest sensitivity.

D

Decoction Solution obtained from boiling a herb in water.

Deep vein thrombosis Blood clot in a deep-lying vein, usually in the leg.

Demulcent Substance that soothes irritated membranes and tissues.

Dermatologist A medical practitioner who specializes in conditions of the skin.

Diastolic blood pressure Lower of the two figures when blood pressure is measured.

Diuretic Chemical that stimulates urine production.

Dorsal root ganglia Groups of cells clustered at the point where the 12 dorsal nerves emerge from the spinal cord.

E

Eicosanoids Chemicals, derived from omega-6 fatty acids, that help regulate inflammation and the flow of blood.

Echocardiography Ultrasound scanning of the heart.

Edema Tissue swollen with fluid.

Electromyographic (EMG) biofeedback Relaxation therapy in which biofeedback sensors, when placed on back or shoulder muscles, emit a rhythmic sound or flashing light in response to the strength of the muscle tension.

Embrocation Lotion for soothing a sore or pulled muscle.

Emollient Softening or smoothing the skin.

Endorphins Morphinelike substances produced by the body to relieve pain. Also known as the body's natural opiates.

Endoscopy Examination of a body cavity, such as the stomach, by means of a tubelike viewing instrument called an endoscope.

Endotoxin Toxin produced inside the body.

Enzyme Protein that speeds up a biochemical reaction.

Enthesitis Inflammation where a tendon attaches to a bone.

Epidermal Relating to the epidermis, or the outer layer of skin.

Epididymides Tightly coiled tubes that lie above and behind each testes where sperm are stored and mature.

Epidural space Space surrounding the membranes that envelop the spinal cord.

Essential fatty acid Polyunsaturated fatty acids that must be supplied in the diet because they are not made in the body. Two main types are omega-6 and omega-3.

Estrogenic Describes chemicals that have an estrogen-like action.

Erythrocyte Red blood cell.

Etiology Cause of a particular disease.

Exfoliant Skin remover.

Exposure therapy Psychological technique designed to help a patient overcome the anxiety of a trauma or fear by carefully managed exposure to the trauma or fear.

Eye movement desensitization and reprocessing (EMDR) Psychological technique that combines elements of exposure therapy and cognitive behavioral therapy.

F

Fistula An abnormal channel between organs or body cavities that normally do not connect, or between an organ or cavity and the skin.

Fatty acid The basic chemical building block of fats and oils.

Flavonoids Antioxidant chemicals, which are thought to help prevent certain forms of cancer. In nature, flavonoids are found in fruits such as lemons, plums, and blackcurrants.

Fluorescein angiography Photographic technique that makes use of a fluorescent dye (fluorescein) to study the blood vessels of the eye.

Food allergen Food that initiates an immune reaction.

Free radicals Potentially harmful molecules produced by the body that can damage DNA and cause a range of physiological problems.

G

Ganglion Cluster of nerve cells.

Gastric Relating to or involving the stomach.

Gestalt therapy Method of psychotherapy that helps clients gain self-awareness through analyzing their thoughts, feelings, and behavior with the therapist in a variety of situations and scenarios.

Glycemic Relating to the level of sugar in the blood.

Guided imagery Psychological technique that involves a patient concentrating his or her imagination on a particular part of the body.

H

H₂ blockers Antiulcer drugs that help healing by preventing the release of histamine in the stomach, reducing acid production.

Hatha yoga A form of yoga that uses physical postures (*asanas*) and breathing to help relieve mental stress while increasing suppleness and fitness.

Heberden's nodes Bony spurs on the end joints of the fingers.

Hernia/herniation Protrusion of an internal organ through a ruptured cavity wall.

Histamine Chemical that is essential to the body's immune system and central to the body's allergic reactions.

Holistic Term used to describe an approach to treatment in which the "whole" person is taken into account, rather than just the symptoms.

Homeostasis Constant state of the body's functions, such as temperature and blood acidity, which feedback mechanisms will restore to normal if disturbed.

Hydrogenation Process by which edible oils are treated to become solid.

Hydrolysates Protein molecules within milk.

Hydrotherapy Techniques in which water is used to stimulate the body and promote self-healing.

Hyperventilation Breathing too deeply or too rapidly so that the carbon dioxide level of the blood falls. It causes numbness of the hands and feet, faintness, muscle spasms, and twitches.

Hypnotherapy Technique in which a patient is hypnotized and temporarily hands over control to a therapist, who initiates mental and physical changes in the patient.

Hypo-allergenic Containing minimal levels of potential allergens

Hypoglycemia Low blood sugar.

I

Imagery Psychological technique that uses positive images and thought processes to invoke the senses and bring about healing.

Immunosuppressants Drugs that suppress the activity of the immune system.

Infusion Herbal tea.

Interpersonal therapy Psychological technique in which individuals are encouraged to examine and change the way they relate to other people.

Ischemic Lack of blood supply.

IU (International Unit) A unit of potency for a vitamin or other biologically active substance accepted as an international standard.

KL

Keratolytic Loosening of dead and hardened cells on the surface of the skin.

Kinesiology Method of detecting body system imbalances, as well as food and environmental sensitivities, by testing muscle resistance.

Lactose A form of sugar found in milk.

Lens capsule Thin layer that encloses the lens.

Lesion Change in a tissue or organ due to a disease.

Leukocyte White blood cell.

Libido Sexual urge.

Lidocaine (lignocaine) Anesthetic that is also used to combat arrhythmia and itching.

Liniment Oily cream for soothing muscle pain.

Liposuction A surgical procedure in which fatty tissue is removed through an incision in the skin.

Liver-tonifying Invigorating the liver.

Loin perineum Region between the anus and the scrotum in men.

Lutein One of a group of yellow carotenoid pigments.

Lymphatic pump techniques Gentle manipulation techniques used by massage and other therapists to encourage the flow of lymph fluid through the body's lymphatic system.

Lymphocytes White blood cells that recognize the antigens of invading bacteria and then produce antibodies.

Lymphocytes (T, or T-cells) White blood cells that recognize the antigens of viruses, parasites, and cancer cells, and then multiply to fight them.

Lysine An essential amino acid that the body extracts from food. Thought to help prevent and treat cold sores and herpes infections.

M

McKenzie-concept exercises Self-treatment exercises to relieve back pain, particularly of the low back. Developed by Robin McKenzie, they focus on improving the structure and metabolism of the soft tissues, such as the disks between the vertebrae of the spine.

Magnetic resonance imaging *See* MRI scans.

Meditation Self-help technique for mastering your thoughts and feelings, bringing relaxation to both mind and body.

Meninges Membranes that cover the brain and spinal cord.

Mensendieck exercises Exercises developed by Bess Mensendieck to train the musculoskeletal system.

Meridians Term used in Traditional Chinese Medicine. The meridians are the energy channels in the body through which *Qi* (energy) flows.

Meta-analysis Systematic review of a number of research studies and clinical trials that provides a more accurate assessment of the available evidence.

Metabolism General term for the chemical processes that govern all the functions of the body.

Microflora Term to describe the "friendly" bacteria in the intestine.

Mind–body therapies Techniques and approaches that harness thoughts, feelings, imagination, and actions in order to influence biochemical and structural processes.

Mono-amine oxidase inhibitors (MAOIs) Antidepressant drugs that increase levels of serotonin and other mood-enhancing brain chemicals.

Motility Term applied to the ability of sperm to swim along.

MRI (Magnetic Resonance Imaging) scans Diagnostic technique that uses high-frequency radio waves to examine the structures of the body, particularly the central nervous system.

Mucilage Gumlike substance found in plants that becomes slippery and viscous in water. Used to soothe tissues.

Myocardial infarction Medical term for a heart attack.

Myofascial Relating to deep muscle tissues.

N

Nebulizer Device that turns a liquid drug into a fine spray, or aerosol. Used to treat asthma.

Neonate Newborn child.

Neurological Relating to the nerves.

Neuromuscular therapy (NMT) Term used to describe manipulation therapy that enhances the mechanics of the body, releases endorphins, and restores the healthy relationship between nerves and the musculoskeletal system.

Neuropathy Disrupted function of one or more nerves.

Neurotransmitter A chemical that is released from the end of a nerve which transmits impulses to another nerve or to a muscle cell.

Neurotoxic Poisonous to nerves.

Nodules Small, red swellings.

Nosodes Homeopathic remedy made from a disease product.

NSAIDs Nonsteroidal anti-inflammatory drugs that relieve pain, stiffness, and painful inflammation in the muscles, bones, and joints.

O

Oral Relating to or involving the mouth.

Orthodontic Relating to the alignment of teeth and jaws.

Orthotic Shock-absorbing foot support device.

Ossicles Tiny bones of the middle ear.

Osteopathy Manipulation therapy that diagnoses and treats structural and biomechanical problems in the body's musculoskeletal framework.

Oxidative attack Damage by free radicals.

P

Papules Inflamed spots.

Pathogenic Disease-causing.

PENS (Percutaneous Electrical Nerve Stimulation) Similar to TENS, except the pulses of low-voltage electricity are delivered into the soft tissue via needles that puncture the skin.

PET (Positron Emission Tomography) scans Diagnostic technique in conventional medicine that uses injected radioactive substances to detect chemical activity in a tissue or organ and assess blood flow.

Photochemical Relating to a reaction that either needs light or UV radiation or else produces light

Phytoestrogens Chemicals from plants, such as the soy bean and other legumes, with properties similar to estrogen.

Pilates Conditioning technique that increases the body's flexibility and strength.

Placebo Chemically inert substance given in place of a drug. Used in medical drug trials as a control.

Plantar fasciitis Injury to the sole of the foot.

Platelets Blood-cell fragments involved in clotting.

Postpartum primapara Term used to describe a woman who has just given birth to her first child.

Probiotics "Friendly," disease-destroying bacteria in the gut that help in the manufacture of vitamins and enzymes, aiding digestion.

Progressive relaxation (also Jacobson's Progressive Relaxation) Technique developed by Edmund Jacobson that alternately tenses and relaxes muscles of the body in an orderly sequence from the toes to the head.

Prophylaxis Preventive measures.

Prostaglandins Drugs or naturally occurring substances within the body that cause muscle contractions and produce mucus in the lining of the stomach.

Prosthesis Artificial body part.

Proteolytic Protein-digesting.

Psychodynamic therapy Psychological technique that encourages an individual to actively bring painful feelings from their subconscious and consciously face them.

Psycho-education Psychological technique aimed at increasing an individual's knowledge and insight into his or her particular mental illness.

Psychotherapy Psychological technique in which an individual discusses his or her personal feelings, experiences, and behavior with a counselor trained to help draw out and resolve any mental problems.

Psychotropic Term used to describe a substance that influences behavior by affecting the mind.

Pulse-testing Traditional Chinese diagnostic technique in which nine pulse points are monitored to check the quality of *Qi* (energy).

Pustules Raised, pus-filled spots with a white center.

QR

Qi (also chi) Life energy force of Traditional Chinese Medicine that flows through the body along meridians and can be accessed at acupoints. It is said to be inherited at conception and to be derived from fresh food and air.

Radiation therapy Use of radioactivity to treat cancer and, occasionally, other diseases.

Range of motion The normal amount that a joint can be moved in certain directions withhout causing pain.

Referred pain Sensation experienced as a result of spinal problems that can affect nerves and muscles linked to other parts of the body, causing problems in those areas.

Reflexology Therapy that treats various ailments by massaging particular "reflex areas" on the feet (or, more rarely, the hands) with a thumb or fingers.

Renal Relating to the kidney.

Resorption Breaking down and absorbing a substance.

S

Sensitizer Chemical that sensitizes the immune system to a specific allergen.

Serotonin Neurotransmitter that calms the mind and helps induce sleep.

Selective serotonin reuptake inhibitors (SSRIs) Antidepressants that keep serotonin levels high.

Sick building syndrome Condition in which fatigue, lack of concentration, and recurrent infections are attributed to poor ventilation and chemical fumes from furnishings and office machines.

Sleep apnea Temporary but repeated interruption of breathing during sleep.

Sp. Abbreviation for species.

Spondylolisthesis Condition in which one vertebra slips forward over the vertebra beneath.

Statins Drugs that lower blood cholesterol. Used to prevent stroke and heart attack.

Stagnation Term applied to *Qi* (energy) when it ceases to flow through the body.

Steroidal Relating to a steroid.

Stress hormones Hormones, such as epinephrine and cortisol, which are released under stress.

Stroke Interruption in the brain's blood supply.

Sub-fertile Term applied to men when they are unable to produce normal sperm.

Supplements Nutrients, such as vitamins, minerals, and trace elements, that can be taken with food to ensure a complete day's nutrients.

Synovial Relating to the fluid secreted by the lining of a joint.

Systematic desensitization Psychological technique that combines relaxation and exposure to images of a feared object (e.g. a picture of a spider) to help the person conquer his or her fears.

Systemic therapy Class of talking therapies that combine cybernetics and anthropology to help resolve psychological problems within a "system," such as a family or group.

T

Tendinitis Painful inflammation of a tendon.

Tenosynovitis Painful swelling of a tendon and the synovial membrane of a joint.

TENS (Transcutaneous Electrical Nerve Stimulation) Stimulation of body tissue with pulses of low-voltage electricity for relieving pain.

Thrombolytic Breaking down a thrombus, or blood clot.

Tincture Herb extract in alcohol.

Topical Applied externally to the skin.

Traction Steady extension of a limb or muscle.

Trans-fatty acids Fats that occur naturally in meat and dairy products, and also in man-made foods such as margarines, where edible oils are treated to become solid (hydrogenation).

Trial, clinical Research which is used to establish scientific proof of a therapy or treatment — for example, the efficacy and safety of a new pharmaceutical drug or herbal remedy.

Trial, controlled A method of testing a treatment in which an experimental group receives the treatment and the control group receives none.

Trial, placebo controlled A method of testing a drug or treatment in which the treatment must be shown to make a significant difference compared to a placebo (an inactive medicine or treatment).

Trial, randomized A clinical scientific trial in which large numbers of patients participate in order to cancel out individual differences.

Trial, randomized double-blind In this type of trial neither the patients nor the practitioners know who is receiving the treatment and who is not.

Tricyclic antidepressants Drugs that raise the levels of neurotransmitters, such as serotonin and norepinephrine, involved in mood.

Triglyceride One of the major fats in the blood and in the cells of fat (adipose) tissue.

Trigger point A knot of tense muscle, which feels like a hard nodule when pressed. Trigger points may be caused by pain from the spine and connective tissue.

UV

Ultrasound High-frequency sound technique used to scan internal organs and the fetus in the womb, and to treat soft-tissue injuries.

UV light Light containing ultraviolet wavelengths, which has antiviral, antifungal, and antibacterial properties.

Vas deferens Tubes that transport sperm away from the epididymides toward the urethra.

Vascular disease Disease of the blood vessels.

Vasodilators Drugs that widen blood vessels. They are used to treat angina and high blood pressure.

Ventricles The lower heart chambers.

Vesicles Small blisters containing serum.

Viability Ability of sperm to fertilize the egg.

Visualization Psychological therapy in which an individual is encouraged to consciously imagine positive and beneficial events as a way of preventing self-fulfilling, negative patterns of behavior.

WXYZ

Yin and yang Opposing but complementary energies in Traditional Chinese Medicine. All things are said to be a manifestation of *yin* and *yang*.

FINDING A PRACTITIONER

Being able to trust your practitioner and having rapport with him or her are vital factors in the healing process and should always be considered when you are looking for a alternative or complementary practitioner. Competence is another key factor. Finding a good practitioner can be a matter of trial and error; consequently, many people prefer word-of-mouth recommendations. Establishing adequate standards of training, ethical practice, and disciplinary procedures for alternative and complementary therapies has always been a problem, particularly since different states require different levels of training and they do not necessarily license the same therapies. Although some practitioners complete three to four years of full or part-time degree studies, others have only a weekend correspondence course.

This lack of regulation means you have little legal recourse should anything go wrong or should you be dissatisfied with your treatment. At the very least, you need to feel confident that any undiagnosed serious condition would be recognized by the practioner and that you would be advised to seek medical help if your practitioner suspected the problem lay beyond his or her expertise.

If you are considering trying chiropractic, osteopathy, acupuncture, psychotherapy, counseling, or hypnotherapy, it is worth asking your doctor whether he or she can recommend a practitioner, because these therapies are becoming more accepted in mainstream medicine. Some medical practices even include practitioners from these fields. Additionally, some conventional health professionals may be qualified in acupuncture or homeopathy.

If you are choosing an alternative or a complementary practitioner for yourself, you should always consider the following issues.

Training and credentials

Always ensure that the practitioner is adequately trained and reputable, especially if the therapy involves the use of either physical manipulation or invasive techniques (e.g. if you swallow medication or have needles inserted into you). Ask the following questions:

- What are the practitioner's qualifications?

- What sort of training was undertaken, and for how long?

- For how many years has the practitioner been in practice?

- Will the practitioner advise your doctor of any treatment?

Professional organizations

Some disciplines have professional associations that regulate training and practice. These associations provide a code of conduct and maintain a register of members. For other disciplines, particularly noninvasive therapies, standards vary greatly and there may not be a single representative body. For these therapies, you should be sure to ask the following questions:

- Is the practitioner registered with a recognized organization, and does this organization have a public register of practitioners?

- Does the organization have a code of practice specifying the professional conduct required?

- Does the organization have a complaints system and an effective disciplinary procedure and sanctions?

- Can the practitioner give you the address and telephone number of his or her professional organization?

Financial considerations

When choosing any form of health care, financial considerations are important. A lengthy course of therapy could be very expensive. Is the treatment available at little or no personal cost on referral by your doctor? Note that some therapies — for example, chiropractic, osteopathy, homeopathy, acupuncture, and psychotherapy — may be available through mainstream health practices.

- Can you claim for the treatment through your private health insurance plan if you have one?

- What is the cost (both short- and long-term) of the treatment?

- How many treatments might you expect to require?

- Does the practitioner have professional indemnity insurance so that you receive compensation if he or she is negligent?

Precautions

Avoid any practitioner with whom you feel uncomfortable. Trust and empathy are important when you are being treated by someone, and indeed treatment is unlikely to succeed without them. Treatment is often conducted on a one-to-one basis, and may involve removing clothes and being touched. You should also avoid any practitioner who seems to be making excessive claims about the treatment or who guarantees that a particular treatment will bring about a cure. No form of treatment — conventional, alternative, or complementary — is perfect, and miracles should neither be expected by the client nor promised by the practitioner. After your initial consultation, you should ask yourself the following questions:

- Was the practitioner's conduct and demeanor entirely professional?

- Did the practitioner answer any questions clearly and thoroughly?

- Were you given further information to read in your own time?

- Were you told how many treatments you might need?

- What was the practitioner's attitude toward any conventional medical treatment you may be receiving? You should avoid any practitioner who suggests changing (or abandoning) your conventional medicine without first consulting your doctor.

USEFUL WEBSITES AND ADDRESSES

Knowing where to go for information and help enables you to become more involved in your own healthcare. When you understand the causes of illness, the meaning of symptoms, and the available treatment options, you may feel more in control of your well-being — and this is therapeutic in itself.

Hundreds of associations and organizations are dedicated to helping people deal with a wide variety of medical and emotional conditions. Sources of information range from government agencies, such as the Department of Health, to nonprofit organizations, such as the American Red Cross. Only a limited sample could be included in this list. Most listings are the headquarters of national groups and organizations. Information on a wide range of such organizations is usually available from libraries as well as from your local hospital and your own doctor.

Most organizations provide information about resources for the management of specific conditions. Many have

support groups to help people with a medical or emotional condition, or they can provide information about local groups in your area. Online sites are given for the US self-help groups. Most online sites provide links to related sites.

Although the web is brimming with advice on health matters, much of it can be ill-informed, biased, or downright wrong. This is especially true of interactive sites. If you ask an "expert" a health question, to be sure to check their credentials and know how much privacy you can expect. You should always be suspicious of "miracle cures" and should note any sponsorship or advertising deals that could indicate a bias in the advice that is given.

> **Caution**
> The publishers cannot accept responsibility for the quality of any information that may be provided by the organizations listed below.

General health information

Aetna Intelihealth
www.intelihealth.com

Alternative Health News Online
www.altmedicine.com

American College of Physicians
www.acponline.org
190 North Independence Mall West
Philadelphia, PA 19106-1572
Tel: (215) 351-2600 / (800) 523-2600

American College of Surgeons
www.facs.org
633 North Saint Clair Street
Chicago, IL 60611
Tel: (312) 202-5000 /(800) 621-4111

American Medical Association
www.ama-assn.org
515 North State Street
Chicago, IL 60610
Tel: (800) 621-8335

Centers for Disease Control and Prevention
www.cdc.gov
1600 Clifton Road
Atlanta, GA 30333
Tel: (404) 639-3311 / (800) 311-3435

Health On the Net Foundation
www.hon.ch

Healthfinder®
www.healthfinder.gov

Medic Alert Foundation International
www.medicalert.org
2323 Colorado Avenue
Turlock, CA 9382
Tel: (888) 633-4298 / (209) 668-3333

MEDLINE Plus
www.medlineplus.gov

National Institutes of Health
www.nih.gov
9000 Rockville Pike
Bethesda, MD 20892
Tel: (301) 496-4000

National Library of Medicine
www.nlm.nih.gov
8600 Rockville Pike
Bethesda, MD 20894
Tel: (888) 346-3656

Office of Rare Diseases
rarediseases.info.nih.gov
National Institutes of Health
6100 Executive Boulevard
Bethesda, Maryland 20892-7518
Tel: (301) 402-4336

Department of Health and Human Services
www.hhs.gov
200 Independence Avenue, SW
Washington, DC 20201
Tel: (202) 619-0257

Food and Drug Administration (FDA)
www.fda.gov
5600 Fishers Lane
Rockville, MD 20857-0001
Tel: (888) 463-6332

World Health Organization
www.who.int

Alcohol, smoking, and drug dependence

Alateen Family Group Headquarters
www.al-anon.alateen.org
1600 Corporate Landing Parkway
Virginia Beach, VA 23454-5617
Tel: (757) 563-1600

Alcoholics Anonymous
www.alcoholics-anonymous.org
Grand Central Station
PO Box 459
New York, NY 10163
Tel: (212) 870-3400

American Council for Drug Education
164 West 74th Street
New York, NY 10023
Tel: (800) 488-DRUG

National Clearinghouse for Alcohol and Drug Information
www.health.org
PO Box 2345
Rockville, MD 20847-2345

National Institute on Alcohol Abuse and Alcoholism
www.niaaa.nih.gov
5635 Fishers Lane, MSC 9304
Bethesda, MD 20892-9304

Narcotics Anonymous
www.na.org
PO Box 9999
Van Nuys, CA 91409
Tel: (818) 773-9999

National Council on Alcoholism and Drug Dependence
www.ncadd.org
22 Cortlandt Street, Suite 801
New York, NY 10007-3128
Tel: (212) 269-7797
HOPE LINE: (800) NCA-CALL

Partnership for a Drug-Free America
www.drugfree.org
405 Lexington Avenue, Suite 1601
New York, NY 10174
Tel: (212) 922-1560

Phoenix House
www.phoenixhouse.org

SAMHSA's National Clearinghouse for Alcohol and Drug Information
www.health.org
PO Box 2345
Rockville, MD 20847-2345
Tel: (800) 729-6686

Smokefree.gov
www.smokefree.gov

CDC Office on Smoking and Health
www.cdc.gov/tobacco
Mail Stop K-50
4770 Buford Highway, NE
Atlanta, GA 30341-3724
Tel: (770) 488-5705

ADHD

Attention Deficit Disorder Association
www.add.org
PO Box 543
Pottstown, PA 19464
Tel: (484) 945-2101

Children and Adults with Attention Deficit/Hyperactivity Disorder
www.chadd.org
8181 Professional Place, Suite 150
Landover, MD 20785

National Resource Center on ADHD
www.help4adhd.org
Tel: (800) 233-4050

Attention Deficit Disorder
www.add.org
PO Box 543
Pottstown, PA 19464
Tel: (484) 945-2101

Allergies

Asthma and Allergy Foundation of America
www.aafa.org
1233 Twentieth Street, NW Suite 402
Washington, DC 20036
Tel: (202) 466-7643

National Institute of Allergy and Infectious Disease
www.niaid.nih.gov
6610 Rockledge Drive, MSC 6612
Bethesda, MD 20892-6612

Food Allergy and Anaphylaxis Alliance
www.foodallergyalliance.org

Alzheimer's disease

Alzheimer's Association
www.alz.org
225 North Michigan Avenue, Floor 17
Chicago, IL 60601
Tel: (800) 272-3900

Alzheimer's Disease Education and Referral Center
www.alzheimers.org
PO Box 8250
Silver Spring, MD 20907-8250
Tel: (800) 438-4380

Ankylosing spondylitis

Spondylitis Association of America
www.spondylitis.org
PO Box 5872
Sherman Oaks, CA 91413
Tel: (818) 981-1616 / (800) 777-8189

Arthritis and rheumatism

American College of Rheumatology
www.rheumatology.org
1800 Century Place, Suite 250
Atlanta, GA 30345-4300
Tel: (404) 633-3777

Arthritis Foundation and American Juvenile Arthritis Organization
www.arthritis.org
PO Box 7669
Atlanta, GA 30357-0669
Tel: (404) 872-7100 / (800) 568-4045

National Institute of Arthritis and Musculoskeletal and Skin Diseases
www.niams.nih.gov
National Institutes of Health
Building 31, Room 4C02
31 Center Drive, MSC 2350
Bethesda, MD 20892-2350
Tel: (301) 496-8190

Asthma

Asthma and Allergy Foundation of America
www.aafa.org
1233 Twentieth Street, NW, Suite 402
Washington, DC 20036
Tel: (202) 466-7643

American Lung Association
www.lungusa.org
61 Broadway, 6th Floor
New York, NY 10006
Tel: (800) LUNGUSA

Back pain

www.allaboutbackandneckpain.com
www.backandneck.about.com
www.spine-health.com
www.spineuniverse.com

Bereavement

The Compassionate Friends
www.compassionatefriends.org
PO Box 3696
Oak Brook, IL 60522-3696
Tel: (630) 990-0010 / (877) 969-0010

GriefNet
www.griefnet.org

Brain and nervous system

American Brain Tumor Foundation
www.abta.org
2720 River Road
Des Plaines, IL 60018
Tel: (800) 886-2282

Brain Research Foundation
brainresearchfdn.org
5812 South Ellis Avenue
MC 7112 Room J-141
Chicago, IL 60637

Brain Tumor Society
www.tbts.org
124 Watertown Street, Suite 3H
Watertown, MA 02472
Tel: (617) 924-9997

National Brain Tumor Foundation
www.braintumor.org
22 Battery Street, Suite 612
San Francisco, CA 94111-5520
Tel: (800) 934-CURE

Pediatric Brain Tumor Foundation
www.pbtfus.org
302 Ridgefield Court
Asheville, NC 28806
Tel: (800) 253-6530

See also
Alzheimer's disease
Headache and migraine
Pain
Chronic fatigue syndrome
Multiple sclerosis

Care and support

Hospice Information Service
www.hospicefoundation.org
Tel: (800) 854-3402

National Center on Caregiving
www.caregiver.org
180 Montgomery Street, Suite 1100
San Francisco, CA 94104
Tel: (800) 445-8106

National Family Caregivers Association
www.thefamilycaregiver.org
10400 Connecticut Avenue, Suite 500
Kensington, MD 20895-3944
Tel: (800) 896-3650

National Organization for Empowering Caregivers
www.nofec.org
425 West 23rd Street, Suite 9B
New York, NY 10011
Tel: (212) 807-1204

Cancer

American Cancer Society
www.cancer.org
Tel: 800-ACS-2345

The Susan G. Komen Breast Cancer Organization
www.komen.org
PO Box 650309
Dallas, TX 75265-0309
Tel: Breast Care Helpline (800) I'M AWARE

Y-ME National Breast Cancer Organization
www.y-me.org
212 West Van Buren, Suite 1000
Chicago, IL 60607-3908
Tel: (312) 986-8338
Tel: Breast Cancer Hotline (800) 221-2141

National Breast Cancer Coalition
www.natlbcc.org
1101 Seventeenth Street, NW, Suite 1300
Washington, DC 20036
Tel: (800) 622-2838

CancerCare
www.cancercare.org
275 Seventh Avenue
New York, NY 10001
Tel: (800) 813-HOPE

American Cancer Research Center
 www.amc.org
1600 Pierce Street
Denver, CO 80214
Tel: (800) 321-1557 / (800) 525-3777

The Leukemia and Lymphoma Society
www.leukemia.org
1311 Mamaroneck Avenue
White Plains, NY 10605
Tel: (800) 955-4572

National Cancer Institute
www.cancer.gov
Tel: 1-800-4-CANCER

National Coalition for Cancer Survivorship
www.canceradvocacy.org
1010 Wayne Avenue, Suite 770
Silver Spring, MD 20910
Tel: (877) NCCS-YES

Patient Advocates for Advanced Cancer Treatments
www.paactusa.org

The Wellness Community
www.thewellnesscommunity.org
919 Eighteenth Street, NW, Suite 54
Washington, DC 20006
Tel: (888) 793-WELL

Prostate Cancer Foundation
www.prostatecancerfondation.org
1250 Fourth Street
Santa Monica, CA 90401
Tel: (310) 570-4700 / (800) 757-CURE

National Ovarian Cancer Coalition
www.ovarian.org
500 NE Spanish River Boulevard, Suite 8
Boca Raton, FL 33431
Tel: (888) OVARIAN

Children's health

American Academy of Pediatrics
www.aap.org
141 Northwest Point Boulevard
Elk Grove Village, IL 60007
Tel: (847) 434-4000

Department of Health and Human Services
www.os.dhhs.gov
200 Independence Avenue, SW
Washington, DC 20201
Tel: (202) 619-0257 / (877) 696-6775

Federation for Children with Special Needs
www.fcsn.org
1135 Tremont Street, Suite 420
Boston, MA 02120
Tel: (617) 236-7210

Chronic fatigue syndrome

Chronic Fatigue and Immune Dysfunction Syndrome (CFIDS) Association of America
www.cfids.org
PO Box 220398
Charlotte, NC 28222-0398
Tel: (704) 365-2343

Complementary therapies

American Academy of Medical Acupuncture
www.medicalacupuncture.org
4929 Wilshire Boulevard, Suite 428
Los Angeles, CA 90010
Tel: (323) 937-5514

American Academy of Osteopathy
www.academyofosteopathy.org
3500 DePauw Boulevard, Suite 1080
Indianapolis, IN 46268
Tel: (317) 879-1881

American Chiropractic Association
www.amerchiro.org
1701 Clarendon Boulevard
Arlington, VA 22209
Tel: (800) 986-4636

American Herbal Products Association
www.ahpa.org
8484 Georgia Avenue, Suite 370
Silver Spring, MD 20910
Tel: (301) 588-1171

American Society for the Alexander Technique
www.alexandertech.com
PO Box 60008
Florence, MA 01062
Tel: (413) 584-2359 / (800) 473-0620

The American Tai Chi Association
www.americantaichi.net
13130 Thornapple Place
Herndon, VA 20171

North American Society of Homeopaths
www.homeopathy.org
PO Box 450039
Sunrise, FL 33345-0039
Tel: (206) 720-7000

Counseling and psychological therapies

American Association for Marriage and Family Therapy
www.aamft.org
112 South Alfred Street
Alexandria, VA 22314-3061
Tel: (703) 838-9808

American Association of Sex Educators, Counselors, and Therapists
www.aasect.org
PO Box 1960
Ashland, VA 23005-1960
Tel: (804) 752-0026

American Counseling Association
www.counseling.org
5999 Stevenson Avenue
Alexandria, VA 22304-3300
Tel: (703) 823-6862 / (800) 347-6647

American Psychoanalytical Association
www.apsa.org
309 East 49th Street
New York, NY 10017
Tel: (212) 752-0450

Diabetes

American Diabetes Association
www.diabetes.org.
1701 North Beauregard Street
Alexandria, VA 22311
Tel: (800) DIABETES

Hypoglycemia Support Foundation
www. hypogylcemia.org
PO Box 451778
Sunrise, FL 33345
Tel: (518) 272-7154

Juvenile Diabetes Research Foundation International
www.jdrf.org
120 Wall Street
New York, NY 10005-4001
Tel: (800) 533-CURE

Digestive disorders

Crohn's and Colitis Foundation of America
www.ccfa.org
386 Park Avenue South, 17th Floor
New York, NY 10016-8804
(800) 932-2423

Digestive Disease National Coalition
www.ddnc.org
507 Capital Court, NE, Suite 200
Washington, DC 20002
Tel: (202) 544-7497

International Foundation for Functional Gastrointestinal Disorders
www.iffgd.org
PO Box 170864
Milwaukee, WI 53217-8076
Tel: (414) 964-1799

Office of Rare Diseases
rarediseases.info.nih.gov
National Institute of Health
6100 Executive Boulevard
Room 3B01, MSC 7518
Bethesda, MD 20892-7518
Tel: (301) 402-4336

See also
Nutrition

Ear and hearing disorders

American Academy of Otolaryngology
www.entnet.org
One Prince Street
Alexandria, VA 22314-3357
Tel: (703) 836-4444

Alexander Graham Bell Association for the Deaf and Hard of Hearing
www.agbell.org
3417 Volta Place, NW
Washington, DC 20007
Tel: (202) 337-5220; (202) 337-5221 (TTY)

American Tinnitus Association
www.ata.org
PO Box 5
Portland, OR 97207-0005
Tel: (800) 634-8978

Deafness Research Foundation
www.drf.org
8201 Greensboro Drive, Suite 300
McLean, VA 22102
Tel: (800) 829-5934

Helen Keller National Center for Deaf-Blind Youths and Adults
www.helenkeller.org/national
141 Middle Neck Road
Sands Point, NY 11050
Tel: (516) 944-8900

Eating disorders

The National Eating Disorder Association
www.nationaleatingdisorders.org
603 Stewart Street, Suite 803
Seattle, WA 98101
Tel: (206) 382-3587

Laureate Eating Disorders Program
www.eatingdisorders/laureate.com
6655 South Yale Avenue
Tulsa, OK 74136
Tel: (918) 491-5600

National Association of Anorexia Nervosa and Associated Disorders
www.anad.org
PO Box 7
Highland Park, IL 60035
Tel: (847) 831-3438

Overeaters Anonymous
www.oa.org
World Service Office
PO Box 44020
Rio Rancho, NM 87174-4020
Tel: (505) 891-2664

Exercise and fitness

American Council on Exercise
www.acefitness.org
4851 Paramount Drive
San Diego, CA 92123
Tel: (800) 825-3636

American Council for Fitness and Nutrition
www.acfn.org
PO Box 33396
Washington, DC 20033-3396
Tel: (800) 953-1700

Eye disorders

American Council of the Blind
www.acb.org
1155 Fifteenth Street, NW, Suite 1004
Washington, DC 20005
Tel: (800) 424-8666

American Foundation for the Blind
www.afb.org
11 Penn Plaza, Suite 300
New York, NY 10001
Tel: (212) 502-7600 / (800) AFB-LINE

American Optometric Association
www.aoanet.org
243 North Lindbergh Boulevard
St. Louis, MO 63141
Tel: (314) 991-4100

Association for the Education and Rehabilitation of the Blind and the Visually Impaired
www.aerbvi.org
1703 North Beauregard Street, Suite 440
Alexandria, VA 22311
Tel: (703) 671-4500 / (877) 492-2708

Association for Macular Disease
www.macula.org
210 East 64th Street
New York, NY 10021
Tel: (212) 605-3777

Glaucoma Research Foundation
www.glaucoma.org
490 Post Street, Suite 1427
San Francisco, CA 94102
Tel: (800) 826-6693

Helen Keller Services for the Blind
www.helenkeller.org
141 Middle Neck Road
Sands Point, N.Y. 11050
Tel: (516) 944-8900

The Lighthouse Foundation
www.lighthouse.org
111 East 59th Street
New York, NY 10022-1202
Tel: (800) 829-0500

National Association for the Visually Handicapped
www.navh.org
22 West 21st Street
New York, NY 10010
Tel: (212) 255-2804

National Eye Institute
www.nei.nih.gov
31 Center Drive MSC 2510
Bethesda, MD 20892-2510
Tel: (301) 496-5248

Prevent Blindness America
www.preventblindness.org
211 West Wacker Drive, Suite 1700
Chicago, IL 60606
Tel: (800) 331-2020

Other Websites:
www.ascrs.org
www.macular.org
www.mdsupport.org

Fibromyalgia

The American Fibromyalgia Syndrome Association
www.afsafund.org
6380 East Tanque Verde, Suite D
Tucson, AZ 85715
Tel: (520) 733-1570

National Fibromyalgia Association
www.nfra.net
PO Box 500
Salem, OR 97308

Other websites:
www.fmnetnew.com
www.fmaware.org

Gout

American College of Rheumatology
www.rhuemotology.org
1800 Century Place, Suite 250
Atlanta, GA 30345-4300
Tel: (404) 633 3777

Headache and migraine

American Migraine Center
www.americanmigrainecenter.com
29001 Cedar Road, Suite 303
Lyndhurst, OH 44124
Tel: (800) 442-6804

National Headache Foundation
www.headache.org
820 North Orleans, Suite 217
Chicago, IL 60610
Tel: (888) NHF-5552

American Council for Headache Education
www.achenet.org
19 Mantua Road
Mt. Royal, NJ 08061
Tel: (856) 423-0258

Heart and circulation disorders

American Heart Association
www.americanheart.org
7272 Greenville Avenue
Dallas, TX 75231
Tel: 1-800-AHA-USA-1

National Heart, Lung and Blood Institute
www.nhlbi.nih.gov
PO Box 30105
Bethesda, MD 20824-0105
Tel: (301) 592-8573

Vascular Disease Foundation
www.vdf.org
1075 South Yukon, Suite 320
Lakewood, Colorado 80226
Tel: (303) 989-0500 / (866) PAD-INFO

Other websites:
www.circ.ahajournals.org
www.coronary-artery.com
www.heartpoint.com

HIV and AIDS

AIDS Action Council
www.aidsaction.org
1906 Sunderland Place NW
Washington, DC 20036
Tel: (202) 530-8030

CDC National HIV/AIDS Hotline
www.cdc.gov
1600 Clifton Road
Atlanta, GA 30333
Tel: (800) 342-2437

Gay Men's Health Crisis
www.gmhc.org
119 West 24th Street
New York, NY 10011
Tel: (212) 367-1000 / (800) AIDS-NYC

HIV/AIDS Treatment Information
www.aidsinfo.nih.gov
PO Box 6303
Rockville, MD 20849-6303
Tel: (800) HIV-0440

Project Inform
www.projinf.org
205 Thirteenth Street, #2001
San Francisco, CA 94103
Tel: (800) 822-7422

Women Alive
www.women-alive.org
1566 Burnside Avenue
Los Angeles, CA 90019
Tel: (800) 554-4876

Infertility

Ferre Institute, Inc.
www.ferre.org
124 Front Street
Binghamton, NY 13905
Tel: (607) 724-4308

Resolve, Inc.
7910 Woodmont Avenue, Suite 1350
Bethesda, MD 20814
Tel: (301) 652-8585

Internet Health Resources
www.ihr.com

Men's health

Men and Father's Resource Center
www.fathers.org
807 Brazos Street, Suite 315
Austin, TX 78701-2508
Tel: (512) 472-3237

Men's Health Network
www.menshealthnetwork.org
PO Box 75972
Washington, DC 20013
Tel: (202) 543-MHN-1, ext. 101

Impotence Sponsored by The American Foundation for Urologic Disease
www.impotence.org
1000 Corporate Boulevard, Suite 410
Linthicum, Maryland 21090
Tel: (410) 689-3990

Prostate Cancer Foundation
www.prostatecancerfoundation.org
1250 Fourth Street
Santa Monica, CA 90401
Tel: (310) 570-4700 /(800) 757-CURE

See also
Infertility

Mind and emotions

American Psychological Association
www.apa.org
750 First Street, NE
Washington, DC 20002-4242
Tel: (800) 374-2721

Depression and Bipolar Support Alliance
www.www.ndmda.org
730 North Franklin Street
Chicago, IL 60610-7204
Tel: (800) 826-3632

National Institute of Mental Health
www.nimh.nih.gov
6001 Executive Boulevard
Room 8184, MSC 9663
Bethesda, MD 20892-9663
Tel: (866) 615-6464

National Alliance for the Mentally Ill
www.nami.org
2107 Wilson Boulevard, Suite 300
Arlington, VA 22201-3042
Tel: (703) 524-7600 / (800) 950-NAMI

National Mental Health Association
www.nmha.org
2001 North Beauregard Street, 12th Floor
Alexandria, Virginia 22311
Tel: (703) 684-7722 / (800) 969-NMHA

See also
Counseling and psychological therapies
Obsessive–compulsive disorder (OCD)
Schizophrenia
Phobias and other anxiety disorders
Post–traumatic stress disorder (PTSD)
Seasonal affective disorder
Stress

Multiple sclerosis (MS)

National Multiple Sclerosis Society
www.mssociety.org.uk
733 Third Avenue
New York, NY 10017
Tel: (800) FIGHT-MS

Nutrition

American Dietetic Association
www.eatright.org
120 South Riverside Plaza, Suite 2000
Chicago, IL 60606-6995
Tel: (800) 877-1600

Food and Drug Administration
www.fda.gov
5600 Fishers Lane
Rockville, Maryland 20857
Tel: 888-INFO-FDA

Obesity

American Obesity Association
www.obesity.org
1250 Twenty-fourth Street, NW, Suite 300
Washington, DC 20037
Tel: 202-776-7711

North American Assoiation for the Study of Obesity
www.obesityresearch.org
8630 Fenton Street, Suite 918
Silver Spring, MD 20910
Tel: (301) 563-6526

Association for Morbid Obesity Support
www.obesityhelp.org
8001 Irvine Center Drive, Suite 1270
Irvine , CA 92618
Tel: (866) WLS-INFO

Obsessive–Compulsive Disorder (OCD)

Obsessive–Compulsive Foundation
www.ocfoundation.org
676 State Street
New Haven, CT 06511
Tel: (203) 401-2070

See also
Counseling and psychological therapies
Mind and emotions

Osteoporosis

Foundation for Osteoporosis Research and Education
www.fore.org
300 Twenty-seventh Street, Suite 103
Oakland, CA 94612
Tel: (888) 266-3015

National Osteoporosis Foundation
www.nof.org
1232 Twenty-second Street NW
Washington, DC 20037-1292
Tel: (202) 223-2226

Osteoporosis and Related Bone Diseases National Resource Center
www.osteo.org
2 AMS Circle
Bethesda, MD 20892-3676
Tel: (202) 223-0344 / (800) 624-BONE

Pain

American Chronic Pain Association
www.theacpa.org
PO Box 850
Rocklin, CA 95677
Tel: (800) 533-3231

National Chronic Pain Outreach Association
www.chronicpain.org
PO Box 274
Millboro, VA 24460
Tel: (540) 862-9437

See also
Brain and nervous system
Fibromyalgia

Phobias and other anxiety disorders

Anxiety Disorders Association of America
www.adaa.org
8730 Georgia Avenue, Suite 600
Silver Spring, MD 20910
Tel: (240) 485-1001

See also
Counseling and psychological therapies
Mind and emotions
Post–traumatic stress disorder (PTSD)

Post–traumatic Stress Disorder

Department of Veterans Affairs National Center for PTSD
www.ncptsd.va.gov
Palo Alto Health Care System
3801 Miranda Avenue
Palo Alto, CA 94304
Tel: (802) 296-6300

PTSD Alliance
www.ptsdalliance.org
Tel: (877) 507-PTSD

Sidran Institute
www.sidran.org
200 East Joppa Road, Suite 207
Towson, MD 21286
Tel: (410) 825-8888

See also
Counseling and psychological therapies
Mind and emotions

Pregnancy and childbirth

American College of Obstetricians and Gynecologists
www.acog.org
PO Box 96920
Washington, DC 20090-6920
Tel: (202) 638-5577

National Healthy Mothers, Healthy Babies Coalition
www.hmhb.org
121 North Washington Street, Suite 300
Alexandria, VA 22314
Tel: (703) 836-6110

Safety and health

National Safety Council
www.nsc.org
1121 Spring Lake Drive
Itasca, IL 60143-3201
Tel: (630) 285-1121

Occupational Safety and Health Administration
www.osha.org
200 Constitution Avenue
Washington, DC 20210
Tel: (800) 321-OSHA

US Consumer Product Safety Commission
www.cpsc.gov
4330 East-West Highway
Bethesda, Maryland 20814-4408
Tel: (800) 638-2772

Schizophrenia

National Alliance for Research on Schizophrenia and Depression
www.narsad.org
60 Cutter Mill Road, Suite 404,
Great Neck, NY 11021
Tel: (800) 829-8289

See also
Counseling and psychological therapies
Mind and emotions

Seasonal affective disorder

National Mental Health Association
www.nmha.org
2001 North Beauregard Street, 12th Floor
Alexandria, VA 22311
Tel: (703) 684-7722 / (800) 969-NMHA

See also
Mind and emotions

Skin disorders

American Academy of Dermatology
www.aad.org
1350 I Street NW, Suite 870
Washington, DC 20005-4355
Tel: (202) 842-3555

National Eczema Association for Science and Education
www.nationaleczema.org
4460 Redwood Highway, Suite 16-D
San Rafael, CA 94903-1953
Tel: (800) 818-7546

National Psoriasis Foundation
www.psoriasis.org
6600 SW 92nd Avenue, Suite 300
Portland, OR 97223-7195
Tel: (800) 723-9166

Sleep Disorders

American Sleep Apnea Association
1424 K Street NW, Suite 302
Washington, DC 20005
Tel: (202) 293-3650

Other websites:
www.narcolepsynetwork.org
www.sleepfoundation.org

Stuttering

National Stuttering Association
www.nsastutter.org
119 West 40th Street, 14th Floor
New York, NY 10018
Tel: (800) We Stutter (937-8888)

Urinary system disorders

American Association of Kidney Patients
www.aakp.org
3505 East Frontage Road, Suite 315
Tampa, FL 33607-1796
Tel: (800) 749-2257

American Foundation for Urologic Disease
www.afud.org
1000 Corporate Boulevard, Suite 410
Linthicum, Maryland 21090
Tel: (800) 828-7866

Interstitial Cystitis Association
www.ichelp.org
110 North Washington Street, Suite 340
Rockville, MD 20850
Tel: (301) 610-5300 / (800) HELP-ICA

Women's health

Center for Menstrual Disorders and Reproductive Choice
www.cmdrc.org
2020 South Clinton Avenue
Rochester, NY 14618
Tel: (888) 272-7990

National Women's Health Network
www.womenshealthnetwork.org
514 Tenth Street NW, Suite 400
Washington DC 20004
Tel: (202) 628-7814

National Women's Health Resource Center
www.healthywomen.org
157 Broad Street, Suite 315
Red Bank, NJ 07701
Tel: (877) 986-9472

See also
Infertility
Pregnancy and childbirth

PRIMARY TREATMENT REFERENCES

This is an evidence-based book and the authors haved cited scientific references whenever possible for all treatments. The references for the complementary primary treatments are as follows. The references for the conventional medical treatments were too numerous to list here. The authors of the conventional medicial text took the Cochrane Library's (www.cochrane.co.uk) reviews of scientific research and other medical databases into account when rating treatments. (For an explanation of how treatments are rated, see p.111.)

A full list of all the authors' references for the treaments in this book may be found by visiting our website at www.dk.com/newmedicine.

Brain and Nervous System

HEADACHES
Gauthier JG, Ivers H, Carrier S. *Nonpharmacological approaches in the management of recurrent headache disorders and their comparison and combination with pharmacotherapy.* Clinical Psychology Review. 1996;16(6):543–571.

Mauskop A, et al. *Intravenous magnesium sulfate rapidly alleviates headaches of various types.* Headache. 1996;36:154–160.

Savi L, et al. *Food and headache attacks. A comparison of patients with migraine and tension-type headache.* Panminerva Med. 2002;44(1):27–31.

MIGRAINE
Awang DVC *Feverfew fever—headache for the consumer.* Herbalgram. 1993;29:34–36.

Egger J, et al. *Is migraine food allergy? A double-blind trial of oligoantigenic diet treatment.* Lancet. 1983;2:865–869.

Facchinetti F, et al. *Magnesium prophylaxis of menstrual migraine: effects on intracellular magnesium.* Headache. 1991;31:298–301.

Gallai V, et al. *Serum and salivary magnesium levels in migraine. Results in a group of juvenile patients.* Headache. 1992;32:132–135.

Hernandez-Reif M, et al. *Migraine headaches are reduced by massage therapy.* Intl J Neurosci. 1998;96:1–11.

Hughs EC, et al. *Migraine: a diagnostic test for etiology of food sensitivity by a nutritionally supported fast and confirmed by long–term report.* Ann Allergy. 1985;55:28–32.

Simons D, Travell J, Simons L. *Myofascial Pain and Dysfunction: The Trigger Point Manual.* Vol 1. 2nd ed. Baltimore: Williams and Wilkins, 1999.

MEMORY IMPAIRMENT
Brush JA, Camp CJ. *Using spaced retrieval as an intervention during speech-language therapy.* Clinical Gerontologist 1998;19:51–64.

Camp CJ, Stevens AB. *Spaced retrieval: A memory intervention for dementia of the Alzheimers type.* Clinical Gerontologist. 1990;10,58–61.

MULTIPLE SCLEROSIS
Swank RL, et al. *Effect of a low saturated fat diet in early and late cases of multiple sclerosis.* Lancet. 1990;336:37–39.

STROKE
Cochrane Outpatient Service Trialists. *Therapy-based rehabilitation services for stroke patients at home.* Cochrane Database of Systematic Reviews. 2003;1:CD002925.

Green J, et al. *Physiotherapy for patients with mobility problems more than 1 year after stroke: a randomised controlled trial.* Lancet. 2002;359(9302):199–203.

Hesse S, et al. *Treadmill training with partial body weight support after stroke.* Physical Medicine And Rehabilitation Clinics Of North America. February 14, 2003;1(suppl):S111–23.

Woessner R, et al. *Stroke therapy. What is established, what is new?* [in German]. MMW Fortschritte Der Medizin. 2002;144(26):29–34.

CARPAL TUNNEL SYNDROME
Dobrusin R. *Osteopathic approach to conservative management of thoracic outlet syndromes.* Journal American Osteopathic Association. 1989;8:1046.

Garfinkel M. *Yoga-based intervention for carpal tunnel syndrome: a randomized trial.* JAMA. 1998;280:1601–1603.

Sequeira W. *Yoga in treatment of carpal-tunnel syndrome.* Lancet. 1999;353(9154):689–690.

Sucher B. *Myofascial manipulative release of carpal tunnel syndrome: documentation with MRI.* J Am Osteopathic Ass. 1994;94:647–663.

Skin Ailments

HERPES SIMPLEX
Flodin NW. *The metabolic roles, pharmacology, and toxicology of lysine.* J Am Coll Nutr. 1997;16:7–21.

ECZEMA AND CONTACT DERMATITIS
Atherton DJ. *Diet and atopic eczema.* Clin Allerg. 1988;18:215–228.

Gimenez-Arnau A, et al. *Effects of linoleic acid supplements on atopic dermatitis.* Adv Exp Med Biol. 1997;443:285–289.

Horrobin DF. *Essential fatty acid metabolism and its modification in atopic eczema.* Am J Clin Nutr. 2000;71(supp):367S–372S.

Niggemann B, et al. *Outcome of double-blind, placebo-controlled food challenge tests in 107 children with atopic dermatitis.* Clin Exp Allergy. 1999;29:91–96.

Sullivan JB, Krieger GR. *Clinical Environmental Health and Toxic Exposures.* 2nd ed. Philadelphia: Lippincott, Williams, & Wilkins; 2001.

PSORIASIS
Kuwano S, Yamauchi K. *Effect of berberine on tyrosine decarboxylase activity of Streptococcus faecalis.* Chem Pharm Bull. 1960;8:491–496.

Rosenberg E, Belew P. *Microbial factors in psoriasis.* Arch Dermatol. 1982;118:1434–1444.

Thurmon FM. *The treatment of psoriasis with sarsaparilla compound.* N Engl J Med. 1942;227:128–133.

URTICARIA

Henz BM, Zuberbier T. *Most chronic urticaria is food-dependent, and not idiopathic.* Exp Dermatol. 1998;7(4):139–142.

Juhlin L. *Additives and chronic urticaria.* Ann Allergy. 1987;59:119–23.

Kulczycki A. *Aspartame-induced urticaria.* Ann Int Med. 1986;104:207–208.

Lessof MH. *Reactions to food additives.* Clin Exp Allergy. 1995;25(suppl 1):27–8.

Eye Ailments

MACULAR DEGENERATION

Age-Related Eye Disease Study Research Group. *A randomized, placebo-controlled, clinical trial of high-dose supplementation with vitamins C and E, beta carotene, and zinc for age-related macular degeneration and vision loss: AREDS Report No. 8.* Arch Ophthalmol. 2001;119:1417–1436.

TINNITUS

Andersson G. *Psychological aspects of tinnitus and the application of cognitive-behavioral therapy.* Clinical Psychology Review. 2002;22(7):977–90.

Kröner-Herwig B, et al. *The management of chronic tinnitus—comparison of a cognitive-behavioural group training with yoga.* J Psychosomatic Res. 1995;39(2):153–165.

EARACHE

Arroyave CM. *Recurrent otitis media with effusion and food allergy in pediatric patients* [in Spanish]. Rev Alerg Mex. 2001;48:141–144.

Nsouli TM, et al. *Role of food allergy in serous otitis media.* Ann Allergy. 1994;73:215–219.

Sanchez A, et al. *Role of sugars in human neutrophilic phagocytosis.* Am J Clinical Nutrition. 1973;26(11):1180–1184.

Respiratory Ailments

COLDS AND FLU

Garland ML, Hagmeyer KO. *The role of zinc lozenges in treatment of the common cold.* Ann Pharmacother. 1998;32:63–69.

Gorton HC, et al. *The effectiveness of vitamin C in preventing and relieving the symptoms of virus-induced respiratory infections.* J Manipulative Physiol Ther. 1999;22(8):530–3.

Hirt M, Nobel S, Barron E. *Zinc nasal gel for the treatment of common cold symptoms: a double-blind, placebo controlled trial.* Ear Nose Throat J. 2000;79:778–80.

Jackson JL, Lesho E, Peterson C. *Zinc and the common cold: a meta-analysis revisited.* J Nutr. 2000;130:1512S–1515S.

Melchart D., et al. *Echinacea for the prevention an dtreatment of the common cold.* Update Software. Cochrane Library. 2000;4:1–23.

Mossad SB, et al. *Zinc gluconate lozenges for treating the common cold. A randomized, double-blind, placebo-controlled study.* Ann Intern Med. 1996,125(2):81–88.

Prasad AS, et al. *Duration of symptoms and plasma cytokine levels in patients with the common cold treated with zinc acetate: a randomized, double-blind, placebo-controlled trail.* Ann Intern Med. 2000;133(4):245–252.

Van Straten M, Josling P. *Preventing the common cold with a vitamin C supplement: a double-blind, placebo-controlled survey.* Adv Ther. 2002;19:151–159.

Vickers AJ, Smith C. *Homoeopathic Oscillococcinum for preventing and treating influenza and influenza-like syndromes.* Cochrane Library. 2001;1:1–10.

ASTHMA

Bowler S, Green A, Mitchell C. *Buteyko breathing techniques in asthma : a blinded randomised controlled trial.* Med J of Australia. 1998;169:575–578.

Fluge T, Richter J, Fabel H., et al. *Long–term effects of breathing exercises and yoga in patients with bronchial asthma.* [in German]. Pneumologie. 1994;48:484–490.

Hockemeyer J, Smyth J. *Evaluating the feasibility and efficacy of a self-administered manual-based stress management intervention for individuals with asthma: results from a controlled study.* Behavioral Medicine. 2002;27(4):161–172.

Kilpelainen M, Koskenvuo M, Helenius H, Terho EO. *Stressful life events promote the manifestation of asthma and atopic diseases.* Clinical and Experimental Allergy. 2002;32(2):256–263.

Liu LY, Coe CL, Swenson CA, Kelly EA, Kita H, Busse WW. *School examinations enhance airway inflammation to antigen challenge.* Am J Respiratory Critical Care Medicine. 2002;165(8):1062–1067.

Rietveld S, Van Beest I, Everaerd W. *Stress-induced breathlessness in asthma.* Psychological Medicine. 1999;29(6):1359–1366.

Stetter F, Kupper S. *Autogenic training: A meta-analysis of clinical outcome studies.* Applied Psychophysiology and Biofeedback. 2002;27(1):45–98.

Tisp B, Burns M, Kro D. *Pursed Lip breathing using ear oximetry.* Chest. 1986;90:218–221.

Wilson AF, Honsberger RW, Chiu JT, Novey SH. *Transcendental meditation and asthma.* Respiration. 1975;32:74–80.

Digestion and Urinary Systems

IRRITABLE BOWEL SYNDROME

Bohmer CJ, Tuynman HA. *The effect of a lactose-restricted diet in patients with a positive lactose tolerance test, earlier diagnosed as irritable bowel syndrome: a five-year follow-up study.* Eur J Gastroenterol Hepatol. 2001;13(8):941–944.

Brown D, et al. *Irritable bowel syndrome.* Quarterly Review of Natural Medicine. 1997;Winter:333–345.

Fernandez-Banares F, et al. *Sugar malabsorption in functional bowel disease: clinical implications.* Am J Gastroenterol. 1993;88:2044–2050.

Jones AV, et al. *Food intolerance: a major factor in the pathogenesis of irritable bowel syndrome.* Lancet. 1982;2:1115–1117.

King TS, et al. *Abnormal colonic fermentation in irritable bowel syndrome.* Lancet. 1998;352:1187–1189.

Keefer L, Blanchard EB. *A one year follow-up of relaxation response meditation as a treatment for irritable bowel syndrome.* Behavior Research & Therapy. 2002;40:541–546.

Ledochowski M, et al. *Fructose- and sorbitol-reduced diet improves mood and gastrointestinal disturbances in fructose malabsorbers.* Scand J Gastroenterol.

2000;35(10):1048–52.

Niec AM, et al. *Are adverse food reactions linked to irritable bowel syndrome?* Am J Gastroenterol. 1998;93:2184–2190.

Parker TJ, et al. *Management of patients with food intolerance in irritable bowel syndrome: the development and use of an exclusion diet.* J Human Nutr Diet. 1995;8:159–166.

Smith MA, et al. *Food intolerance, atopy, and irritable bowel syndrome.* Lancet. 1985;2:1064.

ULCERATIVE COLITIS

Aslan A, Triadafilopoulos G. *Fish oil fatty acid supplementation in active ulcerative colitis: a double-blind, placebo-controlled, crossover study.* Am J Gastroenterol. 1992;87(4):432–7.

Hawthorne AB, et al. *Treatment of ulcerative colitis with fish oil supplementation: a prospective 12 month randomised controlled trial.* Gut. 1992;33(7):922–928.

GALLSTONES

Erlinger S. *Gallstones in obesity and weight loss.* Eur J Gastroenterol Hepatol. 2000;12(12):1347–52.

Everhart JE. *Contributions of obesity and weight loss to gallstone disease.* Ann Intern Med. 1993;119(10):1029–1035.

Kern F Jr. *Epidemiology and natural history of gallstones.* Semin Liver Dis. 1983;3:87–96.

Stampfer MJ, et al. *Risk of symptomatic gallstones in women with severe obesity.* Am J Clin Nutr. 1992;55:652–658.

Thornton JR. *Gallstone disappearance associated with weight loss* [letter]. Lancet. 1992;ii:478.

Wudel LJ Jr, et al. *Prevention of gallstone formation in morbidly obese patients undergoing rapid weight loss: results of a randomized controlled pilot study.* J Surg Res. 2002;102(1):50–6.

CYSTITIS

Foo LY, Lu Y, Howell AB, Vorsa N. *The structure of cranberry proanthocyanidins which inhibit adherence of uropathogenic P-fimbriated Escherichia coli in vitro.* Phytochemistry. 2000;54(2)173–181.

Howell AB, et al. *Inhibition of the adherence of P fimbriated Escherichia coli to uroepithelial-cell surfaces by proanthocyanidin extracts from cranberries.* N Engl J Med.

Jepson RG, Mihaljevic L, Craig J. *Cranberries for treating urinary tract infections.* Cochrane Database Syst Rev. 2000;(2):CD001322.

Jepson RG, Mihaljevic L, Craig J. *Cranberries for preventing urinary tract infections.* Cochrane Database Syst Rev. 2001;(3):CD001321.

Kiel RJ, Nashelsky J, Robbins B. *Does cranberry juice prevent or treat urinary tract infection?* J Fam Pract. 2003;52(2):154–155.

Kingwatanakul P, Alon US. *Cranberries and urinary tract infection.* Child Hosp Q. 1996;8:69–62.

Lowe FC, Fagelman E. *Cranberry juice and urinary tract infections: what is the evidence?* Urology. 2001;57:407–413.

Reid G. *The role of cranberry and probiotics in intestinal and urogenital tract health.* Crit Rev Food Sci Nutr. 2002;42(suppl 3):293–300.

Stothers L. *A randomized trial to evaluate effectiveness and cost effectiveness of naturopathic cranberry products as prophylaxis against urinary tract infection in women.* Can J Urol. 2002;9(3):1558–1562.

Circulatory System

CORONARY ARTERY DISEASE

Ascherio A. *Epidemiologic studies on dietary fats and coronary heart disease.* Am J Med. December 30, 2002;113(suppl 9B):9S–12S.

Cui J, Juhasz B, Tosaki A, Maulik N, Das DK. *Cardioprotection with grapes.* J Cardiovasc Pharmacol. 2002;40(5):762–9.

Folts JD. *Potential health benefits from the flavonoids in grape products on vascular disease.* Adv Exp Med Biol. 2002;505:95–111.

Heber D. *Herbs and atherosclerosis.* Curr Atheroscler Rep. 2001;3(1):93–6.

Hu FB, Willett WC. *Optimal diets for prevention of coronary heart disease.* JAMA. 2002;288(20):2569–78.

Khaw KT, et al. for the European Prospective Investigation into Cancer and Nutrition. *Relation between plasma ascorbic acid and mortality in men and women in EPIC-Norfolk prospective study:a prospective population study.* Lancet. 2001;357:657–663.

Losonczy KG, et al. *Vitamin E and vitamin C supplement use and risk of all-cause and coronary heart disease mortality in older persons: the established populations for epidemiologic studies of the elderly.* Am J Clin Nutr. 1996;64:190–196.

Patrick L, Uzick M. *Cardiovascular disease: C-reactive protein and the inflammatory disease paradigm: HMG-CoA reductase inhibitors, alpha-tocopherol, red yeast rice, and olive oil polyphenols. A review of the literature.* Altern Med Rev. 2001;6(3):248–71.

Rimm EB, et al. *Folate and vitamin B6 from diet and supplements in relation to risk of coronary heart disease among women.* JAMA. 1998;279:359–364.

VARICOSE VEINS

Häfner H, et al. *Medical compression therapy.* Zentralblatt Fur Chirurgie. 2001a;126(7):551–556.

Häfner J. *Conservative therapy in varicose symptom complex.* Revue Suisse De Medecine Praxis. 2001b;90(6):197–204.

Ibegbuna V, et al. *Effect of lightweight compression stockings on venous haemodynamics.* International Angiology: a Journal of The International Union of Angiology. 1997;16(3):185–188.

Muscle, Bone and Joint Ailments

BACK AND NECK PAIN

Blomberg S, et al. *Controlled multicentre trial of manual therapy in low back pain: initial status, sick leave and pain score during follow up.* Orthopaedic medicine. 1994;16:1.

Meade T, et al. *Randomised comparison of chiropractic and hospital outpatient management of low back pain—results from extended follow-up.* BMJ. 1995;11:349.

Triano J, et al. *Manipulative Therapy versus education programmes in chronic low back pain.* Spine. 1995;20:948.

SCIATICA

Cherkin D, et al. *A comparison of physical therapy, chiropractic manipulation, and provision of an educational booklet for the treatment of patients with low back pain.* N Engl J Med. 1998;339(15):1021–1029.

SPORTS INJURIES

Allen R. Sports Medicine. In: Ward R, ed. *Foundations of Osteopath.* Baltimore: Williams & Wilkins; 1997.

Feinberg E. Sports Chiropractic. In: Redwood D, ed. *Contemporary Chiropractic.* New York: Churchill Livingstone; 1997.

TEMPOROMANDIBULAR JOINT DISORDER

Nguyen P, et al. *A randomized double-blind clinical trial of the effect of chondroitin sulfate and glucosamine hydrochloride on temporomandibular joint disorders: a pilot study.* Cranio. 2001;19(2):130–139.

Shankland WE. *The effects of glucosamine and chondroitin sulfate on osteoarthritis of the TMJ: a preliminary report of 50 patients.* Cranio. 1998;16(4):230–235.

FROZEN SHOULDER

Liebenson C, ed. *Rehabilitation of the Spine.* Baltimore: Williams & Wilkins; 2006.

Simons J, Travell J, Simons L. *Myofascial pain and dysfunction: the trigger point manual.* Vol 1, Upper Body. 2nd ed. Baltimore: Williams & Wilkins; 1999:604–612.

Strong J, et al. *Pain: a textbook for therapists.* Edinburgh: Churchill Livingstone; 2002.

OSTEOARTHRITIS

Leeb BF, et al. *A meta-analysis of chondroitin sulfate in the treatment of osteoarthritis.* J Rheumatol. 2000;27(1):205–211.

Lorig K, et al. *The beneficial outcomes of the arthritis self-management course are inadequately explained by behavior change.* Arthritis Rheum. 1989;31(1):91–95.

Lorig K, Mazonson P, Holman HR. *Evidence suggesting that health education for self-management in patients with chronic arthritis has sustained health benefits while reducing health care costs.* Arthritis Rheum. 1993;36(4r):439–446.

Marks R. *Efficacy theory and its utility in arthritis rehabilitation: review and recommendations.* Disabil Rehabil. May 10, 2001;23(7):271–280.

McAlindon TE, et al. *Glucosamine and chondroitin for treatment of osteoarthritis: a systematic quality assessment and meta-analysis.* JAMA. 2000;283:1469–1475.

Mullen PD, et al. *Efficacy of psycho-educational interventions on pain, depression and disability with arthritic adults: a meta-analysis.* J of Rheumatology. 1987;14(15):33–39.

Qiu GX, et al. *Efficacy and safety of glucosamine sulfate versus ibuprofen in patients with knee osteoarthritis.* Arzneimittelforschung. 1998;48:469–474.

Stanford Patient Education Research Center. *The chronic disease self-management workshop leaders manual.* Stanford University, 1999.

Young LD, Bradley LA, Turner RA. *Decreases in health care resource utilization in patients with rheumatoid arthritis following a cognitive behavioral intervention.* Biofeedback and Self-Regulation. 1995;20(3):259–268.

FIBROMYALGIA

Bell IR, et al. *Improved clinical status in fibromyalgia patients treated with individualized homeopathic remedies versus placebo.* Rheumatology. 2004;43:577–582.

Buckelew SP, Conway R, et al. *Biofeedback/Relaxation training and exercise interventions for fibromyalgia: a prospective trial.* Arthritis Care Res. 1998;11(3):196–209.

Fisher P, et al. *Effect of homoeopathic treatment on fibrositis (primary fibromyalgia).* BMJ. 1989;299:365–366.

Hadhazy VA, et al. *Mind-body therapies for the treatment of fibromyalgia: a systematic review.* J Rheumatol. 2000;27(12):2922–2928.

Kaplan KH, Goldenberg DL, Galvin-Nadeau M. *The impact of a meditation-based stress reducton program on fibromyalgia.* Gen Hosp Psychiatry. 1993;15(5):284–289.

GOUT

Emmerson BT. *The management of gout.* N Engl J Med. 1996;334:445–51.

Yu T-F. *Milestones in the treatment of gout.* Am J Med. 1974;56:676–85.

ANKYLOSING SPONDYLITIS

Helliwell P, Abbott CA, Chamberlain MA. *A randomised trial of three different physiotherapy regimes in ankylosing spondylitis.* Physiotherapy. 1996;82:85–90.

OSTEOPOROSIS

Chapuy MC, et al. *Vitamin D and calcium to prevent hip fractures in elderly women.* N Engl J Med. 1992;327:1637–1642.

Dawson-Hughes B, et al. *Effect of calcium and vitamin D supplementation on bone density in men and women 65 years of age or older.* N Engl J Med. 1997;337:670–676.

Eastell R, Lambert H. *Strategies for skeletal health in the elderly.* Proc Nutr Soc. 2002;61:173–180.

Feskanich D, et al. *Calcium, vitamin D, milk consumption, and hip fractures: a prospective study among postmenopausal women.* Am J Clin Nutr. 2003;77(2):504–511.

Minne HW, et al. *Vitamin D and calcium supplementation reduces falls in elderly women via improvement of body sway and normalisation of blood pressure: a prospective, randomised and double-blind study.* Osteoporosis International. 2000;11:S115.

New SA, et al. *Positive associations between net endogenous non-carbonic acid production (NEAP) and bone health: further support for the importance of the skeleton to acid-base balance.* Bone. 2001;28:S94.

Papadimitropoulos E, et al. *Meta-analyses of therapies for postmenopausal osteoporosis. VIII: Meta-analysis of the efficacy of vitamin D treatment in preventing osteoporosis in postmenopausal women.* Endocr Rev. 2002;23(4):560–569.

Women's Health

PREMENSTRUAL SYNDROME

Lauritzen C, Reuter HD, et al. *Treatment of premenstrual tension syndrome with Vitex agnus-castus. Controlled, double-blind study versus pyridoxine.* Phytomed. 1997;4:183–9.

Schellenberg R. *Treatment for the premenstrual syndrome with agnus castus fruit extract: prospective, randomised, placebo controlled study.*

MENSTRUAL PAIN

Butler EB, et al. *Vitamin E in the treatment of primary dysmenorrhoea.* Lancet. 1955;1:844–847.

Deutch B, et al. *Menstrual discomfort in Danish women reduced by dietary supplements of omega-3 PUFA and B^{12} (fish oil or seal oil capsules).* Nutr Res. 2000;20:621–631.

Harel Z, et al. *Supplementation with omega-3 polyunsaturated fatty acides in the management of dysmenorrhea in adolescents.* Amer J Obstet Gynecol. 1996;174(4):1335–1338.

Ziaei S, et al. *A randomised placebo-controlled trial to determine the effect of vitamin E in treatment of primary dysmenorrhoea.* BJOG. 2001;108:1181–1183.

POLYCYSTIC OVARY SYNDROME

Dunaif A. *Insulin resistance and the polycystic ovary syndrome: mechanism and implications for pathogenesis.* Endocr Rev. 1997;18:774–800.

Legro RS, et al. *Prevalence and predictors of risk for type 2 diabetes mellitus and impaired glucose tolerance in polycystic ovary syndrome: a prospective controlled study in 254 affected women.* J Clin Endocrinol Metab. 1999;84:165–169.

Norman RJ, et al. *Metabolic approaches to the subclassification of polycystic ovary syndrome.* Fertil Steril. 1995;63:329–335.

MENOPAUSE

McKenna DJ, Jones K, Humphrey S, Hughes K. *Black cohosh: efficacy, safety, and use in clinical and preclinical applications.* Alternative Therapy Health Medicine. 2001;7(3):93–100.

VAGINAL YEAST

Hilton E, et al. *Ingestion of yogurt containing Lactobacillus acidophilus as prophylaxis for candidal vaginitis.* Ann Intern Med. 1992;116(5):353–357.

SEXUAL PROBLEMS

De Amicis MP. *Clinical follow-up of coupes treated for sexual dysfunction.* Arch Sex Behav. 1985;14:467–489.

Hawton K, Catalan J. *Prognostic factors in sex therapy.* Behav Res & Ther. 1986;24:377–385.

Hawton K, Catalan J. *Sex therapy for*

vaginismus: characteristics of couples and treatment outcome. Sex & Marital Ther. 1990;5:39–48.

Macabe MP. *Evaluation of a cognitive behavior therapy program for people with sexual dysfunction.* J Sex & Marital Ther. 2001;27(3):259–271.

Whitehead A, et al. *The treatment of sexually unresponsive women: A comparative evauation.* Behav Res & Ther. 1987;25:195–205.

Pregnancy and Childbirth

MORNING SICKNESS

Belluomini J, et al. *Acupressure for nausea and vomiting of pregnancy: randomized double-blinded study.* Obstetrics and Gynaecology. 1994;84(2):245–248.

De Aloysio D, Pennacchioni P. *Morning sickness control in early pregnancy by Neiguan point acupressure.* Obstetrics & Gynaecology. 1992;80(5):852–854.

Iatrakis GM, et al. *Vomiting and nausea in the first 12 weeks of pregnancy.* Psychotherapy & psychosomatics. 1988;49:22–24.

Smith C, Crowther C, Beilby J. *Acupuncture to treat nausea and vomiting in early pregnancy: a randomized controlled trial.* Birth. March 2002;29(1):1–9.

LABOR

Martin AA, et al. *The effects of hypnosis on the labor processes and birth outcomes of pregnant adolescents.* J Family Practice. 2001;50(5):441–443.

Mehl LE. *Hypnosis and conversion of the breech to the vertex presentation.* Arch Fam Med. 1994;3:881–87.

Schauble PG, et al. *Childbirth preparation through hypnosis: the hypnorefelexogenous protocol.* Am J Clin Hypnosis. 1998;40:273–83.

POSTPARTUM DEPRESSION

Cooper PJ, Murrary L. The impact of psychological treatments of postnatal depression on maternal mood and infant development. In: Murray L, Cooper PJ eds. *Postpartum depression and child development.* New York, London: Guildford Press; 1997:201–220.

Holden JM, et al. *Counselling in a general*

practice setting: a controlled study of health visitor intervention in treatment of postnatal depression. BMJ. 1989;298:223–6.

Wickberg B, Hwang CP. *Counselling of postnatal depression: controlled study on a population based Swedish sample.* J Affective Disorders. 1996;39:209–16.

Men's Health

BENIGN PROSTATIC HYPERTROPHY (PROSTATE ENLARGEMENT)

Gutrierez M, et al. *Spasmolytic activity of lipid extract from Sabal serrulata fruits; further studies of the mechanisms underlying this activity.* Planta Med. 1996;62:507–511.

Koch E. *Extracts from fruits of saw palmetto (Sabal serrulata) and roots of stinging nettle (Urtica dioica): viable alternatives in the medical treatment of benign prostatic hyperplasia and associated lower urinary tracts symptoms.* Planta Med. 2001(Aug);67(6):489–500.

McCaleb R. *Phytomedicines outperform synthetics in treating enlarged prostate.* Herbalgram. 1997;40.

Sokeland J. *Combined sabal and urtica extract compared with finasteride in men with benign prostatic hyperplasia: analysis of prostate volume and therapeutic outcome.* BJU Int. 2000(Sep);86(4):439–442.

Wagner H, Flachsbarth H. *A new antiphlogistic principle from Sabal serrulata, 1.* Planta Med. 1966;14:402–407.

ERECTILE DYSFUNCTION

Deyama T, Nishibe S, Nakazawa Y. *Constituents and pharmacological effects of Eucommia and Siberian ginseng.* Review. Acta Pharmacol Sin. 2001(Dec);22(12):1057–1070.

Hong B, Ji YH, Hong JH, et al. *A double-blind crossover study evaluating the efficacy of Korean red ginseng in patients with erectile dysfunction: a preliminary report.* J Urol. 2002;168:2070–2073.

Li TB, et al. *Effects of ginsenosides, lectins and Momordica charantia insulin like peptide on corticosterone production by isolated rat adrenal cells.* J Ethnopharmacol. 1987;21:21–29.

Price A, Gazewood J. *Korean red ginseng*

effective for treatment of erectile dysfunction. J Fam Pract. 2003(Jan);52(1):20–21.

Children's Health

HEAD LICE

Charles V, Charles SX. *The use and efficacy of Azadirachta indica ADR ("Neem") and Curcuma longa ("Turmeric") in scabies. A pilot study.* Trop Geogr Med. 1992;44(1–2):178–81.

Jensen O, Nielsen AO, Bjerregaard P. *Pediculosis capitis treated with quassia tincture.* Acta Derm Venereol. 1978;58(6):557–9.

Puri H, ed. *Neem: Medicinal and Aromatic Plants—Industrial Profiles.* London: Taylor and Francis; 1999.

GLUE EAR

Arroyave CM. *Recurrent otitis media with effusion and food allergy in pediatric patients* [in Spanish]. Rev Alerg Mex. 2001;48:141–144.

Nsouli TM, et al. *Role of food allergy in serous otitis media.* Ann Allergy. 1994;73:215–219.

COLIC

Jakobsson I, et al. *Cow's milk proteins cause infantile colic in breast-fed infants: a double-blind crossover study.* Pediatr. 1983;71(2):268–271.

Lothe L, et al. *Cow's milk as a cause of infantile colic: A double-blind study.* Pediatr. 1982;70(1):7–10

Lothe L, et al. *Cow's milk whey protein elicits symptoms of infantile colic in colicky formula-fed infants: A double-blind crossover study.* Pediatr. 1989;83(2):262–266.

TONSILLITIS

Kempe C, et al. *Icelandic moss lozenges in the prevention or treatment of oral mucosa irritation and dried out throat mucosa* [in German]. Laryngorhinootologie. 1997;76(3):186–8.

ADHD

Abikoff H. *Cognitive training in ADHD children: less to it than meets the eye.* J Learning Disability. 1991;65:749–757.

Barkley RA, et al. *A comparison of*

three family therapy programs for treating family conflicts in adolescents with attention-deficit hyperactivity disorders. J Consulting & Clin Psychology. 1992;60:450–462.

DuPaul G, Eckert TL. *The effects of school-based interventions for attention deficit hyperactivity disorder: a meta-analysis.* School Psychology Review. 1997;26:5–27.

Pfiffner LJ, McBurnett K. *Social skills training with parent generalization: treatment effects for children with attention deficit disorder.* J Consulting & Clin Psychology. 1997;65:749–757.

Pisterman S, et al. *The role of parent training in treatment of preschoolers with ADDH.* Amer J Orthopsychiatry. 1992;62:397–408.

Webster-Stratton C, Hammond M. *Predictors of treatment outcome in parent training for families with conduct problem children.* Behavior Therapy. 1990;21:319–337.

Mind and Emotions

STRESS

Baider L, Uziely B, De Nour AK. *Progressive muscle relaxation and guided imagery in cancer patients.* General Hospital Psychiatry. 1994;16:340–347.

Crowther JH. *Stress management training and relaxation imagery in the treatment of essential hypertension.* J Behavioral Med. 1983;6(2):169–187.

Holden-Lund C. *Effects of relaxation with guided imagery on surgical stress and wound healing.* Res in Nursing & Health. 1988;11(4):235–244.

Tsai SL, Crockett MS. *Effects of relaxation training combining imagery and meditation on the stress level of Chinese nurses working in modern hospitals in Taiwan.* Issues in Mental Health Nursing. 1993;14:51–56.

Wynd CA. *Relaxation imagery used for stress reduction in the prevention of smoking relapse.* J Advanced Nursing. 1992;17:294–302.

PHOBIAS

Emmelkamp PMG. *Behavior therapy with adults.* In: Garfield SL, Bergin AE, eds. *Handbook of psychotherapy and behavior change.* 4th ed. New York: John Wiley & Sons Ltd; 1994:79–427.

Gilroy LJ, et al. *Controlled comparison of*

computer-aided vicarious exposure versus live exposure in the treatment of spider phobia. Behavior Therapy. 2003;31:733–744.

Liddell A, et al. *Long–term follow-up of treated dental phobics.* Behaviour Research And Therapy. 1994;32(6):605–610.

Marshall WL. *The effects of variable exposure in flooding therapy.* Behavior Therapy. 1985;16:117–135.

Marshall WL. *The treatment of agoraphobia.* Paper at the Australia Behavior Modification Association, Perth, Western Australia, March 1985.

Ost LG. *Acquisition of blood ad injection phobia and anxiety response pattern in clinical patients.* Behaviour Research & Therapy. 1991;29(4):323–332.

Smith TA, et al. *Evaluating a behavioral method to manage dental fear: A two-year study of dental practices.* J Amer Dent Assoc. 1990;121:525–530.

Wiederhold BK, et al. An investigation into physiological responses in virtual environments: an objective measurement of presence. In: Riva G, Calimberti C, eds. *Toward cyberpsychology: Mind, cognition and society in the internet age.* Amsterdam: IOS Press; 2001.

ANXIETY

Aitken JR, Benson JW. *The use of relaxation/desensitization in treating anxiety associated with flying.* Aviat Space Environ Med. 1984;55(3):196–199.

Ashton C Jr, et al. *Self-hypnosis reduces anxiety following coronary artery bypass surgery. A prospective, randomized trial.* J Cardiovasc Surg (Torino). 1997;38(1):69–75.

Basco MR, et al. *Cognitive-behavioral therapy for anxiety disorders: why and how it works.* Bull Menninger Clin. 2000;64(supp A, pt 3):52–70.

Benson H, et al. *Treatment of anxiety: A comparison of the usefulness of self-hypnosis and a meditational relaxation technique. An overview.* Psychother Psychosom. 1978;30(3–4):229–242.

Borkoved TD, Ruscio AM. *Psychotherapy for generalized anxiety disorder.* J Clin Psychiatry. 2001;62(supp 11):37–42; discussion 43–45.

Butler G, et al. *Comparison of behavior*

therapy and cognitive behavior therapy in the treatment of generalized anxiety disorder. J Consult Clin Psychol. 1991;59(1):167–175.

Clark ME, Hirschman R. *Effects of paced respiration on anxiety reduction in a clinical population.* Biofeedback Self Regul. 1990;15(3):273–284.

Davidson GP, Farnbach RW, Richardson, BA. *Self-hypnosis training in anxiety reduction.* Aust Fam Physician. 1978;7(7):905–910.

Eppley KR, Abrams AI, Shear J. *Differential effects of relaxation techniques on trait anxiety: a meta-analysis.* J Clin Psychol. 1989;45(6):957–974.

Hana J, Stegena K, et al. *Influence of breathing therapy on complaints, anxiety and breathing pattern in patients with hyperventilation syndrome and anxiety disorders.* J Psychosomatic Res. 1999;41(5):481–493

Kabat-Zinn J, et al. *Effectiveness of a meditation-based stress reduction program in the treatment of anxiety disorders.* Am J Psychiatry. 1992;149(7):936–943.

Lenz G, Demal U. *Quality of life in depression and anxiety disorders: an exploratory follow-up study after intensive inpatient cognitive behaviour therapy.* Psychopathology. 2000;33(6):297–302.

Mathew RJ, et al. *Anxiety and platelet MAO levels after relaxation training.* Am J Psychiatry. 1981;138(3):371–373.

Pender NJ. *Effects of progressive muscle relaxation training on anxiety and health locus of control among hypertensive adults.* Res Nurs Health. 1985;8(1):67–72.

Rees BL. *Effect of relaxation with guided imagery on anxiety, depression, and self-esteem in primiparas.* J Holist Nurs. September 1995;13(3):255–267.

Reibel DK, et al. *Mindfulness-based stress reduction and health-related qualify of life in a heterogeneous patient population.* Gen Hosp Psychiatry. 2001;23(4):183–192.

Rice KM, Blanchard EB, Purcell M. *Biofeedback treatments of generalized anxiety disorder: preliminary results.* Biofeedback Self Regul. 1993;18(2):93–105.

Silverman WK, et al. *Treating anxiety*

disorders in children with group cognitive-behavioral therapy: a randomized clinical trial.* J Consult Clin Psychol. 1999;67(6):995–1003.

Stetter F, et al. *Ambulatory short-term therapy of anxiety patients with autogenic training and hypnosis. Results of treatment and 3 month follow-up.* Psychother Psychosom Med Psychol. 1994;44(7):226–234.

Toren P, et al. *Case series: brief parent-child group therapy for childhood anxiety disorders using a manual-based cognitive-behavioral technique.* J Am Acad Child Adolesc Psychiatry. 2000;39(10):1309–1312.

Tusek DL, Cwynar R, Cosgrove DM. *Effect of guided imagery on length of stay, pain and anxiety in cardiac surgery patients.* J Cardiovasc Manag. 1999;10(2):22–28.

Wachelka D, Katz RC. *Reducing test anxiety and improving academic self-esteem in high school and college students with learning disabilities.* J Behav Ther Exp Psychiatry. 1999;30(3):191–198.

Weber S. *The effects of relaxation exercises on anxiety levels in psychiatric inpatients.* J Holist Nurs. 1996;14(3):196–205.

OBSESSIVE–COMPULSIVE DISORDER (OCD)

Abramowitz JS, Brigidi BD, Roche KR. *Cognitive-behavioral therapy for obsessive–compulsive disorder: A review of the treatment literature.* Res on Social Work Practice. 2001;11(3):357–372.

Foa EB, Franklin ME. Psychotherapies for obsessive–compulsive disorder: A review. In: Maj M, Sartorius N, eds. *Obsessive–compulsive disorder. WPA series evidence and experience in psychiatry.* 4th ed. New York: John Wiley & Sons Ltd; 2000:93–146.

Warren R, Thomas JC. *Cognitive-behavior therapy of obsessive–compulsive disorder in private practice: An effectiveness study.* J Anxiety Disorders. 2001;15(4):277–285.

POST-TRAUMATIC STRESS DISORDER

Brom D, Kleber RJ, Defares PB. *Brief psychotherapy for PTSD.* J Consulting & Clinical Psychology. 1989;57:607–612.

Foa EB, Davidson J, Rothbaum BO.

Treatment of PTSD. In: Gabbard GO, ed. *Treatment of Psychiatric Disorders: the DSM.* 4th ed. Washington DC: Amer Psychiatric Press; 1995.

Foa EB, Rothbaum BO, Riggs DS, Murdoch TB. *Treatment of PTSD rape victims: A comparison between cognitive-behavioral procedures and counselling.* J Consulting & Clinical Psychology. 1991;59, 715–723.

Frank E, Stewart R. *Depressive symptoms in rape vitims.* J Affective Disorders. 1984;1:269–277.

Johnson CH, Gilmore JD, Shenoy RZ. *Use of a feeding procedure in the treatment of a stress related anxiety disorder.* J Behaviour Therapy & Experimental Psychiatry. 1982;13:298–301.

Keane TM, Fairbank JA, Caddell JM, Zimering RT. *Implosive therapy reduces symptoms of PTSD in Vietnam veterans.* Behavior Therapy. 1989;20:245–260.

Lindy JD, Green BL, Grace M, Tucker J. *Survivors of the Beverly Hills supper-club fire.* Amer J Psychotherapy. 1983;4:590–610.

Thompson JA, Charlton PFC, Kerry R, Lee D, Turner SW. *An open trial of exposure therapy based on deconditioning for post traumatic stress disorder.* Br J Clinical Psychology. 1995;34:407–416.

Resick PA, Jordan CG, Girelli SA, Hutter CK, Marhoefer-Dvorak S. *A comparative study of behavioral group therapy for sexual assault victims.* Behavior Therapy. 1988;19:385–401.

ADDICTIONS

Project MATCH Research Group. *Matching alcoholism treatment to client heterogeneity: Project MATCH three-year drinking outcomes.* Alcoholism: Clinical & Experimental Research. 1998;22(6):1300–1311.

DEPRESSION

Linde K, et al. *St. John's Wort for depression—an overview and meta-analysis of randomised clinical trials.* BMJ. 1996;313:253–258.

Liske E, et al. *Menopause—Combination product for psycho-vegetative complaints.* TW-Gynakol. 1997;10;4:172–175.

EATING DISORDERS

Crisp AH, et al. *A controlled study of the effect of therapies aimed at adolescent and family psychopathology in anorexia nervosa.* British Journal of Psychiatry. 1991;159:325–333.

Jaeger B, et al. *Psychotherapy and bulimia nervosa: Evaluation and long-term follow-up of two conflict orientated treatment conditions.* Acta Psychiatrica Scandinavica. 1996;93(4):268–278.

Leung N, Waller G, Thomas G. *Group cognitive-behavioural therapy for anorexia nervosa: A case for treatment?* European Eating Disorders Review. 1999;7(5):351–361.

Mitchell K, Carr A. Anorexia and bulimia. In: Carr A, ed. *What works with children and adolescents? A critical review of psychological interventions with children, adolescents and their families.* Florence, Kentucky: Taylor & Francis/Routledge; 2000:233–257.

Whittal ML, Agras WS, Gould RA. *Bulimia nervosa: A meta-analysis of psychosocial and pharmacological treatments.* Behavior Therapy. 1999;30(1):117–135.

Wilfley DE, et al. *A randomized comparison of group cognitive-behavioral therapy and group interpersonal psychotherapy for the treatment of overweight individuals with binge-eating disorder.* Arch General Psychiatry. 2002;59(8):713–721.

Wilson GT, et al. *Cognitive behavioral therapy for bulimia nervosa: Time course and mechanisms of change.* J Consulting & Clin Psychology. 2002;70(2):267–274.

OBESITY

Anderson R, et al. *Effects of lifestyle activity vs structured aerobic exercise in obese women.* J Am Med Assoc. 1999;281(4):335–340.

Ramadan J, et al. *Low-frequency physical activity insufficient for aerobic conditioning is associated with lower body fat than sedentary conditions.* Nutrition. 2001;17(3):225–229.

Riebe D, et al. *Evaluation of a Healthy-Lifestyle Approach to Weight Management.* Preventive Medicine. 2003;36(1):45–54.

McWhorter J, et al. *The obese child: Motivation as a tool for exercise.* J Pediatric Health Care. 2003;17(1):11–17.

Votruba S, et al. *The role of exercise in the treatment of obesity.* Nutrition. 2000;16(3)179–188.

SLEEPING DISORDERS

Backhaus J, et al. *Long-term effectiveness of a short-term cognitive-behavioral group treatment for primary insomnia.* Eur Arch Psychiatry Clin Neurosci. 2001;251(1):35–41.

Bonnet MH, Arand DL. *Caffeine use as a model of acute and chronic insomnia.* Sleep. 1992;15:526–536.

Dashevsky BA, Kramer, M. *Behavioral treatment of chronic insomnia in psychiatrically ill patients.* J Clin Psychiatry. 1998(Dec);59(12):693–699.

Holbrook AM, et al. *The diagnosis and management of insomnia in clinical practice: a practical evidence based approach.* CMAJ. 2000;162(2).

Hollingworth HL, et al. *The influence of caffeine on mental and motor efficiency.* Arch Psychol. 1912;20:1–66.

Lindahl O, Lindwall L. *Double blind study of a Valerian preparation.* Pharmacol Biochem Behav. 1989;32(4):1065–6.

McClusky HY, et al. *Efficacy of behavioral versus triazolam treatment in persistent sleep-onset insomnia.* Am J Psychiatry. 1991(Jan);148(1):121–126.

Morin CM, Mimeault V, Gagne AJ. *Nonpharmacological treatment of late-life insomnia.* Psychosom Res. 1999(Feb);46(2):103–116.

Shirlow MJ, Mathers CD. *A study of caffeine consumption and symptoms; indigestion, palpitations, tremor, headache and insomnia.* J Epidemiol. 1985;14:239–248.

Systemic Disorders

ALLERGIC RHINITIS

Ogle KA, Bullock JD. *Children with allergic rhinitis and/or bronchial asthma treated with elimination diet.* Ann Allergy. 1977;39:8–11.

CANCER SUPPORT

Meyer TJ, Mark MM. *Effects of psychosocial interventions with adult cancer patients: a meta-analysis of randomized experiments.* Health Psychology. 1995;14:101–8.

Spiegel D, Kraemer HC, Bloom JR, Gottheil E. *Effect of psychosocial treatment on survival of patients with metastatic breast cancer.* Lancet. 1989;14:888–891.

CHRONIC FATIGUE SYNDROME

Agency for Healthcare Research and Quality. *Defining and Managing Chronic Fatigue Syndrome.* Evidence Report/Technology Assessment: Number 42. 2001;01-E061. Available at: http://ahrq.gov/clinic/epcsums/cfssum.htm. Accessed August 8, 2006.

Butler S, Chalder T, et al. *Cognitive behavior therapy in chronic fatigue syndrome.* J Neuro Neurosurg Psychiatry. 1991;54(2):153–8.

Clauw DJ, et al. *Magnesium deficiency in the eosinophilia-myalgia syndrome.* Arth Rheum. 1994;9:1331–1334.

Cox IM, et al. *Red blood cell magnesium and chronic fatigue syndrome.* Lancet. 1991;337(8744):757–760.

Deale A, Husain K, et al. *Long-term outcome of cognitive behavior therapy versus relaxation therapy for chronic fatigue syndrome: a five-year follow-up study.* Am J Psychiatry. 2001;158(12):2038–2.

Grant JE, et al. *Analysis of dietary intake and selected nutrient concentrations in patients with chronic fatigue syndrome.* J Am Diet Assoc. 1996;96:383–386.

Heap LC, et al. *Vitamin B status in patients with chronic fatigue syndrome.* J Soc Med. 1999;92:183–185.

Howard JM, et al. *Magnesium and chronic fatigue syndrome.* Lancet. 1992;340:426.

Inbar O, et al. *Physiological responses to incremental exercise in patients with chronic fatigue syndrome.* Med Science Sports Exercise. 2001;33(9):1463–1470.

Price JR, Couper J. *Cognitive behavior therapy for adults with chronic fatigue syndrome.* Cochrane Database Syst Rev. 2000;2:CD001027.

Prins JB, Bleijenberg G, et al. *Cognitive behavior therapy for chronic fatigue syndrome: a multicenter randomized controlled trial.* Lancet. 2001;357(9259):841–7.

INDEX

Page numbers in **bold** type refer to main entries in the ailments section. These include details of the ailment, the factors causing it, the treatment options, suggestions for self-help, and relevant case studies and precautions.

ACKNOWLEDGMENTS

Author Acknowledgments

This book has been a huge collaborative effort and has been a long time in the making. From the initial concept, the book grew and developed with the input and creativity of a great number of people. In particular, we would like to thank the following for their invaluable expert knowledge and assistance: Daniel Firer and Joshua Holexa, Research Assistants, Program in Integrative Medicine, University of Arizona College of Medicine; David Casson BA, MBBS, MRCPI; Austin McCormick MbChB MROpth; Sue Davidson MB BS MRCP, MRCGP. Many thanks are also due to Adriane Fugh-Berman MD and her team, and to Charlea Massion MD for reviewing the photographs and illustrations.

This book would not have been possible without the hard work and combined design and editorial ingenuity of the team at Dorling Kindersley, for which an enormous thank you to everyone, in particular to Mary-Clare Jerram and Penny Warren.

Publisher Acknowledgments

DK Publishing would like to thank Professor Irving Gottesman for permission to base the chart on p.426 on information from his book *Schizophrenia Genius* (1990); to Jennie Brand-Miller and Thomas Wolever for permission to base information on p.43 on information from their book *The Glucose Revolution*; and to NAM Publications for permission to base the illustration on p.471 on material from their website.

DK would also like to thank Laura Knox for specially commissioned photography; Sophia Atcha for hair and make up; Mark Cavanagh for design assistance and PhotoShop imaging; Nicola Erdpresser for DTP assistance; Daphne Razazan for editorial advice; Jenny Lane for editorial assistance; Alyson Lacewing and Jane Perlmutter for proofreading; Nicola Turney for help on the bibliography and Useful Addresses, and Sue Bosanko for the index.

Picture Credits

The publisher would like to thank the following for permission to reproduce images:

Alamy pp 78l/Martyn Vickery, 186/BananaStock; **Bubbles Photo Library** p 382/Lois Joy Thurston; Courtesy of Bruckhoff, Hannover p 189; **Getty Images** pp 50r /Peter Scholey, 82c/Tim Flach; **Nature Picture Library** p 15 /Aflo; **Pulse Picture Library** p 246; Punchstock/Photodisk 32l, 82, 104; **Science Photo Library** pp 12r/Tek Image, 12c/David Mack, 12l/Tek Image, 19/Andrew Syred, 22/Colin Cuthbert, 27/Andrew Syred, 29/ Tek Image, 30/BSIP, Laurent, 35/John Pacy, 46/Eye of Science, 48, 48/Biophoto Associates, 53t/Stefanie Reichelt, 59/SteveGschmeissner, 73/Chris Knapton, 76/Eye of Science, 92/Nasa, 96, 98/AJ Photo/Hop American, 110/Eamonn McNulty, 122/Dr. Arthur Tucker, 134/Alfred Pasieka, 145/Faye Norman, 149/CNRI, 156/VVG, 172/Dr. P.Marazzi, 173/Alexander Tsiaras, 176/Dr. P.Marazzi, 178, 179/Eye of Science, 180/Ralph Eagle, 182/Western Opthalmic Hospital, 185/Omikron, 194/Innerspace Imaging, 201/NIBSC, 202/Dr. Gary Settles, 210/Innerspace Imaging, 215/David McCarthy, 217, 228, 231/Dr. M.A. Ansary, 232/Zephyr, 240/Dr. Linda Stannard, UCT, 250/Zephyr, 264/Dr. P.Marazzi, 266/Alfred Pasieka, 275/Sovereign ISM, 291r/CNRI, 291l/Zephyr, 297/CNRI, 303/Dr. Gilbert Faure, 310l & r /Prof. P.Motta/Dept. of Anatomy/University "La Sapienza", Rome, 312/Alfred Pasieka, 322/Zephyr, 345/Dr. E. Walker, 347/BSIP, DR LR, 354/Dr. M.A. Ansary, 371/BSIP VEM, 374r/VVG, 374l/Manfred Kage, 380/CNRI, 383/Dr. P.Marazzi, 386l/Sinclair Stammers, 386r/VVG, 395, 396/Lowell Georgia, 398/Dr. P.Marazzi, 400/Eamonn McNulty, 406/Tim Beddow, 433/BSIP/Laurent/Laetitia, 454/Chris Bjornberg, 114-155/Volker Steger, 158-179/Andrew Syred, 182-193/Omikron, 196-209/CNRI, 212-241 /CNRI, 244-265/Susuma Nishinaga, 268-311/Dr. P.Marazzi, 314-321/John Burbidge, 324-353/BSIP VEM, 356-367/CC Studio, 370-379/John Walsh, 382-405/CNRI, 456-479/Steve Gschmeissner

Illustration p. 91 by John Woodcock.

All other images © Dorling Kindersley
For further information see: www.dkimages.com